ACCP Critical Care Board Review

Course Syllabus | 2006

The American Board of Internal Medicine (ABIM) is not affiliated with, nor does it endorse, preparatory examination review programs or other continuing medical education. The content of the ACCP Critical Care Board Review Course 2006 Syllabus is developed independently by the American College of Chest Physicians (ACCP), which has no knowledge of or access to ABIM examination material.

The views expressed herein are those of the authors and do not necessarily reflect the views of the ACCP. Use of trade names or names of commercial sources is for information only and does not imply endorsement by the ACCP. The authors and the publisher have exercised great care to ensure that drug dosages, formulas, and other information presented in this book are accurate and in accord with the professional standards in effect at the time of publication. However, readers are advised to always check the manufacturer's product information sheet packaged with the respective products to be fully informed of changes in recommended dosages, contraindications, etc, before prescribing or administering any drug.

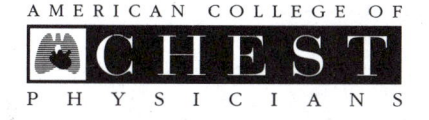

AMERICAN COLLEGE OF CHEST PHYSICIANS

Copyright © 2006 by the AMERICAN COLLEGE OF CHEST PHYSICIANS.
Copyright not claimed on material authored by the US Government. All rights reserved.
No part of this book may be reproduced in any manner without permission of the publisher.

American College of Chest Physicians
3300 Dundee Road
Northbrook, Illinois 60062-2348

Printed in the United States of America. July 2006.
ISBN-10: 0-916609-56-1
ISBN-13: 978-0-916609-56-6

Contents

Bradycardia: Diagnosis and Management 1
    Laurent Lewkowiez, MD

Tachyarrhythmias: Diagnosis and Management 13
    Laurent Lewkowiez, MD

Hypertensive Emergencies and Urgencies 29
    R. Phillip Dellinger, MD, FCCP

Shock 37
    John P. Kress, MD, FCCP

Transplantation 49
    Joshua O. Benditt, MD, FCCP

Myocardial Infarction 59
    Steven M. Hollenberg, MD, FCCP

Heart Failure and Cardiac Pulmonary Edema 75
    Steven M. Hollenberg, MD, FCCP

Thromboembolic Disease 89
    R. Phillip Dellinger, MD, FCCP

Endocrine Emergencies 107
    James A. Kruse, MD

Obesity and Critical Illness 117
    Brian K. Gehlbach, MD

Nervous System Infections and Catheter Infections 123
    George H. Karam, MD, FCCP

Upper Gastrointestinal Bleeding, Lower Gastrointestinal Bleeding, and Hepatic Failure 159
    Gregory T. Everson, MD

Infections in AIDS Patients and Other Immunocompromised Hosts 173
    George H. Karam, MD, FCCP

Nutritional Support in the Critically Ill Patient 201
    Gregory M. Susla, PharmD

Acute Renal Failure in the Critically Ill 215
    Richard S. Muther, MD

Poisonings and Overdoses 233
    Janice Zimmerman, MD, FCCP

Electrolyte Disorders: Derangements of Serum Sodium, Calcium, Magnesium, and Potassium 247
    Richard S. Muther, MD

Hemodynamic Monitoring 265
    Jesse B. Hall, MD, FCCP

Hypothermia, Hyperthermia, and Rhabdomyolysis 275
    Janice L. Zimmerman, MD, FCCP

Pulmonary Hypertension and Critical Illness 289
    Brian K. Gehlbach, MD

Acute Respiratory Distress Syndrome 295
    Jesse B. Hall, MD, FCCP

Weaning From Mechanical Ventilation 307
    James K. Stoller, MD, MS, FCCP

Trauma and Thermal Injury 323
    David J. Dries, MSE, MD, FCCP

Mechanical Ventilation 355
    Gregory A. Schmidt, MD, FCCP

Abdominal Problems in the ICU 367
    David J. Dries, MD, MSE, FCCP

Coma and Delirium 385
    Thomas P. Bleck, MD, FCCP

Acid-Base Disorders 397
    Gregory A. Schmidt, MD, FCCP

Obstetric Issues in Critical Care 407
    Mary E. Strek, MD

Severe Airflow Obstruction 427
    Gregory A. Schmidt, MD, FCCP

Issues in Sedation, Paralytic Agents, and Airway Management 437
    Michael A. Gropper, MD, PhD, FCCP

Blood Products in the Critical Care Setting 451
    Aryeh Shander, MD, FCCP

Issues in Postoperative Management: Postoperative Pain Management and Intensive Glycemic Control 463
    Michael A. Gropper, MD, PhD, FCCP

Perioperative Evaluation and Management of Pulmonary Disease 471
    Jeanine P. Wiener-Kronish, MD, FCCP

Perioperative Evaluation and Management of Cardiovascular Disease 481
    Jeanine P. Wiener-Kronish, MD, FCCP

Severe Pneumonia 493
    Michael S. Niederman, MD, FCCP

Bleeding in the ICU 513
    Aryeh Shander, MD, FCCP

Antibiotic Therapy in Critical Illness 523
    Michael S. Niederman, MD, FCCP

Head and Spinal Cord Trauma 533
    Thomas P. Bleck, MD, FCCP

Seizures, Stroke, and Other Neurologic Emergencies 545
    Thomas P. Bleck, MD, FCCP

IV

Faculty

Director
John P. Kress, MD, FCCP
Assistant Professor of Medicine Section of Pulmonary and Critical Care
University of Chicago
Chicago, IL

Joshua O. Benditt, MD, FCCP
*Director of Respiratory Care Services
Division of Pulmonary and Critical Care Medicine*
University of Washington
School of Medicine
Seattle, WA

Thomas P. Bleck, MD, FCCP
*The Louise Nerancy Eminent Scholar in Neurology
Professor of Neurology, Neurological Surgery, and Internal Medicine
Director, Neuroscience ICU
Department of Neurology*
The University of Virginia
Charlottesville, VA

R. Phillip Dellinger, MD, FCCP
Professor of Medicine
Robert Wood Johnson Medical School
Director, Section of Critical Care Medicine
Cooper University Hospital
Camden, NJ

David J. Dries, MD, FCCP
Assistant Medical Director for Surgical Care
HealthPartners Medical Group
*John F. Perry, Jr., Professor
Department of Surgery*
University of Minnesota
Regions Hospital
St. Paul, MN

Gregory T. Everson, MD
*Professor of Medicine
Director of Hepatology
Medical Director of Liver Transplantation*
University of Colorado School of Medicine
Denver, CO

Brian K. Gehlbach, MD
Assistant Professor of Medicine
University of Chicago
Section of Pulmonary and Critical Care
Chicago, IL

Michael A. Gropper, MD, PhD, FCCP
*Director, Critical Care Medicine
Associate Professor of Anesthesia and Physiology*
University of California, San Francisco
San Francisco, CA

Jesse B. Hall, MD, FCCP
Professor of Medicine, Anesthesia and Critical Care
The University of Chicago
The Pritzker School of Medicine
Chicago, IL

Steven M. Hollenberg, MD, FCCP
Director, Coronary Care Unit
Cooper Health Systems
Camden, NJ

George Karam, MD, FCCP
*Paula Garvey Manship
Professor of Medicine*
Louisiana State University
School of Medicine
New Orleans, LA
Head, Department of Internal Medicine
Earl K. Long Medical Center
Baton Rouge, LA

James A. Kruse, MD
Chief, Critical Care Services
Bassett Hospital
Cooperstown, NY

Laurent Lewkowiez, MD
*Assistant Professor of Medicine
Director Electrophysiology*
Denver Health and Hospitals
Denver Medical Center
Denver, CO

Richard S. Muther, MD
*Medical Director
Division of Nephrology*
Research Medical Center
Kidney Associates of Kansas City, PC
Kansas City, MO

Michael S. Niederman, MD, FCCP
Chairman, Department of Medicine
Winthrop University Hospital
*Professor of Medicine
Vice-Chairman, Department of Medicine*
State University of New York
(SUNY) at Stony Brook
Mineola, NY

Gregory A. Schmidt, MD, FCCP
Professor, Division of Pulmonary, Critical Care & Occupational Medicine
Department of Internal Medicine
University of Iowa
Iowa City, IA

Aryeh Shander, MD, FCCP
*Chief, Department of Anesthesiology
Critical Care Medicine, Pain Management and Hyperbaric Medicine*
Englewood Hospital and Medical Center
Englewood, NJ
Clinical Professor of Anesthesiology, Medicine and Surgery
Mt. Sinai School of Medicine
Mount Sinai Hospital
New York, NY

James K. Stoller, MD, FCCP
Professor of Medicine
Cleveland Clinic, Lerner College of Medicine
*Associate Chief of Staff
Vice Chairman
Division of Medicine*
Cleveland Clinic Foundation
Cleveland, OH

Mary Strek, MD
*Associate Professor of Medicine
Section of Pulmonary and Critical Care*
University of Chicago
Chicago, IL

Gregory M. Susla, PharmD
Pharmacy Manager
VHA, Inc.
Frederick, MD

Jeanine P. Wiener-Kronish, MD, FCCP
*Professor of Anesthesia and Medicine
Vice-Chair, Department of Anesthesia, Critical Care, and Perioperative Care
Investigator, Cardiovascular Research Institute*
University of California, San Francisco, School of Medicine
San Francisco, CA

Janice L. Zimmerman, MD, FCCP
Professor of Medicine
Baylor College of Medicine
Associate Chief, Medical Service
Ben Taub General Hospital
Houston, TX

DISCLOSURE OF FACULTY CONFLICT OF INTEREST

The American College of Chest Physicians (ACCP) remains strongly committed to providing the best available evidence-based clinical information to participants of this educational activity and requires an open disclosure of any potential conflict of interest identified by our faculty members. It is not the intent of the ACCP to eliminate all situations of potential conflict of interest, but rather to enable those who are working with the ACCP to recognize situations that may be subject to question by others. All disclosed conflicts of interest are reviewed by the educational activity course director/chair, the Continuing Education Committee, or the Conflict of Interest Review Committee to ensure that such situations are properly evaluated and, if necessary, resolved. The ACCP educational standards pertaining to conflict of interest are intended to maintain the professional autonomy of the clinical experts inherent in promoting a balanced presentation of science. Through our review process, all ACCP CME activities are ensured of independent, objective, scientifically balanced presentations of information. Disclosure of any or no relationships will be made available on-site during all educational activities.

The following faculty members of the ACCP Critical Care Board Review Course 2006 have disclosed to the ACCP that a relationship does exist with the respective company/organization as it relates to their presentation of material and should be communicated to the participants of this educational activity:

Thomas P. Bleck, MD, FCCP
Research Support: Novo Nordisk, NINDS and NIAID, Actilion

Steven M. Hollenberg, MD, FCCP
Speakers Bureau: Novartis-Makers of Valsartan

George H. Karam, MD, FCCP
Speakers Bureau: Merck & Co., Inc., Pfizer Inc.

Michael S. Niederman, MD, FCCP
Speakers Bureau: Pfizer, Inc. Schering-Plough Corporation, Merck & Co., Inc., Elan, Chiron Corporation, AstraZeneca LP, Aventis Pharmaceuticals, Wyeth

Aryeh Shander, MD, FCCP
Consultant Fee: Biopure, Ortho Biotech, Novo Nordisk
Speakers Bureau: Ortho Biotech, Novo Nordisk, Hospira, Abbott Laboratories
Advisory Committee: Biopure, Ortho Biotech

Mary E. Strek, MD
Grant monies: AstraZeneca LP, GlaxoSmithKline

The following faculty members of the ACCP Critical Care Board Review Course 2006 have disclosed to the ACCP that he or she may be discussing information about a product/procedure/technique that is considered research and is not yet approved for any purpose:

Aryeh Shander, MD, FCCP
Novo VII, EPO

Janice Zimmerman, MD, FCCP
Glucagon and Insulin for beta-blockers and calcium channel blocker overdose

The following faculty members of the ACCP Critical Care Board Review Course 2006 have indicated to the ACCP that no potential conflict of interest exists with any respective company/organization, and this should be communicated to the participants of this educational activity:

Joshua O. Benditt, MD, FCCP
R. Phillip Dellinger, MD, FCCP
David J. Dries, MD, FCCP
Gregory T. Everson, MD
Brian K. Gehlbach, MD
Michael A. Gropper, MD, PhD, FCCP
Jesse B. Hall, MD, FCCP
John P. Kress, MD, FCCP
James A. Kruse, MD
Laurent Lewkowiez, MD
Richard S. Muther, MD
Gregory A. Schmidt, MD, FCCP
James K. Stoller, MD, FCCP
Gregory M. Susla, PharmD
Jeanine P. Wiener-Kronish, MD, FCCP

Needs Assessment/Target Audience

ACCP Critical Care Board Review Course 2006

Review the type of information you should know for the ABIM Critical Care Medicine Subspecialty Examination by attending the ACCP Critical Care Board Review Course 2006. This premier course offers a comprehensive, exam-focused review, ideal for anyone who needs to certify, recertify, or simply review the current practice of critical care medicine. Physicians, surgeons, advanced practice critical care nurses, physician assistants, respiratory therapists, and pharmacists will all benefit. The entire critical care team can rely on this course for an essential update in critical care medicine.

Accreditation Statement

The American College of Chest Physicians is accredited by the Accreditation Council for Continuing Medical Education to provide continuing medical education for physicians.

Continuing Medical Education (CME) is not offered for the Board Review Course Syllabus alone. CME is offered for attending the ACCP Board Review course.

General Publications Disclaimer

The American College of Chest Physicians ("ACCP") and its officers, regents, executive committee, members, and employees are not responsible in any capacity for, do not warrant and expressly disclaim all liability for any content whatsoever in, and in particular without limiting the foregoing, the accuracy, completeness, effectiveness, quality, appearance, ideas, or products, as the case may be, of or resulting from any statements, references, articles, positions, claimed diagnosis, claimed possible treatments, services, or advertising, express or implied, contained in any ACCP publication, all such responsibility being solely that of the authors or the advertisers, as the case may be. All responsibility and liability for any of the foregoing for any claimed injury or damages to any person or property alleged to have resulted from any of the foregoing, whether based on warranty, contract, tort, or any other legal theory, and whether or not any claimant was advised of the possibility of such damages, is expressly disclaimed and denied by ACCP, its officers, regents, executive committee, members, and employees. For any possible specific medical condition whatsoever, all persons should consult a qualified health-care professional of their own choice for advice.

AMERICAN COLLEGE OF CHEST PHYSICIANS

Working for You.

As a member of our multidisciplinary society, you have access to diverse benefits that can enhance every aspect of your career.

Communications

- *CHEST*, the largest circulation respiratory and critical care journal in the world, available in print and online at www.chestjournal.org
- *CHEST Physician*, a monthly news publication providing relevant clinical information, updates on ACCP matters and events, a *Pulmonary Perspectives* article, and more
- The ACCP Web site, featuring education opportunities, advocacy information, membership and NetWork activities, physician resources, career services, and more at www.chestnet.org

Educational Resources

- Discounted tuition for all CME courses and educational products
- Discounted tuition for the annual CHEST meeting, offering essential updates in pulmonary and critical care medicine
    - CHEST benefits for ACCP members only:
        – Free abstract submission
        – Topic proposal submission
- Opportunities to conduct joint local educational programs with the ACCP
- Free CME online via Pulmonary and Critical Care Update (PCCU) articles
- Evidence-based practice guidelines, outlining new protocols in chest medicine
- Patient education tools and teaching materials
- Tools for making presentations to communities about lung health and smoking

Advocacy

- A unified voice to policymakers on medical and payment issues
- Internet access to updates on socioeconomic and political issues affecting practice and research
- Access to electronic tools for contacting Congress about issues affecting your patients, practice, and profession
- Timely alerts on legislation that impact chest and critical care medicine

NetWorks

- Special interest groups focusing on specific areas of chest medicine to develop, exchange, and disseminate relevant information
- Opportunities to form alliances with respected leaders in your field
- Opportunities to plan ACCP educational programs that meet your specific needs
- A position to influence ACCP policies and procedures
- Involvement with ACCP committees and leadership
- Participation in the development of national health-care policies

Other

- Discounts up to 40% off Apple Computer products purchased through the Apple Store online at www.apple.com/edu/accp (US delivery only)

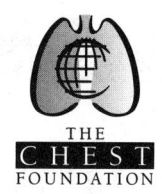

Working for Others.

The CHEST Foundation undertakes initiatives to help you
help your patients live and breathe easier.

Tobacco Prevention

- Antismoking programs sparing children tobacco-related disease
- Lung Lessons™ curriculum teaching elementary school-age children the negative health effects of smoking
- Evils of Tobacco CD-ROM and videotape for children and women in India
- The Speakers Kit on Women & Girls, Tobacco, & Lung Cancer

Critical Care

- The Critical Care Family Assistance Program and replication tool kit to improve coordination of care and communication with ICU staff, patients, and families
- *Stories at the End of Life* booklet series to comfort patient and their families

Humanitarian Awards

- Nearly $700,000 awarded from 1998-2005 to recognize and support volunteer service of ACCP members worldwide

Clinical Research Awards

- Over $3 million conferred from 1998-2005 to support promising clinical research
- Distinguished Scholar awards to foster innovation in clinical care and to address public health related to chest and critical care medicine:
    - Eli Lilly and Company Distinguished Scholar in Critical Care Medicine
    - GlaxoSmithKline Distinguished Scholar in Respiratory Health
    - Organon Sanofi~Synthélabo LLC Distinguished Scholar in Thrombosis
- Clinical research awards in asthma, COPD, critical care, pulmonary fibrosis, and women's health
- Roger C. Bone Award for Advances in End-of-life Care
- Association of Specialty Professors and The CHEST Foundation of the ACCP Geriatric Development Research Award
- Scientific abstract-related awards

You can support these programs and projects through a thoughtful donation to The CHEST Foundation. Your gift can help develop new programs and resources to help you help your patients live and breathe easier.

Donate anytime at www.chestfoundation.org.

Point. Click. Access.

Link to the resources you need.

www.chestnet.org

Education

- Calendar of upcoming courses, including the annual CHEST meeting
- Online education opportunities
- Self-study products

Membership and NetWorks

- Membership information and applications
- ACCP NetWorks and their activities
- Join NetWorks online

Other Resources

- Downloads of consensus statements, ACCP publications, and more
- Practice management information
- Career Connection employment services
- ACCP product catalog

www.chestfoundation.org

- Award and grant information and applications
- Professional resources
- Patient education products

www.chestjournal.org

- Full articles online
- Article submission information
- Subscription information

Critical Care Institute
American College of Chest Physicians

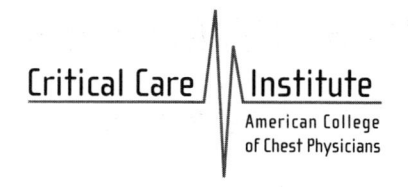

Promoting Excellence in the Care of the Critically Ill

The ACCP Critical Care Institute (ACCP-CCI) focuses and coordinates information and tools from a variety of sources to empower patient care in critical care. Drawing from the work of the ACCP, The CHEST Foundation, partnering societies, patient groups, and industry representatives, the ACCP-CCI actively collaborates to offer a complete repository of resources you can use to advance your knowledge and enhance your clinical skills.

Products currently available under the ACCP-CCI umbrella include:

- The Critical Care Family Assistance Program Replication Toolkit
- *Stories at the End of Life* booklet set
- 2005 ACCP Critical Care Board Review Syllabus
- E-EPEC Training Program—CD-ROM
- Irwin & Rippe's *Intensive Care Medicine* 5th Edition
- *Appropriate Coding for Critical Care Services and Pulmonary Medicine* coding manual
- Best of PCCU—Critical Care
- Clinical practice guidelines
    - ACCP Conference on Antithrombotic and Thrombolytic Therapy
    - Weaning From Mechanical Ventilation
    - Ventilator-Associated Pneumonia

The ACCP-CCI also supports critical care-related education courses through the ACCP, opportunities for research awards from The CHEST Foundation, advocacy initiatives, involvement with the Critical Care NetWork, and more.

Learn about ACCP-CCI resources that can help you in your practice.
www.chestnet.org/institutes/

Bradycardia: Diagnosis and Management

Laurent Lewkowiez, MD

Objectives:

- To describe the cardiac conduction system and its vascular supply
- To describe the mechanisms leading to bradycardia
- To describe various causes of symptomatic bradycardia, as well as their treatment

Key words: atrial fibrillation; AV node; chronotropic incompetence; complete heart block; His Purkinje system; sick sinus syndrome; sinus node

Introduction

Bradycardia is defined as a heart rate of <60 beats per minute (bpm). The causes of bradycardia are numerous. Bradycardia may be a normal underlying rhythm for many, or it may herald impending conduction failure and/or syncope or sudden death. It may be intrinsic or extrinsic, relating to disease processes or drug effects. Bradyarrhythmia may arise from failure of impulse formation or failure of impulse conduction. The significance of the underlying bradycardia—its contribution to symptoms and/or pathology—must be closely scrutinized because its relationship to symptoms and its significance are frequently far from straightforward.

The Cardiac Conduction System

The cardiac conduction system comprises the sinoatrial node (SA node), the atrioventricular node (AV node), the His bundle, and the His Purkinje system, which includes the left and right bundle branches. The SA node is located at the junction of the superior vena cava and right atrium. It initiates the normal heartbeat with rapid rate of depolarization. The vascular supply to the sinus node is provided by the right coronary artery in 55% of the population, by the circumflex coronary artery in 35%, and by both in 10%. The sinus node is innervated heavily by both parasympathetic and sympathetic nerves, which exert a profound effect on its underlying rate of depolarization.

The AV node is located in the anterior interatrial septum superior and anterior to the coronary sinus. The vascular supply of the AV node is provided by the AV nodal artery, which is supplied by the right coronary artery in 85% of the population and the circumflex in 15%. In addition, septal perforators from the left anterior descending artery frequently supply the AV node. The AV node is also extensively innervated by both sympathetic and parasympathetic inputs. Importantly, the conduction of the AV node is decremental. This trait causes the refractoriness of the AV node to increase with increasing stimulation, allowing the AV node to limit input into the ventricular chamber, which protects against ventricular fibrillation.

The His Purkinje system is comprised of the bundle of His, the right and left bundle branches, and the distal Purkinje fibers. The common His bundle is immediately anterior to the AV node and dives into the central fibrous body. The His bundle divides into the right and left bundle branch systems. The vascular supply of the His bundle is dually supplied by both anterior and posterior septal perforators. The right bundle branch travels along the interventricular septum in the subendocardium towards the base of the anterior papillary muscle. It receives its blood supply from both the AV nodal artery and anterior septal perforators from the left anterior descending artery (LAD). The left bundle branch is not as well defined. It is more of a fan-like structure that is roughly divided into a left anterior fascicle and left posterior fascicle. The anterior fascicle passes anteriorly toward the left anterior papillary muscle of the left ventricle. The left posterior fascicle passes posteriomedially along the interventricular septum toward the posterior papillary muscle. Blood supply to the left anterior fascicle is derived from septal perforators from the LAD. Septal perforators from both the LAD and the posterior descending artery feed the left posterior fascicle, which is the larger of the two.

Bradycardia

The etiology of bradyarrhythmias may be divided into extrinsic or intrinsic types. Abnormal impulse formation or conduction occurring as a result of drugs, systemic diseases, or effects from extracardiac pathology is extrinsic in nature. Processes involving abnormalities in cardiac impulse formation and conduction related to primary cardiac degeneration or damage are intrinsic. The vast majority of bradyarrhythmias derive from SA node dysfunction and/or AV nodal block, resulting from either intrinsic or extrinsic causes.

Extrinsic Causes of Bradycardia

Drugs

The extrinsic causes of bradyarrhythmias are varied and most frequently involve the effects of drugs that suppress SA node and AV node function (Table 1). Toxic doses of β-blockers, calcium channel blockers, and digoxin frequently precipitate symptomatic bradycardia. Therapeutic doses of these same drugs can cause symptomatic bradycardia in patients with underlying SA node and/or AV node disease. Patients with digoxin toxicity may present with a variety of cardiac rhythms, including atrial arrhythmias with AV nodal block, regularization of atrial fibrillation, accelerated junctional tachycardia, and ventricular tachycardia. With the presentation of atrial arrhythmias, such as atrial tachycardia with AV block, one must initially consider digoxin toxicity, particularly in the elderly and in patients with renal dysfunction. However, many class I and III antiarrhythmics predispose patients to sinus node dysfunction and AV conduction block, especially when subclinical underlying disease is present. In particular, amiodarone and sotalol are known for exacerbating these conditions. Other drugs that are not primarily used for cardiac rate control express significant effects on cardiac impulse formation and conduction, particularly when underlying cardiac disease is already present. These include many centrally acting antihypertensives that diminish central sympathetic output such as reserpine, alphamethyldopa, and clonidine. In addition, many antidepressants, antipsychotics, and antiseizure medications also may exert negative effects on SA and/or AV nodal function, including tricyclic antidepressants, thioridazine, phenothiazines, lithium, phenytoin, and carbamazepine. Exposure to organophosphates

Table 1. *Extrinsic Causes of Bradyarrhythmias*

Drugs	Situational reflex bradycardia	Metabolic
β-Blocking agents	Neurocardiogenic syncope	Hypokalemia
Calcium channel blockers	Maxillofacial reflex	Hyperkalemia
Lithium	Micturition syncope	Hypothyroidism
Digoxin	Oculocardiac reflex	Hyperthyroidism
$α_2$-Agonists	Cough syncope	Hypercalcemia
Tricyclic antidepressants	Pain syncope	Hypoxia
Cholinergic agents	Defecation syncope	Hypermagnesemia
Chloroquine	Vomiting-induced syncope	Rheumatologic
Class I antiarrhythmic agents	Swallow syncope	SLE
Amantadine	Infection	Reiter's syndrome
Carbamazepine	Viral	RA
Amiodarone	Varicella	Systemic sclerosis
Sotalol	Mononucleosis	Infiltrative processes
Propoxyphene	Hepatitis	Sarcoid
Alphamethyldopa	Mumps	Amyloid
Organophosphate overdose	Rubella	Other
Cholinesterase inhibitors	Rubeola	Obstructive sleep apnea
Phenothiazines	Respiratory syncytial virus	Congenital heart block
Thioridazine	Bacterial	Postsurgical heart block
Phenytoin	Endocarditis	Myotonic dystrophy
Cimetidine	Diphtheria	Hypothyroidism
Reserpine	Lyme disease	
	Parasitic	
	Chagas' disease	

and cholinesterase inhibitors may also be manifested by bradyarrhythmia.

Reflexes

Bradyarrhythmias associated with significant symptoms are frequently secondary to vagally mediated reflexes. The most common vagal reflex is neurocardiogenic syncope, which occurs frequently in young, otherwise healthy individuals. Neurocardiogenic syncope presents as a sudden loss of consciousness (*syncope*) with dramatic episodes of bradycardia and occasionally asystole precipitated by upright posture; it is frequently associated with a prodrome of nausea or sensation of heat. Syncope may also occur without dramatic bradycardia when a predominant vasodepressor component is causative. These episodes are usually diagnosed clinically, but may also be diagnosed with upright tilt table testing. Treatment may include tilt training, anticholinergics, midodrine, β-blocker therapy, salt therapy, fludrocortisone, selective serotonin reuptake inhibitors, and occasionally rate drop pacing. Other reflexes that may also involve bradycardia are situational reflexes such as micturition syncope, cough syncope, defecation syncope, swallow syncope, pain syncope, vomiting-induced syncope, the maxillofacial reflex during surgery, and the oculocardiac reflex. Bradyarrhythmias, of special concern, are associated with intracranial pathology such as hemorrhage, large stroke, and elevated intracranial pressure. Reflex tachycardia and bradycardia may also be seen after spinal cord trauma for up to 4 to 6 weeks after injury.

Metabolic Disturbances

Metabolic disturbances are also a common and generally reversible cause of bradycardia. In particular, hypoxia, hyperkalemia, hypokalemia, hypercalcemia, and hypermagnesemia should be sought. Hypo- and hyperthyroidism should also be ruled out, particularly in the elderly.

Rheumatologic Diseases

Rheumatologic diseases can cause bradycardia and heart block. Although all connective disease processes may, on occasion, involve the cardiac conduction system, overt conduction disorders with these disease processes are the exception rather than the rule. However, rheumatoid arthritis (RA), systemic lupus erythematosus (SLE), and systemic sclerosis rarely involve AV block. Up to 10% of RA patients present with some form of conduction block resulting from rheumatoid nodules' involvement with the conduction system. Reiter's syndrome deserves special note, as heart block may be present in up to 25% of cases. Sarcoid patients also frequently present with some form of conduction block and/or delay in addition to increased risk of sudden death from ventricular arrhythmia.

Infection

Infectious causes of bradycardia and heart block are uncommon in the western world with exceptions. Viral myocarditis, which is frequently caused by coxsackie B virus, is common; it may cause transient heart block or, rarely, permanent heart block. Other viral causes of bradycardia are mononucleosis, mumps, rubella, rubeola, respiratory syncytial virus, and varicella. Bradycardia from bacterial causes is uncommon, but can occur with local extension of endocarditis involving the cardiac conduction system. Diphtheria, rickettsial diseases, and fungal and helminthic infections infrequently cause AV block. Of note in Central and South America is trypanosomiasis; it is generally associated with cardiomyopathy and ventricular arrhythmia, but conduction disorders may also be seen. In the northeastern United States, Lyme disease, a spirochetal disease, causes a significant incidence of AV block. In ≤10% of patients with Lyme disease, cardiac involvement may develop; AV block is the most common presentation, usually occurring within the first 5 months after a tick bite. Conduction block is typically transient, but occasionally persists.

Other Causes

Other unusual causes of bradycardia include trauma, postoperative heart block (particularly after AV valve repair or replacement), and muscular myotonic dystrophy.

Intrinsic Causes of Bradycardia

Intrinsic causes of bradycardia include degeneration of the cardiac conduction system with fibrotic replacement of the SA node, Lev's disease (the spread of fibrosis and calcification from the adjacent cardiac skeleton), Lenègre's disease (an idiopathic fibrotic degeneration of the His Purkinje system), ischemia, and infarction. The infranodal conduction system is particularly susceptible to infarction owing to its discrete location and its function as the only electrical connection between the atria and the ventricles.

Sinus Node Dysfunction

Sinus node dysfunction, also known as sick sinus syndrome, is a common disorder that encompasses patients with tachycardia-bradycardia syndrome, chronotropic incompetence, and inappropriate bradycardia. This spectrum of disorders has been increasing in prevalence among the elderly. Its occurrence is estimated to be 1 in 600 among those older than 65 years. Sinus node dysfunction accounts for >50% of pacemaker implantations in western countries. It may be manifeted by a failure of adequate impulse generation (ie, sinus arrest or sinoatrial block) or as an abnormal transmission within the atria, which may lead to atrial arrhythmias and fibrillation. Patients may also present with excessive overdrive inhibition by arrhythmias, which may lead to prolonged sinus pauses and inability to achieve adequate heart rate with exertion.

Common causes of SA node dysfunction include many of the medications previously mentioned (Table 2). These medications are frequently necessary for treatment of other comorbidities in elderly patients, which would be a reasonable indication for pacemaker implantation. Metabolic disturbances, especially hyperkalemia, and endocrine disorders such as hyper- and hypothyroidism may also lead to or exacerbate SA node dysfunction. Incidents of sinus arrest, severe sinus bradycardia, and AV block have been documented to occur in patients with obstructive sleep apnea. Such incidents have been shown to resolve with successful treatment of the sleep apnea. One must be particularly cautious when diagnosing SA node and AV node dysfunction in the young. Brodsky et al documented significant episodes of high-grade AV block, sinus pauses, and sinus arrest in asymptomatic male medical students by 24-h monitoring. Among well-trained athletes, a resting sinus bradycardia and a junctional rhythm with sinus suppression are generally regarded as normal.

Table 2. Drugs Affecting Sinus Node Function

Amiodarone
Flecainide
Propafenone
Sotalol
Procainamide
Disopyramide
Quinidine (less frequently)
Alphamethyldopa
Clonidine
Reserpine
β-Blockers
Pindolol
Acebutolol (less so, secondary to ISA)
Verapamil
Diltiazem
Cimetidine
Phenytoin
Carbamazepine
Lithium

*ISA = intrinsic sympathomimetic activity

Intrinsic Causes of Sinus Node Dysfunction

Fibrotic degeneration of the SA node in the elderly is common and likely is responsible for a large portion of SA node dysfunction, as is underlying coronary disease. As both of these processes occur with increasing incidence in the elderly, ascertaining which one is causing the SA node dysfunction is difficult. The diagnosis of sinus node dysfunction remains inexact. Practically speaking, however, sinus pauses lasting >3 s while awake are relatively rare and may trigger further evaluation. First-degree sinus node block cannot be discerned from a surface ECG. Wenckebach periodicity to sinus block can be seen as a shortening of the PP interval prior to loss of the P wave. Chronotropic incompetence also lacks an accepted definition, but some use the inability to reach 90% of the age-predicted maximal heart rate as a definition. Patients with tachycardia-bradycardia syndrome manifest both atrial arrhythmias and excessive sinus node suppression. These patients are at increased risk of comorbidity secondary to thromboembolism.

The diagnosis of sinus node dysfunction is clinical, with symptoms of fatigue, dizziness, presyncope, syncope, and exercise intolerance with or without the symptoms of transient tachycardia.

It is supported by findings of sinus bradycardia, exit block, or arrest while awake, and is frequently associated with intermittent atrial fibrillation. Because symptoms are frequently intermittent, evaluation with continuous-loop monitors or implantable loop monitors may be required. Intracardiac evaluation of sinus node function and the sinus node recovery time after rapid atrial pacing has relatively good specificity in the 90% range and sensitivity in the 60 to 70% range. Evaluation with exercise treadmill testing may be very helpful for the diagnosis of chronotropic incompetence.

Treatment of sinus node dysfunction is directed at alleviation of symptoms as well as preventing complications of the syndrome. In previous studies, dual-chamber pacing reduced the risk of new-onset atrial fibrillation from 5% per year to 1.2% per year. The incidence of thromboembolism was reduced from nearly 15% at 38 months to 1.6% in atrial-paced patients. In a review of multiple nonrandomized studies, atrial-based pacing reduced the incidence of atrial fibrillation by 74% in comparison with ventricular pacing; however, anticoagulation is still necessary in patients with atrial fibrillation. Treatment with pacing is extremely effective when bradyarrhythmias are causing symptoms (see Table 3). In addition, rate-adaptive pacing may be extremely effective in treatment of chronotropic incompetence. The removal of an offending extrinsic drug may significantly improve symptoms. However, pacing has not been proven to improve mortality rates in sinus node dysfunction. Catheter ablation of focal atrial arrhythmias may have a larger role in the future with the advent of spatial mapping systems and pulmonary vein ablation.

AV Conduction Disturbances

AV conduction involves conduction from the atrium through the AV node, common His bundle, and bundle branch system. A conduction block that occurs in the AV node and common His bundle will result in complete AV block. A conduction block that occurs below the His bundle will result in either bundle branch block or a fascicular block with AV conduction maintained through the remaining fascicles unless extensive infranodal conduction disease exists. Similar to the SA node, both extrinsic and intrinsic causes of conduction block may occur. In addition, because these specialized areas of conduction are discretely defined anatomically, they are susceptible to injury from trauma and, even more commonly, from infarction and ischemia. The location of the

Table 3. *Indications for Pacing**

Indications for Pacing in Sinus Node Dysfunction:

Class I = Evidence or agreement that treatment is beneficial and effective.
1. Sinus node dysfunction with documented symptomatic bradycardia, including frequent sinus pauses that produce symptoms. Inpatients with iatrogenic sinus dysfunction caused by drugs essential to their care without acceptable alternative.
2. Symptomatic chronotropic incompetence.

Class III = Evidence or agreement that treatment is not useful or effective and may be harmful. Not recommended.
1. Sinus node dysfunction in asymptomatic patient, including heart rate <40 bpm when caused by drug therapy.
2. Sinus node dysfunction in patients with symptoms that are suggestive of bradycardia and are clearly not related to underlying rate.
3. Sinus node dysfunction with symptomatic bradycardia due to nonessential drugs.

Indications for Pacing in Neurocardiogenic Syncope and Carotid Hypersensitivity:

Class I
1. Recurrent syncope caused by carotid sinus stimulation; minimal carotid pressure induces >3 s asystole in absence of drug effect.

Class III
1. Hyperactive cardioinhibitory response to carotid stimulation without symptoms.
2. Hyperactive cardioinhibitory response to carotid stimulation with vague symptoms, such as dizziness or lightheadedness.
3. Recurrent syncope, lightheadedness, or dizziness in absence of hyperactive cardioinhibitory response.
4. Situational vasovagal syncope where avoidance behavior is effective.

* Note: Class II covers all conflicting evidence–not included.

conduction block can frequently be determined by examining the remaining pattern of cardiac activation and/or the etiology of the block. The prognostic significance of the conduction block depends upon the location of the disturbance—nodal vs infranodal—as well as the etiology. AV block located in the supranodal or nodal region generally does not progress rapidly to complete heart block. However, an AV block located in the infranodal region may frequently demonstrate unpredictable conduction owing to an all-or-nothing conduction, which may rapidly progress to complete heart block. In addition, an escape rhythm with nodal block is generally located in the AV junction, which has a stable escape rate between 40 and 60 bpm. Escape rhythms originating below the AV junction generally have a much slower escape rate and are frequently unreliable.

Atrial Fibrillation

Special consideration must be given to bradycardia associated with an underlying atrial fibrillation. A conservative approach should be entertained when evaluating pauses in this population because heart rate variability among patients with atrial fibrillation dramatically exceeds that of sinus rhythm. Implantation of pacemakers for symptomatic bradycardia in this condition is relatively common; however, a review of Holter-monitor data from asymptomatic patients with atrial fibrillation revealed frequent and prolonged pauses. Pauses >2 s were found to occur in two thirds of the patients and pauses >3 s in 20% of the patients. Therefore, daytime pauses up to 2.8 s and nighttime pauses up to 4 s during atrial fibrillation may be considered within normal limits.

First-Degree AV Block

By definition, first-degree AV block represents a PR interval >200 ms (equal to one large block on ECG at a standard speed of 25 mm/s). There is maintenance of AV conduction with each beat. In general, first-degree AV block arises from delayed AV nodal conduction, although it may also be due in part to slow intra-atrial conduction and occasionally to delayed conduction below the AV node when a wide ventricular complex is seen.

Second-Degree AV Block

Second-degree AV block implies continued conduction of supraventricular stimuli to the ventricle with some organized atrial activation that fails to conduct to the ventricle. There are two distinct subtypes.

Mobitz Type I Pattern (Wenckebach): Mobitz type I (Wenckebach) appears as a progressive conduction delay prior to the blocked beat. It presents with a lengthening PR interval. The greatest increment in PR prolongation is seen in the second PR interval in a classic Wenckebach sequence. The degree of lengthening between atrial and ventricular depolarization lessens with each beat, resulting in a narrowing of the RR interval. The PR interval usually shortens after the blocked beat and the pattern may repeat itself. A classic Wenckebach pattern is present only 30% of the time. Wenckebach periodicity more commonly presents as an atypical Wenckebach pattern in which the PR prolongation may not be progressive or may be variable due to the additional effect of sinus arrhythmia. The presence of a Wenckebach conduction block, classic or atypical, generally implies that the AV node is the site of the block. However, a block in the His Purkinje system may occasionally present in this fashion (but rarely does) when significant disease is present. The underlying ventricular complex is generally narrow unless underlying bundle branch block or intraventricular conduction delay is present.

Mobitz Type II: Mobitz type II block is defined as AV nodal conduction with intermittent failure to conduct without evidence of progressive PR interval prolongation prior to block. Mobitz type II block is most often associated with His-Purkinje disease. The QRS complex is usually wide.

2:1 AV Block

Block location in 2:1 AV block cannot be known with certainty. Certain findings, however, may suggest nodal or infranodal AV block. An underlying narrow complex rhythm suggests nodal disease, although His bundle disease cannot be excluded. A PR interval that is >300 ms suggests an AV nodal location of the block. AV block associated with slowing sinus rate suggests a vagally mediated etiology, also suggesting an AV nodal level of block.

Third-Degree AV Block (Complete Heart Block)

Third-degree AV block or complete heart block occurs when atrial and ventricular activity are independent, with atrial activity faster than ventricular activity. The location of the block, though generally infranodal, may be implied by the width of the QRS escape rhythm. A rate of 40 to 60 bpm is consistent with a junctional or AV nodal escape rhythm. A wide complex rhythm that is <40 bpm suggests an infranodal level of block.

Bradycardia With Acute Myocardial Infarction

Acute myocardial infarction (MI) presents with significant bradyarrhythmias approximately 25 to 30% of the time. Forty percent of these bradyarrhythmias are sinus bradycardia; 20% present as a junctional rhythm, and 15% present as an idioventricular rhythm. Junctional and ventricular escape rhythms occur with failure of higher pacemaker sites. The remaining 35% are due to AV block—first- or second-degree AV block in 27% and complete heart block in 8%.

The location and pathophysiology of the AV block as well as the symptom status of the patient are essential considerations in the decision to proceed with temporary pacing and/or aggressive pharmacologic therapy. Patients with acute inferior MI and AV block frequently have AV nodal ischemia with high levels of local adenosine, causing AV block. This generally is responsive to pharmacologic therapy such as atropine or methylxanthines and the long-term prognosis for recovery of conduction is quite good.

Acute necrosis of the AV node is rare because of the dual blood supply from the LAD and right coronary artery distributions. In contrast, high-grade AV block in acute anterior MI is typically associated with necrosis of the local conduction system. Patients with AV block and anterior MI have increased mortality resulting from complications of the conduction block and, mainly, from their larger extent of infarction. The AV block in these patients rarely responds to pharmacologic therapy; patients generally would benefit from prophylactic temporary pacing and have an indication for permanent pacing.

Table 4. *Scoring Risk in Patients With Complete Heart Block**

Risk Scale for Complete Heart Block With Acute MI

Conduction Defect	Points
First-degree AV block	1
Second-degree type I, II	1
Right bundle branch block	1
Left bundle branch block	1
Left anterior fascicular block	1
Left posterior fascicular block	1

Risk Score for Complete Heart Block

Score	Heart Block
0	1.2%
1	7.8%
2	25%
3 or more	36.4%

*Adapted from Lamas, et al.

Risk Progression for Complete Heart Block

The risk of progression to complete heart block in acute myocardial infarction may be predicted by scoring based on the presenting underlying conduction disease (Table 4). The risk of progression to complete heart block in acute MI depends on the extent of infranodal conduction defects as opposed to symptoms. The survival of patients with acute MI and AV block is determined largely by the extent of myocardial damage and the degree of infranodal conduction system disease. This is due to the unfavorable short- and long-term prognosis of patients with acute MI and intraventricular conduction defects with the exception of left anterior fascicular block. The increased risk of death is not necessarily a result of the AV block, although risk of block in these patients is increased as shown in Table 4. Pacing in these patients is aimed at treating AV block and reducing the risk of sudden death. Reduction in mortality with pacing in these patients is thought to be masked by increases in mortality due to the extensive area of infarction; thus, pacing is still recommended.

Therapy for AV Block With Acute MI

Therapy for AV block that accompanies acute MI is guided by the etiology and location of the AV block (nodal or infranodal), type of MI (anterior or inferior), and associated symptoms. For inferior MI and nodal AV block, atropine is an excellent initial therapy, particularly in the first 6 h after presentation. Doses should be administered in 0.5-mg increments with a maximal dose of 0.04 mg/kg. Doses of <0.5 mg should be avoided because of the risk of paradoxical bradycardic response. Increasing emphasis is being placed on the use of temporary transcutaneous pacing in light of the low risk of complications and relatively high effectiveness. Patches may be placed prophylactically on patients who are considered

Table 5. *Treatment Indications for Various Bradyarrhythmias*

Indications for Placement of a Transcutaneous Patch in Acute MI

Class I
1. Symptomatic sinus bradycardia.
2. Mobitz type II block.
3. Third-degree AV block.
4. Alternating bundle branch block and/or right bundle branch block with alternating left anterior fascicular and left posterior fascicular block.
5. Newly acquired bifascicular block.
6. Right bundle branch block and first-degree AV block.

Indications for Atropine With Bradycardia and Acute MI

Class I
1. Symptomatic bradycardia with heart rate <50/bpm associated with hypertension, ischemia, or a ventricular escape rhythm.
2. Asystole.
3. Symptomatic AV block at the AV nodal level type I, second-degree AV block, or high-grade AV block with narrow escape rhythm.

Class III
1. AV block at an infranodal level, second-degree type II or third-degree AV block, or AV block with a wide complex rhythm due to MI.
2. Asymptomatic sinus bradycardia.

General Indications for Permanent Pacing

Class I
1. Third-degree AV block at any level when associated with symptoms.
2. Third-degree AV block with asystole ≥3 s or escape rate <40 bpm in an awake, symptom-free patient.
3. After an AV junctional ablation.
4. Postoperative AV block that is not expected to resolve.
5. Neuromuscular disease with AV block, such as myotonic dystrophy, Kearns-Sayre syndrome, Erbs dystrophy, and peroneal muscular atrophy.
6. Second-degree AV block, regardless of location, with symptoms.
7. Intermittent third-degree AV block with bifascicular or trifascicular block.
8. Type II second-degree AV block with bifascicular or trifascicular block.
9. Bilateral bundle branch block.

Class III
1. Asymptomatic first-degree AV block.
2. Asymptomatic type I second-degree AV block, not known to be intrahisian or infrahisian.
3. AV block expected to resolve.
4. Bifascicular block without AV block or symptoms.
5. Bifascicular block with first-degree AV block without symptoms.

Permanent Pacing After Acute Phase of MI

Class I
1. Persistent second-degree AV block in the His Purkinje system with bilateral bundle branch block or third-degree AV block within or below the His Purkinje system.
2. Transient advanced second- or third-degree infranodal block AV block with associated bundle branch block. If site uncertain, electrophysiologic study may be indicated.
3. Persistent and symptomatic second- and third-degree AV block.

to have only a moderate risk of development of AV block. Transcutaneous patches also may be placed and used while waiting for placement of a temporary transvenous pacemaker. Indications for temporary transvenous pacemaker placement include symptomatic bradycardia, unresponsiveness to pharmacologic therapy, alternating bundle branch block, bifascicular block with first-degree AV block, and Mobitz type II second-degree block. Access should generally be obtained via the right internal jugular or left subclavian vein to reduce the risk of complications and to ensure safe placement and stability. An adequate pacing safety margin of three times the threshold is recommended. See Table 5 for a therapeutic summary.

Conclusion

The evaluation and treatment of bradycardia is, to a large extent, determined by the company it keeps. In the emergency department, only 15% of bradyarrhythmias are attributed to primary conduction system disorders. Elderly patients are much more likely to present with primary conduction disorders and are much less likely to respond to pharmacologic therapy. The clinician must astutely assess the etiology of bradycardia (extrinsic vs intrinsic causes) as well as the location of the conduction defect (sinus, AV node, or His Purkinje system) in order to assess the reversibility and the risk of progression to a life-threatening rhythm. In addition, one must be cognizant that bradycardia is a frequent finding in asymptomatic individuals and may be unassociated with the patient's presenting symptoms. There are few indications for permanent pacing in an asymptomatic individual. However, regardless of location, symptomatic bradycardia, which is unlikely to resolve and not due to an easily reversible cause, is an indication for pacing. Bradycardia occurring only during sleep should prompt investigation for obstructive sleep apnea but is not an indication for pacing. In symptomatic individuals in whom the relationship to bradycardia is unclear, a loop monitor or implantable loop monitor may be helpful in discerning cause and effect. Patients presenting with AV block and infranodal conduction disease are at greater risk of progressing to complete heart block. Patients with sick sinus syndrome will likely benefit from dual-chamber pacing to reduce the risk of thromboembolism as well as symptomatic improvement. Finally, patients with neurocardiogenic or vagally mediated bradycardia should avoid the aggravating stimulus. In those patients in whom the aggravating stimulus (*eg*, upright posture) is unavoidable, treatment with various pharmacologic therapy, tilt training, and rate-drop pacing appear effective and promising.

Annotated Bibliography

Andersen HR, Nielsen JC, Thomsen PE, et al. Long-term follow-up of patients from a randomised trial of atrial versus ventricular pacing for sick-sinus syndrome. Lancet 1997; 350:1210–1216.
Trial documenting benefits of atrial pacing vs ventricular pacing in patients with sick sinus syndrome: reduced mortality, reduced atrial fibrillation, and reduced incidence of thromboembolism were observed.

Brady WJ Jr, Harrigan RA. Evaluation and management of bradyarrhythmias in the emergency department. Emerg Med Clin North Am 1998; 16(2):361–388
A thorough review of the various causes of bradycardia, as well as a reasonable discussion of the relevant therapies.

Brodsky M, Wu D, Denes P, et al. Arrhythmias documented by 24 hour continuous electrocardiographic monitoring in 50 male medical students without apparent heart disease. Am J Cardiol 1977; 39:390–395
An important paper revealing the range of rhythm disturbances found in healthy volunteers by Holter moniter.

Gregoratos G, Abrams J, Epstein AE, et al. ACC/AHA/NASPE 2002 guideline update for implantation of cardiac pacemakers and antiarrhythmia devices: summary article: a report of the American College of Cardiology/American Heart Association Task Force on Practice Guidelines (ACC/AHA/NASPE Committee to Update the 1998 Pacemaker Guidelines). Circulation 2002; 106:2145–2161

Gregoratos G, Cheitlin MD, Conill A, et al. ACC/AHA guidelines for implantation of cardiac pacemakers and antiarrhythmia devices: a report of the American College of Cardiology/American Heart Association Task Force on Practice Guidelines (Committee on Pacemaker Implantation). J Am Coll Cardiol 1998; 31:1175–1209
A complete review of indications for implantation of permanent pacing devices and antitachycardic devices.

Lamas GA, Muller JE, Turi ZG, et al. A simplified method to predict occurrence of complete heart block during acute myocardial infarction. Am J Cardiol 1986; 57:1213–1219

Mangrum JM, DiMarco JP. The evaluation and management of bradycardia. N Engl J Med 2000; 342:703–709
An excellent review of bradycardia, its classification, and management.

Prystowsky EN, Benson DW Jr, Fuster V, et al. Management of patients with atrial fibrillation: a Statement for Healthcare Professionals; From the Subcommittee on Electrocardiography and Electrophysiology, American Heart Association. Circulation 1996; 93:1262–1277
An excellent and thorough review of this extensive subject, including pathophysiology, treatment options, and a critical review of current data regarding anticoagulation and rhythm and rate control.

Ryan TJ, Antman EM, Brooks NH, et al. 1999 update: ACC/AHA Guidelines for the Management of Patients With Acute Myocardial Infarction: Executive Summary and Recommendations; A report of the American College of Cardiology/American Heart Association Task Force on Practice Guidelines (Committee on Management of Acute Myocardial Infarction). Circulation 1999; 100: 1016–1030
Discussion of post-MI management, including acute and chronic pacing after MI.

Stegman SS, Burroughs JM, Henthorn RW. Asymptomatic bradyarrhythmias as a marker for sleep apnea: appropriate recognition and treatment may reduce the need for pacemaker therapy. Pacing Clin Electrophysiol 1996; 19:899–904
A discussion of marked rhythm disturbances noted in patients with sleep apnea.

Notes

Notes

Tachyarrhythmias: Diagnosis and Management

Laurent Lewkowiez, MD

Objectives:

- To understand the basic mechanisms of arrhythmias
- To understand the basic types of supraventricular arrhythmias and their treatments
- To understand the basic assessment of wide-complex tachycardias
- To understand the basic management of atrial fibrillation
- To understand the basic treatment of ventricular tachycardia and fibrillation

Key words: atrial fibrillation; atrial flutter; atrioventricular nodal reentrant tachycardia; orthodromic reciprocating tachycardia; ventricular fibrillation; ventricular tachycardia; Wolff-Parkinson-White syndrome

Introduction

The assessment, diagnosis, and management of tachyarrhythmias is a complex and sometimes difficult task. These arrhythmias share many basic similarities, however. When approached with a logical and organized algorithm, they may be accurately diagnosed and managed successfully. It is helpful to separate supraventricular arrhythmias from ventricular arrhythmias as they have markedly different treatments and risks of death.

The mechanisms of arrhythmia include abnormal automaticity, triggered arrhythmias, and reentry arrhythmias. Abnormal automaticity is defined as automatic impulse generation from cells that do not normally demonstrate this behavior or when the automaticity of these cells overtakes the sinus node, the primary site of automatic depolarization.

Triggered arrhythmias are generally due to secondary depolarizations that arise early during repolarization or immediately following repolarization. They typically are described as early after depolarization, the presumptive cause of torsades de pointes, and delayed after depolarizations, the presumptive cause of digoxin toxicity-induced proarrhythmia.

Reentry is the most commonly encountered mechanism of arrhythmia. The primary requirements of reentrant arrhythmias are an area of slow or delayed conduction, an anatomical or functional separate path of conduction, and unidirectional block.

Clinically arrhythmias caused by various mechanisms act quite differently with pharmacologic and electrical intervention. Automatic arrhythmias are usually either transiently suppressed by external stimulation, as in pacing, or are unaffected. In general, they cannot be pace-terminated or terminated with electrical cardioversion and are frequently resistant to pharmacologic therapy. They are amenable to catheter ablation. Reentry arrhythmias are amenable to pace termination, cardioversion, ablation, and pharmacologic intervention. Finally, the activity of triggered arrhythmias, although difficult to prove in vivo, behaves in a fashion that is somewhere in between that of automatic and reentrant arrhythmias.

Supraventricular Tachycardias

Diagnosis

Supraventricular tachycardias (SVTs) are a common clinical problem. The ECG is the cornerstone of diagnosis. In particular, it should be appreciated that the zones of transition frequently lead to the diagnosis of the underlying arrhythmia. These zones are typically onset, termination, and slowing or bundle branch block during tachycardia. It is at these points that information regarding the arrhythmia is acquired. During the tachycardia, it is difficult to know if the atria are driving the ventricles or vice versa.

Types

The types of SVTs and their prevalence are dependent on the age of the population studied. In young infants and children, atrial tachycardia and junctional tachycardia are common. In adolescents and adults, the majority of SVT cases are of the reentrant variety. Approximately 90% of regular narrow complex tachycardias are of reentrant etiology. The common supraventricular arrhythmias (and their prevalence in adults) include the following: AV nodal reentrant tachycardia (60%), orthodromic reciprocating tachycardia (ORT; 30%), and atrial tachycardia (10%). Approximately 2 to 5% of SVT is associated with the well-publicized Wolff-Parkinson-White (WPW) syndrome.

The clinical importance in their differentiation lies mainly in determining the response to various pharmacologic treatments and catheter-based interventions. SVTs are best assessed by the relationship of the P wave to the R wave. If the P wave is closer to the previous R wave than the subsequent R wave, the arrhythmia is considered a short-RP tachycardia. If the P wave is closer to the subsequent R wave, then the arrhythmia is considered a long-RP tachycardia.

Short-RP Tachycardias

AV Nodal Reentrant Tachycardia

AV nodal reentrant tachycardia (AVNRT) is a narrow-complex tachycardia in which the pathways involved are thought to be within the AV node itself or limited to the perinodal tissue. One pathway has fast conduction and the other pathway conducts slowly.

The onset of this arrhythmia, when captured, frequently begins with a premature atrial contraction that conducts with a dramatically lengthened PR interval. This ECG finding is the surface manifestation of a block in forward conduction down the usually fast-conducting AV nodal pathway and subsequent conduction down a slowly conducting AV nodal pathway found in these patients. The onset of this arrhythmia requires the recovery of the fast-conducting pathway allowing for retrograde conduction. This completes the circuit and meets the requirements for reentry.

AVNRT is characterized on ECG by a very short RP conduction interval with a retrograde P wave visible in only one third of the cases. In these cases, close inspection of lead V_1 for a pseudo R' and of inferior leads for a pseudo S wave may be confirmatory. In the remaining two thirds of the cases, the P wave is buried within the QRS complex.

AVNRT is extremely responsive to AV nodal blocking agents and may be acutely terminated with vagal maneuvers in about one third of the cases. Patients are nearly always responsive to adenosine, β-blockers, or calcium channel blockers administered acutely. However, medical therapy is rarely 100% effective and recurrences are the norm. Catheter ablation of this arrhythmia is 95% successful with major complications occurring in <1% of cases.

Orthodromic Reciprocating Tachycardia

ORT is also a short-RP and narrow-complex tachycardia. Anterograde (forward) conduction occurs via the normal AV nodal conduction system, with retrograde conduction via a concealed accessory pathway. The RP interval is forcibly longer than with AVNRT because it requires some conduction through the ventricle before returning up the accessory pathway.

Patients with the WPW syndrome frequently present with ORT as a narrow-complex tachycardia without evidence of preexcitation. Importantly, if the associated tachycardia rate slows with the onset of a bundle branch block, then this is a strong indicator that the tachycardia is ORT with the accessory pathway located on the side of the bundle branch block that is present.

Because the AV node must be used for anterograde conduction in ORT, this tachycardia is amenable to acute and chronic therapy with AV nodal blocking agents. Although ORT utilizes an accessory pathway, its lack of forward conduction allows the safe use of AV nodal blocking agents, in contrast to WPW syndrome. However, pharmacologic therapy is frequently less than adequately effective and recurrences during medical therapy are common. This arrhythmia is also well suited to catheter ablation, which has a 95% success rate and a low complication rate.

Long-RP Tachycardias

Long-RP tachycardias are less commonly encountered. They include sinus tachycardia, sinus node reentrant tachycardia, syndrome of inappropriate sinus tachycardia, and atrial tachycardia. Some cases include atrial flutter, although the flutter wave generally falls midway between the R-wave complexes. Other less common arrhythmias that also present as long-RP tachycardias include atypical AVNRT, permanent form of junctional reciprocating tachycardia (an ORT with a slowly conducting, retrograde-only accessory pathway), and, more rarely, junctional tachycardia.

Sinus Tachycardia

Sinus tachycardia is generally described as a long-RP tachycardia that usually occurs in response to physiologic etiologies such as pain or hypovolemia. The P-wave morphology is generally upright in leads I, II, and aVF, which is consistent with its origin at the superior vena cava and right atrial junction, with subsequent spread laterally and inferiorly. Sinus tachycardia is differentiated from sinus node reentrant tachycardia by its onset and termination rather than P-wave morphology, which is similar in both conditions.

Sinus Node Reentrant Tachycardia

Sinus node reentrant tachycardia has an abrupt onset and termination as opposed to the gradual onset and termination of sinus tachycardia. It is amenable to calcium channel blockers, such as diltiazem and verapamil, and to adenosine for acute termination, but is much less well-controlled by β-blocker therapy. In addition, it has been treated very successfully with catheter ablation.

Syndrome of Inappropriate Sinus Tachycardia

The syndrome of inappropriate sinus tachycardia is generally diagnosed by history and Holter monitoring after other causes of resting sinus tachycardia have been excluded. It presents with typical sinus complex and a lower heart rate, ≥130 beats per minute (bpm). It frequently presents in young women. It is treated with β-blockers, although high doses may be needed for control. Catheter ablation of this arrhythmia has met with disappointing results because of a high rate of recurrence.

Atrial Tachycardia

Atrial tachycardia is generally described as a long-RP tachycardia, with a heart rate between 150 and 250 bpm. It may, however, present as a short-RP tachycardia when associated with first-degree AV block, although this is rare. As implied by its name, this arrhythmia generally does not require AV nodal or infranodal tissue for its maintenance. The P-wave complex is generally different from that seen in tachycardia of sinus origin. The PR interval is >0.12 ms, which differentiates this arrhythmia from junctional tachycardia with retrograde conduction. The origin of the atrial tachycardia may be inferred with some accuracy by evaluating its morphology in leads V_1 and aVL. An upright P wave in lead V_1 and negative wave in aVL implies a left atrial tachycardia, while the reverse implies a right atrial source.

The diagnosis of atrial tachycardia, aside from its ECG appearance, may be aided by the use of adenosine. If IV adenosine leads to AV block with continued atrial arrhythmia, then ORT is excluded and AVNRT is significantly less likely. The response of sinus tachycardia to adenosine is one of general slowing or transient arrest. However, in some published series, as many as 70 to 80% of atrial tachycardias may also be transiently terminated with adenosine.

The mechanism of atrial tachycardia is frequently related to associated comorbidities. Patients with increased catecholamine state may present with automatic and triggered mechanisms. Patients with previous cardiac surgery may present more often with scar reentry tachycardia. The arrhythmia circumnavigates the surgical scar, forming separate functional or anatomic limbs of the tachycardia. Slow conduction and unidirectional block induced by a premature beat complete the triad leading to reentry.

Therapy for atrial tachycardia is complex and controversial. The automatic atrial tachycardia that is frequently found in children may spontaneously regress. Atrial tachycardia in adults is frequently treated with antiarrhythmic therapy. Rate control of these rhythms may be difficult despite use of calcium channel blockers and β-blockers. The use of digoxin may exacerbate triggered causes of atrial tachycardia. Class Ia agents such as procainamide and class Ic agents such as flecainide and propafenone may be used in patients without structural heart disease or coronary artery disease. However, the GI side effects of procainamide and its frequent association with drug-induced lupus limit its utility. Class III agents such as sotalol and amiodarone are used frequently in these patients for rhythm control as well. However, the need to initiate sotalol as an inpatient in order to monitor the patient for dramatic QT prolongation, sotalol's potential for causing torsades de pointes, and amiodarone's high side-effect profile limit enthusiasm for their use. Factors such as comorbidities, drug side effects, reluctance to undertake lifelong drug therapy, and the fact that the drugs are only moderately effective have led many to pursue ablation therapy. Catheter ablation has up to an 80% cure rate.

Atrial Flutter

An arrhythmia related to reentrant atrial tachycardia is the commonly encountered atrial flutter. Patients with atrial flutter generally have atrial rates between 250 and 350 bpm and ventricular rates of 75 to 150 bpm. Occasionally, atrial flutter presents with a variable ventricular response. Atrial flutter typically rotates in a counterclockwise fashion around the right atrium, bounded anteriorly by a narrow isthmus of tissue located between the tricuspid valve and posteriorly by the Eustachian ridge. Typically, it has negative sawtooth pattern in inferior leads II and aVF and positive flutter waves in lead V_1. It may occasionally travel in a clockwise rotation with reversed ECG presentation but with an identical atrial rate.

The treatment of atrial flutter is similar to that of atrial fibrillation, but rate control in flutter is substantially more difficult to obtain. Atrial flutter may respond to direct current (DC) cardioversion or may be pace-terminated by pacing in the atrium at increasing rates above that of the intrinsic arrhythmia. Atrial flutter may be associated with a lower rate of thromboembolism than atrial fibrillation. However, it has been associated with multiple documented episodes of stroke after cardioversion. The indications for anticoagulation are considered the same as for atrial fibrillation. Radiofrequency ablation targeting the isthmus of tissue is highly effective in patients with primarily atrial flutter without concomitant atrial fibrillation. When bidirectional conduction block is obtained in the isthmus (inability to conduct in the isthmus), typical atrial flutter is no longer possible. The success rate of atrial flutter ablation, in experienced hands, is in the 80 to 90% range.

WPW Syndrome

WPW syndrome is estimated to be present in 0.3% of the population, with an estimated risk of sudden death of 1 per 1,000 patient-years. As previously mentioned, WPW syndrome may present with the narrow-complex tachycardia ORT. However, much of the discussion regarding this syndrome is associated with atrial fibrillation (see "Atrial Fibrillation" for more information). WPW syndrome may also present as a regular wide-complex tachycardia, indicating anterograde conduction over the accessory pathway. The differentiation of the wide-complex manifestations of this syndrome is beyond the scope of this discussion.

The ECG presentation of WPW syndrome is an accelerated AV conduction with a short PR interval and a QRS duration >120 ms (3 small boxes on ECG) with an abnormal bizarre initial upstroke and frequently abnormal repolarization. In addition, patients with WPW syndrome frequently have pseudoinfarction on ECG secondary to their abnormal origin of ventricular depolarization.

The cause of this abnormal ventricular depolarization is the presence of one or more accessory pathways. These accessory pathways are small bands of tissue that failed to separate during development, allowing continued electrical conduction between the atria and ventricles at sites other than at the AV node. The accessory pathway conduction circumvents the usual conduction delay between the atria and ventricles that occurs within the AV node. This leads to early eccentric activation of the ventricles and subsequent fusion with the usual AV nodal conduction. These pathways may allow rapid conduction from the atria to the ventricle, which can predispose patients to a risk of sudden death from ventricular fibrillation.

Atrial Fibrillation

Atrial fibrillation is the most common arrhythmia and affects 2 to 4% of the population. Its prevalence increases markedly with age, increasing to as much as 5 to 10% of people >80 years old. Atrial fibrillation remains one of the more complex and challenging cardiac arrhythmias to manage. It is associated with significant comorbidities and an increased risk of death. Patients with atrial fibrillation have double the mortality of those without atrial fibrillation. Patients may have no symptoms or may experience syncope, dizziness, palpitations, worsening heart failure, and angina.

Atrial fibrillation is characterized by a lack of organized atrial activity on surface ECG, manifesting as a lack of clear P waves between QRS complexes. It also presents with an irregularly irregular ventricular response.

The mechanisms of atrial fibrillation are now more clearly understood and new management strategies continue to evolve. Atrial fibrillation has now been shown to result from multiple reentrant wavelets conducting between the right and left atrium. Factors that increase the number of wavelets that can exist at any one time increase the likelihood that atrial fibrillation will be sustained. Likewise, factors that diminish the number of wavelets increase the likelihood that atrial fibrillation will spontaneously terminate. Thus, increased atrial size, slow intra-atrial conduction, and a shortened atrial refractory period all lead to an increased number of wavelets and increase the likelihood that atrial fibrillation will be sustained. Conversely, pharmacologic treatment frequently prolongs the refractory period of atrial tissue. A prolonged refractory period increases the path length of the reentrant wavelet, thereby decreasing the number of possible wavelets that can occupy the atria. This renders the arrhythmia more likely to self-terminate. The aim of nonpharmacologic treatment of atrial fibrillation with a catheter and the surgical maze procedures is to electrically isolate the atria into small areas that are not capable of maintaining numerous wavelets, thereby preventing maintenance of atrial fibrillation.

Management of atrial fibrillation involves more than symptom relief. Atrial fibrillation is known to be associated with increased risk of stroke and death. The risk of thromboembolism in patients who are not taking an anticoagulant is 5 to 6% per year, but may be as high as 20% in certain populations, including the elderly and those with certain valvular lesions (ie, mitral stenosis). In addition, atrial fibrillation with rapid ventricular response has been shown to lead to a tachycardia-mediated cardiomyopathy (a rate-induced form of progressive left ventricular dysfunction) that is reversible if maintenance of sinus rhythm and/or rate control is attained. Improvement in left ventricular function has been shown to occur with pharmacologic control as well as after AV nodal ablation with pacing in patients with tachycardia-induced cardiomyopathy.

Acute Management of Atrial Fibrillation

Acute management of atrial fibrillation initially focuses on rate control and anticoagulation. Rate control is usually accomplished through the use of calcium channel blockers, β-blockers, amiodarone, and rarely with digoxin alone to slow the ventricular response. The use of acute β-blocker therapy for rate control in patients with left ventricular dysfunction and decompensated congestive heart failure should be avoided. In these patients, calcium channel blockers may be used with caution. Digoxin and amiodarone may be particularly effective in light of their lack of negative inotropic effect. Patients in whom atrial fibrillation lasts <48 h may generally undergo DC cardioversion to normal sinus rhythm with minimal risk of thromboembolism. The rate of embolism with cardioversion within 48 h without prior anticoagulation is estimated to be approximately 0.8%. Pharmacologic therapy for acute conversion to sinus rhythm may also be performed within 48 h. After that time, conversion should be performed only with extreme caution unless previous anticoagulation has been documented. Cardioversion may be performed in extreme cases such as severe refractory congestive heart failure, intractable angina, or refractory hypotension when ventricular response cannot be controlled. Such cases are, however, extremely rare.

Patients with atrial fibrillation that has lasted >48 h who have not received anticoagulants may undergo transesophageal echocardiography and subsequent cardioversion if no thrombus is seen within the left atria or appendage, followed by anticoagulation for >1 month as an alternative to prolonged preconversion anticoagulation. This method was associated with a low incidence of thromboembolism in a small pilot study; a larger study compared conventional anticoagulation and transesophageal guided cardioversion with short-term anticoagulation. Regardless of prior anticoagulation, 4 weeks of anticoagulant therapy is required, attaining an international normalized ratio of 2 to 3. This is to prevent thrombus formation and embolization before recovery of normal atrial function.

It is important to realize, prior to initiation of immediate cardioversion, that 50% of patients with paroxysmal atrial fibrillation will spontaneously convert without electrical or pharmacologic intervention.

Digoxin, which in the past was used heavily for the prevention and conversion of atrial fibrillation, is ineffective for both and may actually be profibrillatory by shortening the atrial refractory period.

After cardioversion, calcium channel blockers have been shown to decrease the incidence of early recurrence of atrial fibrillation. Certain studies have shown a greater propensity of spontaneous conversion with β-blocker therapy than with calcium channel blocker therapy.

Chronic Management of Atrial Fibrillation

Chronic therapy of atrial fibrillation may focus on rhythm or rate control as well as anticoagulation.

Patients who have atrial fibrillation, paroxysmal or sustained, along with diabetes, hypertension, valvular heart disease, congestive heart failure, hyperthyroid state, or age >65 years, should take anticoagulants to decrease the risk of thromboembolism chronically.

The fervor with which maintenance of sinus rhythm is pursued should be based on the severity of symptoms as well as the associated comorbidities (eg, congestive heart failure).

Chronic ventricular rate control, similar to acute treatment, may generally be attained in atrial fibrillation with calcium channel blockers (diltiazem and verapamil) or β-blockers such as esmolol, metoprolol, atenolol, or propranolol.

Digoxin was traditionally used in the past, but it is effective mainly in bed-bound patients and is easily overcome with sympathetic stimulation. Digoxin is particularly helpful in patients who present with congestive heart failure due to left ventricular dysfunction, in whom the negative inotropic effects of β-blockers and calcium channel blockers may be detrimental. In patients in whom digoxin, calcium channel blockers, and β-blockers are ineffective or inapplicable, amiodarone may be used a for rate control and to aid in future maintenance of sinus rhythm. This is particularly helpful in congestive heart failure but is unlikely to acutely convert the patient.

The benefit of chronic maintenance of sinus rhythm vs ventricular rate control alone is an unsettled debate. Numerous clinical risk factors militate against the successful maintenance of sinus rhythm. Prolonged atrial fibrillation, enlarged left atrial size >5.0 cm, and advanced age all make lasting sinus rhythm less likely. However, at least one attempt at cardioversion and maintenance of sinus rhythm should be entertained. Preliminary results from studies comparing rhythm vs rate control have thus far failed to show benefit.

Pharmacologic Maintenance of Sinus Rhythm

In patients in whom maintenance of sinus rhythm is desired and pharmacologic assistance is required, a variety of antiarrhythmic drugs may be helpful; however, the patient's underlying comorbidities are important in selection of the appropriate drug class. Maintenance of sinus rhythm with pharmacologic therapy is similar for class I and III drugs. Average recurrence of atrial fibrillation approaches 50% with medication vs 80% with placebo at 1 year.

Some evidence exists that amiodarone, a class III drug, may have slightly higher success rate, as may dofetilide, a new class III drug. Both amiodarone and dofetilide have been shown to also be safe in coronary artery disease and left ventricular dysfunction. Class 1C agents, such as flecainide and propafenone, are safe in the absence of structural heart disease and coronary artery disease. Many experts have touted these as the drugs of choice in patients who have atrial dysrhythmias and no structural heart disease. However, these drugs have the ability to convert atrial fibrillation to atrial flutter with 1-to-1 ventricular conduction. This can lead to extremely rapid ventricular rates and subsequent cardiovascular collapse. Therefore, with class IC drugs, an AV nodal blocking agent should also be used. Exercise testing while taking medication is advocated by some as use dependence associated with these drugs (increasing drug effect at increasing heart rates) can lead to proarrhythmia at rapid heart rates.

It is important to realize that reversion to atrial fibrillation during medical therapy does not represent failure. Indeed, if the patient improves symptomatically and remains in sinus rhythm for a reasonable period of time, recurrent cardioversion and pharmacologic maintenance are a reasonable treatment plan (determined by the willingness of the physician and patient to undergo subsequent cardioversion). Currently, randomized trials have failed to demonstrate a mortality benefit of rhythm control over rate-control paradigms.

When pharmacologic maintenance of sinus rhythm is ineffective and rate control is inadequate for symptom relief, new therapies on the horizon may help. The success of the surgical maze procedure approaches a 90% rate of freedom from recurrent atrial fibrillation. The maze procedure involves a thoracotomy with substantial morbidity and a mortality of approximately 2%. These risks have prompted investigation of a percutaneous maze procedure, which appears difficult.

There is new enthusiasm for pulmonary vein isolation and linear left atrial ablation. In atrial fibrillation, ablations targeting the exit sites of initiating areas (which are frequently found in the pulmonary veins), or reducing the ability to sustain atrial fibrillation with circular lesions, are being carried out with a catheter approach. These procedures appear to be a promising alternative to medical therapy.

Rate Control in Atrial Fibrillation

Rate control with AV nodal blocking agents is relatively effective for control of symptoms in many patients. Amiodarone may be considered for rate control in patients with severe left ventricular dysfunction who cannot tolerate the negative inotropic effect of calcium channel blockers and β-blockers. In some patients, maintenance of sinus rhythm is not feasible and AV nodal blockade with adequate rate control is impossible to obtain through pharmacologic treatment. For such patients, several nonpharmacologic treatments are available.

Significant experience with AV nodal ablation and subsequent pacemaker implantation has demonstrated significant improvement in symptoms, but the need for anticoagulation is not avoided as the atrial fibrillation continues. In addition, an increased incidence of sudden death has been noted immediately after ablation, which is thought to be related to pause-dependent arrhythmic death secondary to torsades de pointes. Long-term outcomes in these patients have been shown to be similar to those for medical therapy with regard to mortality, with improved quality of life and symptoms.

Management of Atrial Fibrillation with WPW

Management of atrial fibrillation in a patient with WPW syndrome is a special situation. The use of AV nodal blocking agents as the primary therapy for rate control should be avoided because they may paradoxically increase AV nodal conduction and heart rate due to removal of a concealed retrograde conduction in the accessory pathway. This may lead to an increased rate of ventricular response, ventricular fibrillation, and possibly death.

IV procainamide or ibutilide is the initial drug of choice to slow conduction down the accessory pathway and to facilitate possible conversion and maintenance of sinus rhythm. IV amiodarone is the drug of choice in patients who have a rapid ventricular response with diminished left ventricular function and/or heart failure. DC cardioversion should be undertaken in patients who have a rapid ventricular response with symptomatic hypotension.

All atrial fibrillation patients with symptomatic WPW syndrome should undergo electrophysiologic evaluation. Patients with rapid ventricular conduction over the accessory pathway at a rate >240 bpm and any preexcited ventricular complex with an RR interval shorter than 250 ms may be at increased risk of sudden death as compared with the general population and should undergo radiofrequency ablation. Patients who have symptomatic WPW syndrome without the above findings should also be studied and undergo ablation rather than receive medical treatment if inducible arrhythmias utilizing the pathway are found. Asymptomatic patients with WPW syndrome do not generally require electrophysiologic study unless they are in high-risk professions, such as airline pilot or professional climber.

Wide-Complex Arrhythmias

The assessment of wide-complex tachyarrhythmias can be confusing and challenging. The diagnosis of wide-complex tachycardia depends on a ventricular rate of >100 bpm and QRS duration >120 ms. The differential diagnosis of wide-complex tachyarrhythmia is ventricular tachycardia, SVT with bundle branch block or with functional bundle branch block (aberrancy), and preexcited tachycardias with anterograde accessory pathway conduction with a supraventricular arrhythmia. Metabolic disorders, such as extreme hyperkalemia, and occasionally large anterior myocardial infarction (MI) may mimic wide-complex arrhythmias. The majority of patients seen with wide-complex tachycardias present with sinus tachycardia and bundle branch block. Higher-risk populations, which include patients with depressed left ventricular function and patients with previous MI, overwhelmingly present with ventricular arrhythmias as a cause of their wide-complex tachyarrhythmias. Indeed, diagnosis by history in these patients has been shown to work nearly as well as more complex algorithms.

It is important to differentiate SVT with bundle branch block from ventricular tachycardia (VT) in order to avoid delays in appropriate therapy and prevent use of contraindicated medications (such as verapamil, which was used historically with SVT). Verapamil has precipitated numerous episodes of hemodynamic collapse in patients with VT. Evaluation by a 12-lead ECG determines whether the wide complex is typical for a bundle branch block. If the complex is not typical for a bundle branch block, then the diagnosis defaults to VT. Although this sounds simple, the algorithms developed may be complicated and cumbersome.

The Brugada Criteria

A frequently used diagnostic algorithm presented by Brugada et al incorporates many previously published morphology criteria in a stepwise algorithm and has been demonstrated to be very sensitive and specific in the absence of preexisting intraventricular conduction abnormalities. Wide-complex tachycardias are divided into right and left bundle branch types. If the complex is upright in lead V_1 of a standard 12-lead ECG, it is defined as a right bundle branch type. If the complex is negative in lead V_1, it is defined as a left bundle branch type. (See Tables 1 and 2.)

Once the diagnosis of VT has been made, therapy depends on the clinical condition of the patient and the presence or absence of left ventricular dysfunction. If the patient is unstable, DC cardioversion is indicated. If the patient appears stable, has minimal symptoms with no heart failure or angina, and has adequate blood pressure, pharmacologic treatment may be used. The choice of agent depends greatly on the presence or absence of left ventricular dysfunction.

New Guidelines for Advanced Cardiac Life Support

There have been significant changes in published guidelines for advanced cardiac life support, in particular regarding monomorphic ventricular tachycardia and ventricular fibrillation. The results of out-of-hospital arrest trials have shown significant efficacy for amiodarone.

Table 1. *Diagnosis of Wide QRS–Complex Tachycardia With a Regular Rhythm*

Step 1. Is there absence of an RS complex in all precordial leads V_1 to V_6?

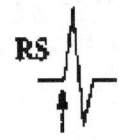

If yes, then the rhythm is VT.
- Sensitivity, 0.21; specificity, 1.0

Step 2. Is the interval from the onset of the R wave to the nadir of the S wave >100 ms in any precordial leads?

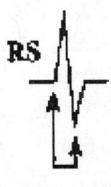

If yes, then the rhythm is VT.
- Sensitivity, 0.66; specificity, 0.98

Step 3. Is there AV dissociation?
If yes, then the rhythm is VT.
- Sensitivity, 0.82; specificity, 0.98

Step 4. Are morphology criteria for VT present?
See Table 2.

Table 2. *Morphology Criteria for VT*

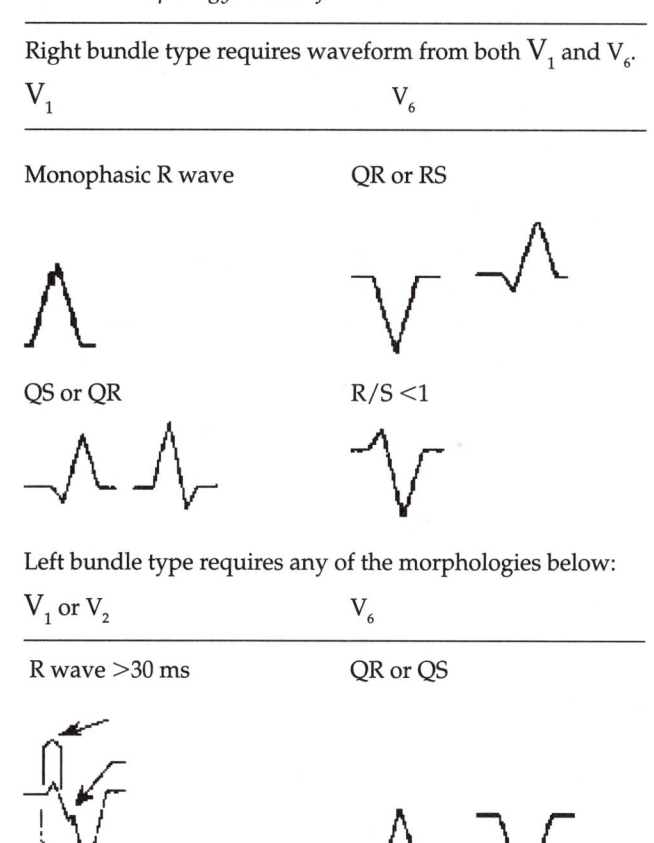

Right bundle type requires waveform from both V_1 and V_6.

V_1	V_6
Monophasic R wave	QR or RS
QS or QR	R/S <1

Left bundle type requires any of the morphologies below:

V_1 or V_2	V_6
R wave >30 ms	QR or QS
Notched downstroke S wave. >60 ms nadir S wave.	

Adapted from Brugada et al.

Multiple studies have shown a neutral effect on mortality or trend toward benefit in patients who are treated with amiodarone post-MI as well as patients with congestive heart failure, particularly in the nonischemic population. As a result, amiodarone has replaced many formerly heavily used antiarrhythmics as the primary therapy. In addition, it should be noted that the use of combination antiarrhythmic therapy is strongly discouraged because of a proarrhythmic potential and limited efficacy.

New emphasis in the advanced cardiac life support guidelines is placed on the differentiation of treatment in patients with normal left ventricular function from those with diminished function. For patients with depressed left ventricular function, amiodarone is the agent of choice. In patients with preserved left ventricular function and wide-complex arrhythmia of unknown etiology or VT, acceptable choices for therapy include DC cardioversion, amiodarone, or procainamide.

For every tachyarrhythmia, amiodarone may be used as a primary or secondary choice. Lidocaine is now considered secondary in therapy as a result of its limited effectiveness in VT in nonischemic tissue.

For wide-complex tachycardias, DC cardioversion is a universally acceptable treatment option and should be considered the primary choice. Proper sedation should always be provided prior to cardioversion. DC cardioversion is always indicated for unstable rhythms.

Polymorphic VT—in which the ventricular complex changes morphology or axis throughout the arrhythmia—and ventricular fibrillation should receive rapid treatment with DC cardioversion. The pharmacologic treatment of choice is IV amiodarone administered as a 150-mg bolus over 10 min, but it has been used successfully for out-of-hospital arrests with a 300-mg IV bolus. These rhythms are generally the result of severe metabolic disturbance and cardiac ischemia. However, polymorphic VT is rarely associated with a prolonged QT interval presenting as torsades de pointes.

Ventricular Tachycardia in Patients With Normal Left Ventricular Function

In addition to monomorphic ventricular tachycardia (in which ventricular complexes are stable from beat to beat with regard to morphology) due to coronary artery disease and nonischemic cardiomyopathies, VT also occurs rarely in patients without structural heart disease. These VTs present frequently as palpitations, and extremely rarely as sudden death. The morphology may be a left bundle-branch type with inferior axis in patients with right ventricular outflow-tract tachycardia. This type of VT is adenosine sensitive and responds to calcium channel blockers and occasionally β-blockers. It frequently is erroneously diagnosed as having a supraventricular origin. Right bundle-branch morphology superior axis VT originating from the left ventricle may also present in patients without structural heart disease. This type of VT is responsive to verapamil. Both types of VT are also amenable to catheter ablation, which has a curative rate of >90%.

Torsades de Pointes

Torsades de pointes has been described as appearing to twist around its baseline. It is polymorphic VT defined by its association the QT-segment prolongation. This rhythm is adversely affected by bradycardia and is frequently pause dependent (initiated after a pause). An assessment should be made for causative agents, which include many noncardiac medications. In addition, many antiarrhythmics that prolong cardiac repolarization such as Vaughn-Williams class Ia and class III drugs will exacerbate this arrhythmia.

Most cases of torsades de pointes are acquired by a combination of iatrogenic prolongation of ventricular repolarization from drugs (see Table 3), hypokalemia, or hypomagnesemia and an underlying mild repolarization abnormality.

Because the QT interval lengthens with decreasing heart rate, a measurement of a rate-independent QT interval may be calculated. The standard correction for rate is the QT interval by divided the square root of the RR interval measured in milliseconds. The presence of a corrected QT interval of >440 to 460 ms should be considered abnormal. Patients with QT intervals corrected for rate >500 ms and certainly >600 ms have been shown to be at increased risk for torsades de pointes.

Treatment of acquired long-QT syndrome leading to torsades de pointes consists of removal of the offending agents or conditions. Further therapy includes treatment with IV magnesium, which prevents the onset of torsades de pointes. Temporary pacing or administration of isoproterenol increases the underlying heart rate and shortens the QT interval, diminishing the risk of arrhythmia.

Congenital Long-QT Syndrome

Some patients present with syncope or sudden death and are found to have pause-dependent polymorphic VT, torsades de pointes, and a prolonged QT interval without any offending agent or condition. These patients have congenital long-QT syndrome. The majority of patients with congenital long-QT syndrome have long-QT syndrome 1. These patients have an abnormality in a potassium ion channel, leading to prolonged ventricular repolarization and an increased risk of sudden death, particularly with exercise. Patients with long-QT syndrome 3 have an abnormality involving a sodium channel that also leads to prolonged repolarization and increased risk of death. These patients, paradoxically, have an increased risk of death while sleeping. Therapy for congenital long-QT syndrome patients with symptoms of dizziness, syncope, or sudden death consists of β-blocker therapy and pacing. Some advocate a left stellate ganglionectomy in addition.

Many experts feel that the addition of an implantable cardiodefibrillator (ICD) rather than surgery in combination with β-blocker therapy is optimal. β-Blocker therapy has been shown to decrease the risk of death by approximately 50%. In addition, it is believed that pacing reduces mortality by approximately 25%. β-Blocker therapy is particularly effective for patients with long-QT syndrome 1, and a smaller subgroup of patients

Table 3. *QT-Prolonging or Torsadogenic Drugs*

The following drugs have been shown to prolong the QT interval or have documented clinical torsades de pointes reported in the literature:

Amantadine	Ketoconazole
Aminophylline	Levofloxacin
Amiodarone	Levomethadyl
Barium	Mesoridazine
Bepridil	Hydrochlorothiazide
Chloral hydrate	Moxifloxacin
Chloroquine	Naratriptan
Chlorpromazine	Nicardipine
Ciprofloxacin	Octreotide
Cisapride	Pentamidine
Clarithromycin	Pimozide
Desipramine	Probucol
Disopyramide	Quetiapine
Dofetilide	Quinidine
Doxepine	Risperdone
Droperidol	Salmeterol
Erythromycin Felbamate	Sertraline
Flecainide	Sotalol
Fluoxetine	Sparfloxacin
Foscarnet	Sumatriptan
Fosphenytoin	Tacrolimus
Gatifloxacin	Tamoxifen
Halofantrine	Terfenadine
Haloperidol	Thioridazine
Hydroxyzine	Tizanidine
Ibutilide	Trimethoprim/ sulfamethoxazole
Imipramine	
Indapamide	Venlafaxine
Isradipine	Zolmitriptan

with a potassium channel abnormality known as long-QT syndrome 2. Patients with long-QT syndrome 3 do not respond to β-blocker therapy; this may explain why some patients in the past appeared to benefit from β-blockers, while others in the population did not. These patients may be treated with some efficacy using mexiletine (a sodium channel blocker) but would also require an ICD if syncope or resuscitation after sudden death has occurred.

Sudden Death in Patients With Normal Left Ventricular Function

In addition to long-QT syndrome, patients with normal left ventricular function may also present with ventricular fibrillation and cardiac arrest. This patient population may have some rare syndromes of which clinicians should be aware. The Brugada syndrome is characterized by syncope and sudden death. These patients frequently present with ECG findings consistent with incomplete right bundle branch block ST elevations in leads V_1 and V_2 that may be exacerbated with IV procainamide and flecainide. These drugs increase the degree of ST-segment elevation. The degree of ST-segment elevation may also vary over time. This may complicate the diagnosis, as patients may at times have a normal resting ECG. Treatment in patients with cardiac arrest or syncope with the above ECG finding consists of ICD implantation.

Right Ventricular Dysplasia

Right ventricular dysplasia is a common cause of arrest in young patients, particularly in Europe. The ECG presentation is delayed right ventricular activation presenting as incomplete or complete right bundle branch block. An epsilon wave seen as a positive deflection following the R wave and deep T wave inversion in the anterior precordium are classic ECG findings. The diagnosis is commonly confirmed with an MRI revealing fatty infiltration of the right ventricle. It may also be confirmed with echocardiography, although that is insensitive, or with right ventricular angiography. It presents with ventricular arrhythmias originating from the right ventricle and is exacerbated by exercise. Although sotalol has been shown to be effective at suppressing inducible arrhythmias with right ventricular dysplasia, ICD therapy is recommended. Patients occasionally die from progressive right ventricular mechanical failure.

Hypertrophic Cardiomyopathy

Sudden death or syncope in patients with significant left ventricular hypertrophy should alert the physician to the possibility of hypertrophic cardiomyopathy. These patients are frequently asymptomatic prior to their arrest, which is frequently related to exertion. This syndrome accounts for the majority of sudden cardiac death in young adults in the United States. Risks for sudden death among patients with suspected hypertrophic cardiomyopathy are extreme ventricular hypertrophy, exertional hypotension, documented nonsustained VT, and previous syncope and family history of sudden death. Although ICDs have been shown to be effective therapy, screening and appropriate selection of asymptomatic patients remains problematic.

Implantable Cardiodefibrillators

Since the 1983 Food and Drug Administration approval of ICDs for human use, the indications for ICD implantation continue to expand. Technical advances allow increasing ease of implantation with diminishing size. ICDs are now placed almost entirely without thoracotomy, and the risk of death with implantation is <1%. The devices frequently include many of the features of pacemakers, including dual-chamber pacing and sensing. They may have rate-responsive abilities in addition to impressive intracardiac electrogram monitoring, including some Holter-monitoring abilities. In addition, they have complex algorithms that aid in decreasing spurious electrical therapy for rapid SVT, which may overlap in rate with dangerous ventricular arrhythmias. ICDs are extremely effective at preventing arrhythmic death. Many studies report that the risk of death due to arrhythmia is reduced to 2% per year. Increasing evidence is mounting as to the superiority of ICD therapy in patients with cardiac arrest and inducible ventricular arrhythmias with coronary artery disease.

The Amiodarone Versus the Implantable Defibrillator (AVID) study demonstrated the superiority of the ICD in patients with cardiac arrest or poorly tolerated VT, with an ejection fraction of <35%. In addition, primary prevention studies in high-risk patients (*eg*, those with ejection fraction <40% plus coronary artery disease, those found to have inducible arrhythmias in electrophysiology study) have demonstrated the benefit of the ICD over medical therapy with a dramatic reduction in overall mortality. Patients receiving ICDs in this population achieved relative mortality reductions approaching 50%! Recent data have also demonstrated a benefit for ICD, compared with conventional therapy, in primary prevention of sudden death in patients with severely reduced ejection fraction (<30%) and a history of previous MI, as well as patients with nonischemic cardiomyopathies and ejection fraction <35%. Patients with prolonged QRS duration >120 ms and class III or IV CHF have also demonstrated significant improvement in heart failure symptoms with biventricular pacing, in addition to improvement in combined endpoint of heart failure admissions and mortality.

As a result of these advances and the increase in implantation, the critical care physician is increasingly likely to encounter patients with ICDs and ICD-related complications and/or emergencies. In order to understand the emergency, one must realize that the ICD mainly treats arrhythmias based on the ventricular rate. Preprogrammed heart rate zones trigger the device to intervene with therapy such as automatic pacing or low- or high-energy shocks. Complex algorithms to prevent therapy for SVT and atrial fibrillation exist, but are not always utilized due to fear of withholding appropriate therapy for ventricular arrhythmias that could be misclassified as SVT or sinus tachycardia.

Complications Associated with ICDs

Complications of ICD therapy include inappropriate shocks secondary to lead fracture, atrial fibrillation with rapid ventricular response, failure to treat as a result of undersensing or inappropriate therapy because of oversensing of intrinsic cardiac signal, or external noise such as electronic theft devices. Patients receiving more than two or three ICD discharges in a 24-h period should be treated as having a medical emergency.

Treatment

ICD shocks are extremely painful and can be very traumatic, which can result in posttraumatic stress disorder. Patients presenting with incessant shocks that are appropriately delivered should be admitted to ICU. They frequently require sedation and antiadrenergic therapy, as well as antiarrhythmic therapy and correction of any underlying electrolyte abnormalities. A search for exacerbating conditions such as congestive heart failure or increasing ischemia should be undertaken. An emergent consultation with an electrophysiologist should be obtained to interrogate the device for the possibility of malfunction. If an electrophysiology consultation is not available and the patient appears to be receiving spurious shocks without evidence of ventricular arrhythmia, the placement of a strong magnet over the device will impede its ability to sense and thereby prevent further device intervention.

Troubleshooting

If the ICD fails to terminate arrhythmias, one should look for migration of the ventricular lead or pharmacologic causes of increased defibrillation threshold such as amiodarone or certain class I agents (*eg*, flecainide). If a device completes all of its therapy without terminating the arrhythmia, it will generally not reinitiate therapy unless sinus rhythm has been detected again. Occasionally, in patients with incessant arrhythmias, the device will terminate the arrhythmia with each output; however, the reinitiation of arrhythmia occurs before success has been detected. In this situation, the device may withhold further therapy after completing the maximal number of interventions.

When a device produces ineffective defibrillation, patients should be externally defibrillated. Paddles or patches should not be placed directly on the device. Subsequent to external defibrillation, the device should be interrogated to ensure that no changes in programming occurred.

Problems Associated With Tests/Procedures in ICD Patients

Patients with ICDs are problematic with regard to various tests and procedures. In general, with few exceptions, patients with ICDs should not undergo MRI scanning. The strong magnetic field will impair the sensing ability of the device and may damage internal circuits.

Electrocautery during surgery frequently will be interpreted by the device as a rapid tachyarrhythmia. This leads to inappropriate discharges to the patient, with disconcerting but harmless shocks to the surgeon. Patients with ICD frequently must have their device detection algorithms turned off or placed on monitor during surgery if electrocautery is planned. The problem of electrical oversensing is increased in pacer-dependent patients with ICDs that also function as pacemakers. In these patients, a temporary pacer may need to be placed in asynchronous mode during electrocautery because electrocautery will lead to inhibition of pacing and possible asystole. If only limited electrocautery is needed, then monitoring the patient's rhythm for prolonged pauses may suffice, along with limitations on the length of surgical radiofrequency application.

Finally, as patients receiving ICDs frequently have other severe comorbid diseases, end-of-life issues frequently arise. If a patient is clearly terminal or the decision to withdraw care has been made, it is reasonable to turn off the ICD to avoid therapy for terminal arrhythmias. The device must be removed prior to cremation to avoid explosion of the battery. Because of the complex and specialized nature of ICDs and their programming, the input of an electrophysiologist should be obtained as soon as possible.

Conclusion

The diagnosis of tachyarrhythmias depends heavily on ECG assessment. Treatment depends mainly on differentiation of supraventricular and ventricular arrhythmias, as well as the presence or absence of left ventricular dysfunction. Patients with unstable rhythms should immediately undergo DC cardioversion or defibrillation. Patients with stable symptoms may be treated pharmacologically. Patients with stable ventricular arrhythmias should still be considered for electrical therapy because of the low risk of proarrhythmia associated with such treatment.

Class Ia drugs (eg, procainamide, quinidine, and disopyramide), class Ic drugs (eg, propafenone), and flecainide should be avoided in patients with left ventricular dysfunction and/or coronary artery disease due to their increased mortality with the use of these drugs. In this population, amiodarone is the pharmacologic treatment of choice.

Once the ventricular arrhythmia is controlled, ICD therapy is frequently indicated. ICDs are more effective at preventing death in patients with depressed left ventricular function with previous arrest and/or sustained monomorphic VT with coronary artery disease.

Patients with SVT may be controlled with a variety of antiarrhythmics and AV nodal blocking agents. An increasing number of patients are definitively treated with catheter ablation.

Atrial fibrillation continues to be troublesome, but new catheter-based modalities promise to offer new therapeutic options in the near future. Until then, rate control and rhythm control remain reasonable treatment strategies depending on patient symptoms. Patients at moderate or high risk for thromboembolism—including those with diabetes, hypertension, valvular disease, congestive heart failure, previous stroke, or age >65 years—should receive anticoagulant therapy with warfarin to reduce the risk of stroke, with a target international normalized ratio of 2.0 to 3.0.

Patients with WPW syndrome should be screened for symptoms. Asymptomatic patients generally do not need further evaluation. Patients with palpitations or syncope should undergo electrophysiologic study with ablation for inducible arrhythmias or rapid accessory pathway conduction faster than 250 bpm.

Annotated References

A comparison of antiarrhythmic drug therapy with implantable defibrillators in patients resuscitated from near-fatal ventricular arrhythmias: the Antiarrhythmics versus Implantable Defibrillators (AVID) Investigators. N Engl J Med 1997; 337:1576–1583
First major study to demonstrate benefit of ICD over drugs in patients with sustained arrhythmias or arrest.

Bristow MR, Saxon LA, Boehmer J, et al. Cardiac-resynchronization therapy with or without an implantable defibrillator in advanced chronic heart failure. N Engl J Med 2004; 350:2140–2150

Study demonstrating additional benefit of both biventricular pacing and biventricular pacing with defibrillation in heart failure patients over optimal medical therapy.

Brugada P, Brugada J, Mont L, et al. A new approach to the differential diagnosis of a regular tachycardia with a wide QRS complex. Circulation 1991; 83:1649–1659

A classic article illustrating an algorithmic and reproducible approach to differentiating wide-complex tachycardia.

Effect of prophylactic amiodarone on mortality after acute myocardial infarction and in congestive heart failure: meta-analysis of individual data from 6500 patients in randomised trials; Amiodarone Trials Meta-Analysis Investigators. Lancet 1997; 350:1417–1424

A meta-analysis suggesting that amiodarone improves survival after MI and in congestive heart failure.

Fuster V, Ryden LE, Asinger RW, et al. ACC/AHA/ESC Guidelines for the Management of Patients With Atrial Fibrillation: Executive Summary; A Report of the American College of Cardiology/American Heart Association Task Force on Practice Guidelines and the European Society of Cardiology Committee for Practice Guidelines and Policy Conferences (Committee to Develop Guidelines for the Management of Patients With Atrial Fibrillation) Developed in Collaboration With the North American Society of Pacing and Electrophysiology. Circulation 2001; 104:2118–2150

Current updated recommendations for management of atrial fibrillation.

Gregoratos G, Cheitlin MD, Conill A, et al. ACC/AHA guidelines for implantation of cardiac pacemakers and antiarrhythmia devices: a report of the American College of Cardiology/American Heart Association Task Force on Practice Guidelines (Committee on Pacemaker Implantation). J Am Coll Cardiol 1998; 31:1175–1209

Review of indications for implantation of pacemakers and ICD.

Guidelines 2000 for Cardiopulmonary Resuscitation and Emergency Cardiovascular Care. Part 6: advanced cardiovascular life support: section 4: devices to assist circulation. The American Heart Association in collaboration with the International Liaison Committee on Resuscitation. Circulation 2000; 102(8 Suppl):I105–I111

Updated guidelines for resuscitation and an explanation of the supportive data.

Moss AJ, Zareba W, Hall WJ, et al. Prophylactic implantation of a defibrillator in patients with myocardial infarction and reduced ejection fraction. N Engl J Med 2002; 346:877–883

Study revealing primary prevention mortality benefit of ICD vs control therapy in depressed left ventricular function and previous MI without arrhythmia induction.

Myerburg RJ, Mitrani R, Interian A Jr, et al. Interpretation of outcomes of antiarrhythmic clinical trials: design features and population impact. Circulation 1998; 97:1514–1521

An excellent discussion on confounding factors that influence the design and interpretation of antiarrhythmic studies.

Preliminary report: effect of encainide and flecainide on mortality in a randomized trial of arrhythmia suppression after myocardial infarction; the Cardiac Arrhythmia Suppression Trial (CAST) Investigators. N Engl J Med 1989; 321:406–412

Seminal study that showed dramatically increased mortality in patients treated with encainide and flecainide in a post-MI population despite arrhythmia suppression.

Prystowsky EN, Benson DW Jr, Fuster V, et al. Management of patients with atrial fibrillation: from the Subcommittee on Electrocardiography and Electrophysiology, American Heart Association. Circulation 1996; 93:1262–1277

An exhaustive review on the subject of atrial fibrillation.

Singh BN. Current antiarrhythmic drugs: an overview of mechanisms of action and potential clinical utility. J Cardiovasc Electrophysiol 1999; 10:283–301

An excellent review of the mechanism of action and application of current antiarrhythmics.

Torp-Pedersen C, Moller M, Bloch-Thomsen PE, et al. Dofetilide in patients with congestive heart failure and left ventricular dysfunction: Danish Investigations of Arrhythmia and Mortality on Dofetilide Study Group. N Engl J Med 1999; 341:857–865

Dofetilide had no adverse mortality effect in a group of patients with congestive heart failure.

Wellens HJJ, Bar FW, Lie KI, et al. The value of the electrocardiogram in the differential diagnosis of a tachycardia with a widened QRS complex. Am J Med 1978; 64:27–33

Classic article helping to differentiate VT from aberrancy.

Notes

Notes

Hypertensive Emergencies and Urgencies

R. Phillip Dellinger, MD, FCCP

Objectives:

- To identify acute end organ dysfunction due to hypertension
- To recognize importance of blood pressure lowering in a timely but finite manner
- To match appropriate drugs for treatment of hypertensive emergencies/urgencies based on patient characteristics
- To appreciate potential toxicities and side effects of drug choice

Key words: hypertensive emergency; hypertensive encephalopathy; hypotensive urgency; postoperative hypertension

Introduction

Severe hypertension with acute organ dysfunction is a reason for admission to the ICU and uncontrolled hypertension may complicate ICU stay for those patients admitted for other reasons. Hypertensive emergencies are typically defined as elevations in blood pressure associated with acute organ dysfunction and identify a circumstance in which immediate blood pressure lowering is indicated. Hypertensive urgencies identify patients at risk for organ dysfunction due to hypertension and in these patients blood pressure lowering needs may be immediate or may be accomplished over hours after assessment of risk.

Identification of End Organ Damage

Most patients with hypertensive emergencies will have a history of poorly controlled essential hypertension. Secondary hypertension (renal artery stenosis, for example) should, however, be considered. Symptoms may be important clues to trigger a search for acute organ dysfunction in hypertensive patients such as headache, confusion, or seizures in hypertensive encephalopathy. Chest pain may signify aortic dissection or myocardial ischemia. Physical examination of chest may reveal rales associated with hypertension-induced pulmonary edema, a murmur of aortic insufficiency associated with proximal aortic dissection or extremity pulse deficits related to aortic dissection. Pertinent laboratory tests in the evaluation of patients with known or suspected hypertensive emergencies or urgencies include a urine analysis in search of glomerulonephritis as a secondary cause of hypertension or creatinine as a marker of hypertension-induced acute renal dysfunction (when baseline value is known). An ECG may reveal myocardial ischemia driven by hypertension and chest radiograph may offer clues to aortic dissection (such as widened mediastinum) or hypertension-induced pulmonary edema.

Hypertensive Encephalopathy

A 52-yr-old man presents with generalized seizures and a blood pressure of 244/160 mm Hg. The patient received lorazepam IV with cessation of seizures. He is intubated and mechanically ventilated. Fundus exam reveals papilledema and supports the diagnosis of hypertensive encephalopathy.

Clinical manifestations of hypertensive encephalopathy-induced increase in intracranial pressure include headache, nausea, vomiting, confusion, lethargy, generalized seizures, and coma. Differential diagnosis of hypertensive encephalopathy includes severe hypertension in association with subarachnoid hemorrhage or stroke. CT scan may be required to assure the absence of these entities. In hypertensive encephalopathy, as well as in most hypertensive emergencies and urgencies, the initial blood pressure therapeutic target is to decrease mean arterial pressure by 15% to 25%. In patients with chronic hypertension the cerebral blood flow autoregulation curve is shifted to the right. In the normotensive patient cerebral blood flow is autoregulated such that cerebral blood flow remains constant between mean arterial pressures of 50 and 150 mm Hg. In chronically hypertensive patients this autoregulation shifts to the right and occurs at a much higher pressure range. Overzealous lowering of mean arterial pressure in hypertensive emergencies to even high normal blood pressures may put the patient at risk for a decrease in cerebral blood flow and may be particularly problematic in patients with underlying cerebral vascular disease, producing iatrogenic strokes.

General Principles of Intravenous Drug Therapy for the Hypertensive Emergencies

In hypertensive encephalopathy as in other causes of hypertensive emergencies the ideal drug is an intravenous vasodilator with quick onset of action and quick offset of action. Drugs that offer these traits include nitroprusside, nicardipine, fenoldopam, and nitroglycerin.

Sodium nitroprusside is begun with an initial infusion of .5 to 1.0 µg/kg/min with a maximum dosage of 10 µg/kg/min for 10 min or maximum sustained dose of 3 µg/kg/min. Cyanide and thiocyanate toxicity are potential problems with nitroprusside infusion. This rarely occurs with recommended infusion rates during 48 h or less of therapy. Even in patients with anuric renal failure nitroprusside used at recommended doses during the initial stabilization of blood pressure is safe. Nitroprusside is nonenzymatically converted to cyanide in the blood and cyanide is converted to thiocyanate in the liver. Thiocyanate is excreted by the kidney. Patients with liver disease are at increase risk of cyanide toxicity and patients with kidney disease at increased risk of thiocyanate toxicity. In patients without renal dysfunction thiocyanate levels can be followed as a marker for risk of cyanide and thiocyanate toxicity. An arterial line is advised with nitroprusside.

Fenoldopam is a drug with a very similar pharmacodynamic profile as nitroprusside. It also offers the potential renal benefit of being a selective dopamine-1 receptor agonist. It has been demonstrated to increase renal blood flow although clinical studies have not been able to demonstrate clinical outcome benefit compared to nitroprusside. Dosing is .01 to .03 µg/kg/min. It is safer than nitroprusside in patients with renal dysfunction but considerably more expensive. Some tachyphylaxis may be seen and it may cause tachycardia.

Nitroglycerin is a direct-acting vasodilator and unlike nitroprusside, which is a balanced arteriolar intravenous acting drug, has predominately venous capacitance effects. It does have the potential to redistribute coronary artery blood flow to actively ischemic myocardium. Primary consideration for nitroglycerin should be in hypertensive emergencies/urgencies associated with congestive heart failure, coronary artery disease, post-coronary artery bypass surgery, and increased left ventricular (LV) filling pressures. It is particularly useful in patients with active myocardial ischemia, high LV filling pressures, and mild to moderate hypertension.

Intravenous nicardipine is an effective titratable continuous infusion calcium-channel blocker for treatment of hypertensive emergencies/urgencies. It has rapid onset and intermediate offset and is an arterial vasodilator that is associated with increased cardiac index and increase coronary artery blood flow. Unlike other calcium-channel blockers, it is unlikely to produce any negative inotropic effect and is unlikely to produce clinically significant tachycardia. It is begun at 5 mg/h and increased 2.5 mg/hq5 min to a maximum of 15 mg/h.

Intravenous labetalol is also an alternative to nitroprusside and is a reliable drug to treat hypertensive encephalopathy as well as other etiologies of hypertensive emergencies. It has quick onset of action but is long-acting. Its combined α/β effect typically produces significant lowering of peripheral vascular resistance with minimal decrease in heart rate and minimal change in cardiac output. A loading dose is given by IV bolus of 20 to 80 mg q10 to 15 min depending on response. Loading by continuous infusion at .5 to 2 mg/min is also possible. Unlike nitroprusside, labetalol may be utilized in some patients without arterial line placement. Although maintenance continuous infusions have been successfully utilized, labetalol was primarily developed for initial control of blood pressure through loading followed by conversion to PO labetalol or other alternative anti-hypertension therapies. Labetalol should not be used in patients with second degree heart block or greater, patients with asthma, or patients with significant systolic cardiac dysfunction.

Hypertensive Crisis With High Pressure Pulmonary Edema

Clinical features of severe hypertension-induced rise in left ventricular end diastolic pressure with associated high pulmonary capillary pressure and pulmonary edema include severe hypoxemia, CO_2 retention, pink frothy sputum, and pulmonary edema on chest radiograph. The typical patient will have chronic left ventricular hypertrophy with diastolic function and normal or increased ejection fraction. Initial therapy includes anything that lowers the left ventricular end diastolic pressure. This will include increase in venous capacitance, decrease in arteriolar resistance and softening of the LV. Diuresis is effective although studies have demonstrated that most patients with this diagnosis do not have increased intravascular blood volume and therefore vasodilatation is the most effective therapy. Since diastolic function is often present β blockers are also very effective. Labetalol may also be very useful as a combination α/β blocker. Acute ischemia, associated with hypertension, may occur during weaning from mechanical ventilation may also produce increase in blood pressure and associated rise in left ventricular end diastolic pressure driving the patient into pulmonary edema as a cause of weaning failure. This presentation may be more insidious than the patient presenting to the emergency department with acute hypertension-induced pulmonary edema since lower ranges of blood pressure elevation may be present with a contribution of ischemia-induced wall stiffness also playing a prominent role in the rise in pulmonary capillary pressure.

Enalaprilat is an intravenous drug with potential to treat hypertension and to improve cardiac function. It is an afterload reducer with onset of action in 15 min in duration of action of 12 h. The dose is .625 to 5 mg administered as a single bolus every 6 h. It may be chosen to treat mild to moderate hypertension in patients with congestive heart failure due to systolic dysfunction or in patients with activation of the renin-angiotensin system, such as scleroderma kidney. It is not usually a "go to" drug to treat severe life-threatening hypertension. Potential disadvantages of enalaprilat include idiopathic angioedema. It should not be used in patients with bilateral renovascular disease or in pregnant women. When used on an ongoing basis in the ICU, creatinine should be followed and the drug discontinued if creatinine begins to rise. It can however be instituted in patients with baseline elevated creatinine.

Hypertension With Acute Central Nervous System Events

An increase in blood pressure is thought to be a normal physiologic response to acute central nervous system ischemic events including bland stroke, hemorrhagic stroke, intracranial hemorrhage, and subarachnoid hemorrhage. Although increased blood pressure is considered to put the patient at risk for increased edema in areas of injury as well as an increased chance of bleeding or re-bleeding, equally important in these patients is watershed areas of brain penumbra at risk for further ischemic injury which might benefit from higher blood pressure-induced collateral flow. There is general agreement that in an unclipped subarachnoid hemorrhage blood pressure should be normalized, and once the aneurysm is clipped that very high blood pressures may be tolerated as there is no significant risk of re-bleed and hypertension may be protective against postbleed vasospasm.

Significant increases in blood pressure should also be tolerated after bland stroke, hemorrhagic stroke, and intracerebral hemorrhage (Table1). Less hypertension is tolerated when thrombolytics are to be given (Table 2). Obviously comfort decreases as one progresses over these three entities. In intracerebral hemorrhage the penumbra issues are very important. Lowering of blood pressure by 20% likely does not put the penumbra at risk after intracerebral hemorrhage and may decrease risk of further bleeding.

Severe Hypertension-Induced Renal Dysfunction

A patient may present with severe hypertension and acute deterioration in renal function. Drugs that may be particularly suited to this group include labetalol and hydralazine where greater preservation of renal blood flow may occur. Dialysis is the treatment of choice for severe hypertension primarily driven by volume overload.

Hydralazine is a direct arteriolar vasodilator with onset of action in 15 to 30 min and duration of effect 2 to 4 h. It is also advocated as a drug of particular benefit in eclampsia. It is associated with reflex tachycardia and should be avoided in

Table 1. *Treatment of Patients Not Eligible for Thrombolytic Therapy**

Blood Pressure (mm Hg)	Treatment
Systolic <220 OR Diastolic <120	Observe unless other end-organ involvement, *eg*, aortic dissection, acute myocardial infarction, pulmonary edema, hypertensive encephalopathy
	Treat other symptoms of stroke, such as haedache, pain, agitation, nausea, and vomiting
	Treat other acute complications of stroke, including hypoxia, increased intracranial pressure, seizures, or hypoglycemia
Systolic >220 OR Diastolic 121–140	Labetalol IV-May repeat or double every 10 min (maximum dose 300 mg) OR
	Nicardipine IV infusion
	Aim for a 10 to 15% reduction in blood pressure
Diastolic >140	Sodium nitroprusside with continuous blood pressure monitoring Aim for a 10 to 15% reduction in blood pressure

*Reprinted with permission from Adams et al. Stroke 2003; 34:1056–1083.

Table 2. *Treatment of Patients Eligible for Thrombolytic Therapy**

Blood Pressure (mm Hg)	Treatment
Pretreatment systolic >185 OR Diastolic >110	Labetalol 10–20 IV over 1–2 min
	May repeat 1X OR nitroglycerin ointment 1–2 inches
	If blood pressure is not reduced and maintained at desired levels (systolic ≤185 and diastolic ≤110), do not administer rtPA
During and after treatment 1. Monitor BP 2. Diastolic >140 3. Systolic >230 OR Diastolic 121–140	Check blood pressure every 15 min for 2 h, then every 30 min for 6 h, and then every hour for 16 h. Sodium nitroprusside 0.5 µg/kg/min IV infusion as initial dose and titrate to desired blood pressure
	Labetalol 10 mg IV over 1–2 min
	May repeat or double labetalol every 10 min to a maximum dose of 300 mg or give the initial labetalol bolus and then start a labetalol drip at 2 to 8 mg/min OR nicardipine 5 mg/h IV infusion as initial dose; titrate to desired effect by increasing 2.5 mg/h every 5 min to maximum of 15 mg/h. If blood pressure is not controlled by labetalol, consider sodium nitroprusside
4. Systolic 180-230 OR Diastolic 105-120	Labetalol 10 mg IV over 1–2 min May repeat or double labetalol every 10 to 12 min to a maximum dose of 300 mg or give the initial labetalol bolus and then start a labetalol drip at 2 to 8 mg/min

*Reprinted with permission from Adams et al. Stroke 2003; 34:1056–1083.

patients with dissecting aortic aneurysm and acute myocardial ischemia.

Hypertension With Eclampsia and Severe Pre-eclampsia

Hypertensive patients with eclampsia and severe pre-eclampsia should be hospitalized in the ICU. As a general rule the blood pressure target is to keep a diastolic BP of around 110 mm Hg. In addition to magnesium, hydralazine has traditionally been the drug of choice. Potential problems include tachycardia and side effects that mimic symptoms of eclampsia (nausea, vomiting, headaches, and anxiety). Excessive hypotension can be dangerous to both mother and fetus. Labetalol and nifedipine are alternative agents for treatment.

Postoperative Hypertension

A diastolic of >110 mm Hg and a systolic >200 mm Hg put patients at risk for postoperative complications. Hypertension-induced postoperative complications include arrhythmias, myocardial ischemia/infarction, stroke, and wound hemorrhage.

A wide variety of drugs may by used to manage postoperative hypertension depending upon particular patient characteristics. These include nitroprusside, nicardipine, hydralazine, labetalol, esmolol, and fenoldopam.

Esmolol is a cardioselective β-adrenergic blocker with quick onset action (peak effects within 5 to 15 min) and short half-life (9 to 10 min). It is a good fit for patients with tachycardia, hypertension, and good systolic function. Either esmolol or intermittent bolus metoprolol may offer advantage to postoperative patients with hypertension, tachycardia, and good systolic function. These drugs should be used with caution in patients with obstructive airways disease and avoided in patients with asthma. When a β-blocker is used in patients with potential side effects of β-blockade, esmolol is preferred over intermittent metoprolol. Table 3 contrasts esmolol with two other intravenous antihypertensive choices.

Aortic Dissection

Dissecting thoracic aorta aneurysms are classified as either involving the arch/descending aorta or involving the ascending aorta. Dissecting thoracic aorta aneurysms involving the arch and descending aorta that do not interfere with major vessel outflow are typically managed medically with blood pressure control. Aneurysms involving the ascending aorta are typically surgically treated. Aneurysms of the ascending aorta may dissect proximally producing a murmur of aortic insufficiency or acute pericardial tamponade. Distal migration may produce obstruction of major vascular outflow vessels or rupture into the thorax. Occasionally a leak may occur into the thorax which is diagnosed in time to allow life-saving surgery. The propagating force for a dissection is the change in pulse over change in time or dp/dt max. This "shearing force" is minimized by a combination of keeping pulse in the low normal range, normalizing blood pressure, and decreasing inotropy. Dissection of the aorta is another circumstance in which normalization of the blood pressure, is indicated. Dissection is usually diagnosed with CT with and without contrast demonstrating a grayish false lumen predominately filled with clot alongside a bright white dye filled true aortic channel.

Suggested Reading

Adams HP, Adams RJ, Brott T, et al. Guidelines for the early management of patients with ischemic stroke: a scientific statement from the Stroke Council of the American Stroke Association. Stroke 2003; 34: 1056–1083

Blumenfeld JD, Laragh JH. Management of hypertensive crises: the scientific basis for treatment decisions. Am J Hypertens 2001; 14:1154–1167

Elliott WJ. Hypertensive emergencies. Crit Care Clin 2001; 17:435–451

Erstad BL, Barletta JF. Treatment of hypertension in the perioperative patient. Ann Pharmacother 2000; 34:66–79

Table 3. *Contrasting Effects of Nicardipine, Esmolol, and Labetalol**

	Nicardipine	Esmolol	Labetalol
Administration	Continuous infusion	Continuous infusion	Bolus continuous infusion
Onset	Rapid	Rapid	Rapid
Offset	Rapid	Rapid	Slower
HR	Minimal increase	Decreased	Minimal decrease
SVR	Decreased	0	Decreased
Cardiac output	Increased	Decreased	No change
Myocardial O$_2$ balance	Positive	Positive	Positive

*HR, heart rate; SVR, systemic vascular resistance.

Frohlich ED. Local hemodynamic changes in hypertension: insights for therapeutic preservation of target organs. Hypertension 2001; 38:1388–1394

Hoshide S, Kario K, Fujikawa H, et al. Hemodynamic cerebral infarction triggered by excessive blood pressure reduction in hypertensive emergencies. J Am Geriatr Soc 1998; 46:1179–1180

IV Nicardipine Study Group. Efficacy and safety of intravenous nicardipine in the control of postoperative hypertension. Chest 1991; 99:393–398

Kitiyakara C, Guzman NJ. Malignant hypertension and hypertensive emergencies. J Am Soc Nephrol 1998; 9:133–142

Lisk DR, Grotta JC, Lamki LM, et al. Should hypertension be treated after acute stroke? Arch Neurol 1993; 50:855–862

McKillion PC, Dellinger RP. Hypertensive emergencies and urgencies. In: Civetta J, Taylor RW, Kirby RR, eds. Critical Care. 3rd ed. Philadelphia, PA: JP Lippincott, 1997; 1811–1822

Murphy MB, Murray C, Shorten GD. Fenoldopam: a selective peripheral dopamine-receptor agonist for the treatment of severe hypertension. N Engl J Med 2001; 345:1548–1557

Neutel JM, Smith DHG, Wallin D, et al. A comparison of intravenous nicardipine and sodium nitroprusside in the immediate treatment of severe hypertension. Am J Hypertens 1994; 7:623–628

Oparil S, Aronson S, Deeb GM, et al. Fenoldopam: a new parenteral antihypertensive: consensus roundtable on the management of perioperative hypertension and hypertensive crises. Am J Hypertens 1999; 12:653–664

Phillips RA, Greenblatt J, Krakoff LR. Hypertensive emergencies: diagnosis and management. Prog Cardiovasc Dis 2002; 45:33–48

Probst BD. Hypertensive disorders of pregnancy. Emerg Med Clin North Am 1994; 12:73–89

Qureshi AI, Tuhrim S, Broderick JP, et al. Spontaneous intracerebral hemorrhage. N Engl J Med 2001; 344:1450–1460

Tietjen CS, Hurn PD, Ulatowski JA, et al. Treatment modalities for hypertensive patients with intracranial pathology: options and risks. Crit Care Med 1996; 24:311–322

Varon J, Marik PE. The diagnosis and management of hypertensive crises. Chest 2000; 118:214–227

Vaughan CJ, Delanty N. Hypertensive emergencies. Lancet 2000; 356:411–417

Vidt DG: Emergency room management of hypertensive urgencies and emergencies. J Clinical Hypertension 2001; 3:158–164

Notes

Notes

Shock

John P. Kress, MD, FCCP

Objectives:

- To describe the clinical evaluation of patients with shock
- To describe the different types of shock
- To describe resuscitation of shock
- To describe new therapies for septic shock
- To describe vasoactive drugs used for treatment of shock

Key words: left ventricular failure; right ventricular failure; sepsis; shock; vasopressors

---

Shock is a common condition necessitating admission to the ICU or occurring in the course of critical care. This chapter discusses the pathophysiology of various shock states, followed by recommendations for the diagnosis and treatment of each category of shock. Lastly a brief review of commonly used vasoactive agents is presented.

Shock Defined

Shock is defined by the presence of multisystem end-organ hypoperfusion. Clinical indicators include reduced mean blood pressure, tachycardia, tachypnea, cool skin and extremities, acute altered mental status, and oliguria. Hypotension is usually, though not always, present. The end result of multiorgan hypoperfusion is tissue hypoxia, often clinically seen as lactic acidosis.

Clinical Evaluation of Patients in Shock

Most patients who present with shock are hypotensive. Since the mean blood pressure is the product of the cardiac output (CO) and the systemic vascular resistance (SVR), reductions in blood pressure can be categorized by decreased CO and/or decreased SVR. Accordingly, the initial evaluation of a hypotensive patient should evaluate the adequacy of the CO. Clinical evidence of diminished CO includes a narrow pulse pressure (a surrogate marker for stroke volume), and cool extremities with delayed capillary refill. Signs of increased CO include a widened pulse pressure (particularly with a reduced diastolic pressure), warm extremities with bounding pulses and rapid capillary refill. If a hypotensive patient has clinical signs of increased CO, one can infer that the reduced blood pressure is a result of decreased SVR.

In hypotensive patients with clinical evidence of reduced CO, an assessment of intravascular and cardiac volume status is appropriate. A hypotensive patient with decreased intravascular and cardiac volume status may have a history suggesting hemorrhage or other volume losses (eg, vomiting, diarrhea, polyuria). The jugular venous pulse is often reduced in such a patient. A hypotensive patient with an increased intravascular and cardiac volume status may have S3 and/or S4 gallops, increased jugular venous pressure (JVP), extremity edema, and crackles on lung auscultation. The chest radiograph may show cardiomegaly, congestion of the vascular pedicle,[1] Kerley B lines and pulmonary edema. Chest pain and electrocardiograph (ECG) changes consistent with ischemia may also be noted.

In hypotensive patients with clinical evidence of increased CO, a search for causes of decreased SVR is appropriate. The most common cause of high cardiac output hypotension is sepsis. Accordingly, one should search for signs of the systemic inflammatory response syndrome (SIRS), which include abnormalities in temperature ($\geq 38°$ C or $\leq 36°$ C), heart rate (≥ 90 beats/min), respiratory rate (≥ 20 breaths/min), and WBC count ($\geq 12,000/mm^3$ or $\leq 4,000/mm^3$ or ≥ 10 bands).[2] A person with SIRS and a presumed or confirmed infectious process fulfills criteria for sepsis. A person with sepsis and one or more organ failures fulfills criteria for severe sepsis. Other causes of high cardiac output hypotension include: liver failure, severe pancreatitis, burns and other trauma which elicit the systemic inflammatory response syndrome, anaphylaxis, thyrotoxicosis and peripheral arteriovenous shunts.

In summary, the three most common categories of shock include cardiogenic, hypovolemic and high CO with decreased SVR. Certainly these categories may overlap and occur simultaneously (*eg*, hypovolemic and septic shock, septic and cardiogenic shock).

The initial assessment of a patient in shock as outlined above should take only a few minutes. It is important that aggressive, early resuscitation is instituted based on the initial assessment, particularly since there are data suggesting that early resuscitation of shock (both septic and cardiogenic) may improve survival.[3,4] If the initial bedside assessment yields equivocal or confounding data, more objective assessments such as echocardiography and/or central venous or pulmonary artery catheterization may be useful. The goal of early resuscitation is to reestablish adequate perfusion to prevent or minimize end organ injury.

During the initial resuscitation of patients in shock, principles of advanced cardiac life support should be followed. Since patients in shock may be obtunded and unable to protect the airway, an early assessment of the patient's airway is mandatory during resuscitation from shock. Early intubation and mechanical ventilation are often required. Reasons for institution of endotracheal intubation and mechanical ventilation include acute hypoxemic respiratory failure as well as ventilatory failure. Acute hypoxemic respiratory failure may occur in cardiogenic shock (pulmonary edema) as well as septic shock (pneumonia or the acute respiratory distress syndrome [ARDS]). Ventilatory failure often occurs as a result of an increased load on the respiratory system. This load may present in the form of acute metabolic acidosis (often lactic acidosis) or decreased compliance of the lungs as a result of pulmonary edema. Inadequate perfusion to respiratory muscles in the setting of shock may be another reason for early intubation and mechanical ventilation. Normally, the respiratory muscles receive a very small percentage of the CO.[5] However, in patients who are in shock with respiratory distress for the reasons listed above, the percentage of cardiac output dedicated to respiratory muscles may increase ten fold or more.[6,7] Mechanical ventilation may relieve the patient of the work of breathing and permit redistribution of a limited cardiac output to other vital organs. Such patients often demonstrate signs of respiratory muscle fatigue including: inability to speak full sentences, accessory respiratory muscle use, paradoxical abdominal muscle activity, extreme tachypnea (>40 breaths/min), and decreasing respiratory rate despite an increasing drive to breathe.

Endotracheal intubation and mechanical ventilation with sedation and, if necessary, muscle paralysis will decrease oxygen demand of the respiratory muscles allowing improved oxygen delivery to other hypoperfused tissue beds.[8] Patients in shock should be intubated before other procedures are performed, since attention to the airway and breathing may wane during such procedures.

Resuscitation

Resuscitation should focus on improving end organ perfusion, not simply raising the blood pressure. Accordingly, a patient with a reduced CO by clinical assessment with a decreased intravascular and cardiac volume status should receive aggressive intravenous resuscitation. The type of intravenous fluid is (colloid [*eg*, albumin] vs crystalloid) controversial.[9,10] Though one study reported improved outcomes in trauma patients whose volume resuscitation was delayed until definite surgical repair (average time to operation ~2 h),[11] aggressive volume resuscitation in patients with reduced intravascular and cardiac volume status is merited in virtually all but perhaps torso trauma patients who can undergo surgical repair quickly. Early administration of vasoactive drugs in hypovolemic patients in order to increase the blood pressure is not recommended. This practice may impair the assessment of the patient's circulatory status and potentially delay definitive treatment. The transfusion of packed red blood cells to anemic patients in order to improve oxygen delivery is physiologically rational; however, recent data suggest that, as long as hemoglobin levels remain greater than 7 g/dL, this practice may not improve outcomes and perhaps even worsen outcomes in select subgroups of patients.[12] Certainly, a conservative transfusion strategy does not apply to hemorrhaging, hypovolemic patients in shock. Blood products should be administered through a blood warmer, in order to minimize hypothermia and subsequent disturbances in coagulation. In summary, it is important to remember that oxygen delivery is the product of cardiac output, oxygen-carrying capacity of the blood, and arterial oxygen saturation. Each of these components must be considered and optimized when addressing resuscitation of patients in shock.

Early reassessment of the patient with purported hypovolemic shock after the initial resuscitation is extremely important. Concrete end points such as increased blood pressure and pulse pressure, improved capillary refill, urine output and mental status should be sought. The absence of a response suggests that the volume challenge may not be adequate. Careful and repeated searches for signs of volume overload (increased JVP, new gallop or extra heart sounds, pulmonary edema) should be done while the resuscitation is ongoing.

If the patient remains in shock despite adequate volume resuscitation, support with vasoactive drugs is appropriate. Occasionally, vasoactive drugs must be started "prematurely" when volume resuscitation needs are large. When severe hypotension and hypovolemia are present, this approach is occasionally needed to "buy time" while volume resuscitation is ongoing. This strategy is only rarely necessary and should only be instituted temporarily until volume resuscitation is accomplished. It is important to remember that vasoactive drugs may obscure hypovolemic shock by raising blood pressure in spite of a low cardiac output state.

Once intravascular volume has been restored, patients who remain in shock may benefit from vasoactive drugs. These drugs should be titrated to end-organ perfusion, rather than an arbitrary blood pressure value. Accordingly, mental status, urine output, lactic acidosis, capillary refill and skin temperature, and venous oxygen saturation are reasonable end points to target in these patients. If evidence of hypoperfusion persists, one should consider inadequate volume resuscitation, impaired cardiac output, inadequate hemoglobin, and/or inadequate oxygen saturation as a likely explanation. If objective information obtained by physical examination is unclear or ambiguous, additional information obtained via invasive monitoring (central venous pressure, pulmonary artery catheterization or echocardiography) may be useful. Echocardiography is a useful adjunct or even replacement to invasive pressure measurements and can be used to distinguish poor ventricular pumping function from hypovolemia; a good study can exclude or confirm tamponade, pulmonary hypertension, or significant valve dysfunction, all of which influence therapy and may supplement or replace the more invasive right heart catheterization. These topics are covered separately in another chapter in the syllabus.

Cardiogenic Shock

The model of the heart as a pump is useful in considering cardiogenic shock. By definition, pump failure is seen when cardiac output is inappropriately low despite adequate input in the form of venous return (determined by right atrial pressure). The specific cause of decreased pump function must be considered. Left and/or right ventricular dysfunction may occur due to by decreased systolic contractility, impaired diastolic relaxation, increases in afterload, valvular dysfunction, or abnormal heart rate and rhythm.

Left Ventricular Failure

Systolic Dysfunction: This is the classic example of cardiogenic shock. When left ventricular (LV) systolic function is impaired, the most common reason is acute coronary ischemia. The result is a reduction of cardiac output relative to increases in preload. Attempted compensation for this impaired pump function occurs via the Frank-Starling mechanism as well as by fluid retention by the kidneys and by increased venous tone mediated by the sympathetic nervous system. Patients present with reduced cardiac output and a resulting increased oxygen extraction ratio by the peripheral tissues. The low mixed venous oxygen saturation may exacerbate hypoxemia, especially in patients with pulmonary edema and intrapulmonary shunt physiology. As mentioned above, acute myocardial infarction or ischemia is the most common cause of LV failure leading to shock. Cardiogenic shock is reported to complicate up to 10% of acute myocardial infarctions.[13] Recent evidence supports the use of early aggressive revascularization using angioplasty or coronary artery bypass grafting in patients with cardiogenic shock.[4] Survival benefit was seen in patients subjected to this strategy compared to medical management of cardiogenic shock, including those given thrombolytic therapy. Treatment of cardiogenic shock due to systolic dysfunction includes the judicious administration of volume if hypovolemia is present. A more precise characterization of the circulation can be obtained with the use of pulmonary artery catheterization and/or echocardiography—topics discussed in more detail in another chapter of the syllabus. Inotropic support includes the use of agents such as dobutamine, milrinone or levosimendan. Intra-aortic balloon counterpulsation may be used to support the circulation as a bridge to coronary artery revascularization.

Diastolic Dysfunction: Increased LV diastolic chamber stiffness and impaired LV filling most commonly occur as a result of myocardial ischemia, though LV hypertrophy and restrictive myocardial diseases may also contribute. Patients usually present with increased cardiac filling pressures despite a small LV end diastolic volume as documented by echocardiography (usually best seen in the short axis view at the level of the papillary muscles). Aside from the management of acute ischemia, this condition may be difficult to treat. Volume administration can be tried, but many times only further increases diastolic pressure with little change in diastolic volume. Inotropic agents are usually ineffective. Aggressive management of tachycardia with volume administration and cautious use of negative chronotropic agents is a rational approach to therapy. Since very little ventricular filling occurs late in diastole in these patients, a very low heart rate (*eg*, sinus bradycardia) may be detrimental. Often, careful titration of chronotropic agents to achieve the "optimal" heart rate which maximizes cardiac output is necessary. The maintenance of a normal sinus rhythm is important to maximize ventricular filling.

Valvular Dysfunction: The management of valvular disease contributing to cardiogenic shock is guided by interventions to counter the specific pathophysiology. Accordingly, aortic stenosis is managed by efforts to decrease heart rate while maintaining sinus rhythm. Preload should be maintained and afterload must not be reduced, since there is a fixed afterload imposed by the aortic stenosis which may not tolerate further reductions in afterload via arteriolar dilation. Surgical evaluation or palliative valvuloplasty are other important considerations in cardiogenic shock complicated by aortic stenosis. Cardiogenic shock due to aortic insufficiency may present acutely and may require urgent surgical repair. Medical management includes the use of chronotropic agents to decrease regurgitant filling time and afterload reducing agents to facilitate forward flow. Mitral regurgitation may occur acutely as a result of ischemic injury to papillary muscles. Medical management includes attempts to establish and maintain sinus rhythm, as well as afterload reduction to decrease the percentage of regurgitant blood flow. This may be accomplished with medications such as nitroprusside or intra-aortic balloon counterpulsation as a bridge to mitral valve repair or replacement. Mitral stenosis contributing to cardiogenic shock is managed by negative chronotropic agents, which seek to maximize diastolic filling time across the stenotic valve. Last, hypertrophic cardiomyopathy may contribute to cardiogenic shock. This lesion is managed by maintenance of preload with volume administration and negative inotropic and chronotropic agents, which serve to decrease the obstruction of the LV outflow tract during systole. Rarely, acute obstruction of the mitral valve by left atrial thrombus or myxoma may also result in cardiogenic shock. These conditions generally require acute surgical interventions.

Cardiac Arrhythmias: Dysrhythmias may exacerbate shock in critically ill patients. Detailed discussion on the management of dysrhythmias is beyond the scope of this chapter and the reader is referred to other sections of the syllabus for further discussion of this topic.

Right Ventricular Failure

Right ventricular (RV) failure resulting in cardiogenic shock is typically associated with increased right atrial pressure and reduced cardiac output.[14] Though the most common reason for RV failure is concomitant LV failure, this section will discuss management of isolated RV failure. Right ventricular infarction may result in RV failure, usually accompanied by inferior myocardial infarction. Elevated JVP in the presence of clear lungs is the classic physical finding seen in acute RV infarction. It is important to distinguish RV infarction from cardiac tamponade. Echocardiography may be helpful in making this distinction. Therapy includes careful volume administration to maintain preload; however, volume overload is common with RV failure, and RV dilation may increase tricuspid regurgitation, leading to worsening hepatic and renal congestion. Dobutamine may be used to increase RV inotropy.[15] and norepinephrine may improve RV endocardial perfusion.

Right ventricular failure as a result of increases in right heart afterload may be due to pulmonary embolism, ARDS and other causes of alveolar hypoxia, hypercapnia and metabolic acidosis. Management is focused at treating the underlying physiologic derangement, with circulatory support again centered around inotropic agents as well as norepinephrine.[16,17] Norepinephrine is more effective at improving RV function and RV coronary perfusion pressure than phenylephrine.[18] Treatment of RV failure is complicated, since volume administration may result in worsening RV function by causing mechanical overstretch and/or by reflex mechanisms that depress contractility.[19] However, some investigators have found volume administration to result in favorable hemodynamics in acute RV failure due to increased RV afterload.[20] Optimal management is often facilitated by echocardiographic or pulmonary artery catheter directed therapy. Thrombolytic therapy for acute pulmonary embolism complicated by cardiogenic shock has been shown to improve survival[21] and is currently accepted as a recommended strategy.[22] Hypoxic pulmonary vasoconstriction may be reduced by improving alveolar and mixed venous oxygenation by administering supplemental oxygen. More aggressive correction of hypercapnia and acidemia may be necessary in patients with acute right heart syndromes. Pulmonary vasodilator therapy (eg, inhaled nitric oxide and prostaglandin E_1) may be considered, though outcome benefits in the acute setting are largely lacking. Recently, levosimendan (the first of a new class of drugs known as calcium sensitizers) has become available. Levosimendan is discussed in more detail in the section *Vasoactive Agents*.

Pericardial Tamponade and Other Syndromes Causing External Compression of the Heart

Cardiac tamponade impairs diastolic filling, resulting in shock. The diagnosis is established by the presence of elevated jugular venous pulse with Kussmaul's sign and pulsus paradoxus. Pulmonary artery catheterization may reveal a decreased cardiac output with equalization of right atrial, left atrial (PCWP) and RV diastolic pressures. Echocardiography reveals pericardial fluid with diastolic collapse of the atria and RV, and right-to-left septal shift during inspiration. Other causes of external cardiac compression include tension pneumothorax, elevated intra-abdominal pressure (*eg*, tense ascites)—so called abdominal tamponade, large pleural effusions and pneumopericardium. Treatment is focused at the underlying cause and includes pericardial drainage with a catheter or surgical "window" in the case of pericardial tamponade. In unstable patients, blind drainage of the pericardial sac with a needle may be necessary. Medical management of the circulatory pathophysiology of tamponade includes the use of aggressive volume administration as well as inotropic and chronotropic support to increase heart rate and thus maintain forward flow.

Decreased Venous Return

Hypovolemia is the most common cause of shock due to decreased venous return. The venous circuit has tremendous capacitance potential and venoconstriction in response to hypovolemia can compensate for initial decreases in intravascular volume. Orthostatic changes in blood pressure and heart rate may be seen early in hypovolemic shock.[23] At a level of approximately 40% loss of intravascular volume, venoconstriction driven by the sympathetic nervous system can no longer maintain mean arterial blood pressure.

In hypovolemic shock, tissue injury (especially gut ischemia) and resulting systemic inflammation may lead to ongoing shock despite replacement of volume losses.[24] This is particularly relevant if resuscitation is delayed and underscores the importance of early aggressive resuscitation of hypovolemic shock. The phenomenon of systemic inflammation as it pertains to shock will be discussed in more detail in the section on septic shock.

Other causes of shock due to decreased venous return include severe neurologic damage or drug exposure resulting in hypotension due to loss of venous tone. The prototypical example of loss of venous tone due to drug exposure is anaphylaxis. This unregulated immunologically-mediated release of histamine can result in profound shock requiring aggressive catecholamine support (epinephrine is the drug of choice). Septic shock is a common cause of shock due to decreased venous tone and is discussed separately in the following section. All of these processes result in decreased venous tone and impaired venous return resulting in decreased cardiac output and blood pressure. Obstruction of veins due to compression (eg, pregnancy, intra-abdominal tumor), thrombus formation, or tumor invasion increases the resistance to venous return and may occasionally result in shock.

The principal therapy of hypovolemic shock and other forms of shock due to decreased venous return is aggressive volume resuscitation while attempting to reverse the underlying problem driving the pathophysiology. This has been described in more detail above. In hemorrhagic shock, resuscitation with packed red blood cells should be done through a blood warmer. The optimal hemoglobin concentration is controversial and transfusion should be paced by the extent of ongoing blood loss. After large volume red blood cell transfusions, dilutional thrombocytopenia and reduction in clotting factors should be anticipated, sought and corrected with platelet and plasma product transfusions as directed by platelet count and coagulation assays.

High Cardiac Output Hypotension

Septic Shock

Septic shock is the most extreme presentation of a spectrum of pathophysiologic responses to an infectious insult. Sepsis is defined by the presence of the systemic inflammatory response syndrome in the presence of known or suspected infection.[2] Severe sepsis occurs when patients with sepsis accrue one or more organ failure(s). Septic shock is seen in patients with severe sepsis who manifest shock as described above. Any infectious organism may result in sepsis and septic shock, including all bacteria, fungi, viruses and parasites. As noted above, patients typically present with evidence of high cardiac output (assuming hypovolemia has been resuscitated). These patients have a widened pulse pressure, warm extremities, brisk capillary refill, and a reduced diastolic and mean blood pressure. A subgroup of patients with septic shock may present with depressed cardiac function. Circulating myocardial depressant factors have been identified in some septic patients,[25-27] but the reason only a small subgroup of patients manifest cardiac depression is not well understood.

Sepsis is a significant problem in the care of critically ill patients. It is the leading cause of death in noncoronary ICUs in the United States.[28] Current estimates suggest that more than 750,000 patients are affected each year[29] and these numbers are expected to increase in the coming years as the population continues to age and a greater percentage of people vulnerable to infection will likely seek medical care.

Decades of research have focused on modifying the pathophysiologic responses of the body to severe infection. For many years, an unregulated pro inflammatory state was thought to be the driving force behind severe sepsis and septic shock. Numerous trials attempting to block a particular inflammatory pathway were conducted without any survival benefits noted.[30] More recently, the pathophysiology behind severe sepsis has become better understood. Currently, the pathophysiology of severe sepsis, is thought to be driven by unregulated inflammation (via cytokines such as interleukin 6 and tumor necrosis factor), coupled to a hypercoagulable state favoring microvascular coagulation and impaired fibrinolysis. Such unregulated microvascular coagulation is thought to lead to impaired tissue perfusion and predispose patients to the multiple organ dysfunction syndrome that is commonly observed in severe sepsis.[31] Activated protein C has a salutary impact on all three pathophysiologic derangements noted in severe sepsis. Recently, a survival benefit was reported in patients with severe sepsis treated with recombinant activated protein C.[32] This study was the first to ever demonstrate a survival benefit from a therapy directed at modifying the underlying pathophysiology of severe sepsis. Because of its anticoagulant properties, there was a small but significant increase in bleeding complications associated with activated protein C.

The mainstay of therapy for septic shock is aggressive supportive care. This includes early identification of the source of infection with eradication by surgical or percutaneous drainage, if possible. Over 80% of patients with severe sepsis will require ventilatory support for respiratory failure, which should be instituted early for reasons outlined earlier in this chapter. Circulatory failure is supported with aggressive volume administration to correct any component of hypovolemia. Objective monitoring using central venous catheterization, pulmonary artery catheterization, and echocardiography should be used early to guide therapy. Vasoactive support is directed by the underlying circulatory derangement. The optimal extent of volume resuscitation is controversial. Some clinicians favor aggressive volume administration, while others favor earlier use of vasoactive drugs (keeping patients "dry"). Trials are ongoing to attempt to better answer this difficult question. Early institution of broad spectrum antibiotic therapy focused on potential pathogens has been shown to improve survival.[33,34] Acute renal failure in septic shock carries a poor prognosis. Recent literature supports the use of an aggressive approach to renal replacement therapy, with a survival benefit demonstrated with daily hemodialysis compared to alternate day hemodialysis.[35] The use of low-dose dopamine as a renal protective strategy was recently found to be of no benefit in preventing acute tubular necrosis in patients with SIRS and acute renal insufficiency.[36] Other therapeutic interventions in severe sepsis await further evaluation. Early trials evaluating the utility of high dose corticosteroids in septic shock failed to demonstrate a survival benefit.[37,38] Corticosteroid therapy remains controversial and further studies are needed before it can be recommended for widespread use. Recent data suggest that the response to an ACTH stimulation test may have important prognostic implications.[39] Furthermore, a recent multicenter trial found that a combination of low dose hydrocortisone and fludrocortisone improved survival in patients with septic shock who had relative adrenal insufficiency.[40]

Other Types of Shock

Adrenal insufficiency is often viewed as a rare occurrence in critically patients. However, a recent study reported a 54% incidence of blunted adrenal response to ACTH in patients with septic shock.[39] This number may be a generous estimate since the parameters for defining adrenal insufficiency are not universally agreed upon;[41] nevertheless, adrenal insufficiency may not be as rare as previously thought. It is reasonable to consider testing all patients who present with septic or other occult reasons for shock with an ACTH stimulation test. Conventionally, this test is performed in the morning with a baseline cortisol level drawn and then 250 µg of ACTH administered intravenously. Thirty- and sixty-minute cortisol levels are then drawn. A level > 20 µg/dL is viewed as an appropriate response. If adrenal insufficiency is suspected, dexamethasone (does not cross react with the cortisol laboratory assay) should be administered while the ACTH stimulation test is performed.

Neurogenic shock typically occurs as a result of severe injury to the central nervous system. The loss of sympathetic tone results in venodilation and with venous blood pooling. Mainstays of therapy include volume repletion and vasoactive support with drugs that have venoconstricting properties

Severe hypothyroidism or hyperthyroidism may result in shock. Myxedema presenting as shock should be treated with administration of intravenous thyroid hormone. One should watch carefully for myocardial ischemia and/or infarction which may complicate aggressive thyroid replacement. Thyroid storm requires urgent therapy with Lugol's solution, propylthiouracil, steroids, propranolol, fluid resuscitation, and identification of the precipitating cause. Pheochromocytoma often presents with a paradoxical hypertension despite a state of shock and impaired tissue perfusion. Intravascular volume depletion is masked by extreme venoconstriction from endogenous catecholamines in pheochromocytoma. The increase in afterload caused by endogenous catecholamines may also precipitate a shock-like state. Treatment includes aggressive volume replacement as well as alpha and beta adrenergic blockade. A search for the location of the pheochromocytoma with subsequent surgical removal is indicated.

Vasoactive Agents

The choice of vasoactive medications should be based upon the underlying pathophysiology of the circulation as gleaned by the physical examination and supplemented by more sophisticated measurements. It is sobering to realize that despite widespread use of these agents for many decades, there are no outcomes studies to guide clinicians with regard to a particular agent in the management of shock.

Dobutamine

Dobutamine is a powerful inotrope which stimulates both β_1- and β_2-receptors. The end result is typically an increase in cardiac output with diminished systemic vascular resistance. This reduction in afterload may benefit patients with LV systolic dysfunction.

Milrinone

Milrinone is an inotropic agent that induces a positive inotropic state via phosphodiesterase inhibition. It has potent vasodilating properties that decrease both systemic and pulmonary vascular resistance. A recent study of patients with acute exacerbations of congestive heart failure did not demonstrate a benefit with regard to days hospitalized for cardiovascular causes, in-hospital mortality, 60-day mortality, or the composite incidence of death or hospital readmission. Rather, hypotension and new atrial arrhythmias were found to occur more frequently in patients who received milrinone compared to placebo.[42]

Levosimendan

Levosimendan is the first clinically available agent from a new class of drugs known as calcium sensitizers. Calcium sensitizers improve myocardial contractility without significantly increasing intracellular calcium levels. Levosimendan increases the sensitivity of the cardiac myofilaments to calcium during systole, which increases the force and rate of contraction. It appears to enhance cardiac output without increasing myocardial oxygen consumption. These drugs may improve diastolic relaxation or at least are neutral with regard to diastolic function.[43,44] Levosimendan causes dilation of systemic, pulmonary and coronary arteries.[45,46] Studies have shown levosimendan to be superior to placebo and dobutamine in patients with chronic congestive heart failure.[47,48] Preliminary studies suggest that levosimendan may improve RV mechanical efficiency.[44] The role of levosimendan in the management of shock or RV failure has not been studied extensively.

Dopamine

Dopamine is purported to have varying physiologic effects at different doses. Classically, "low-dose" dopamine (1-3 µg/kg/min) is thought to stimulate dopaminergic receptors and increase renal and mesenteric blood flow. This notion has recently been disproven, however.[36,49] Indeed, there is evidence that dopamine may impair mesenteric perfusion to a greater degree than norepinephrine.[50] As data are accumulating reporting the ill effects of dopamine in shock, this agent has recently fallen out of favor in the view of many clinicians, with other agents such as norepinephrine being more widely used (see below).[51]

Norepinephrine

Norepinephrine stimulates β_1- as well as α-receptors. Data are now accumulating suggesting norepinephrine may be a preferred drug in septic and other vasodilatory types of shock. It appears to have a lesser propensity to cause renal injury[52] and provides a more reliable increase in blood pressure compared to dopamine.[53] A recent prospective observational cohort study found a significant reduction in mortality when compared to dopamine and/or epinephrine in patients with septic shock.[54]

Phenylephrine

Phenylephrine is a pure α_1-agonist, which results in veno- and arteriolar constriction. It often elicits a reflex bradycardia mediated via baroreceptors. This may prove useful in patients with tachydysrhythmias accompanied by hypotension. In a prospective observational study of patients with septic shock, phenylephrine was found to increase blood pressure, SVR and cardiac index when added to low-dose dopamine or dobutamine after volume resuscitation.[55] There is a theoretical concern that α-agonism may precipitate myocardial ischemia, though are few objective data to support or refute this concern.

Epinephrine

Epinephrine has both β- as well as α-agonist properties. It has potent inotropic as well as vasoconstricting properties. It appears to have a higher propensity toward precipitating mesenteric ischemia,[56] a property which limits its utility as a first-line agent for the management of shock, regardless of the underlying etiology.

Vasopressin

The use of vasopressin as a vasoactive agent has increased tremendously in the last few years. Patients who present with septic shock or late-phase hemorrhagic shock have been shown to have a relative deficiency of vasopressin. A recent study found patients with septic shock to demonstrate an increase in blood pressure and urine output without evidence of impaired cardiac, mesenteric or skin perfusion when treated with "low-dose" (40 milliunits per minute) vasopressin.[57] The exact role of vasopressin in various shock states requires further investigation.

References

1. Ely EW, Smith AC, Chiles C, et al. Radiologic determination of intravascular volume status using portable, digital chest radiography: a prospective investigation in 100 patients. Crit Care Med 2001; 29:1502-1512
2. Bone RC, Balk RA, Cerra FB, et al. Definitions for sepsis and organ failure and guidelines for the use of innovative therapies in sepsis. The ACCP/SCCM Consensus Conference Committee. American College of Chest Physicians/Society of Critical Care Medicine. Chest 1992; 101:1644-1655
3. Rivers E, Nguyen B, Havstad S, et al. Early goal directed therapy in the treatment of severe sepsis and septic shock. N Engl J Med 2001; 345: 1368-1377
4. Hochman JS, Sleeper LA, Webb JG, et al. Early revascularization in acute myocardial infarction complicated by cardiogenic shock. SHOCK Investigators. Should we emergently revascularize occluded coronaries for cardiogenic shock. N Engl J Med 1999; 341:625-634
5. Rochester DF, Pradel-Guena M. Measurement of diaphragmatic blood flow in dogs from xenon 133 clearance. J Appl Physiol 1973; 34:68-74
6. Hussain SNA, Roussos C. Distribution of respiratory muscle and organ blood flow during endotoxic shock in dogs. J Appl Physiol 1985; 59:1802-1808
7. Robertson CH Jr, Foster GH, Johnson RL Jr. The relationship of respiratory failure to the oxygen consumption of, lactate production by, and distribution of blood flow among respiratory muscles during increasing inspiratory resistance. J Clin Invest 1977; 59:31-42
8. Hall JB, Wood LDH. Liberation of the patient from mechanical ventilation. JAMA 1987; 257:1621-1628
9. Human albumin administration in critically ill patients: systematic review of randomised controlled trials. Cochrane Injuries Group Albumin Reviewers. BMJ 1998; 317:235-240
10. Finfer S, Bellomo R, Boyce N, et al. A comparison of albumin and saline for fluid resuscitation in the intensive care unit. N Engl J Med 2004; 350:2247-2256
11. Bickell WH, Wall MJ Jr, Pepe PE, et al. Immediate versus delayed fluid resuscitation for hypotensive patients with penetrating torso injuries. N Engl J Med 1994; 331:1105-1109
12. Hebert PC, Wells G, Blajchman MA, et al. A multicenter, randomized, controlled clinical trial of transfusion requirements in critical care. Transfusion Requirements in Critical Care Investigators, Canadian Critical Care Trials Group. N Engl J Med 1999; 340:1056
13. Goldberg RJ, Gore JM, Alpert JS, et al. Cardiogenic shock after acute myocardial infarction: incidence and mortality from a community-wide perspective, 1975 to 1988. N Engl J Med 1991; 325:1117-1122
14. Mebazaa A, Karpati P, Renaud E, et al. Acute right ventricular failure—from pathophysiology to new treatments. Intensive Care Med 2004; 30:185-196
15. Dell'Italia LJ, Starling MR, Blumhardt R, et al. Comparative effects of volume loading, dobutamine and nitroprusside in patients with predominant right ventricular infarction. Circulation 1985; 72:1327-1335

16. Hirsch LJ, Rooney MW, Wat SS, et al. Norepinephrine and phenylephrine effects on right ventricular function in experimental canine pulmonary embolism. Chest 1991; 100:796-801
17. Layish DT, Tapson VF. Pharmacologic hemodynamic support in massive pulmonary embolism. Chest 1997; 111:218-224
18. Hirsch LJ, Rooney MW, Wat SS, et al. Norepinephrine and phenylephrine effects on right ventricular function in experimental canine pulmonary embolism. Chest 1991; 100:796-801
19. Ghignone M, Girling L, Prewitt RM. Volume expansion versus norepinephrine in treatment of a low cardiac output complicating an acute increase in right ventricular afterload in dogs. Anesthesiology 1984; 60:132-135
20. Mathru M, Venus B, Smith R, et al. Treatment of low cardiac output complicating acute pulmonary hypertension in normovolemic goats. Crit Care Med 1986; 14:120-124
21. Jerjes-Sanchez C, Ramirez-Rivera A, Gareia M de L, et al. Streptokinase and heparin versus heparin alone in massive pulmonary embolism: a randomized controlled trial. J Thromb Thrombolysis 1995; 2:227-229
22. Arcasoy SM, Kreit JW. Thrombolytic therapy of pulmonary embolism: a comprehensive review of current evidence. Chest 1999; 115:1695-1707
23. Knopp R, Claypool R, Leonardi D. Use of the tilt test in measuring acute blood loss. Ann Emerg Med 1980; 9:72-75
24. Barroso-Aranda J, Schmid-Schonbein GW, Zweifach BW, et al. Granulocytes and no-reflow phenomenon in irreversible hemorrhagic shock. Circ Res 1988; 63:437-447
25. Parker MM, Shelhamer JH, Bacharach SL, et al. Profound but reversible myocardial depression in patients with septic shock. Ann Intern Med 1984; 100:483-490
26. Schremmer B, Dhainault JF. Heart failure in septic shock: effects of inotropic support. Crit Care Med 1990; 18:S49-S55
27. Parrillo JE, Burch C, Shelhamer JH, et al. A circulating myocardial depressant substance in humans with septic shock. J Clin Invest 1985; 76:1539-1553
28. Sands KE, Bates DW, Lanken PN, et al. Epidemiology of sepsis syndrome in eight academic medical centers. JAMA 1997; 278:234-240
29. Angus DC, Linde-Zwirble WT, Lidicker J, et al. Epidemiology of severe sepsis in the United States: analysis of incidence, outcome, and associated costs of care. Crit Care Med 2001; 29:1303-1310
30. Bone RC. Why sepsis trials fail. JAMA 1996; 276:565-566
31. Kidokoro A, Iba T, Fukunaga M, et al. Alterations in coagulation and fibrinolysis during sepsis. Shock 1996; 5:223-228
32. Bernard GR, Vincent JL, Laterre PF. Efficacy and safety of recombinant human activated protein C for severe sepsis. N Engl J Med 2001; 344:699-709
33. Ibrahim EH, Sherman G, Ward S, et al. The influence of inadequate antimicrobial treatment of bloodstream infections on patient outcomes in the ICU setting. Chest 2000; 118:146-155
34. Kollef MH, Sherman G, Ward S, et al. Inadequate antimicrobial treatment of infections: a risk factor for hospital mortality among critically ill patients. Chest 1999; 115:462-474
35. Schiffl H, Lang SM, Fischer R. Daily hemodialysis and the outcome of acute renal failure. N Engl J Med 2002; 346:305-310
36. Bellomo R, Chapman M, Finfer S, et al. Low-dose dopamine in patients with early renal dysfunction: a placebo-controlled randomised trial. Australian and New Zealand Intensive Care Society (ANZICS) Clinical Trials Group. Lancet 2000; 356:2139-2143
37. Bone RC, Fisher CJ, Clemmer TP, et al. A controlled clinical trial of high-dose methylprednisolone in the treatment of severe sepsis and septic shock. N Engl J Med 1987; 317:653-658
38. Effect of high-dose glucocorticoid therapy on mortality in patients with clinical signs of systemic sepsis. The Veterans Administration Systemic Sepsis Cooperative Study Group. N Engl J Med 1987; 317:659-665
39. Annane D, Sebille V, Troche G, et al. A 3-level prognostic classification in septic shock based on cortisol levels and cortisol response to corticotropin. JAMA 2000; 283:1038-1045
40. Annane D, Sebille V, Charpentier C, et al. Effect of treatment with low doses of hydrocortisone and fludrocortisone on mortality in patients with septic shock. JAMA 2002; 288:862-871
41. Zaloga GP. Sepsis-induced adrenal deficiency syndrome. Crit Care Med 2001; 29:688-690
42. Cuffe MS, Califf RM, Adams KF, et al. Short-term intravenous milrinone for acute exacerbation of chronic heart failure: a randomized controlled trial. JAMA 2002; 287:1541-1547

43. Haikala H, Nissinen E, Etemadzadeh E, et al. Troponin C-mediated calcium sensitization induced by levosimendan does not impair relaxation. J Cardiovasc Pharmacol 1995; 25:794-801
44. Ukkonen H, Saraste M, Akkila J, et al. Myocardial efficiency during levosimendan infusion in congestive heart failure. Clin Pharmacol Ther 2000; 68:522-531
45. Yokoshiki H, Katsube Y, Sunagawa M, et al. Levosimendan, a novel calcium sensitizer, activates the glibenclamide-sensitive K$^+$ channel in rat arterial myocytes. Eur J Pharmacol 1997; 333:249-259
46. Slawsky MT, Colucci WS, Gottlieb SS. Acute hemodynamic and clinical effects of levosimendan in patients with severe heart failure. Circulation 2000; 102:2222-2227
47. Follath F, Cleland JG, Just H, et al. Efficacy and safety of intravenous levosimendan compared with dobutamine in severe low-output heart failure (the LIDO study): a randomised double-blind trial. Lancet 2002; 20:196-202
48. Moiseyev VS, Poder P, Andrejevs N, et al. Safety and efficacy of a novel calcium sensitizer, levosimendan, in patients with left ventricular failure due to an acute myocardial infarction: a randomized, placebo-controlled, double-blind study (RUSSLAN). Eur Heart J 2002; 23:1422-1432
49. Hannemann L, Reinhart K, Grenzer O, et al. Comparison of dopamine to dobutamine and norepinephrine for oxygen delivery and uptake in septic shock. Crit Care Med 1995; 23:1962-1970
50. Marik PE, Mohedin M. The contrasting effects of dopamine and norepinephrine on systemic and splanchnic oxygen utilization in hyperdynamic sepsis. JAMA 1994; 272:1354-1357
51. Nasraway SA. Norepinephrine: no more "leave 'em dead"? Crit Care Med 2000; 28:3096-3098
52. Desjars P, Pinaud M, Bugnon D, et al. Norepinephrine therapy has no deleterious renal effects in human septic shock. Crit Care Med 1989; 17:426-429
53. Martin C, Papazian L, Perrin G, et al. Norepinephrine or dopamine for the treatment of hyperdynamic septic shock? Chest 1993; 103:1826-1831
54. Martin C, Viviand X, Leone M, et al. Effect of norepinephrine on the outcome of septic shock. Crit Care Med 2000; 28:2758-2765
55. Gregory JS, Bonfiglio MF, Dasta JF, et al. Experience with phenylephrine as a component of the pharmacologic support of septic shock. Crit Care Med 1991; 19:1395-1400
56. Levy B, Bollaert PE, Charpentier C, et al. Comparison of norepinephrine and dobutamine to epinephrine for hemodynamics, lactate metabolism, and gastric tonometric variables in septic shock: a prospective, randomized study. Intensive Care Med 1997; 23:282-287
57. Tsuneyoshi I, Yamada H, Kakihana Y, et al. Hemodynamic and metabolic effects of low-dose vasopressin infusions in vasodilatory septic shock. Crit Care Med 2001; 29:487-493

Notes

Transplantation

Joshua O. Benditt, MD, FCCP

Objectives:

- To identify general principles and common themes of organ transplantation
- To review the clinical course and serious complications of liver transplantation
- To identify common problems associated with heart, heart-lung, and lung transplantation
- To outline major complications of kidney and kidney-pancreas transplantation

Key words: heart transplantation; heart-lung transplantation; kidney transplantation; liver transplantation; lung transplantation; pancreas transplantation

General Principles

The number of transplants performed each year is increasing steadily. Approximately 23,000 organs were transplanted in the United States in 2000, and nearly 80,000 patients are currently on waiting lists. Intensivists are likely to face transplant-related problems in the preoperative support of transplant candidates with end-stage organ failure, in the routine postoperative care of transplant recipients, and in the management of life-threatening complications of transplantation.

Temporal Organization of Complications

The complications of transplantation are related to the underlying disease and premorbid condition of the patient, the transplant procedure, rejection of the graft or host, and the consequences of immunosuppression. These complications occur in temporal patterns.

Noninfectious problems in the first few weeks after solid organ transplantation include (1) surgical complications; (2) graft dysfunction related to ischemia, preservation, and reperfusion; and (3) rejection. After the first few months, chronic rejection is a significant problem.

Infectious complications also exhibit temporal patterns. Nosocomial infections are prominent in the early posttransplant course, followed by the reactivation of latent infection in the graft or host and new opportunistic infections related to the intensity and duration of immunosuppression. Staphylococci and Gram-negative bacilli are the most common early bacterial pathogens, followed later by infections caused by Legionella, Nocardia, Mycobacteria, and Listeria. Candidiasis and aspergillosis are the major fungal infections occurring in the first few months after transplantation, but reactivation of endemic mycoses and cryptococcosis may present later. Herpes simplex virus (HSV) often reactivates in the initial weeks after transplantation, and herpesvirus-6 is increasingly recognized 2 to 4 weeks posttransplant. Cytomegalovirus (CMV) and hepatitis C infections typically present after the first month. The peak incidence of Epstein-Barr virus (EBV)-related posttransplant lymphoproliferative disorder (PTLD) is 3 to 6 months after transplant. Dermatomal reactivation of varicella zoster virus (VZV) also occurs in this time frame. Toxoplasmosis and Pneumocystis carinii pneumonia may develop after the first posttransplant month.

Immunosuppression

Immunosuppression is required to prevent rejection of the transplanted organ or, in the case of bone marrow transplantation, to prevent graft-vs-host disease. The approaches to induction and maintenance immunosuppression, as well as the treatment of established rejection, vary significantly from one institution to another. Most centers use a combination of agents in low doses to minimize the toxicity of individual drugs.

Cyclosporine is a fungal cyclic peptide that inhibits transcription of interleukin-2 (IL-2) and the expression of IL-2 receptors, resulting in blockade of T-cell activation. There are marked individual variations in the absorption and metabolism of cyclosporine; precise timing of dosages and monitoring of drug levels are essential. Cyclosporine is metabolized by the hepatic cytochrome p450 system and is subject to many drug interactions. Drugs that increase cyclosporine levels include erythromycin, ketoconazole, itraconazole, cimetidine, and diltiazem. Agents that decrease cyclosporine levels include phenytoin, phenobarbital, trimethoprim, rifampin, and isoniazid. Important side effects include nephrotoxicity, hypertension, neurotoxicity (tremors, paresthesias, seizures, etc.), gingival hyperplasia, hyperlipidemia, and hypertrichosis.

Tacrolimus (FK506) is a macrolide that has essentially the same mechanism of action as cyclosporine. In liver, kidney, and lung transplant recipients, tacrolimus is more effective than cyclosporine in preventing acute and chronic rejection, and is effective in the treatment of acute rejection. In comparison with cylosporine, tacrolimus is associated with more neurotoxicity, nephrotoxicity, and glucose intolerance, but less hypertension, dyslipidemia, gingival hyperplasia, or hirsutism.

Azathioprine is a purine analog that inhibits lymphocyte proliferation. Leukopenia, hepatitis, and cholestasis are important toxicities. Mycophenolate mofetil is a more selective inhibitor of purine synthesis that appears to be more effective than azathioprine at preventing acute rejection. Diarrhea, emesis, and leukopenia are the principal side effects of mycophenolate mofetil.

Corticosteroids are nonspecific antiinflammatory agents that inhibit cytokine production, antigen recognition, and T-cell proliferation. The familiar side effects of corticosteroids include Cushing's syndrome, hyperglycemia, hyperlipidemia, osteoporosis, myopathy, and cataracts.

Polyclonal and monoclonal antibodies are used to deplete the T cells that mediate acute rejection. Antithymocyte and antilymphocyte globulin may cause serum sickness, thrombocytopenia, and leukopenia. Initial treatment with OKT3, a murine monoclonal antibody to the T-cell receptor, often elicits fever, chills, and a capillary leak syndrome resulting in hypotension and pulmonary edema. OKT3 also increases the risks of CMV infection and EBV-related PTLD. Newer mouse/human chimeric monoclonal antibodies to IL-2 receptors (basiliximab, daclizumab) are associated with less toxicity.

Rejection

Several patterns of rejection have been described in solid organ transplantation. Hyperacute rejection is seen within minutes to hours of transplantation, and is mediated by preformed antibodies that cause vascular injury. The kidney and heart are particularly susceptible, but the liver is resistant to hyperacute rejection. There is no treatment, but this form of rejection often can be avoided by pretransplant cross-matching. Accelerated rejection is an uncommon form of antibody-mediated rejection that is seen several days after transplantation and characterized histologically by vascular necrosis. Acute rejection is the most common cause of graft failure, and is mediated by T cells. Acute rejection may be seen as early as the first week, and any time thereafter. Chronic rejection appears >3 months after transplantation, is characterized by a slowly progressive course associated with histologic fibrosis, and often is refractory to treatment.

Infection

Pretransplant identification of latent infections in the donor and recipient is essential in defining risks. Routine testing includes serologies for CMV, HSV, EBV, VZV, hepatitis A, B, and C, HIV, toxoplasmosis, and relevant endemic mycoses such as histoplasmosis and coccidioidomycosis. A tuberculin test should be placed and the chest radiograph evaluated for granulomatous disease. Indolent infection of the oral cavity and sinuses should be excluded, and immunizations should be brought up to date. Prophylaxis is effective against many latent and some acquired infections. Routine surveillance is helpful for the preemptive management of CMV infections, and possibly others. Suspected infection should be approached with an assessment of risks and an aggressive effort at specific diagnosis.

CMV is the bane of transplantation. Primary infection occurs when a seronegative patient receives an organ from a seropositive donor; secondary or reactivation infection develops in seropositive recipients. Active infection (viral replication) will develop in most patients at risk, and is diagnosed by antigen detection, nucleic acid identification, or culture. Symptomatic disease develops in 40 to 60% of primary infections and approximately 20% of secondary infections. The manifestations of CMV disease vary with the organ transplanted. The risk of CMV disease is increased in patients who are treated with antithymocyte globulin or OKT3. CMV disease is treated with ganciclovir, with or without CMV immune globulin. CMV disease can be prevented by the use of screened blood products, oral valacyclovir prophylaxis, and by prophylactic or preemptive (at the earliest sign of viral replication) treatment with ganciclovir and hyperimmune globulin.

The PTLD is caused by EBV infection and occurs in 6 to 9% of lung transplants, 3 to 5% of heart transplants, 2 to 4% of liver transplants, and <1% of kidney transplants. The risk of PTLD is increased by treatment with anti-T-cell antibodies. PTLD presents 6 to 24 weeks after transplantation with an infectious mononucleosislike syndrome or diverse local manifestations that may involve any lymphatic tissue, the GI tract, lungs, kidneys, or brain. The diagnosis is made by demonstrating the EBV genome in association with benign or malignant lymphatic proliferation. Treatment strategies include reduced immunosuppression, interferon-α, and cytotoxic chemotherapy. Local resection may be helpful and there is an uncertain role for acyclovir or ganciclovir.

Liver Transplantation

Perspective

There were 5,326 liver transplants performed in the United States in 2002. The most common indications are chronic active hepatitis C, alcoholic cirrhosis, cryptogenic cirrhosis, primary biliary cirrhosis, and sclerosing cholangitis. For patients who received transplants over the last 10 years, graft and patient survival rates are 73% and 82%, respectively, at 1 year, and 63% and 73% at 4 years.

Usual Clinical Course

Liver transplant recipients require ICU care for 2 to 4 days after surgery. The cardiac output is generally high and the systemic vascular resistance low; circulatory instability is common and usually volume-responsive. Myocardial depression is a poor prognostic sign. Calcium may be depleted by the citrate in blood products. Hyperglycemia is common and potassium levels may be high or low. A mild metabolic acidosis may be present initially, but metabolic alkalosis develops as the liver metabolizes citrate. Deficient clotting factors and thrombocytopenia contribute to a significant bleeding diathesis. Blood products are usually replaced empirically (for evident bleeding and a fall in hematocrit), although many centers monitor coagulation with thromboelastography, a rapid measure of the time to onset of clotting, the rate of clot formation, and maximum clot elasticity. Important signs of a functioning graft are the production of golden-brown bile, the restoration of clotting, the absence of a metabolic acidosis, and the resolution of encephalopathy. Patients should be awake and alert within 12 h. The serum bilirubin may rise initially because of hemolysis, but liver enzymes should fall each day. The prothrombin time and partial thromboplastin time should improve daily and be normal within 72 h. Most patients can be extubated within 48 h.

Noninfectious Complications

Hemorrhage in the first 48 h usually is caused by diffuse oozing in the setting of a coagulopathy and is managed with blood products. Later, intraabdominal bleeding may be related to necrosis of a vascular anastamosis. GI hemorrhage may result from stress ulceration or the development of portal hypertension.

Primary graft failure occurs in 1 to 5% of liver transplants and usually is a consequence of ischemic injury. The signs of graft failure include poor bile formation, metabolic acidosis, and failure to resolve encephalopathy and coagulopathy. The treatment is retransplantation within 48 h, before brainstem herniation from cerebral edema.

Vascular complications include thromboses of the hepatic artery, hepatic vein, or portal vein. Hepatic artery thrombosis occurs in about 5% of patients and presents in one of four ways: massive liver necrosis (fever, rising enzymes, deterioration in mental status, renal insufficiency, shock); a bile leak with or without evidence of liver injury; recurrent bacteremia from hepatic abscesses; or as an asymptomatic finding on routine ultrasound. The diagnosis is made by duplex ultrasonography, and the treatment is operative repair or retransplantation. Portal vein thrombosis is less common, and presents with ascites and variceal hemorrhage, with or without graft dysfunction. Hepatic vein thrombosis is rare and presents with liver failure and massive ascites.

Biliary complications occur in up to 28% of patients. Bile leaks are caused by traumatic or ischemic injury to the common bile duct. Biliary obstruction may be caused by kinking or displacement of drainage tubes, dysfunction of the sphincter of Oddi, or strictures. Biliary complications are diagnosed by cholangiography, and are managed with surgical or endoscopic repair.

Acute rejection is the most common cause of liver dysfunction after transplantation. Most patients experience at least one episode, usually 4 to 14 days after transplantation. The clinical signs (fever, tenderness and enlargement of graft) and laboratory features (elevated hepatocellular enzymes and bilirubin) are nonspecific. The diagnosis is confirmed with liver biopsy demonstrating mononuclear cell portal infiltration, ductular injury, and venulitis. Most patients respond to pulse steroids or anti-T-cell antibodies. ICU readmission is rarely required.

Common noninfectious pulmonary complications of liver transplantation include atelectasis, pleural effusions, and pulmonary edema. In most cases, preoperative shunting caused by the hepatopulmonary syndrome improves over days to months posttransplant. Respiratory muscle weakness, the abdominal wound, impaired mental status, and severe metabolic alkalosis may contribute to delayed weaning. ARDS occurs in <10% of liver graft recipients, usually as a consequence of sepsis.

Neurologic dysfunction after liver transplantation may be caused by hepatic encephalopathy, hypoglycemia, intracranial hemorrhage, air embolism, drug toxicity, or infection.

Infection

Bacteria are the most important causes of infection after liver transplantation, particularly in the first 6 weeks after grafting. Gram-positive cocci and Gram-negative bacilli are the predominant pathogens, and the site of infection often involves the transplanted liver or the reconstructed biliary tree. Intra-abdominal abscesses, peritonitis, cholangitis, and surgical wound infections are the most common foci of bacterial infection, followed by pneumonia, catheter sepsis, and urinary tract infections. Prophylactic systemic and topical antibiotics are commonly used but are of unproven value.

CMV infection will be evident in approximately 50% of liver transplant recipients, and half of these cases will be symptomatic. A seropositive donor is the most important risk factor for CMV disease. The peak onset of CMV infection is 28 days after transplantation. A mononucleosislike syndrome characterized by fever, malaise, myalgias, and neutropenia is the most common manifestation. Hepatitis is the most common organ involvement. Anecdotal reports suggest that treatment of CMV disease with ganciclovir is beneficial. CMV disease can be prevented in high-risk patients by long-term (100-day) ganciclovir prophylaxis or by preemptive treatment at the first sign of viral replication. HSV mucositis reactivates in 40 to 50% of seropositive patients and can be prevented or treated with acyclovir.

Fungal infections complicate 10 to 40% of liver transplants, usually in the first 2 months, and are more common than with other organ transplants. Candidemia, from an abdominal or vascular source, is the leading mycosis, followed by pulmonary aspergillosis. Pneumocystis infections are rare in patients receiving prophylaxis.

Heart Transplantation

Perspective

In 2002, 2,153 heart transplants were performed in the United States. Ischemic cardiomyopathy, idiopathic cardiomyopathy, and congenital heart disease are the leading indications, together accounting for >80% of procedures. Patient survival is 83% at 1 year, and 72% at 4 years.

Usual Clinical Course

Cardiac function is depressed for several days postoperatively, and the right ventricle recovers more slowly than the left. Cardiac output is initially rate-dependent in the denervated heart, and low-dose isoproterenol or pacing is often required for 2 to 4 days. Patients are routinely extubated within 24 h and discharged from the ICU within 48 h.

Noninfectious Complications

The early complications of heart transplantation include those of cardiac surgery in general. Most patients develop left lower-lobe atelectasis that may persist for weeks. Pleural, pericardial, and mediastinal fluid collections are common, but hemorrhage is unusual. Pulmonary edema is a frequent occurrence because of pretransplant congestion, postoperative left ventricular dysfunction, and volume overload; heparin-protamine reactions and reperfusion injury may alter lung permeability. Persistent pulmonary hypertension is an important early problem that may lead to right ventricular failure. Prostaglandin E_1, nitric oxide, inotropes, and assist devices may be effective.

Rejection may occur any time after heart transplantation and is diagnosed histologically from routine surveillance endomyocardial biopsies. Clinical signs of rejection such as fever, heart failure, arrhythmias, and pericardial friction rubs are unreliable. The severity of rejection is graded by the degree of lymphocytic infiltration and myocyte necrosis. Mild cases may resolve spontaneously; about one third of patients require treatment for rejection. Most episodes respond to pulse corticosteroids and/or increased doses of cyclosporine. Refractory cases usually respond to anti-T-cell treatment.

Accelerated coronary atherosclerosis is the leading cause of death >1 year after heart transplantation. The cumulative incidence is approximately 10% *per annum*. Calcium channel blockers and HMG-CoA reductase inhibitors may slow the development of allograft vasculopathy.

Infection

Nosocomial bacterial pneumonia, mediastinitis, empyema, and catheter-related infections are common in the first month after transplantation. Gram-negative bacilli and *Staphylococcus aureus* are frequent pathogens. Legionella pneumonia and wound infections are important in the first 3 months after heart transplantation, particularly in hospitals with contaminated water supplies. Nocardia infection of the lung may present any time after the first postoperative month, and may disseminate to brain or bone. Atypical mycobacterial infections have been reported in 3% of heart transplant recipients, usually involving the lung, mediastinum, or soft tissues.

Aspergillosis is the most common fungal infection after heart transplantation, developing in 5 to 10% of recipients, usually in the first month. The lung is the primary site of infection, but dissemination is evident in half the cases at diagnosis.

Toxoplasmosis is an important consideration when a seronegative recipient receives a heart from a seropositive donor. Primary infection presents 4 to 6 weeks after transplantation with fever and nonspecific signs involving the heart, brain, eyes, lungs, and/or liver; myocardial infection may mimic rejection. The diagnosis is supported by seroconversion and confirmed by the demonstration of tachyzoites in tissue. Treatment with pyrimethamine and sulfadiazine is effective if instituted promptly. Pyrimethamine also may be effective in preventing primary infection. Reactivation of latent toxoplasmosis in seropositive recipients is not clinically significant. *P carinii* pneumonia develops in 3% of cardiac transplant patients without prophylaxis, but is now rare.

Active CMV infection will develop in most seropositive patients and seronegative recipients of hearts from seropositive donors. One third of these infections will be symptomatic, usually with a mononucleosislike syndrome. CMV pneumonia develops in 10% of infected patients. Serious morbidity and mortality are largely limited to patients with primary infection. Ganciclovir appears to be effective in the treatment of CMV disease in heart transplant patients. The role of ganciclovir in prophylaxis is uncertain. Reactivation of oral and genital HSV infection is common in the first few months after heart transplantation. VZV typically reactivates in a dermatomal distribution 3 to 6 months after transplantation. HSV and VZV infections usually remain localized and respond to acyclovir.

PTLD develops in 2 to 7% of heart transplant recipients, usually presenting 3 to 6 months after transplantation. PTLD is probably caused by EBV and the risk is markedly increased by treatment with OKT3. Any lymphatic tissue may be involved, as well as the GI tract, lungs, kidneys, or brain. Most cases respond to a reduction in immunosuppressive therapy. Resection of localized tumors and treatment with acyclovir may be helpful.

Lung and Heart-Lung Transplantation

Perspective

There were 1,042 lung transplants and 48 heart-lung transplants are performed in the United States in 2002. The leading indications for single-lung transplantation are COPD, idiopathic pulmonary fibrosis, and α_1-antitrypsin deficiency. Double-lung transplants usually are performed mainly for septic lung disease (cystic fibrosis or bronchiectasis). The leading indications for heart-lung transplants are Eisenmenger's complex and primary pulmonary hypertension. The survival rates for grafts and patients after lung transplantation are 73% and 74%, respectively, at 1 year, and 47% and 50% at 4 years. The survival of heart-lung transplants is 65% at 1 year and 46% at 5 years.

Usual Clinical Course

Volume overload and pulmonary edema are common early problems. Cardiac function may be impaired if cardiopulmonary bypass was required (all heart-lung transplants, some lung transplants). Cardiac output is rate-dependent in denervated hearts, and responds to isoproterenol. Care must be taken to avoid air trapping in an emphysematous native lung. Independent lung ventilation through a double-lumen endotracheal tube may be necessary in some single-lung transplants to improve ventilation-perfusion matching or reduce air trapping. Most patients can be extubated within 36 h. Patients receiving single-lung transplants for primary pulmonary hypertension often are heavily sedated for 48 to 72 h before extubation to reduce pulmonary arterial hypertensive crises. Reflexive coughing is lost in the denervated lung, and pulmonary toilet is critical for secretion management. Lymphatics are severed in the transplanted lung, impairing extravascular fluid clearance and rendering the graft particularly susceptible to edema.

Noninfectious Complications

Hemorrhage early after lung transplantation is usually from the mediastinum or pleura. Bleeding is particularly common in heart-lung transplants because of the extensive mediastinal dissection and the need for heparinization during bypass. Patients with cystic fibrosis also are at increased risk of hemorrhage because pleural adhesions often must be severed to remove the native lungs. Bilateral bronchial anastomoses require less mediastinal dissection and are associated with less bleeding than tracheal anastomoses.

The pulmonary reimplantation response is evident in most patients. This is a form of reperfusion injury that results in noncardiogenic pulmonary edema. The clinical features include alveolar and interstitial infiltrates on chest radiograph, a decline in lung compliance, and impaired gas exchange. The response peaks 2 to 4 days after transplantation and resolves gradually thereafter with careful fluid management and diuresis. The diagnosis is made by the clinical presentation and time course, and the exclusion of infection, rejection, and cardiogenic pulmonary edema.

Airway dehiscence, stenosis, and bronchomalacia were major causes of morbidity and mortality in the early years of lung transplantation. The use of omental wraps or telescoping bronchial anastomoses has markedly reduced the incidence of airway complications. Strictures now develop in about 10% of cases, and stents are occasionally required for the management of stenoses.

Phrenic nerve paralysis resulting from thermal or mechanical injury occurs in <5% of patients. The injury is often temporary, with gradual recovery over several weeks.

Acute rejection occurs as early as 3 days after lung transplantation and most patients will experience at least one episode within the first postoperative month. Lung rejection is more common than heart rejection in heart-lung transplants. The clinical manifestations are nonspecific and include low-grade fever, dyspnea, cough, fatigue, hypoxemia, a fall in FEV_1, and new or changing infiltrates on chest radiograph (the chest radiograph is usually normal when rejection occurs >1 month after transplantation). Infection and edema are the major alternative considerations in the first few weeks after transplantation; later, CMV is the principal concern. Bronchoscopy is helpful in excluding infection and confirming rejection. Transbronchial biopsies demonstrate the characteristic perivascular mononuclear infiltrates with a sensitivity of 70 to 90% and specificity of >90%. There may be a role for identifying donor-sensitized lymphocytes by BAL. Most patients respond promptly to pulse corticosteroids; nonresponders are treated with anti-T-cell antibodies.

Obliterative bronchiolitis is the major manifestation of chronic rejection in the transplanted lung and a leading cause of late mortality. The incidence of obliterative bronchiolitis increases over time and is found in 60 to 70% of patients who survive for 5 years after transplantation. Repeated episodes of acute rejection and CMV infection are possible risk factors. Obliterative bronchiolitis may present any time after the second postoperative month, with half the cases presenting in the first year. Patients may complain of dyspnea or cough, and chest radiographs are usually normal. The clinical diagnosis hinges on spirometric demonstration of significant declines in FEV_1 and forced expiratory flow, midexpiratory phase. Some centers have found transbronchial biopsies to be helpful. Treatment is with increased immunosuppression, but no strategy has been demonstrated to be effective. Pulmonary function may stabilize with treatment, but rarely improves. The mortality of obliterative bronchiolitis is 40% within 2 years of diagnosis.

Infection

Infection is the leading cause of death after lung transplantation, and most infections are located in the thorax. Most centers advocate an aggressive approach to etiologic diagnosis, relying heavily on bronchoscopy. In single-lung transplant recipients, infection in the native lung is a significant problem.

Bacteria are the most common agents of infection after lung transplantation. Bacterial pneumonia is most frequent in the early postoperative period, but purulent bronchitis often presents weeks to months after transplantation; late bacterial infections are particularly common in patients with obliterative bronchiolitis. Typical nosocomial pathogens are the usual culprits, although native strains of *Pseudomonas cepacia* and *Pseudomonas aeruginosa* are problematic in patients with cystic fibrosis. Prophylactic broad-spectrum antibiotics are routinely administered for the first 48 to 72 h after transplantation, empirically or guided by cultures from the donor and recipient respiratory tracts; the validity of this practice has not been tested by controlled trial. Bacterial infections usually respond to antibiotics.

CMV disease is more common in lung allograft recipients than in other solid-organ transplant patients. Most seropositive recipients will develop positive blood and BAL cultures (active infection) a median of 40 days after transplantation in the absence of prophylaxis, but the risk and severity of symptomatic CMV disease are highest in seronegative patients who receive a lung from a seropositive donor (*ie*, those with primary infection). Treatment with OKT3 is an additional risk for CMV disease. CMV pneumonitis is the most common manifestation of CMV disease in lung allograft recipients. The chest radiograph is nonspecific and a positive BAL culture is predictive of histologic evidence of infection only in the highest-risk patients (seronegative recipient, seropositive donor). Transbronchial biopsies are required to identify viral inclusions and to exclude rejection. Treatment of CMV pneumonitis in lung transplant recipients with ganciclovir is probably effective, but has not been prospectively studied. The direct mortality from CMV disease in treated patients is about 1%, but CMV infection may increase the risk of acute and chronic rejection. Prophylaxis with ganciclovir may be effective in preventing or delaying CMV disease in at-risk patients, but the optimal regimen has not been defined.

HSV mucositis develops in 30% of seropositive lung transplant recipients in the absence of acyclovir prophylaxis, and half of these patients develop pneumonia. Primary HSV infections are rare. Acyclovir appears to be effective in preventing reactivation of HSV. EBV-related PTLD occurs in approximately 6% of lung allograft recipients. The typical case presents within the first 4 months after transplantation with nodular infiltrates in the lung allograft, although any lymphoid tissue may be involved. Most patients respond to a reduction in the immunosuppressive regimen.

Fungal infections occur in 15 to 35% of lung transplant recipients. Candidiasis is the most common mycosis, and may involve the mediastinum, the airway anastomosis, or dissemination from a cutaneous or vascular site. Invasive aspergillosis typically presents as a focal pneumonia or necrotizing airway infection. The reported mortality of fungal infections after lung transplantation has ranged from 20 to 80%. The roles for antifungal prophylaxis and aggressive treatment of mucosal isolates are unclear.

Kidney Transplantation

Perspective

There were 14,731 kidney transplants performed in the United States in 2002. The leading indications are diabetes mellitus, hypertensive nephroclerosis, and chronic glomerulonephritis. The current survival rates for grafts and patients after cadaveric transplant are 88% and 95% at 1 year, respectively, and 67% and 85% at 4 years. After living donor transplants, the survival rates of grafts and patients are 92% and 97% at 1 year, respectively, and 81% and 92% at 4 years. Graft survival is influenced by human leukocyte antigen matching. Postoperatively, urine output, volume status, and electrolytes must be followed closely, but most renal transplant recipients have a stable course and require intensive care for <24 h.

Noninfectious Complications

Serious noninfectious complications are uncommon after renal transplantation. Volume overload and graft dysfunction occasionally lead to pulmonary edema. Surgical complications such as renal artery thrombosis, renal vein thrombosis, urine leaks, and lymphoceles occur in <5% of patients. Hyperacute rejection from preformed antibodies causes immediate graft failure and is usually detected in the operating room. Acute rejection occurs in 50 to 60% of cases within the first 3 months and is suspected by a rise in creatinine not attributable to cyclosporine toxicity. Acute rejection is empirically treated with corticosteroids; refractory cases are confirmed by renal biopsy. Chronic rejection develops in 8 to 10% of patients and causes steady deterioration of graft function.

Infection

Urinary tract infections are common early after renal transplantation and can be prevented with prophylactic antibiotics. Bacterial infections of the wound, IV catheter sites, and the respiratory tract also may complicate the early postoperative course. Opportunistic infections caused by Legionella, Nocardia, and Listeria usually occur 1 to 6 months after transplantation. Fungal infections are less common in renal graft recipients than in other organ transplant patients.

Primary CMV infection develops in 70 to 90% of seronegative recipients of a kidney from a seropositive donor, and 50% to 60% of these patients will be symptomatic. CMV infection develops in 50 to 80% of seropositive recipients and 20 to 40% of these patients will have clinical disease. The onset of infection is usually 1 to 6 months after transplant. The mononucleosislike CMV syndrome is the most common manifestation of CMV disease in renal transplant recipients; about 25% of symptomatic patients will develop CMV pneumonia. Ganciclovir appears to be effective in treating CMV disease in the setting of renal transplantation.

Kidney-Pancreas Transplantation

Perspective

In 2002, 546 pancreas transplants were performed in the United States; of these, most were in association with kidney transplants for diabetic nephropathy. Pancreas transplantation normalizes glucose metabolism and reduces the recurrence of vascular disease in the renal graft. The exocrine output of the transplanted pancreas is drained to the bladder via a duodenocystostomy. Current survival rates for grafts and patients after pancreas transplantation are 77% and 92% at 1 year, respectively, and 64% and 84% at 4 years.

Usual Clinical Course

Patients require ICU monitoring of fluids and electrolytes, and tight glucose control with an insulin drip to keep the pancreas at rest. Glucose regulation may normalize within hours, but several days are often required for full graft function.

Noninfectious Complications

Complications are more common after kidney-pancreas transplantation than after renal grafting alone. Surgical complications include vascular thrombosis, hematuria, perforation of the duodenal segment, and urethral stricture. Loss of sodium bicarbonate in the urine may cause significant dehydration and metabolic acidosis. Acute pancreatic rejection occurs in >85% of cases, more commonly than kidney rejection, and is more refractory to corticosteroids. Pancreatic rejection is diagnosed by an abrupt fall in urinary amylase; some centers confirm rejection histologically by cystoscopic biopsy. Most cases of pancreatic rejection fail to respond to corticosteroids and require repeated courses of OKT3.

Infection

Infections also are more common in patients with kidney-pancreas transplants than in recipients of a renal allograft alone because of the additional surgery and the need for more immunosuppression. Wound infections, urinary tract infections, and abdominal abscesses caused by bacteria or fungi are particularly frequent in the first month after transplant, but may appear a year or more postoperatively. Active CMV infection will develop in most patients at risk, and the majority of these infections will be symptomatic with a viremic syndrome; hepatitis is the most common site of tissue infection.

Further Reading

Arcasoy SM, Kotloff RM. Lung transplantation. N Engl J Med 1999; 340:1081–1091
An informative and concise review.

Duarte AG, Lick S. Perioperative care of the lung transplant patient. Chest Surg Clin North Am 2002; 12:397–416
A good and complete review of postoperative management.

Judson MA, Sahn SA. The pleural space and organ transplantation. Am J Respir Crit Care Med 1996; 153:1153–1165
A very thorough review of pre- and posttransplant pleural complications associated with marrow and organ transplantation.

Larsen J, Lane J, Mack-Shipman L. Pancreas and kidney transplantation. Curr Diab Rep 2002; 2:359–364
General overview of these transplants.

McGilvray ID, Greig PD. Critical care of the liver transplant patient: an update. Curr Opin Crit Care 2002; 8:178–182
Excellent overview including pre- and postoperative management.

Rubin RH. Infection in transplantation. Infect Dis Clin North Am 1995; 9:811–1092
Excellent articles covering every aspect of infection in organ and marrow transplantation.

Trulock EP. Lung transplantation. Am J Respir Crit Care Med 1997; 155:789–818
A very thorough review based on the Washington University experience.

Wiesner RH, Rakela J, Ishitani MB, et al. Recent advances in liver transplantation. Mayo Clin Proc 2003; 78:197–210
An excellent review, including a discussion of pretransplant considerations.

Winkel E, DiSesa VJ, Costanzo MR, et al. Advances in transplantation. Dis Mon 1999; 45:60–114
Discussions of heart, pancreas, and liver transplantation.

Notes

Myocardial Infarction

Steven M. Hollenberg, MD, FCCP

Objectives:

- To review the diagnosis of myocardial infarction, with emphasis on diagnostic pitfalls
- To understand indications, contraindications, and use of thrombolytic therapy
- To understand the role of cardiac catheterization, angioplasty, and surgical revascularization
- To review adjunctive medical therapy of acute myocardial infarction
- To review complications of acute myocardial infarction

Definitions

Ischemic heart disease results from an inadequate level of coronary blood flow to meet myocardial oxygen demand. The heart is an aerobic organ with only a limited capacity for anaerobic glycolysis and it makes use of oxygen avidly and efficiently, extracting 70 to 80% of the oxygen from coronary arterial blood. Because the heart extracts oxygen nearly maximally independent of demand, and increases in demand must be met by commensurate increases in coronary blood flow. Myocardial infarction (MI) occurs when prolonged ischemia causes myocardial necrosis.

Myocardial ischemia is associated almost immediately with failure of contraction. Although this can result in part from myocardial necrosis, areas of nonfunctional but viable myocardium can also cause or contribute to the development of systolic dysfunction. This reversibly dysfunctional myocardium comes under two main categories: stunning and hibernation. *Stunned myocardium* is muscle that has been reperfused after ischemia but still exhibits profound contractile dysfunction despite restoration of normal blood flow. *Myocardial hibernation* can be seen as an adaptive response in which segments with severely reduced coronary blood flow reduce their contractile function to restore equilibrium between flow and function, minimizing the potential for ischemia or necrosis. Both stunned and hibernating myocardium retain contractile reserve, and function of both may improve with time and/or revascularization.

Pathogenesis

Myocardial infarction is usually due to thrombus formation within a coronary artery, most often resulting from rupture of an atherosclerotic plaque. Classification of infarctions into those which are transmural and those which are nontransmural has been largely abandoned due to the recognition that electrocardiographic criteria are neither sensitive nor specific to make this distinction. Acute coronary syndromes have traditionally been classified into Q-wave myocardial infarction, non-Q wave myocardial infarction (NQMI), and unstable angina. More recently, classification has shifted and has become based on the initial electrocardiogram: patients are divided into those with ST-elevation (STEMI), without ST elevation (non-ST elevation acute coronary syndrome). Within the latter category, patients with evidence of myocardial damage are deemed to have non-ST elevation MI (or NSTEMI), and those with normal enzyme levels have unstable angina. Classification according to presenting electrocardiogram coincides with current treatment strategies, since patients presenting with ST elevation benefit from immediate reperfusion and should be treated with thrombolytic therapy or urgent revascularization, whereas fibrinolytic agents are not effective in other patients with acute coronary syndromes.

Distributions of the Major Coronary Arteries

The left anterior descending coronary artery (LAD) supplies the anterior left ventricle, anterior septum and usually the left ventricular apex; the LAD has septal and diagonal branches. Anterior infarction is seen in electrocardiographic (ECG) leads V_1 to V_5. The right coronary artery (RCA) supplies the inferior left ventricular wall, usually the inferior septum, most of the right ventricle and the sinus node. The RCA is dominant (that is, it gives rise to a posterior descending artery and so supplies left ventricular myocardium in the inferior septal region) in 80% of patients. Inferior infarction is seen in ECG leads II, III, and aVF. The circumflex coronary artery runs in the atrioventricular (A-V) groove; obtuse marginal (OM) branches supply the lateral and posterolateral left ventricle. Lateral infarction is seen in ECG leads I, aVL, V_5, and V_6.

Diagnosis of Acute Infarction

The diagnosis of acute myocardial infarction is made on the basis of a compatible clinical presentation, electrocardiographic changes, and a rise and fall in enzymes indicative of myocardial damage. The differential diagnosis of acute infarction includes dissecting aortic aneurysm, pericarditis, pleuritis, pulmonary processes such as pulmonary embolism, pneumonia, and pneumothorax, gastrointestinal processes such as esophageal or peptic ulcer disease and cholecystitis, musculoskeletal pain, and costochondritis. Other heart diseases (valvular heart disease, cardiomyopathies, myocarditis) not attributable to coronary artery stenosis may also cause substernal chest tightness and should also be included in the differential diagnosis.

The classic electrocardiographic feature of acute infarction is ST segment elevation, followed by T wave inversion and ultimate development of Q waves. The diagnosis can be limited in the presence of pre-existing left bundle-branch block (LBBB) or permanent pacemaker. Nonetheless, new LBBB with a compatible clinical presentation should be treated as acute myocardial infarction and treated accordingly. Criteria for diagnosing acute infarction in the setting of LBBB exist and are fairly specific but not especially sensitive. True posterior MI, which usually accompanies inferior infarction, can be subtle; hallmarks include prominent R waves, tall upright T waves and depressed ST segments in leads V_1 and V_2. The clinician must also beware or electrocardiographic "imposters" of acute infarction, which include pericarditis, J-point elevation, Wolff-Parkinson-White syndrome, and hypertrophic cardiomyopathy.

The classic biochemical marker of acute myocardial infarction has been elevation of creatine phosphokinase (CPK) MB isoenzyme levels, which appear in the plasma 4 to 8 h after onset of infarction, and its level peak at 12 to 24 h, and return to baseline at 2 to 4 days. To be diagnostic for MI, the total plasma CK value must exceed the upper limit of normal, and the fraction consisting of the MB isoenzyme must exceed a certain value (which depends on the CK-MB assay used; usually >5%).

CPK levels have now been largely superseded by measurement of cardiac troponins, constituents of the contractile protein apparatus of cardiac muscle that are much more specific for the detection of myocardial damage. Troponins are also more sensitive than CPK for the detection of myocardial damage, and troponin elevation in patients without ST elevation (or in fact, without elevation of CPK-MB) identifies a subpopulation at increased risk for complications. Rapid point-of-care troponin assays, have further extended the clinical utility of this marker. Troponins may not be elevated until 6 hours after an acute event, and so critical therapeutic interventions should not be delayed pending assay results. Once elevated, troponin levels can remain high for days to weeks, limiting their utility to detect late reinfarction.

Thrombolytic Therapy for Acute Myocardial Infarction

Early reperfusion of an occluded coronary artery is indicated for all eligible candidates. Thrombolytic therapy has been proven to decrease mortality in patients with ST segment elevation; patients treated early derive the most benefit. Indications and contraindications for thrombolytic therapy are listed below (Table 1).

Thrombolytic Agents

Streptokinase (SK) is a single-chain protein produced by α-hemolytic streptococci. SK is given as a 1.5 million unit IV infusion over 1 h, which produces a systemic lytic state for about 24 h. Hypotension with infusion usually responds to fluids and a decreased infusion rate, but allergic reactions are possible. Hemorrhagic complications are the most feared side effect, with a rate of

Table 1. *Indications and Contraindications for Thrombolytic Therapy*

Indications
- Symptoms consistent with acute myocardial infarction
- ECG showing 1-mm (0.1 mV) ST elevation in at least two contiguous leads, or new left bundle-branch block
- Presentation within 12 h of symptom onset
- Absence of contraindications

Contraindications
- Absolute
  - Active internal bleeding
  - Intracranial neoplasm, aneurysm, or A-V malformation
  - Stroke or neurosurgery within 6 weeks
  - Trauma or major surgery within 2 weeks which could be a potential source of serious rebleeding
  - Aortic dissection
- Relative
  - Prolonged (>10 minutes) or clearly traumatic cardiopulmonary resuscitation*
  - Severe uncontrolled hypertension (>200/110 mm Hg)*
  - Trauma or major surgery within 6 weeks (but more than 2 weeks)
  - Pre-existing coagulopathy or current use of anticoagulants with INR >2-3
  - Noncompressible vascular punctures
  - Active peptic ulcer
  - Infective endocarditis
  - Pregnancy
  - Chronic severe hypertension

* Could be an absolute contraindication in low-risk patients with myocardial infarction

intracranial hemorrhage of approximately 0.5%. Streptokinase produces coronary arterial patency approximately 50 to 60% of the time, and has been shown to decrease mortality 18% compared to placebo.

Tissue plasminogen activator (t-PA) is a recombinant protein that is more fibrin-selective than streptokinase and produces a higher early coronary patency rate (70 to 80%). The Global Utilization of Streptokinase and Tissue Plasminogen Activator for Occluded Coronary Arteries (GUSTO) trial compared SK to t-PA in 41,021 patients with STEMI, and demonstrated a small but significant survival benefit for t-PA (1.1% absolute, 15% relative reduction). The GUSTO angiographic substudy showed that the difference in patency rates explains the difference in clinical efficacy between these two agents. t-PA is usually given in an accelerated regimen consisting of a 15 mg bolus, 0.75 mg/kg (up to 50 mg) IV over the initial 30 minutes, and 0.5 mg/kg (up to 35 mg) over the next 60 minutes. Allergic reactions do not occur because t-PA is not antigenic, but the rate of intracranial hemorrhage may be slightly higher than that with SK, around 0.7%.

Reteplase (r-PA) is a deletion mutant of t-PA with and extended half-life, and is given as two 10 mg boluses 30 minutes apart. Reteplase was originally evaluated in angiographic trials which demonstrated improved coronary flow at 90 minutes compared to t-PA, but subsequent trials showed similar 30-day mortality rates. Why enhanced patency with r-PA did not translate into lower mortality is uncertain.

Tenecteplase (TNK-tPA) is a genetically engineered t-PA mutant with amino acid substitutions that result in prolonged half-life, resistance to plasminogen-activator inhibitor-1, and increased fibrin specificity. TNK-tPA is given as a single bolus, adjusted for weight. A single bolus of TNK-tPA has been shown to produce coronary flow rates identical to those seen with accelerated t-PA, with equivalent 30-day mortality and bleeding rates. Based on these results, single-bolus TNK-tPA is an acceptable alternative to t-PA that can be given as a single bolus.

Because these newer agents in general have equivalent efficacy, side effect profiles, at no current additional cost compared to t-PA, and because they are simpler to administer, they have gained popularity. The ideal thrombolytic agent has not yet been developed. Newer recombinant agents with greater fibrin specificity, slower clearance from the circulation, and more resistance to plasma protease inhibitors are being studied.

In contrast to the treatment of STEMI, thrombolytics have shown no benefit to increased risk of adverse events when used for the treatment of unstable angina/NSTEMI. Based on these findings, there is currently no role for thrombolytic agents in these latter syndromes.

Adjunctive Anticoagulant and Antiplatelet Therapy With Fibrinolytic Agents in ST-Elevation Myocardial Infarction

Normal (TIMI grade 3) flow is achieved in only 50% to 60% of cases with fibrinolytic therapy alone. Furthermore, fibrinolysis activates platelets, which causes further thrombus formation and subsequent reocclusion and reinfarction in a significant number of patients. There has thus been great interest in combining full-dose platelet glycoprotein IIb/IIIa inhibition with reduced doses of fibrinolytics. Although some early studies showed improved rates of TIMI 3 flow with this approach, the large GUSTO V trial using abciximab showed no difference in mortality, and increased rates of major bleeding. Reinfarction and nonhemorrhagic stroke were decreased, however.

Administration of full doses of unfractionated heparin is standard after thrombolytic therapy. Low-molecular-weight heparin (LMWH) may be an alternative. The LMWH enoxaparin decreased the combined endpoint of death, MI, and stroke compared to unfractionated heparin, but no benefit was observed in patients >75 and in diabetics. These results await confirmation in additional studies.

Primary Percutaneous Coronary Intervention

As many as one-half to two-thirds of patients presenting with acute myocardial infarction may be ineligible for thrombolytic therapy, and these patients should be considered for primary percutaneous coronary intervention (PCI). The major advantages of primary PCI over thrombolytic therapy include a higher rate of normal (TIMI grade 3) flow, lower risk of intracranial hemorrhage and the ability to stratify risk based on the severity and distribution of coronary artery disease.

Data from several randomized trials have suggested that PCI is preferable to thrombolytic therapy for acute MI patients at higher risk, including those over 75 years old, those with anterior infarctions, and those with hemodynamic instability. The largest of these trials is the GUSTO-IIb Angioplasty Substudy, which randomized 1,138 patients to angioplasty or t-PA and noted a decrease. At 30 days, there was a clinical benefit in the combined primary endpoints of death, nonfatal reinfarction, and nonfatal disabling stroke in the patients treated with percutnaeous transluminal coronary angioplasty (PTCA) compared to t-PA, but no difference in the "hard" endpoints of death and myocardial infarction at 30 days, and no difference in the combined endpoint at 6 months. The recent CAPTIM trial compared prehospital thrombolysis with t-PA to primary PCI in 840 pts; the combined endpoint of death, MI, or stroke at 30 days occurred in 8.2% or the lytic group and 6.2% of the PCI group, but this was not statistically different (RR 1.96, CI −1.53-5.46, p = 0.29). It should be noted that mortality rates were quite low in both groups. The recent C-PORT trial 451 patients randomized 451 patients to t-PA or primary PTCA in hospitals without on-site cardiac surgery, and found a significant decrease in the primary endpoint of death, MI, and stroke at 6 months from 19.9% of lytic group vs 12.4% PTCA (p = 0.03). The most recent and largest study in this area is the DANAMI trial, which randomized 1,572 patients in Denmark to t-PA or PCI. Patients randomized to PCI at a site without interventional capability were transferred emergently to a PCI center. The combined endpoint of death, recurrent MI, and stroke was decreased in both PCI centers (from 12.3% to 6.7%, p = 0.05), and also in patients transferred for PCI (from 14.2% to 8.5%, p = 0.002). A recent meta-analysis showed both improved short and long-term outcomes with PCI compared to thrombolytic therapy. It should be noted that this analysis included lysis with both SK and t-PA, and that the differences are less marked when only trials using newer thrombolytic agents are considered.

It should be noted that both time to revascularization and procedural volume is important as well. Recent analyses show higher mortality when door-to-needle time exceeds 120 min, and lower mortality in hospitals performing primary PCI more than 3 times/month. Thus, direct angioplasty, if performed in a timely manner (ideally within 90 min) by highly experienced personnel, may be the preferred method of revascularization since it offers more complete revascularization with improved restoration of normal coronary blood flow and detailed information about coronary anatomy. When performing PTCA will require a substantial time delay, and in less experienced hands, thrombolytic therapy may be preferable. There are certain subpopulations, however, in which primary PCI is preferred. These subsets are listed in Table 2. Revascularization for patients with cardiogenic shock is discussed in

Table 2. *Considerations for PTCA or Thrombolytic Agents Among Subsets of Patients With AMI*

Situations in which PTCA is preferable to thrombolytics in AMI
- Contraindications to thrombolytic therapy
- Cardiogenic shock
- Patients in whom uncertain diagnosis prompted cardiac catheterization which revealed coronary occlusion

Situations in which PTCA *may be* preferable to thrombolytics in AMI
- Elderly patients (>75 years)
- Hemodynamic instability
- Prior coronary artery bypass grafting
- Large anterior infarction
- Patients with a prior myocardial infarction

---

the Heart Failure and Cardiac Pulmonary Edema chapter.

Coronary Stenting and Glycoprotein IIb/IIIa Antagonists

Primary angioplasty for acute myocardial infarction results in a significant reduction in mortality but is limited by the possibility of abrupt vessel closure, recurrent in-hospital ischemia, reocclusion of the infarct related artery, and restenosis. The use of coronary stents has been shown to reduce restenosis and adverse cardiac outcomes in both routine and high-risk PCI. Coronary stenting has now been accepted as superior to balloon angioplasty alone in acute MI, probably because antegrade flow rates are superior, decreasing reocclusion.

Glycoprotein IIb/IIIa receptor antagonists inhibit the final common pathway of platelet aggregation, blocking crosslinking of activated platelets, and their use in PCI has become routine. The benefits of glycoprotein IIb/IIIa inhibition and coronary stenting appear to be additive. Thus, combining glycoprotein IIb/IIIa antagonism and stenting in acute MI makes theoretical sense, and has now been tested in two large clinical trials. The ADMIRAL trial evaluated abciximab as an adjunct to primary PTCA and stenting in 300 acute MI patients, and showed a nearly 50% relative risk reduction in the incidence of death, recurrent MI, and urgent revascularization at 30 days, although this was associated with an increased incidence of minor bleeding. Administration of glycoprotein IIb/IIIa inhibitors during stenting for acute MI has become routine

Other Indications for Angioplasty in Acute Myocardial Infarction

In patients who fail thrombolytic therapy, rescue PTCA improves outcomes, although the initial success rate is lower than that of primary angioplasty, reocclusion is more common, and mortality is higher than primary PCI.

There is no convincing evidence to support empirical delayed PTCA in patients without evidence of recurrent or provokable ischemia after thrombolytic therapy. The TIMI IIB trial and others studies suggest that a strategy of "watchful waiting" allows for identification of patients who will benefit from revascularization.

"Facilitated" PCI refers to planned percutaneous coronary intervention after reduced dose pharmacological reperfusion therapy. Rather than rescuing only those patients with failed thrombolysis, all patients would have prompt (even prehospital) admnistration of lytic agents, followed by catheterization with intervention if appropriate. The hope is that such an approach would optimize early patency and allow for management of residual stenosis. This strategy is has been shown to be feasible with an acceptable safety profile. Studies are currently underway to determine whether this combined approach could provide the optimal reperfusion strategy.

Adjunctive Therapies in ST-Elevation Myocardial Infarction

Aspirin

Unless contraindicated, all patients with suspected myocardial infarction should be given aspirin, 160 to 325 mg. This should be accomplished within the first 10 min of hospital evaluation and the aspirin should be chewed to accelerate absorption. Aspirin has been shown to reduce mortality in acute infarction to the same degree as thrombolytic therapy, and its effects are additive to thrombolytics. In addition, aspirin reduces the risk of reinfarction.

Once begun, aspirin should probably be continued indefinitely. Aspirin irreversibly inactivates platelet cyclooxygenase, inhibiting platelet aggregation and reducing the release of platelet-derived vasoconstrictors such as serotonin and thromboxane A$_2$. Recent data suggest that the anti-inflammatory effects of aspirin may play a role in inhibiting plaque rupture as well. Toxicity with aspirin is mostly gastrointestinal; enteric-coated preparations may minimize these side effects.

Heparin

Administration of full-dose heparin after thrombolytic therapy with t-PA is essential to diminish reocclusion after successful reperfusion. Dosing should be adjusted to weight (and doses in conjunction with lytics are lower than for other indications), with a bolus of 60 U/kg up to a maximum of 4,000 U and an initial infusion rate of 12 U/kg/h up to a maximum of 1000 U/h, with adjustment to keep the partial thromboplastin time (PTT) between 50 and 70 s. Heparin should be continued for 24 to 48 h.

Nitrates

Nitrates reduce myocardial oxygen demand by decreasing preload and afterload, and may also improve myocardial oxygen supply by increasing subendocardial perfusion and collateral blood flow to the ischemic region. Occasional patients with ST elevation due to occlusive coronary artery spasm may have dramatic resolution of ischemia with nitrates. In addition to their hemodynamic effects, nitrates also reduce platelet aggregation. Despite these benefits, the GISSI-3 and ISIS-4 trials failed to show a significant reduction in mortality from routine acute and chronic nitrate therapy. Nonetheless, nitrates are still first-line agents for the symptomatic relief of angina pectoris and when myocardial infarction is complicated by congestive heart failure.

Our practice is to administer sublingual nitroglycerin to all patients presenting with chest pain, unless the systolic blood pressure is <100 mm Hg or evidence of right ventricular infarction is present. For patients with persistent chest pain, intravenous nitroglycerin is infused at 10 μg/min and increased in increments of 5 to 10 μg/min every 5 min until the pain resolves.

The major adverse effects of nitrates are hypotension and headache. Nitrates should be used with great caution in patients with right ventricular infarction, who may not tolerate decreases in filling pressure. Similarly, precipitous decreases in blood pressure in patients presenting with inferior myocardial infarction should raise the suspicion of right ventricular involvement. Nitrate-induced hypotension is usually caused by vasodilation and is treated with rapid bolus infusion of intravenous fluids.

β-Blockers

β-blockers are beneficial both in the early management of myocardial infarction and as long-term therapy. In the pre-thrombolytic era, early intravenous atenolol was shown to significantly reduce reinfarction, cardiac arrest, cardiac rupture, and death. In conjunction with thrombolytic therapy with t-PA, immediate β-blockade with metoprolol resulted in a significant reduction in recurrent ischemia and reinfarction, although mortality was not decreased. In the most recent trial, the CAPRICORN study, the nonselective β-blocker carvedilol decreased mortality from 15 to 12% in patients with MI and ejection fraction less than 40% (p = 0.03), although the primary endpoint (death or hospitalization) was unchanged.

Administration of intravenous β-blockade should be considered for all patients presenting with acute myocardial infarction, especially those with continued ischemic discomfort and sympathetic hyperactivity manifested by hypertension or tachycardia. Therapy should be avoided in patients with moderate or severe heart failure, hypotension, severe bradycardia or heart block, and severe bronchospastic disease. Metoprolol can be given as a 5 mg IV bolus, repeated every 5 minutes for a total of 3 doses. Because of its brief half-life, esmolol may be advantageous in situations were precise control or the heart rate is necessary or rapid drug withdrawal may be needed if adverse effects occur.

Oral β-blockade has been clearly demonstrated to decrease mortality after acute MI, and should be initiated in all patients who can tolerate it, even if they have not been treated with intravenous β-blockers. Diabetes mellitus is not a contraindication.

Angiotensin-Converting Enzyme inhibitors

Angiotensin-converting enzyme (ACE) inhibitors have been shown unequivocally to improve hemodynamics, functional capacity and symptoms, and survival in patients with chronic congestive heart failure. Moreover, ACE inhibitors prevent the development of congestive heart failure in patients with asymptomatic left ventricular dysfunction. This information was the spur for trials evaluating the benefit the prophylactic administration of ACE inhibitors in the post-MI period. The SAVE trial showed that patients with left ventricular dysfunction (ejection fraction <40%) after MI had a 21% improvement in survival after treatment with the ACE inhibitor captopril. A smaller but still significant reduction in mortality was seen when all patients were treated with captopril in the ISIS-4 study. The HOPE study demonstrated improved survival additive to the benefits of aspirin and β-blockers with the ACE inhibitor ramipril used as secondary prevention. The mechanisms responsible for the benefits of ACE inhibitors probably include limitation in the progressive left ventricular dysfunction and enlargement (remodeling) that often occur after infarction, but a reduction in ischemic events was seen as well. Recent studies have suggested that ACE inhibition can ameliorate endothelial dysfunction in atherosclerosis.

ACE inhibition should be started early, preferably within the first 24 hours after infarction. Immediate intravenous ACE inhibition with enalaprilat has not been shown to be beneficial. Patients should be started on low doses of oral agents (captopril 6.25 mg three times daily) and rapidly increased to the range demonstrated beneficial in clinical trials (captopril 50 mg three times daily, enalapril 10 to 20 mg twice daily, lisinopril 10 to 20 mg once daily, or ramipril 10 mg once daily).

Angiotensin Receptor Blockers

Angiotensin receptor blockers (ARBs) have hemodynamic effects similar to those of ACE inhibitors. The recent VALIANT trial compared valsartan to captopril and the found equivalent outcomes in patients with LV dysfunction after MI. The combination of valsartan and captopril was not more effective but did produce more side effects. On the basis of these data, valsartan is an alternative to ACE inhibition, particularly in patients who do not tolerate ACE inhibitors.

Calcium Antagonists

Randomized clinical trials have not demonstrated that routine use of calcium channel blockers improves survival after myocardial infarction. In fact, meta-analyses suggest that high doses of the short-acting dihydropyridine nifedipine increase mortality in myocardial infarction. Adverse effects of calcium-channel blockers include bradycardia, atrioventricular block, and exacerbation of heart failure. The relative vasodilating, negative inotropic effects, and conduction system effects of the various agents must be considered when they are employed in this setting. Diltiazem is the only calcium channel blocker that has been proven to have tangible benefits, reducing reinfarction and recurrent ischemia in patients with patients with non-Q-wave infarctions who do not have evidence of congestive heart failure.

Calcium channel blockers may be useful for patients whose postinfarction course is complicated by recurrent angina, because these agents not only reduce myocardial oxygen demand but inhibit coronary vasoconstriction. For hemodynamically stable patients, diltiazem can be given, starting at 60 to 90 mg orally every 6 to 8 h. In patients with severe left ventricular dysfunction, long-acting dihydropyridines without prominent negative inotropic effects such as amlodipine, nicardipine, or the long-acting preparation of nifedipine may be preferable; increased mortality with these agents has *not* been demonstrated.

Antiarrhythmic Agents

Even though lidocaine increases the frequency of premature ventricular contractions and of early ventricular fibrillation, overall mortality is not decreased. In fact, meta-analyses of pooled data have demonstrated increased mortality from the routine use of lidocaine and so its routine prophylactic administration is no longer recommended. Nonetheless, lidocaine may be used after an episode of sustained ventricular tachycardia or ventricular fibrillation, and considered in patients with nonsustained ventricular tachycardia.

Lidocaine is administered as a bolus of 1 mg/kg (not to exceed 100 mg), followed by a second bolus of 0.5 mg/kg 10 min later, along with an infusion at 1 to 3 mg/min. Lidocaine is metabolized by the liver, and so lower doses should be given in the presence of liver disease, in the elderly, and in patients who have congestive heart failure severe enough to compromise hepatic perfusion. Toxic manifestations primarily involve the central nervous system, and can include confusion, lethargy, slurred speech, and seizures. Because the risk of malignant ventricular arrhythmias decreases after 24 h, lidocaine is usually discontinued after this point. For prolonged infusions, monitoring of lidocaine levels (therapeutic between 1.5 and 5 g/mL) is sometimes useful.

Intravenous amiodarone is an alternative to lidocaine for ventricular arrhythmias. Amiodarone is given as a 150 mg IV bolus over 10 min, followed by 1 mg/min for 6 h, then 0.5 mg/min for 18 h.

Perhaps the most important point in the prevention and management of arrhythmias after acute myocardial infarction is correcting hypoxemia, and maintaining normal serum potassium and magnesium levels. Serum electrolytes should be followed closely, particularly after diuretic therapy. Magnesium depletion is also a frequently overlooked cause of persistent ectopy. The serum magnesium level, even if it is within normal limits, may not reflect myocardial concentrations. Routine administration of magnesium has not been shown to reduce mortality after acute myocardial infarction, but empiric administration of 2 grams of intravenous magnesium in patients with early ventricular ectopy is probably a good idea.

Complications of Acute Myocardial Infarction

Postinfarction Angina and Infarct Extension

Causes of ischemia after infarction include decreased myocardial oxygen supply due to coronary reocclusion or spasm, mechanical problems which increase myocardial oxygen demand, and extracardiac factors such as hypertension, anemia, hypotension, or hypermetabolic states. Nonischemic causes of chest pain, such as postinfarction pericarditis and acute pulmonary embolism, should also be considered.

Immediate management includes aspirin, β-blockade, IV nitroglycerin, heparin, consideration of calcium-channel blockers, and diagnostic coronary angiography. Post-infarction angina is an indication for revascularization. PCI can be performed if the culprit lesion is suitable. Coronary artery bypass graft (CABG) should be considered for patients with left main disease, three-vessel disease, and those unsuitable for PCI. If the angina cannot be controlled medically or is accompanied by hemodynamic instability, an intra-aortic balloon pump should be inserted.

Ventricular Free Wall Rupture

Ventricular free wall rupture typically occurs during the first week after infarction. The classic patient is elderly, female, and hypertensive. Early use of thrombolytic therapy reduces the incidence of cardiac rupture, but late use may actually increase the risk. Free wall rupture presents as a catastrophic event with shock and electromechanical dissociation. Salvage is possible with prompt recognition, pericardiocentesis to relieve acute tamponade, and thoracotomy with repair. Emergent echocardiography or pulmonary artery catheterization can help make the diagnosis.

Ventricular Septal Rupture

Septal rupture presents as severe heart failure or cardiogenic shock, with a pansystolic murmur and parasternal thrill. The hallmark finding is a left-to-right intracardiac shunt ("step-up" in oxygen saturation from right atrium to right ventricle), but the diagnosis is most easily made with echocardiography.

Rapid institution of intra-aortic balloon pumping and supportive pharmacologic measures is necessary. Operative repair is the only viable option for long-term survival. The timing of surgery has been controversial, but most authorities now suggest that repair should be undertaken early, within 48 h of the rupture.

Acute Mitral Regurgitation

Ischemic mitral regurgitation is usually associated with inferior myocardial infarction and ischemia or infarction of the posterior papillary muscle. Papillary muscle rupture typically occurs 2 to 7 days after acute myocardial infarction and presents dramatically with pulmonary edema, hypotension, and cardiogenic shock. When a papillary muscle ruptures, the murmur of acute mitral regurgitation may be limited to early systole because of rapid equalization of pressures in the left atrium and left ventricle. More importantly, the murmur may be soft or inaudible, especially when cardiac output is low.

Echocardiography is extremely useful in the differential diagnosis, which includes free wall rupture, ventricular septal rupture, and infarct extension with pump failure. Hemodynamic monitoring with pulmonary artery catheterization may also be helpful. Management includes afterload reduction with nitroprusside and intra-aortic balloon pumping as temporizing measures. Inotropic or vasopressor therapy may also be needed to support cardiac output and blood pressure. Definitive therapy, however, is surgical valve repair or replacement, which should be undertaken as soon as possible since clinical deterioration can be sudden.

Right Ventricular Infarction

Right ventricular infarction occurs in up to 30% of patients with inferior infarction and is clinically significant in 10%. The combination of a clear chest x-ray with jugular venous distention in a patient with an inferior wall MI should lead to the suspicion of a coexisting right ventricular infarct. The diagnosis is substantiated by demonstration of ST segment elevation in the right precordial leads (V_{3R} to V_{5R}) or by characteristic hemodynamic findings on right heart catheterization (elevated right atrial and right ventricular end-diastolic pressures with normal to low pulmonary artery occlusion pressure and low cardiac output). Echocardiography can demonstrate depressed right ventricular contractility. Patients with cardiogenic shock on the basis of right ventricular infarction have a better prognosis than those with left-sided pump failure. This may be due in part to the fact that right ventricular function tends to return to normal over time with supportive therapy, although such therapy may need to be prolonged.

In patients with right ventricular infarction, right ventricular preload should be maintained with fluid administration. In some cases, however, fluid resuscitation may increase pulmonary capillary occlusion pressure but may not increase cardiac output, and overdilation of the right ventricle can compromise left ventricular filling and cardiac output. Inotropic therapy with dobutamine may be more effective in increasing cardiac output in some patients, and monitoring with serial echocardiograms may also be useful to detect right ventricular overdistention. Maintenance of atrioventricular synchrony is also important in these patients to optimize right ventricular filling. For patients with continued hemodynamic instability, intra-aortic balloon pumping may be useful, particularly because elevated right ventricular pressures and volumes increase wall stress and oxygen consumption and decrease right coronary perfusion pressure, exacerbating right ventricular ischemia.

Reperfusion of the occluded coronary artery is also crucial. A study using direct angioplasty demonstrated that restoration of normal flow resulted in dramatic recovery of right ventricular function and a mortality rate of only 2%, whereas unsuccessful reperfusion was associated with persistent hemodynamic compromise and a mortality of 58%.

Cardiogenic Shock

Cardiogenic shock as a complication of acute myocardial infarction carries a high mortality rate, approaching 60 to 90% in some series. It is considered in detail in the section on acute heart failure in the intensive care unit. Hemodynamically, cardiogenic shock is defined as a cardiac index <1.8 L/min/m^2 with an elevated PAOP, generally >18 mm Hg. Prompt reperfusion of the occluded coronary artery is the best way to reduce the mortality associated with cardiogenic shock. Because thrombolytic therapy alone does not appear to be very effective in cardiogenic shock, primary PCI is recommended. An intra-aortic balloon pump should be placed before the PCI to stabilize the patient and enhance coronary blood flow and reduce myocardial oxygen demand. Urgent coronary artery bypass surgery may be necessary if left main coronary stenosis is the culprit.

Non-ST Elevation Myocardial Infarction

The key to initial management of patients with acute coronary syndromes who present without ST elevation is risk stratification. The overall risk of a patient is related to both the severity of pre-existing heart disease and the degree of plaque instability. Risk stratification is an ongoing process, which begins with hospital admission and continues through discharge.

Braunwald has proposed a classification for unstable angina based on severity of symptoms and clinical circumstances for risk stratification. The risk of progression to acute MI or death in acute coronary syndromes increases with age. ST segment depression on the electrocardiogram identifies patients at higher risk for clinical events. Conversely, a normal ECG confers an excellent short-term prognosis. Biochemical markers of cardiac injury are also predictive of outcome. Elevated levels of troponin T are associated with an increased risk of cardiac events and a higher 30-day mortality.

Antiplatelet Therapy

Aspirin is a mainstay of therapy for acute coronary syndromes. Aspirin reduces the risk of death or myocardial infarction by approximately 50% in patients with unstable angina or NQMI. Aspirin also reduces events after resolution of an acute coronary syndrome, and should be continued indefinitely.

Clopidogrel or ticlopidine, thienopyridines that inhibit ADP-induced platelet activation and are more potent than aspirin, can be used in place of aspirin if necessary. They are used in combination with aspirin when intracoronary stents are placed. Clopidogrel is generally better tolerated than ticlopidine since the risk of neutropenia is much lower.

The CURE trial randomized 12,562 patients with unstable angina to clopidogrel or placebo in addition to aspirin, and demonstrated a significantly reduced the risk of myocardial infarction, stroke or cardiovascular death (from 11.4 to 9.3%, $p < 0.001$). It should be noted that this benefit came with a 1% absolute increase in major, non-life threatening bleeds ($p = 0.001$) as well as a 2.8% absolute increase in major/life threatening bleeds associated with CABG within 5 days ($p = 0.07$). These data have raised concerns about giving clopidogrel prior to information about the coronary anatomy.

Anticoagulant Therapy

Heparin is an important component of primary therapy for patients with unstable coronary syndromes without ST elevation. When added to aspirin, heparin has been shown to reduce refractory angina, infarction, and the composite end point of death or MI.

Heparin, however, can be difficult to administer, because the anticoagulant effect is unpredictable in individual patients; this is due to heparin binding to heparin-binding proteins, endothelial and other cells, and heparin inhibition by several factors released by activated platelets. Therefore, the APTT (activated partial thromboplastin time) must be monitored closely. The potential for heparin-associated thrombocytopenia is also a safety concern.

Low-molecular-weight heparins (LMWH), which are obtained by depolymerization of standard heparin and selection of fractions with lower molecular weight, have several advantages. Because they bind less avidly to heparin binding proteins, there is less variability in the anticoagulant response and a more predictable dose-response curve, obviating the need to monitor APTT. The incidence of thrombocytopenia is lower (but not absent, and patients with heparin-induced thrombocytopenia with anti-heparin antibodies cannot be switched to LMWH). Finally, LMWHs have longer half-lives, and can be given by subcutaneous injection. These properties make treatment with LMWH at home after hospital discharge feasible.

Several trials have documented beneficial effects of LMWH therapy in unstable coronary syndromes. Both the ESSENCE trial and the TIMI 11B trials showed that the LMWH enoxaparin reduced the combined endpoint of death, MI, or recurrent ischemia at both 14 and 30 days when compared to heparin. Although LMWH are substantially easier to administer than standard heparin, they are also more expensive. Specific considerations with the use of LMWH include decreased clearance in renal insufficiency and the lack of a commercially available test to measure the anticoagulant effect. LMWH should be given strong consideration in high-risk patients, but whether substitution of LMWH for heparin in all patients is cost-effective is uncertain.

Glycoprotein IIb/IIIa Antagonists

Platelet glycoprotein IIb/IIIa antagonists inhibit the final common pathway of platelet aggregation. Three agents are currently available. Abciximab is a chimeric murine-human monoclonal antibody Fab fragment which binds with relatively high affinity to platelet receptors giving it a short plasma half-life (10 to 30 min) but a long duration of biologic action by virtue of the strength of the bond formed with the surface of the activated platelet. As abciximab remains tightly bound to platelets in the event of a major bleeding complication, platelet transfusions may be helpful. Abciximab is currently approved for elective PCI or unstable coronary syndromes with planned PCI. Tirofiban is a small molecule, synthetic nonpeptide agent with a half-life of approximately 2.5 h and a lower receptor affinity than abciximab. This agent is approved for the medical management of unstable angina/NSTEMI with or without planned PCI. Given the large drug to platelet ratio (ie, large plasma pool of free drug) seen with this agent as well as with eptifibatide, platelet transfusions are generally not regarded as helpful in the event of a major bleed. It is recommended that the drug simply be shut off and supportive therapy instituted during the relatively short biologic activity period. Eptifibatide is a small molecule, cyclic heptapeptide with a 2 h half-life. Like tirofiban, it is approved for the medical management of unstable angina with or without subsequent PCI, however it may also be used as adjunctive therapy in elective PCI.

The benefits of glycoprotein IIb/IIIa inhibitors as adjunctive treatment in patients undergoing percutaneous intervention have been substantial and consistently observed. Abciximab has been most extensively studied, but a benefit for eptifibatide has also been demonstrated. In acute coronary syndromes, the evidence supporting the efficacy of GP IIb/IIIa inhibitors is somewhat less impressive. Five major trials have been completed (the "4 P's" and GUSTO-IV). In the PRISM trial, tirofiban reduced death, MI, or refractory ischemia when compared to heparin from 5.6% to 3.8% (p<0.01) at 48 hours, but there was no difference at 30 days (7.1% vs 5.8%, p=0.11). In the subsequent PRISM-PLUS trial, tirofiban added to heparin reduced death, MI, or refractory ischemia at 30 days from 11.9% to 8.7% (p=0.03). In the PURSUIT trial, eptifibatide reduced the rate of death or MI from 15.7% to 14.2% (p=0.04) at 30 days. The PARAGON trial with lamifiban did not show a significant benefit with GP IIb/IIIa inhibition. Abciximab did not produce an improvement in the GUSTO-IV ACS trial, which included patients for whom percutaneous intervention was not planned. when patients with refractory angina and planned angioplasty were randomized to receive abciximab or placebo from 24 hours prior to the procedure through one hour following PTCA in the CAPTURE trial, the primary end point, death, MI or urgent revascularization at 30 days, was reduced by IIb/IIIa inhibition, and the rate of MI before PTCA was reduced as well. When patients were broken down into those with and without increased troponin, the benefit was confined to the positive troponin group.

Recent meta-analyses have found a relative risk reduction of 40% for GP IIb/IIIa therapy adjunctive to PCI, and a reduction of 11% for GP IIb/IIIa inhibitors in NSTEMI acute coronary syndromes. Additional analysis suggests that glycoprotein IIb/IIIa inhibition is most effective in high-risk patients, those with either ECG changes or elevated troponin. The benefits are observed primarily in patients undergoing percutaneous intervention, which may not be entirely surprising.

Interventional Management

Cardiac catheterization may be undertaken in patients presenting with symptoms suggestive of unstable coronary syndromes for one of several reasons: to assist with risk stratification, as a prelude to revascularization, and to exclude significant epicardial coronary stenosis as a cause of symptoms when the diagnosis is uncertain.

An early invasive approach has now been compared to a conservative approach in several prospective studies. Two earlier trials were negative. The TIMI IIIb study randomized 1,473 patients to early angiography or conservative management with angiography and revascularization only for recurrent chest pain or provokable ischemia and found no significant difference in the combined endpoint of death, MI, or positive treadmill test at 6 weeks. There was, however, a high crossover rate (64%) from the conservative to the invasive arm. The VANQWISH trial of 920 patients with non-Q wave MI actually showed an increase in the primary endpoint of death or MI with an invasive strategy, although overall mortality was not significantly different. Difficulties with this trial included the fact that only 44% of patients randomized to the invasive arm underwent revascularization, compared to 33% in the conservative arm, and very high surgical mortality (11.6%). It is important to consider that these trials were performed before widespread use of coronary stenting and platelet glycoprotein IIb/IIIa inhibitors, both of which have now been shown to improve outcomes after angioplasty.

More recently, a substudy of the FRISC II study, which used the LMWH dalteparin, randomized 2457 patients to an early invasive or a noninvasive strategy, and found a significantly lower mortality in the invasive group at 30 days, which was maintained at one year. The TACTICS TIMI-18 trial used aspirin, heparin, and tirofiban in 2,220 patients, and found a significant reduction in the combined endpoint of death, MI, or readmission for acute coronary syndrome with invasive management. It is important to recognize that both of these trials selected high-risk patients (identified either on the basis of ECG changes or enzyme elevations) for inclusion. Addition of adjunctive antiplatelet therapy beyond the use of aspirin alone in conjunction with reperfusion may also have contributed to the improved outcomes with invasive strategies in these more recent trials.

An initial strategy of medical management with attempts at stabilization is warranted in patients with lower risk, but patients at higher risk should be considered for cardiac catheterization. Pharmacologic and mechanical strategies are intertwined in the sense that selection of patients for early revascularization will influence the choice of antiplatelet and anticoagulant medication. When good clinical judgment is employed, early coronary angiography in selected patients with acute coronary syndromes can lead to better management and lower morbidity and mortality.

Annotated Bibliography

Andersen HR, Nielsen TT, Rasmussen K, et al. A comparison of coronary angioplasty with fibrinolytic therapy in acute myocardial infarction. N Engl J Med 2003; 349:733-742

Danish Acute MI (DANAMI) trial in which 1,572 patients were randomized in Denmark to t-PA or PCI (either on-site or by transfer to a PCI center). The combined endpoint of death, recurrent MI, and stroke was decreased in both PCI centers (from 12.3% to 6.7%, p=0.05), and also in patients transferred for PCI (from 14.2% to 8.5%, p=0.002).

Cannon CP, Weintraub WS, Demopoulos LA, et al. Comparison of early invasive and conservative strategies in patients with unstable coronary syndromes treated with the glycoprotein IIb/IIIa inhibitor tirofiban. N Engl J Med 2001; 344:1879-1887

TACTICS-TIMI 18 study, in which 2,220 patients unstable angina or non-ST elevation MI were treated with aspirin, heparin, and tirofiban and randomized to an early invasive strategy of catheterization within 4 to 48 h and revascularization as appropriate, or to a more conservative strategy, in which catheterization was performed only if the patient had objective evidence of recurrent ischemia or an abnormal stress test. The composite of death, MI, and rehospitalization for an acute coronary syndrome at 6 months was decreased significantly, from 19.4% to 15.9%.

Cohen M, Demers C, Gurfinkel EP, et al. A comparison of low-molecular-weight heparin with unfractionated heparin for unstable coronary artery disease. Efficacy and Safety of Subcutaneous Enoxaparin in Non-Q-Wave Coronary Events Study Group. N Engl J Med 1997; 337:447-452

ESSENCE trial of 3,171 patients with angina at rest or NQMI randomized to LMWH (enoxaparin) or unfractionated heparin. At 14 and 30 days the risk of death, myocardial infarction, or recurrent angina was significantly lower with enoxaparin.

Fibrinolytic Therapy Trialists' (FTT) Collaborative Group. Indications for fibrinolytic therapy in suspected acute myocardial infarction: collaborative overview of early mortality and major morbidity results from all randomised trials of more than 1000 patients. Lancet 1994; 343:311-322

Excellent compilation of the randomized trials of thrombolytic therapy in MI, emphasizing the direct relationship between early treatment and improved outcomes.

Grines CL, Browne KF, Marco J, et al. A comparison of immediate angioplasty with thrombolytic therapy for acute myocardial infarction. N Engl J Med 1993; 328:673-679

395 thrombolytic-eligible patients randomized to t-PA or primary angioplasty for myocardial infarction. Primary angioplasty was successfully accomplished in almost 90% of patients. For the group as a whole, mortality was not significantly decreased with angioplasty (2.6% vs 6.5%, p = 0.06), but the combined endpoint of death or reinfarction was decreased (5.1% vs 12%).

Gruppo Italiano per lo Studio della Sopravvinza nell'Infarto Miocardico (GISSI). Effectiveness of intravenous thrombolytic treatment in acute myocardial infarction. Lancet 1986; 2:397-402

The landmark study of 11,712 patients, which demonstrated a 19% reduction in mortality with intravenous streptokinase.

GUSTO Investigators. An international randomized trial comparing four thrombolytic strategies for acute myocardial infarction. N Engl J Med 1993; 329:673-682

A mega-trial of 41,021 patients randomized to accelerated t-PA or streptokinase. Accelerated t-PA reduced mortality from 7.3% to 6.3% (reduction, 14%) compared to streptokinase, with a slight increase (0.2%) in the rate of disabling stroke.

GUSTO Angiographic Investigators. The effects of tissue plasminogen activator, streptokinase, or both on coronary-artery patency, ventricular function, and survival after acute myocardial infarction. N Engl J Med 1993; 329:1615-1622

Angiographic substudy of the GUSTO trial in which patients underwent coronary angiography at 90 min. The degree of coronary flow (TIMI grade) was directly related to outcome, validating the open artery hypothesis. Improved flow was seen with t-PA compared to streptokinase, but normal (TIMI grade 3) flow was present in only 55% of patients at 90 min.

Hochman JS, Sleeper LA, Webb JG, et al. Early revascularization in acute myocardial infarction complicated by cardiogenic shock. N Engl J Med 1999; 341:625-634

Landmark trial of 302 patients with MI and cardiogenic shock randomized to an early invasive strategy or aggressive medical management. The early invasive strategy reduced 30-day mortality from 556.0 to 46.7% (p = 0.11), and, as reported later, 1 year mortality was reduced from 66.4 to 53.3% (p = 0.03).

ISIS-2 Collaborative Group. Randomised trial of intravenous streptokinase, oral aspirin, both, or neither among 17,187 cases of suspected acute myocardial infarction: ISIS-2. Lancet 1988; 2:349-360

Aspirin alone reduced mortality in patients with acute myocardial infarction by 23%, and streptokinase alone reduced mortality by 25%. The combination of the two decreased mortality by 42% without increasing stroke rates. It has become widespread practice since this study to administer aspirin acutely to almost every patient presenting with an acute myocardial infarction.

Keeley EC, Boura JA, Grines CL. Primary angioplasty versus intravenous thrombolytic therapy for acute myocardial infarction: a quantitative review of 23 randomised trials. Lancet 2003; 361:13-20

A meta-analysis of trials comparing fibrinolytic therapy and primary angioplasty, demonstrating decreased mortality, reinfarction, and combined endpoints (death, MI, and target vessel revascularization) with angioplasty.

Libby P, Ridker PM, Maseri A. Inflammation and atherosclerosis. Circulation 2002; 105:1135-1143

An excellent review of the concepts of the pathogenesis of acute ischemic syndromes.

Montalescot G, Barragan P, Wittenberg O, et al. Platelet glycoprotein IIb/IIIa inhibition with coronary stenting for acute myocardial infarction. N Engl J Med 2001; 344:1895-1903

ADMIRAL trial in which 300 patients with acute MI randomized to abciximab plus stenting or placebo plus stenting. Abciximab improved coronary patency before stenting, the success rate of the stenting procedure, the rate of coronary patency at six months, left ventricular function, and clinical outcomes.

Ohman EM, Armstrong PW, Christenson RH, et al. Cardiac troponin T levels for risk stratification in acute myocardial ischemia. N Engl J Med 1996; 335:1333-1341

Cardiac troponin T levels, CK-MB levels, and electrocardiograms were analyzed in 855 patients presenting with acute coronary syndromes. Mortality within 30 days was directly correlated with troponin T levels and troponin T level was an independent risk marker. The study showed that troponin levels allow for further stratification of risk when combined with standard measures.

Pfeffer MA, McMurray JJ, Velazquez EJ, et al. Valsartan, captopril, or both in myocardial infarction complicated by heart failure, left ventricular dysfunction, or both. N Engl J Med 2003; 349:1893-1906

VALIANT trial comparing the ARB valsartan, the ACE inhibitor captopril, or both in patients with MI and systolic dysfunction and/or CHF. Valsartan was as effective as captopril, but not better, and the combination of valsartan and captopril increased the rate of adverse events without improving survival.

Rogers WJ, Canto JG, Lambrew CT, et al. Temporal trends in the treatment of over 1.5 million patients with myocardial infarction in the United States from 1990 to 1999. J Am Coll Cardiol 2000; 36:2056-2063

Results from this registry document the percentage of patients treated with different therapies after myocardial infarction. Care is improving, but some interventions proven to reduce mortality after myocardial infarction are still underutilized.

Ryan TJ, Anderson JL, Antman EM, et al. American College of Cardiology/American Heart Association guidelines for the management of patients with acute myocardial infarction. 1999 Update. A report of the American College of Cardiology/American Heart Association Task Force on Practice Guidelines. J Am Coll Cardiol 1999; 34:890-911

A comprehensive consensus statement regarding the indications for various invasive diagnostic and therapeutic maneuvers, when to consider temporary pacemakers, and the appropriate roles of assorted pharmacologic interventions.

Scandinavian Simvastatin Survival Study Group. Randomised trial of cholesterol lowering in 4,444 patients with coronary heart disease: The Scandinavian Simvastatin Survival Study (4S). Lancet 1994; 344:1383-1389

The first trial to demonstrate a mortality benefit from lipid-lowering therapy. Long-term therapy with simvastatin improved survival and decreased coronary events in patients with coronary artery disease and elevated cholesterol.

Schwartz GG, Olsen AG, Ezekowitz MD. Effects of atorvastatin on early recurrent ischemic events in acute coronary syndromes: The MIRACL study: a randomized controlled trial. JAMA 2000; 285:1711-1718

3,086 patients with unstable angina or non-Q-wave MI randomized to atorvastatin or placebo 1 to days after admission. At 16 weeks, the combination of death, MI, resuscitated cardiac arrest, or recurrent ischemia requiring rehospitalization was decreased significantly from 17.4% to 14.8%. This trial provides a rationale for initiation of statins in-hospital.

Yusuf S, Sleight P, Pogue J, et al. Effects of an angiotensin-converting-enzyme inhibitor, ramipril, on cardiovascular events in high-risk patients. N Engl J Med 2000; 342:145-153

9,297 high-risk patients (55 or older, with vascular disease or diabetes plus one other cardiovascular risk factor) randomized to ramipril or placebo for a mean of 5 years. Ramipril significantly reduced the rates of death, myocardial infarction, and stroke.

Yusuf S, Zhao F, Mehta SR, et al. Effects of clopidogrel in addition to aspirin in patients with acute coronary syndromes without ST-segment elevation. N Engl J Med 2001; 345:494-502

CURE trial of 12,562 patients with non-ST elevation MI randomized to clopidogrel or placebo in addition to aspirin. The composite endpoint (cardiovascular death, MI, or stroke) was reduced by 2.1% (RR 18%), at a cost of a 1% increase in major bleeding.

Notes

Notes

Heart Failure and Cardiac Pulmonary Edema

Steven M. Hollenberg, MD, FCCP

Objectives:

- To review the definition, demographics, and etiology of congestive heart failure diagnosis
- To understand the pathophysiology of the heart failure syndrome
- To review general treatment goals and medical therapy for heart failure, with an emphasis on acute heart failure in the intensive care unit
- To understand the etiology and pathophysiology of cardiogenic shock
- To review initial and definitive management of cardiogenic shock

Definition and Epidemiology

Congestive heart failure (CHF) can be defined as the inability of the heart to provide an adequate cardiac output without invoking maladaptive compensatory mechanisms. CHF affects more than 3 million patients in the US, nearly 1.5% of the adult population. 400,000 patients develop heart failure for the first time every year, cardiovascular death from CHF is estimated at 200,000/year, and CHF results in 1,000,000 hospital admissions per year in the US. CHF is now the most common reason for hospitalization in the elderly, and an estimated $8 billion is spent on heart failure annually.

Table 1 lists the causes of heart failure. The predominant causes, however, are ischemia, hypertension, alcoholic cardiomyopathy, myocarditis, and idiopathic cardiomyopathy. Coronary artery disease is increasing, both as a primary cause and as a complicating factor.

Heart failure can be broken down into several different classifications: acute vs chronic, left-sided vs right-sided, systolic vs diastolic dysfunction. Most patients in the intensive care unit have acute left-sided heart failure and present with pulmonary edema, which is not usually difficult to diagnose. It is important for the clinician, however, to distinguish between systolic and diastolic dysfunction. Although CHF results most commonly from decreased systolic performance, diastolic dysfunction, defined clinically as cardiogenic pulmonary congestion in the presence of normal systolic performance, is becoming more common as a cause of CHF as the US population ages.

Pathophysiology

Heart failure is a syndrome caused not only by the low cardiac output resulting from compromised systolic performance, but also by the effects of compensatory mechanisms. Myocardial damage from any cause can produce myocardial failure. To compensate for the reduced cardiac output of a failing heart, an elevation in ventricular filling pressure occurs in an attempt to maintain output via the Frank-Starling law. These elevated diastolic filling pressures can compromise subendocardial blood flow and cause or worsen ischemia. With continued low cardiac output, additional compensatory

Table 1. *Etiologies of Congestive Heart Failure*

Ischemic
Hypertensive
Idiopathic
Valvular
Peripartum
Familial
Toxic
    Alcoholic
    Radiation
    Drug-related (anthracyclines)
    Heavy metals (cobalt, lead, arsenic)
Metabolic/nutritional
Systemic diseases
    Hypothyroidism
    Connective tissue disease
    Diabetes
    Sarcoidosis
Infiltrative
    Amyloidosis
    Hemochromatosis
Tachycardia-induced
Autoimmune

mechanisms come into play, including sympathetic nervous system stimulation, activation of the renin-angiotensin system, and vasopressin secretion. All of these mechanisms lead to sodium and water retention and venoconstriction, increasing both preload and afterload. These increases in preload and afterload, although initially compensatory, can exacerbate the heart failure, because elevated preload increases pulmonary congestion, and elevated afterload impedes cardiac output. Activation of neurohormonal mechanisms can also engender cardiac remodeling and predispose to arrhythmias.

Diagnosis of Pulmonary Edema

The symptoms and signs of congestive heart failure relate both to low cardiac output and elevated ventricular filling pressures. Low output produces the symptoms of weakness and fatigue and an ashen appearance, sometimes with mottling. Increased left-sided filling pressures result in symptoms of pulmonary congestion such as dyspnea, cough, orthopnea, and paroxysmal nocturnal dyspnea as well as signs which may include tachycardia, pulmonary rales, a diffuse, enlarged and laterally displaced point of maximal impulse, an S_3 and S_4 gallop, a murmur of mitral regurgitation. Elevated right-sided preload can lead to symptoms such as anorexia, nausea, and abdominal pain along with signs of systemic congestion such as jugular venous distension, a right-sided S_3 gallop, a murmur of tricuspid regurgitation, hepatomegaly, ascites, and peripheral edema.

Patients in the intensive care unit often present with acute heart failure and pulmonary edema. Their presentation can be dramatic with sudden onset of shortness of breath and tachypnea with use of accessory muscles. Crackles and often wheezing can be heard throughout the lung fields, at times obscuring some of the cardiac auscultatory findings. Hypotension and evidence of peripheral vasoconstriction and hypoperfusion may be present if cardiac output is decreased. The differential diagnosis of cardiac pulmonary edema includes other causes of acute dyspnea such as pulmonary embolism, pneumothorax, and bronchial asthma and causes of noncardiac pulmonary edema such as aspiration, infection, toxins, or trauma.

Initial evaluation of the patient with pulmonary edema should include an electrocardiogram and chest radiograph. The electrocardiogram may show evidence of myocardial ischemia, infarction, or arrhythmias. The chest radiograph can demonstrate cardiomegaly along with pulmonary infiltrates. Echocardiography can be extremely useful to evaluate systolic performance and the presence of regional wall motion abnormalities suggestive of ischemia. Valvular abnormalities can be diagnosed rapidly as well. Invasive hemodynamic monitoring may be useful, not only to make the diagnosis, but also to guide pharmacologic therapy in the decompensated patient.

General Treatment Goals

The goals of congestive heart failure therapy are to control symptoms, improve exercise tolerance, prolong life, and where possible, to correct the underlying cause. In the critical care setting, control of symptoms and correction of underlying causes are emphasized. Different therapies can have different effects on these goals.

The therapeutic agents can be viewed in the light of the pathophysiologic mechanisms of CHF development. Fluid restriction, diuretics, and venodilators decrease cardiac preload. Angiotensin-converting enzyme (ACE) inhibitors, angiotensin receptor blockers (ARBs), and aldosterone antagonists counteract activation of the renin-angiotensin-aldosterone system and reduce afterload as well. Arterial dilators can also reduce afterload. Inotropic agents can improve cardiac pump function and increase output. Beta blockers can counteract sympathetic activation and are being used more commonly in chronic heart failure management, but have a less prominent role in acute CHF.

Heart Failure Therapy

Diuretics

Diuretics cause renal sodium and water loss, resulting in decreased preload and pulmonary and systemic congestion. In the intensive care unit, loop diuretics such as furosemide are usually chosen initially because of their rapid onset and are given as intravenous boluses. Most of the rapid effect of furosemide is attributable to venodilation.

If intermittent bolus doses of loop diuretics are ineffective or are poorly tolerated due to large fluid shifts and consequent hypotension, continuous infusion may be preferable. The dosage is titrated to the desired effect. Alternatively, another diuretic with a different mechanism of action, such as metolazone or chlorothiazide may be added.

Use of diuretics can lead to significant hypokalemia or hypomagnesemia, which can predispose the patient to arrhythmias. Careful addition of a potassium-sparing diuretic can be considered in some settings.

Nitrates

Nitrates are still first-line agents for the symptomatic relief of angina pectoris and when myocardial infarction is complicated by congestive heart failure. Given the high incidence of coronary artery disease in patients with congestive heart failure, use of nitrates to reduce preload is often desirable. In severely decompensated CHF, intravenous nitroglycerin is preferred because of questionable absorption of oral and transdermal preparations and for ease of titration. Intravenous nitroglycerin should be started at 5 µg/min and increased in increments of 5 µg/min every 3 to 5 min as needed for symptomatic relief. The major adverse effects of nitrates are hypotension and headache.

Angiotensin-Converting Enzyme Inhibitors

Angiotensin-converting enzyme inhibitors have been shown unequivocally to improve hemodynamics, functional capacity and symptoms, and survival in patients with chronic congestive heart failure. The CONSENSUS trial showed a mortality benefit in patients with NYHA class IV heart failure, and the SOLVD treatment trials showed a similar benefit for patients with class II and class III heart failure. Moreover, ACE inhibitors prevent the development of congestive heart failure in patients with asymptomatic left ventricular dysfunction. Several large randomized trials have recently demonstrated that ACE inhibitors decrease mortality after myocardial infarction. The benefits result in part from limitation in progressive left ventricular dysfunction and enlargement (remodeling). Recent studies have suggested that ACE inhibition can ameliorate endothelial dysfunction in atherosclerosis, and the HOPE study demonstrated improved survival with the ACE inhibitor ramipril used as secondary prevention in patients with atherosclerosis multiple cardiac risk factors.

ACE inhibitors can be given intravenously in the acute setting if necessary, or started orally once the patient is more stable. Patients should be started on low doses and titrated upward to the range demonstrated beneficial in clinical trials (captopril 50 mg three times daily, enalapril 10 to 20 mg twice daily, or lisinopril 10 to 40 mg once daily).

Angiotensin Receptor Blockers

An alternative approach to inhibiting the effects of angiotensin II is use of agents that block the angiotensin II receptor (ARBs). Since these agents do not increase bradykinin, the incidence of some side effects, such as cough and angioedema, is greatly reduced. The hemodynamic effects of ARBs have been shown in a number of trials to be similar to those of ACE inhibitors. Trials comparing ACE inhibitors to ARBs in patients with heart failure have suggested similar mortality reductions, but in comparison with ACE inhibitors, the number of heart failure patients treated with ARBs and followed for mortality is still relatively small. The most recent guidelines do not support initiation of ARBs instead of ACE inhibitors to decrease mortality in patients with heart failure. In patients who cannot tolerate ACE inhibitors, however, ARBs are a good alternative.

There is increasing recognition that angiotensin II is produced by pathways other than ACE. Thus, there has been some interest in the combination of ACE inhibitors and ARBs. This approach was tested in the recent Valsartan in Heart Failure (Val-Heft) trial, in which valsartan or placebo was added to usual therapy in patients with heart failure. Although mortality was unchanged, a combined endpoint of mortality and hospital admission for CHF was reduced with valsartan. Provocative results were obtained from analysis of subsets in this study. Patients who were on ACE inhibitors but not β-blockers, and patients on β-blockers but not ACE inhibitors, both had improved mortality with valsartan. Patients who were on both ACE inhibitors and β-blockers and had valsartan added on top of that, however, had *increased* mortality with ARBs. Further studies to elucidate these findings are underway. In the VALIANT trial, which compared valsartan, captopril, and the combination of the two in patients with acute MI and either systolic dysfunction or CHF, an adverse effect of the combination of ACE, ARB, and β-blockers was not seen. The effects of this triple combination thus remain unclear, and it should be used with caution.

Aldosterone Antagonists

Although aldosterone is predominantly known for its role in regulation of renal sodium and potassium excretion, its neurohumoral effects are gaining increasing recognition. The RALES trial randomized 1,653 patients with class III and IV heart failure to spironolactone or placebo, and found a reduction in 24-month mortality from 46% to 35% (RR 30%, p<0.001). Hyperkalemia was uncommon, and the main side effect was gynecomastia.

The recently reported EPHESUS trial randomized 6,632 patients with left ventricular dysfunction after MI to eplerenone or placebo, and found a 15% reduction in mortality (RR 0.85, CI 0.75-0.96, p<0.01). In this trial, hyperkalemia was noted in 5.5% of the eplerenone group compared to 3.9% of the placebo group (p<0.01), but interestingly, hypokalemia was reduced, from 13.1 to 8.4%.

It should be noted that the dosage of aldosterone antagonists used in these heart failure trials were well below those used for diuresis. Nonetheless, careful attention to serum potassium levels is warranted when using these agents for any indication.

Vasodilators

Nitroprusside: Nitroprusside is a balanced arterial and venous vasodilator that causes direct relaxation of smooth muscle by activating guanylate cyclase. The rapid onset and reversibility of action of nitroprusside make it an especially useful drug in the critical care setting. Nitroprusside reduces arteriolar resistance and venous tone to an equivalent extent, lowering both systemic vascular resistance and left and right ventricular filling pressures. Nitroprusside can increase stroke volume in heart failure by means of cardiac unloading. Venodilation decreases filling pressures and can decrease left ventricular wall stress in addition to relieving pulmonary congestion. Nitroprusside is used in acute cardiogenic pulmonary edema, decompensated congestive heart failure, mitral insufficiency, aortic insufficiency, and is a drug of choice for malignant hypertension. Nitroprusside may also be useful in low cardiac output syndromes in conjunction with inotropic therapy.

Nitroprusside is given by continuous intravenous infusion. In heart failure, nitroprusside is started at 10 μg/min and increased by 10 μg/min every 5 to 15 min; a decrease of 20 to 50% in wedge pressure and an increase of 20 to 40% in cardiac output is considered a positive response. Individual responses are highly variable, but most patients show a beneficial effect at 1 to 2 μg/kg/min. In pulmonary edema with hypertension, the starting dose is the same but is increased more rapidly, in increments of 20 μg/kg every 3 to 5 min. Doses required to treat hypertension are generally considerably higher than those used in heart failure.

The major complication of nitroprusside therapy is hypotension. A marked hypotensive response should always prompt consideration of whether the filling pressures are lower than expected. The other major toxicity of nitroprusside therapy results from accumulation of cyanide or thiocyanate. This usually occurs only in patients who have been receiving high doses of nitroprusside for 24 h or more, commonly in patients with renal insufficiency or failure. Cyanide inhibits oxidative phosphorylation and leads to metabolic acidosis. Treatment of cyanide toxicity involves facilitation of its metabolism to thiocyanate with thiosulfate and sodium nitrite. Thiocyanate toxicity may present with confusion, hyperreflexia, and convulsions.

Hydralazine: Hydralazine reduces afterload by directly relaxing smooth muscle. Its effects are almost exclusively confined to the arterial bed. In normal subjects, the hypotensive actions of hydralazine provoke a marked reflex tachycardia, but this response is often blunted in with heart failure. Hydralazine is effective in increasing cardiac output in heart failure, and improves mortality in chronic congestive heart failure when given in conjunction with oral nitrates.

In the critical care unit, intravenous hydralazine is often preferable to oral dosing, infused slowly over 20 min to minimize hypotension. Doses start at 5 to 10 mg and can be increased to 20 mg given every 6 to 8 h. Oral doses range from 25 to 100 mg every 6 h, but some patients may need much higher doses due to malabsorption. Tachycardia develops with hydralazine therapy in some patients. This mandates caution in administering the drug to patients with known or suspected ischemic heart disease. Prolonged administration of hydralazine is attended by the development of a lupus-like syndrome in up to 20% of patients.

Nesiritide: Nesiritide (recombinant human B-type natriuretic peptide, or BNP) is a vasodilator that also has a natriuretic effect. In patients with heart failure, intravenous nesiritide has been shown to increase cardiac output and decrease PCWP, with improvement of symptoms. Nesiritide added to standard care improved hemodynamic function and symptoms compared to nitroglycerin. Studies showing improved outcomes are not yet available. Hypotension is the most common side effect.

Digoxin: Digitalis, which has been used to treat heart failure for more than 200 years, works by inhibiting Na-K-dependent ATPase activity, causing intracellular sodium accumulation and increasing intracellular calcium via the sodium-calcium exchange system. Digoxin improves myocardial contractility and increases cardiac output, but its inotropic effects are mild in comparison to catecholamines. When used chronically for CHF in conjunction with diuretics and ACE inhibitors, digoxin has been shown to reduce symptoms and decrease hospital admissions, but it has no effect on mortality. Digoxin has a slow onset and long half-life (36 h) compared to the catecholamines. It has a narrow toxic/therapeutic ratio and individual hemodynamic responses to acute digitalis administration are highly variable. For these reasons, digoxin has a role for the control of supraventricular tachycardias but is not often useful as an inotrope in the critical care unit.

Inotropic Agents

In severe decompensated heart failure, inotropic support may be initiated. Dobutamine is a selective β_1-adrenergic receptor agonist that can improve myocardial contractility and increase cardiac output. Dobutamine is the initial inotropic agent of choice in patients with decompensated acute heart failure and adequate systolic blood pressure. Dobutamine has a rapid onset of action and a plasma half-life is 2 to 3 min; infusion is usually initiated at 5 μg/kg/min and then titrated. Tolerance to the effect of dobutamine may develop after 48 to 72 h, possibly due to down-regulation of adrenergic receptors. Dobutamine has the potential to exacerbate hypotension in some patients, and can precipitate tachyarrhythmias.

Milrinone is a phosphodiesterase inhibitor milrinone with both positive inotropic and vasodilatory actions. Because milrinone does not stimulate adrenergic receptors directly, it may be effective when added to catecholamines or when β-adrenergic receptors have been downregulated. Compared to catecholamines, phosphodiesterase inhibitors have fewer chronotropic and arrhythmogenic effects.

Although clearly useful to improve hemodynamics in the acute setting, controversy has arisen regarding use of inotropic agents (other than digoxin) as outpatient maintenance therapy for chronic heart failure. Concerns have included exacerbation of arrhythmic complications, either by induction of myocardial ischemia or by independent pathways, and perpetuation of neurohumoral activation which might accelerate the progression of myocardial damage. Milrinone was recently examined in a prospective manner in the OPTIME-CHF trial in order to determine whether its use could reduce hospitalization time following an acute heart failure exacerbation. Although these observations did not demonstrate any advantage for patients treated with milrinone, patients whom the investigators felt "needed" acute inotropic support were not included in the trial, thereby biasing the enrollment toward a less severely afflicted cohort. Therefore, the utilization of such agents today remains at the discretion of the clinician. The proof that these agents have beneficial effects on hard clinical endpoints remains elusive, but their hemodynamic effects are attractive for treating decompensated patients.

Inotropic infusions need to be titrated carefully in patients with ischemic heart disease to maximize coronary perfusion pressure with the least possible increase in myocardial oxygen demand. Invasive hemodynamic monitoring can be extremely useful to allow for optimization of therapy in these unstable patients, because clinical estimates of filling pressure can be unreliable, and because changes in myocardial performance and compliance and therapeutic interventions can change cardiac output and filling pressures precipitously. Optimization of filling pressures and serial measurements of cardiac output (and other parameters, such as mixed venous oxygen saturation) allow for titration of inotropes and vasopressors to the minimum dosage required to achieve the chosen therapeutic goals, thus minimizing the increases in myocardial oxygen demand and arrhythmogenic potential.

β-Blockers

Although perhaps counterintuitive on hemodynamic grounds, there is now compelling evidence that β-blockers are beneficial not only for patients with acute myocardial infarction complicated by heart failure but also with chronic heart failure from all causes. Three different agents have been shown to decrease mortality: metoprolol XL in the MERIT trial, bisoprolol in the CIBIS-2 trial, and carvedilol in several randomized trials. Recent studies with carvedilol suggest that the benefits extend to patients with class IV heart failure. These agents can, however, be problematic during the acute phase of heart failure, as they can depress contractility. When given for heart failure indications per se, β-blockers should be introduced when the patient is in a well compensated and euvolemic state, typically in the ambulatory setting and at minimal doses.

Patients who experience an exacerbation of heart failure while on maintenance β-blocker therapy, particularly at a higher dose, present a previously rare dilemma that is becoming more common. No controlled observations are available to guide therapy, so current practice remains largely at the discretion of individual clinicians. Discontinuing β-blockers, or decreasing their dose, should expose myocardial β-receptors to endogenous catecholamines, and may result in a brief increase in contractility. On the other hand, slow titration of beta blockers will need to begin anew after resolution of acute CHF. Our practice is to attempt to resolve acute episodes of heart failure by diuresis and adjustment of other medications while holding β-blocker doses constant. If heart failure persists, the dose is halved, and if it still does not resolve, β-blockers are discontinued. We attempt to apply the same standards to modification of β-blocker dosage as we do to institution of catecholamine therapy in the management of decompensated heart failure. An innovative alternative which may lessen the risk of acute increase in catecholamine exposure while allowing temporary increase in inotropic state would be to maintain the β-blocker regimen at or near baseline while administering a non-catecholamine inotropic agent such as milrinone. This approach may reduce the risk of deleterious side effects in patients deemed to require inotropic therapy, although there is little supporting data in this regard as yet.

Cardiogenic Shock

Cardiogenic shock can be defined as a state of inadequate tissue and cellular perfusion resulting from cardiac dysfunction. Defined clinically, this includes decreased cardiac output and evidence of tissue hypoxia in the presence of adequate intravascular volume. Hemodynamic criteria include sustained hypotension (systolic blood pressure less than 90 mm Hg or 30 mm Hg below basal levels for at least 30 min) and a reduced cardiac index (less than 2.2 L/min/m^2) in the presence of elevated pulmonary capillary wedge pressure (greater than 15 mm Hg).

Etiology

The most common cause of cardiogenic shock is an extensive acute myocardial infarction, although a smaller infarction in a patient with previously compromised left ventricular function may also precipitate shock. Shock presenting with a delayed onset may result from infarct extension, reocclusion of a previously patent infarct artery, or decompensation of function in the non-infarct zone due to metabolic abnormalities. Cardiogenic shock can also be caused by mechanical complications such as acute mitral regurgitation, rupture of the interventricular septum, or free wall rupture, or by large right ventricular infarctions. Other causes of cardiogenic shock include myocarditis, end-stage cardiomyopathy, valvular heart disease, and myocardial dysfunction after prolonged cardiopulmonary bypass.

Pathophysiology

Cardiac dysfunction in cardiogenic shock is usually initiated by myocardial infarction or ischemia. The myocardial dysfunction resulting from ischemia worsens that ischemia, setting up a vicious cycle. Systolic myocardial dysfunction decreases stroke volume and cardiac output, leading to hypotension which decreases coronary perfusion pressure, which can exacerbate ischemia. The increased ventricular diastolic pressures that result from heart failure reduce the pressure gradient for coronary blood flow, and the additional wall stress elevates myocardial oxygen requirements, also worsening ischemia. Tachycardia reduces the time available for diastolic filling, further compromising coronary blood flow. Decreased cardiac output compromises systemic perfusion, which can lead to lactic acidosis. Compensatory vasoconstriction in response to decreased perfusion can increase afterload, producing further strain on an already compromised left ventricle.

Cardiogenic shock also leads to diastolic myocardial dysfunction. Infarction and ischemia decrease diastolic compliance, increasing left ventricular diastolic pressures and leading to pulmonary edema. Pulmonary congestion can cause hypoxemia, which can also contribute to ischemia.

Diagnosis

After recognizing the presence of cardiogenic shock, the clinician must perform the clinical assessment required to understand its cause while initiating supportive therapy before shock causes irreversible damage to vital organs. The challenge is that since speed is important to achieve a good outcome, evaluation and therapy must begin simultaneously. While the evaluation must be thorough, neither overzealous pursuit of a diagnosis before stabilization has been achieved nor overzealous empiric treatment without establishing the underlying pathophysiology is desirable. A practical approach is to make a rapid evaluation initially, based on a limited history, physical examination, and specific diagnostic procedures. The diagnosis of circulatory shock at the bedside is made by the presence of hypotension along with a combination of clinical signs indicative of poor tissue perfusion, including oliguria, a clouded sensorium, and cool, mottled extremities indicative of reduced blood flow to the skin. Cardiogenic shock is diagnosed after documentation of myocardial dysfunction and exclusion of nonmyocardial factors such as hypovolemia, hypoxia, and acidosis. Patients with cardiogenic shock usually have symptoms and signs of heart disease, including elevated filling pressures, gallop rhythms, and other evidence of heart failure. A murmur of mitral regurgitation, aortic stenosis, or ventricular septal defect may be heard. An electrocardiogram should be performed immediately; other initial diagnostic tests ordinarily include a chest radiograph, arterial blood gas, electrolytes, complete blood count, and cardiac enzymes.

Echocardiography is an excellent initial tool for confirming the diagnosis of cardiogenic shock and for sorting through the differential diagnosis, and should be performed early as a routine. Echocardiography provides information on overall and regional systolic function, and can rapidly diagnose mechanical causes of shock such as papillary muscle rupture and acute mitral regurgitation, acute ventricular septal defect, and free wall rupture and tamponade. In some cases, echocardiography may reveal findings compatible with right ventricular infarction.

Invasive hemodynamic monitoring is critical for confirming the diagnosis and for guiding pharmacologic therapy. The hemodynamic profile of cardiogenic shock includes a pulmonary capillary wedge pressure greater than 15 mm Hg and a cardiac index less than 2.2 L/min/m^2. It should be recognized that optimal filling pressures may be higher than this in individual patients due to left ventricular diastolic dysfunction. Right heart catheterization may reveal an oxygen step-up diagnostic of ventricular septal rupture or a large "v" wave suggestive of severe mitral regurgitation. The hemodynamic profile of right ventricular infarction includes high right-sided filling pressures in the presence of normal of low wedge pressures.

Initial Management

General Considerations: Maintenance of adequate oxygenation and ventilation are critical. Many patients require intubation and mechanical ventilation early in their course, if only to reduce the work of breathing and facilitate sedation and stabilization before cardiac catheterization. Some recent studies have suggested that use of continuous positive airway pressure in patients with cardiogenic pulmonary edema can decrease the need for intubation, but the studies are small and need to be evaluated with some caution; failure of noninvasive ventilation occurred at least half of the time.

Electrolyte abnormalities should be corrected, and morphine (or fentanyl if systolic pressure is compromised) used to relieve pain and anxiety, thus reducing excessive sympathetic activity and decreasing oxygen demand, preload, and afterload. Arrhythmias and heart block may have major effects on cardiac output, and should be corrected promptly with antiarrhythmic drugs, cardioversion, or pacing.

Following initial stabilization and restoration of adequate blood pressure, tissue perfusion should be assessed. If tissue perfusion remains inadequate, inotropic support or intra-aortic balloon pumping should be initiated. If tissue perfusion is adequate but significant pulmonary congestion remains, diuretics may be employed. Vasodilators can be considered as well, depending on the blood pressure.

Fluids: The initial approach to the hypotensive patient should include fluid resuscitation unless frank pulmonary edema is present. Patients are commonly diaphoretic and relative hypovolemia may be present in as many as 20% of patients with cardiogenic shock. Fluid infusion is best initiated with predetermined boluses titrated to clinical endpoints of heart rate, urine output and blood pressure. Ischemia produces diastolic as well as systolic dysfunction, and thus elevated filling pressures may be necessary to maintain stroke volume in patients with cardiogenic shock. Patients who do not respond rapidly to initial fluid boluses or those with poor physiologic reserve should be considered for invasive hemodynamic monitoring.

Optimal filling pressures vary from patient to patient; hemodynamic monitoring can be used to construct a Starling curve at the bedside, identifying the filling pressure at which cardiac output is maximized. Maintenance of adequate preload is particularly important in patients with right ventricular infarction.

Vasopressor Agents: When arterial pressure remains inadequate, therapy with vasopressor agents may be required to maintain coronary perfusion pressure. Maintenance of adequate blood pressure is essential to break the vicious cycle of progressive hypotension with further myocardial ischemia. Dopamine increases both blood pressure and cardiac output, and is usually the initial choice in patients in the presence of systolic pressures less than 80 mm Hg. When hypotension remains refractory, norepinephrine may be necessary to maintain organ perfusion pressure. Phenylephrine, a selective α-1 adrenergic agonist, may be a good choice when tachyarrhythmias limit therapy with other vasopressors. Vasopressor infusions need to be titrated carefully in patients with cardiogenic shock to maximize coronary perfusion pressure with the least possible increase in myocardial oxygen demand. It is also mandatory to ensure that filling pressures are optimal. Hemodynamic monitoring is useful in this regard.

Inotropic Agents: In patients with inadequate tissue perfusion and adequate intravascular volume, cardiovascular support with inotropic agents should be initiated. Dobutamine, a selective β_1-adrenergic receptor agonist, can improve myocardial contractility and increase cardiac output, and is the initial agent of choice in patients with systolic pressures greater than 80 mm Hg. Dobutamine may exacerbate hypotension in some patients, and can precipitate tachyarrhythmias. Use of dopamine may be preferable if systolic pressure is less than 80 mm Hg, although tachycardia and increased peripheral resistance may worsen myocardial ischemia In some situations, a combination of dopamine and dobutamine can be more effective than either agent alone.

Milrinone is a phosphodiesterase inhibitor that increases intracellular cyclic AMP by mechanisms not involving adrenergic receptors, producing both positive inotropic and vasodilatory actions. This effect may be important in patients with chronic heart failure, in whom chronic elevation of circulating catecholamine levels can produce downregulation of β-adrenergic receptors.

Milrinone has minimal chronotropic and arrhythmogenic effects compared to catecholamines. In addition, because milrinone does not stimulate adrenergic receptors directly, its effects may be additive to those of the catecholamines. Milrinone, however, has the potential to cause hypotension and has a long half-life; in patients with tenuous clinical status, its use is often reserved for situations in which other agents have proven ineffective. Standard administration of milrinone calls for a loading dose of 50 µg/kg followed by an infusion of 0.5 µg/kg/min, but many clinicians eschew the loading dose (or halve it) in patients with marginal blood pressure.

Patients With Adequate Tissue Perfusion and Pulmonary Congestion

In patients whose primary abnormality after initial resuscitation from cardiogenic shock is pulmonary congestion but who appear to have adequate tissue perfusion, diuretics may be employed. Bolus doses of loop diuretics are usually employed, but continuous infusion may be more effective in patients with tenuous hemodynamics. Vasodilators should be used with extreme caution in the acute setting due to the risk of precipitating further hypotension and decreasing coronary blood flow.

After blood pressure has been stabilized, however, vasodilator therapy can decrease both preload and afterload. Sodium nitroprusside is a balanced arterial and venous vasodilator that decreases filling pressures and can increase stroke volume in patients with heart failure by reducing afterload. Nitroglycerin is an effective venodilator that reduces the pulmonary capillary occlusion pressure and can decrease ischemia by reducing left ventricular filling pressure and redistributing coronary blood flow to the ischemic zone. Both agents may cause acute and rapid decreases in blood pressure and dosages must be titrated carefully; invasive hemodynamic monitoring can be useful in optimizing filling pressures when these agents are used.

Reperfusion Therapy

Although thrombolytic therapy reduces the likelihood of subsequent development of shock after initial presentation, its role in the management of patients who have already developed shock is less certain. The number of patients in randomized trials is small since most fibrinolytic trials have excluded patients with cardiogenic shock at presentation, but the available trials (have not demonstrated that fibrinolytic therapy reduces mortality in patients with established cardiogenic shock. On the other hand, in the SHOCK Registry, patients treated with fibrinolytic therapy had a lower in-hospital mortality rate than those who were not (54% vs. 64%, p = 0.005), even after adjustment for age and revascularization status (OR 0.70, p = 0.027).

Fibrinolytic therapy is clearly less effective in patients with cardiogenic shock than in those without. The explanation for this lack of efficacy appears to be the low reperfusion rate achieved in this subset of patients. The reasons for decreased thrombolytic efficacy in patients with cardiogenic probably include hemodynamic, mechanical, and metabolic factors that prevent achievement and maintenance of infarct-related artery patency.

Intra-aortic balloon counterpulsation (IABP) reduces systolic afterload and augments diastolic perfusion pressure, increasing cardiac output and improving coronary blood flow. These beneficial effects, in contrast to those of inotropic or vasopressor agents, occur without an increase in oxygen demand. IABP is efficacious for initial stabilization of patients with cardiogenic shock. Small randomized trials in the prethrombolytic era, however, failed to show that IABP alone increases survival, perhaps because IABP alone does not produce a significant improvement in blood flow distal to a critical coronary stenosis. Attempts to increase reperfusion rates by increasing blood pressure with aggressive inotropic and pressor therapy and intra-aortic balloon counterpulsation make theoretic sense, and two small studies support the notion that vasopressor therapy to increase aortic pressure improves thrombolytic efficacy. In hospitals without direct angioplasty capability, stabilization with IABP and thrombolysis followed by transfer to a tertiary care facility may be the best management option. Retrospective studies have shown that patients with cardiogenic shock in the community hospital treated with IABP placement followed by thrombolysis had improved in-hospital survival and improved outcomes after subsequent transfer for revascularization, although selection bias is clearly a confounder.

Pathophysiologic considerations favor aggressive mechanical revascularization for patients with cardiogenic shock due to myocardial infarction. Patients with cardiogenic shock are candidates for direct angioplasty, which can achieve brisk flow in the infarct artery in most patients. An extensive body of observation and registry studies showed consistent benefits from revascularization with angioplasty, but could not be regarded as definitive due to their retrospective design. Two randomized controlled trials have now evaluated revascularization for patients with myocardial infarction.

The recently reported SHOCK trial is a landmark study with randomized, controlled, prospective data addressing revascularization in patients with cardiogenic shock. The SHOCK trial randomly assigned patients with cardiogenic shock to receive optimal medical management – including IABP and thrombolytic therapy– or to cardiac catheterization with revascularization using PTCA or CABG. The trial enrolled 302 patients and was powered to detect a 20% absolute decrease in 30-day all-cause mortality rates. Mortality at 30 days was 46.7% in patients treated with early intervention and 56% in patients treated with initial medical stabilization, but this difference did not reach statistical significance ($p = 0.11$). At 6 months, the absolute risk reduction was 13% (50.3% compared with 63.1%, $p = 0.027$). Subgroup analysis showed a substantial improvement in mortality rates in patients younger than 75 years of age at both 30 days (41.4% versus 56.8%, $p = 0.01$) and 6 months (44.9% vs 65.0%, $p = 0.003$).

It is important to note that the control group (patients who received medical management) had a lower mortality rate than that reported in previous studies; this may reflect the aggressive use of thrombolytic therapy (64%) and balloon pumping (86%) in these controls. These data provide indirect evidence that the combination of thrombolysis and IABP may produce the best outcomes when cardiac catheterization is not immediately available. The trial was underpowered to detect the primary end point, but the improved survival with revascularization at 6 months and in patients younger than 75 years of age strongly supports the superiority of a strategy of early revascularization in most patients with cardiogenic shock.

The SMASH trial was independently conceived and had a very similar design, although a more rigid definition of cardiogenic shock resulted in enrollment of sicker patients and a higher mortality. The trial was terminated early due to difficulties in patient recruitment, and enrolled only 55 patients. In the SMASH trial, a similar trend in 30-day absolute mortality reduction similar to that in the SHOCK trial of 9% was observed (69% mortality in the invasive group vs. 78% in the medically managed group, RR = 0.88, 95% CI = 0.6 – 1.2, $p = NS$). This benefit was also maintained at one year.

When the results of both the SHOCK and SMASH trials are put into perspective with results from other randomized, controlled trials of patients with acute myocardial infarction, an important point emerges: despite the moderate *relative* risk reduction (for the SHOCK trial 0.72, CI 0.54-0.95, for the SMASH trial, 0.88, CI, 0.60-1.20) the *absolute* benefit is important, with 9 lives saved for 100 patients treated at 30 days in both trials, and 13.2 lives saved for 100 patients treated at one year in the SHOCK trial. This latter figure corresponds to a number needed to treat (NNT) of 7.6, one of the lowest figures ever observed in a randomized, controlled trial of cardiovascular disease.

Current practice of primary PCI for acute MI usually involves stenting with adjunctive glycoprotein IIb/IIIa inhibition. Although this has been less well studied in cardiogenic shock, a recent study of direct PTCA in patients with shock reported a success rate of 94%, with placement of stents in 47%; in-hospital mortality was 26%. Reports of consecutive case series have supported the use of GP IIb/IIIa inhibitors as well.

Annotated References

Anderson RD, Ohman EM, Holmes DR, Jr., et al. Use of intraaortic balloon counterpulsation in patients presenting with cardiogenic shock: observations from the GUSTO-I Study. Global Utilization of Streptokinase and TPA for Occluded Coronary Arteries. J Am Coll Cardiol 1997; 30:708-715

72% of the patients in the GUSTO trial had cardiogenic shock; IABP appears to be underutilized in these patients in this analysis.

Antoniucci D, Valenti R, Santoro GM, et al. Systematic direct angioplasty and stent-supported direct angioplasty therapy for cardiogenic shock complicating acute myocardial infarction: In-hospital and long-term survival. J Am Coll Cardiol 1998; 31:294-300
Observational study of direct PTCA for cardiogenic shock. 47% of patients received stents, and open arteries with normal (TIMI grade 3 flow) were achieved in 85% of all patients. In-hospital mortality was 26%, and 6-month mortality was 29%.

Barron HV, Every NR, Parsons, LS. Use of intra-aortic balloon counterpulsation in patients with cardiogenic shock complicating acute myocardial infarction: Data from the National Registry of Myocardial Infarction 2. Am Heart J 2001; 141:933-939
Registry data suggesting improved outcomes with IABP use in patients with cardiogenic shock.

Berger PB, Holmes DR, Jr., Stebbins AL, et al. Impact of an aggressive invasive catheterization and revascularization strategy on mortality in patients with cardiogenic shock in the Global Utilization of Streptokinase and Tissue Plasminogen Activator for Occluded Coronary Arteries (GUSTO-I) trial. An observational study. Circulation 1997; 96:122-127
In the GUSTO trial, a strategy of early angiography and revascularization was associated with decreased mortality in cardiogenic shock.

Cohn JN, Tognoni G. A randomized trial of the angiotensin-receptor blocker valsartan in chronic heart failure. N Engl J Med 2001; 345:1667-1675
Val-Heft trial in which valsartan or placebo was added to usual therapy in patients with heart failure. Mortality was unchanged, but a combined endpoint of mortality and hospital admission for CHF was reduced with valsartan. In the very small group of patients not on ACE inhibitors, valsartan did reduce mortality compared to placebo.

Digitalis Investigation Group. The effect of digoxin on mortality and morbidity in patients with heart failure. N Engl J Med 1997; 336:525-533
A large multicenter randomized, controlled trial of digoxin or placebo added to diuretics and ACE inhibitors in patients with congestive heart failure. Digoxin reduced hospital admissions for CHF, but had no effect on mortality.

Goldberg RJ, Yarbebske J, Lessard, D, Gore JM. A two-decades (1975 to 1995) long experience in the incidence, in- hospital and long-term case-fatality rates of acute myocardial infarction: A community-wide perspective. J Am Coll Cardiol 1999; 33:1533-1539
Results of the Worcester Heart Attack Study showing a consistent incidence of cardiogenic shock; (7.5%), with consistent mortality up to the last 4 years studied, when a decrease was noted.

Hochman JS, Buller CE, Sleeper LA, et al. Cardiogenic shock complicating acute myocardial infarction—Etiologies, management and outcome: a report from the SHOCK Trial Registry. SHould we emergently revascularize Occluded Coronaries for cardiogenic shock? J Am Coll Cardiol 2000; 36:1063-1070
Final results of a registry for the SHOCK trial randomizing patients with cardiogenic shock to immediate catheterization and revascularization or thrombolysis and delayed catheterization

Hochman JS, Sleeper LA, Webb JG et al. Early revascularization in acute myocardial infarction complicated by cardiogenic shock. N Engl J Med 1999; 341:625-634
Landmark study randomizing 302 patients with cardiogenic shock on the basis of left ventricular failure to emergency revascularization or initial medical stabilization. Overall mortality at 30 days was 9.3% lower in the revascularization group (46.7% vs 56.0%), but this did not reach statistical significance. (p=0.11) The difference was significant, however, at 6 months, and in patients less than 75.

Hollenberg SM, Kavinsky CJ, Parrillo, JE. Cardiogenic shock. Ann Intern Med 1999; 131:47-59
A brief review of cardiogenic shock.

Hollenberg SM, Bates ER. Cardiogenic shock. Armonk, NY: Futura Publishing Company, 2002
Everything you always wanted to know.

Kovack PJ, Rasak MA, Bates ER, et al. Thrombolysis plus aortic counterpulsation: improved survival in patients who present to community hospitals with cardiogenic shock. J Am Coll Cardiol 1997; 29:1454-1458
Retrospective analysis; mortality with thrombolytics plus IABP was 33%, significantly better than thrombolytics alone (68%).

Martin SJ, Danziger LH. Continuous infusion of loop diuretic in the critically ill: A review of the literature. Crit Care Med 1994; 22:1323-1329
Review of continuous furosemide infusion in the critical care setting.

Metoprolol CR/XL Randomised Intervention Trial in Congestive Heart Failure Investigators. Effect of metoprolol CR/XL in chronic heart failure: Metoprolol CR/XL Randomised Intervention Trial in Congestive Heart Failure (MERIT-HF). Lancet 1999; 353:2001-2007
3991 patients with class II-IV CHF and EF<40% randomized to metoprolol or placebo. Mortality was decreased with metoprolol from 11% to 7.2%, a 34% reduction. Secondary outcomes were improved as well

Packer M, Coats AJ, Fowler MB. Effect of carvedilol on survival in severe chronic heart failure. N Engl J Med 1999; 344:1651-1658

2,289 patients with EF < 25% and class III or IV heart failure randomized to carvedilol or placebo. Mortality was reduced by 35%, and death or hospitalization decreased by 24%. This trial shows that even patients with severe heart failure may benefit from ß-blockade.

Pitt B, RemmieW, Zannad F. Eplerenone, a selective aldosterone blocker, in patients with left ventricular dysfunction after myocardial infarction. N Engl J Med 2003; 348:1309-1321

6,632 patients with LV dysfunction and heart failure randomized to the aldosterone antagonist eplerenone or placebo in addition to other therapy after acute MI. Mortality was reduced by 15% over 16 months. The incidence of hyperkalemia was higher with eplerenone, but the incidence of hypokalemia was lower

Stevenson LW, Dracup KA, Tillisch JH. Efficacy of medical therapy tailored for severe congestive heart failure in patients transferred for urgent cardiac transplantation. Am J Cardiol 1989; 63:461-464

Hemodynamic-guided therapy in patients referred for transplantation led to clinical improvement in a substantial fraction, obviating the need for transplantation.

VMAC Investigators. Intravenous nesiritide vs nitroglycerin for treatment of decompensated congestive heart failure: a randomized controlled trial. JAMA 2002; 287:1531-1540

When added to standard care in patients hospitalized with acutely decompensated CHF, nesiritide improves hemodynamic function and some self-reported symptoms more effectively than intravenous nitroglycerin or placebo.

Notes

Notes

Thromboembolic Disease

R. Phillip Dellinger, MD, FCCP

Objectives:

- To recognize the risk factors for pulmonary embolism (PE).
- To appreciate the typical clinical presentations of pulmonary embolism.
- To choose rationally among perfusion lung scanning, leg ultrasound, CT scanning, and D-dimers in the diagnostic approach to pulmonary embolism.
- To understand the place of anticoagulation, inferior vena cava filter placement, and thrombolytic therapy in the management of pulmonary embolism.

Key words: anticoagulation; compression ultrasound; deep-vein thrombosis; pulmonary embolism; thromboembolism; thrombolytic therapy; ventilation/perfusion lung scanning

Risk Factors

Major risk factors for pulmonary emboli are processes that predispose a patient to the development of deep-vein thrombosis (DVT) (*ie*, any cause of venous stasis, such as venous valvular insufficiency, right-sided heart failure, the postoperative period, and prolonged bed rest, or immobilization). Abdominal operations requiring general anesthesia of >30 min place the patient at risk for venous thromboembolism (VTE). Orthopedic surgery of the lower extremity has long been recognized as one of the greatest risk factors for VTE. More than 50% of patients who do not received prophylactic therapy undergoing elective total hip replacement and knee replacement surgery develop DVT. Over 90% of proximal thrombi occur in hip replacement patients on the operated side. Since the first controlled trials demonstrating a reduced rate of pulmonary embolism (PE) mortalities with anticoagulant prophylaxis were carried out in this high-risk group, patients with fractures of the pelvis, hip, or femur are of significant historical relevance.

Trauma to the extremities, advanced malignancy (increasingly recognized as a major risk factor), pregnancy, the postpartum state and, to a lesser degree, birth control pills (current formulations have lower estrogen content) are significant risk factors. Long-distance air travel has also been linked to PE. There is an estimated 40% risk of VTE and a 5% incidence of PE in patients with traumatic spinal cord injury and associated paralysis of lower extremities. The period of greatest risk is during the first 2 weeks post-initial injury; death occurs rarely in PE patients after 3 months.

The frequency of VTE increases exponentially between the ages of 20 and 80 years. Although an age of >40 years has often been used as a break point for age-related increase in VTE, increasing age increases risk beginning with adulthood and continues to increase after the age of 40 years, nearly doubling with each decade. One study demonstrated a 23% incidence of PE in 175,730 tertiary-care hospital admissions with linear relation to age. The incidence in women was higher in individuals ≥50 years old, but not in those <50 years old (Stein et al, 1999). In patients with a history of thromboembolic disease who undergo hospitalization, there is nearly an eight-fold increase in acute thromboembolism compared with patients without such a history, therefore making acute thromboembolism one of the more important risk factors for VTE.

Patients with a history of VTE who undergo major surgery, periods of immobility, or who are hospitalized for serious medical illnesses must be aggressively targeted for prophylaxis therapy. Although precise estimates of risk increase in malignancy are difficult to ascertain, advanced cancer is associated with a high risk of VTE. With other risk factors considered equal, surgery for malignant disease results in a two- to three-fold increase in thromboembolism compared with surgery for nonmalignant conditions. Hypercoagulable states secondary to deficiencies of antithrombin III, protein C, or protein S, as well as the presence of anticardiolipin antibody, lupus anticoagulant, prothrombin G20210A mutation or factor V Leiden mutation are predisposing factors for thromboembolic disease. Screening for select hypercoagulable states is appropriate in patients with no obvious risk factors who develop PE. This screening is most appropriate for the three coagulopathies that can be easily and accurately measured accurately in the presence of acute clot burden/anticoagulation and have therapeutic implications: and factor V Leiden (most common hypercoagulable state and would warrant more aggressive prophylaxis), anticardiolipin antibody or lupus anticoagulant (dictates more aggressive warfarin therapy), and hyperhomocysteinemia (may benefit from treatment with B vitamins). Although most pulmonary emboli come from deep veins of the lower extremities, clinically significant emboli also occur from other sites of venous thrombosis including the iliac veins, pelvic veins, and less frequently, the inferior vena cava. Central venous catheters are risk factors for superior vena cava/axillary/subclavian vein thrombosis, as well as femoral vein thrombosis.

Clinical Findings

The clinical diagnosis of PE is difficult. Clinical acumen falters due to both sensitivity and specificity problems. The most common symptoms/signs of dyspnea, tachypnea, and tachycardia are seen with a myriad of other disorders. Tachypnea and tachycardia may be transient. The physical examination is not typically helpful in considering PE, with the exception of the presence of findings to support acute increases of right-sided pressure such as a right-sided S_3, widely split-second heart sound, murmur of tricuspid regurgitation, or an accentuated pulmonary closure sound. Examination of the lower extremity is unreliable for predicting the presence or absence of DVT. Nevertheless, new findings supportive of acute deep-vein obstruction, particularly unilateral leg swelling in the setting of pulmonary symptoms compatible with thromboembolism, should strengthen the possibility of PE.

Pulmonary infarction is the classic presentation of PE and is characterized by a pulmonary infiltrate that is often peripheral and wedge-shaped, pleuritic chest pain, hemoptysis, and, not infrequently, a bloody pleural effusion. These findings represent the "textbook" version of PE that is taught to medical students and seen in only 10% of pulmonary emboli. Pulmonary infarction is rare due to three sources of oxygen and two sources of nutrient supply to the lung; the bronchial and pulmonary arteries and the airways. In addition, back-perfusion from the pulmonary venous system may also be a potential source of oxygen and nutrient supply. Pulmonary infarction is more likely to occur in the face of pre-existing compromise of nutrient or oxygen supply, such as in intrinsic lung disease or in the presence of reduced cardiac output.

A more frequent presentation of PE is acute onset of shortness of breath or hypoxemia in the absence of pulmonary infarction, with or without chest pain (often pleuritic when present). Radiographic infiltrates may or may not be present. This is the most common presentation of PE.

Less frequent, but more lethal, is acute massive PE characterized by a large thromboembolus lodging in the proximal pulmonary circulation resulting in hypotension and possible syncope. Chest pain may be present and is probably due to right ventricular or left ventricular myocardial ischemia. Infiltrates are usually absent in massive PE unless the embolus has fragmented and moved peripherally. Acute pulmonary hypertension with central dilated pulmonary arteries may also be present. Hypoxemia is almost always present, although hypotension is usually the primary clinical concern.

Fever (temperature $\geq$ 100.0°F) has been demonstrated to be present in 14% of angiographically documented PE with no other cause of fever. Only 2 of 228 patients had temperatures $\geq$103.0°F. Leukocytosis may or may not be present.

Tachycardia and nonspecific ST-T changes are the most common electrocardiographic findings in PE. In massive PE, right-heart strain may be indicated by P-wave pulmonale, $S_1Q_3T_3$ pattern, right axis deviation, or right bundle branch block.

Chest radiographic abnormalities due to PE include pulmonary infiltrate, pleural effusion, elevated hemidiaphragm, and atelectasis. A pleural-based, wedge-shaped infiltrate called a Hampton's hump may be seen in some cases of pulmonary infarction. An unremarkable chest radiograph with significant hypoxemia and no obvious cause, such as asthma or exacerbation of COPD, should also raise the concern for PE. Patients who develop PE in the ICU typically have abnormal chest radiographs due to preexisting pulmonary disease. One study found cardiomegaly to be the most common chest radiograph abnormality.

Analysis of pleural fluid in a patient suspected of having PE is useful only to confirm other diagnoses. There are no pathognomonic pleural effusion findings with PE; the effusion may be a transudate or exudate; it may or may not be bloody. A bloody pleural effusion that accompanies PE usually implies pulmonary infarction. Other potential etiologies of bloody pleural effusions include malignancy and trauma.

Echocardiography is most helpful in delineating other etiologies of clinical findings, such as myocardial ischemia or pericardial tamponade. However, findings such as acute right ventricular (RV) dilation and hypokinesis, tricuspid regurgitation, pulmonary hypertension estimated from tricuspid regurgitation jet, pulmonary artery dilation, loss of respiratory variation in inferior vena cava diameter, interventricular septum bulge into the left ventricle (LV), and reduced diastolic-shaped LV size may support the diagnosis of PE, but are not specific enough to establish the diagnosis. A distinct radiograph pattern has recently been noted in patients with large PE in which regional RV dysfunction is noted but the apex is spared. Clinically significant PE may also occur in the absence of any abnormal RV findings on echocardiography. Rarely, a clot may be visualized in the right heart and thus allows a specific diagnosis.

Recent (non-latex agglutination) assays are clinically useful in the evaluation for possible PE since a non-elevated D-dimer makes PE unlikely. A D-dimer measured by enzyme-linked immunosorbent assay (ELISA) was noted to be normal in <10% of angiographically documented PE in one study (Quinn et al). An elevated D-dimer however may be seen in many circumstances other than PE (recent surgery, malignancy, total bilirubin >2 mg/dL, sepsis, late pregnancy, trauma, advanced age). The traditional ELISA assay typically requires 24 hours for results. Newer, second-generation tests, including rapid ELISA, turbidimetric assay, and immunofiltration may offer reliable and rapid bedside testing. The D-dimer assay may be particularly important in the emergency department, in low pretest clinical suspicion scenarios and in combination with other studies in the inpatient population.

A fall in end-tidal CO_2 may also be useful in raising the clinical suspicion of PE, while a decrease in $Paco_2$ may be a marker of success of thrombolytic therapy in patients with PE.

Respiratory alkalosis is a common finding in the tachypneic patient with PE. With massive pulmonary embolus, respiratory acidosis may be present due to increased dead space. Although a room air Pao_2 of >80 mm Hg (>10.7 kPa) or a normal alveolar-arterial gradient makes the diagnosis of PE less likely, neither can be relied on to exclude PE. Patients with PE may have a normal alveolar-arterial (A-a) gradient. This finding is more likely to occur in the presence of previous normal cardiopulmonary status. Hypoxemia and an increase in alveolar-arterial gradient may also be transient. Forty-two patients in the Prospective Investigation of Pulmonary Embolism Diagnosis (PIOPED) trial had suspected PE, no prior cardiopulmonary disease, and fulfilled all of the following criteria: Pao_2 >80 mm Hg (>10.7 kPa), $Paco_2$ >35 mm Hg (>4.7 kPa), and normal alveolar-arterial gradient. Sixteen (38%) patients had angiographically documented PE. In patients who had prior cardiopulmonary disease and who met all three criteria mentioned above, 14% had PE. Therefore, normal arterial blood gases, in general, and in patients with no prior history of cardiopulmonary disease, in particular, do not allow discontinuation of the pursuit of PE.

Nonmassive PE produces hypoxemia by release of bronchoconstrictors, production of atelectasis (surfactant depletion over hours), and perhaps reperfusion injury to the endothelial-epithelial barrier. Massive PE is almost always associated with hypoxemia and frequently with CO_2 retention. In addition to the same causes of hypoxemia as related above for nonmassive PE, the amputation of pulmonary vascular bed in massive PE produces both a large increase in dead space (as a cause of increased $Paco_2$) and a large amount of blood flow diverted to noninvolved areas of the lung, causing a low ventilation/perfusion ($\dot{V}/\dot{Q}$) ratio in those areas due to overperfusion. This low $\dot{V}/\dot{Q}$ ratio in uninvolved areas of the lung is a likely cause of hypoxemia in massive PE. Other potential causes of hypoxemia in massive PE include low mixed venous oxygen due to low cardiac output, as well as the potential for opening of a probe-patent foramen ovale due to high right-sided pressures. A probe-patent foramen ovale is present in a small but significant percentage of the general population. In the presence of very high right-heart pressures, this right-to-left shunt produces hypoxemia unresponsive to oxygen therapy and also places the patient at risk for embolic cerebral vascular events.

Diagnosis

The treatment of PE or DVT is essentially the same as in patients with suspected PE; therefore, either diagnosis is sufficient for decision-making. Less invasive studies are initially used to pursue the possibility of thromboembolic disease, typically either perfusion lung scanning combined with leg ultrasound or spiral CT scanning. Pulmonary angiography may on occasions be needed.

Perfusion Lung Scanning and Lower Extremity Ultrasound

Perfusion lung scanning (usually done in combination with ventilation scanning) is typically classified into high probability, intermediate probability, low probability, and normal. Probability of PE increases with size of perfusion defect, number of moderate-to-large size defects, and perfusion defects that are significantly larger than ventilation defects or present in the absence of ventilation defects. Although ventilation scanning is usually performed in combination with perfusion scanning to quantify ventilation defects, chest radiographs can be used in place of ventilation scanning in patients without chronic pulmonary disease or acute bronchospasm. The use of perfusion scanning alone with classification of abnormal scans into those with wedge-shaped defects (PE+) and those without wedge-shaped defects (PE−) has also been demonstrated to be clinically useful in predicting which abnormal scans actually represent PE. In the United States, the PIOPED study is the most frequently utilized reference document for classification of V̇/Q̇ lung scanning. The PIOPED study supported the following findings:

- Normal lung scans make PE very unlikely.
- Reliability of a high-probability scan increases with:

- The degree of clinical suspicion using history, physical examination, and clinical information
- No underlying cardiopulmonary disease.
- No history of pulmonary emboli.
- A minority of patients have high-probability perfusion scans.
- A low-probability scan does not exclude PE.
- A clinical impression of low likelihood of PE when combined with a low-probability scan increases the predictive value of the low probability scan.
- Intermediate-probability scans cannot be used for definitive decision-making.
- The great majority of patients with suspected PE cannot have PE excluded with perfusion scanning.
- It is best to call low- and intermediate-probability scans "nondiagnostic," with the classification system then becoming high-probability, nondiagnostic, and normal.

Nondiagnostic scans require additional testing. Additional testing typically begins with noninvasive leg studies. Spiral (helical) CT follows if the diagnosis remains in doubt. Pulmonary angiography may be required in patients with high risk and equivocal or conflicting results. No differentiation is made between low- and very low-probability scans. Other pertinent facts in the consideration of PE include the knowledge that pulmonary emboli rarely predominate in upper lobes and are rarely single. In anticipation of a later question of failure of heparin therapy, a baseline perfusion scan should be considered even when the clinical diagnosis of PE is made, based on the presence of DVT. This will allow repeat scanning for the presence or absence of additional perfusion defects if new symptoms develop or symptoms continue.

Leg ultrasound is typically obtained in the following circumstances:

- A nondiagnostic (low-probability or intermediate-probability) perfusion scan in any patient.
- A normal perfusion scan in a high-risk patient.
- A high-probability perfusion scan in a low-risk patient.
- In combination with a negative spiral CT to enhance negative predictive power.

The rationale for combining leg ultrasound with the perfusion scan results is that diagnostic acumen is improved, clinically significant pulmonary emboli are unlikely to occur in the absence of DVT, and morbidity and mortality rates in PE are due to additional emboli.

Compression ultrasound (CUS) combines Doppler venous flow detection with venous imaging and has become the imaging procedure of choice for DVT in most medical centers in the United States. The diagnostic utility of CUS is related to imaging of a venous filling defect that persists with compression of the lesion. Impressive sensitivity and specificity for proximal vein thrombosis are usually obtained with this technique in patients with leg symptoms. This technique does not detect isolated thrombosis in the iliac veins or the superficial femoral veins within the adductor canal. It is, however, unlikely that these areas will be involved unless the thrombus is also present in the more readily imageable popliteal and deep femoral system. Diagnosis of calf vein thrombosis is more challenging, as these veins are smaller, have slower flow, and have more anatomic variability. CUS may also diagnose other etiologies of clinical findings such as Baker's cyst, hematoma, lymphadenopathy, and abscess. CUS cannot be performed if the leg is cast. CUS may also be limited by pain and edema.

Diagnosis of DVT by CUS allows treatment since treatment for PE and DVT are essentially the same. Absence of DVT by CUS, in combination with low-probability perfusion scan and absence of high clinical suspicion, usually allows withholding treatment. One concern in regards to this approach, however, is that the sensitivity of CUS is significantly diminished in high-risk patients without leg symptoms or signs.

Clinically evident pulmonary emboli are even more unlikely in the presence of serial negative noninvasive leg studies (typically repeated 1 to 3 times over a period of 3 to 14 days) and may be performed in this group to further enhance clinical acumen. A negative leg ultrasound in a patient with an intermediate-probability scan usually implies the need for pulmonary angiography or a spiral CT.

Pregnancy

The pursuit of diagnosis of PE in pregnant women is challenging. Ventilation/perfusion scanning is low-risk. Warfarin is an absolute contraindication in the first trimester, and a relative contraindication in the second and third trimesters. Long-term heparin administration in the pregnant woman is a significant risk for osteoporosis. Pulmonary angiographic confirmation of diagnosis may be in the patient's best interest in many cases.

Angiography

Pulmonary angiography is the gold standard for diagnosis of PE, and morbidity and mortality rates are low and acceptable. Angiography is considered positive when a persistent filling defect or cut-off sign is noted. Risk is increased if angiography is followed by thrombolytic therapy. The risk/benefit ratio of pulmonary angiography is usually acceptable and the risk to the patient is usually greater from anticoagulation in the absence of PE or failure to treat PE that is present. The death rate from pulmonary angiogram in the PIOPED study was 0.5% with a low incidence (0.8%) of major nonfatal complications (respiratory failure, renal failure or hematoma necessitating transfusion). Major nonfatal complications were four times more likely to occur in ICU patients.

Despite early studies that suggested a higher incidence of mortality due to pulmonary angiogram in patients with high pulmonary artery pressures, this was not found to be true in the PIOPED study. A pulmonary angiogram done within 1 week of acute symptoms should reliably detect pulmonary emboli even in the presence of anticoagulation. In patients with angiographically proven PE, perfusion defects persist for at least 7 days without resolution, and in the majority, for 14 days. This is an important consideration since patients may be referred to a tertiary-care center with uncertain diagnosis of PE, having received therapy for a considerable period of time.

Computed Tomography

Computed tomography angiography (CTA) (spiral [helical] or electron brain) is of significant value in detecting pulmonary emboli. A negative spiral CT makes pulmonary emboli unlikely when using the most recent CT imaging with digital reconstruction. A positive study assuming this same technology and an experienced well trained reader allows diagnosis and treatment.

The primary concern with the use of CTA in the evaluation for PE is sensitivity and whether, as a single test, a negative study rules out PE. Although specificity (the chance of a positive test being a true positive) is very good, sensitivity in some older studies was suboptimal. It is likely that improved imaging techniques (higher resolution, dramatically faster scanning time, better peripheral visualization and less motion artifact) and more experienced readers have markedly improved sensitivity. CTA also allows identification of other pulmonary processes as the cause of clinical findings

One sensitivity issue with the CTA diagnosis of PE is the decreased ability to detect vessels beyond the segmental arteries. This may be of less clinical significance, since the natural history of pulmonary emboli limited to subsegmental arteries may have a benign course especially in patients with self-limited risk factors. Withholding anticoagulant therapy in patients with a negative CT scan coupled with a negative ultrasonographic study of the legs is a safe strategy, except in those patients who present with a high clinical probability of embolism.

A recent publication in the *New England Journal of Medicine* offers an approach to evaluation for presence or absence of PE based on pre-test probability and choice of CTA or $\dot{V}/\dot{Q}$ scanning as initial test (Figs 1–3). In addition the potential role of D-dimer testing in low-probability pretesting scenarios is outlined (Fig 4).

Treatment

Anticoagulation

Heparin therapy is discontinued after a minimum of 4 to 5 days of therapy, at least 48 hours of warfarin therapy, and a warfarin-induced prolongation of international normalized ratio (INR) for prothrombin time of >2.0. The activated partial thromboplastin time (aPTT) should be maintained at 1.5 to 2 times control with heparin therapy.

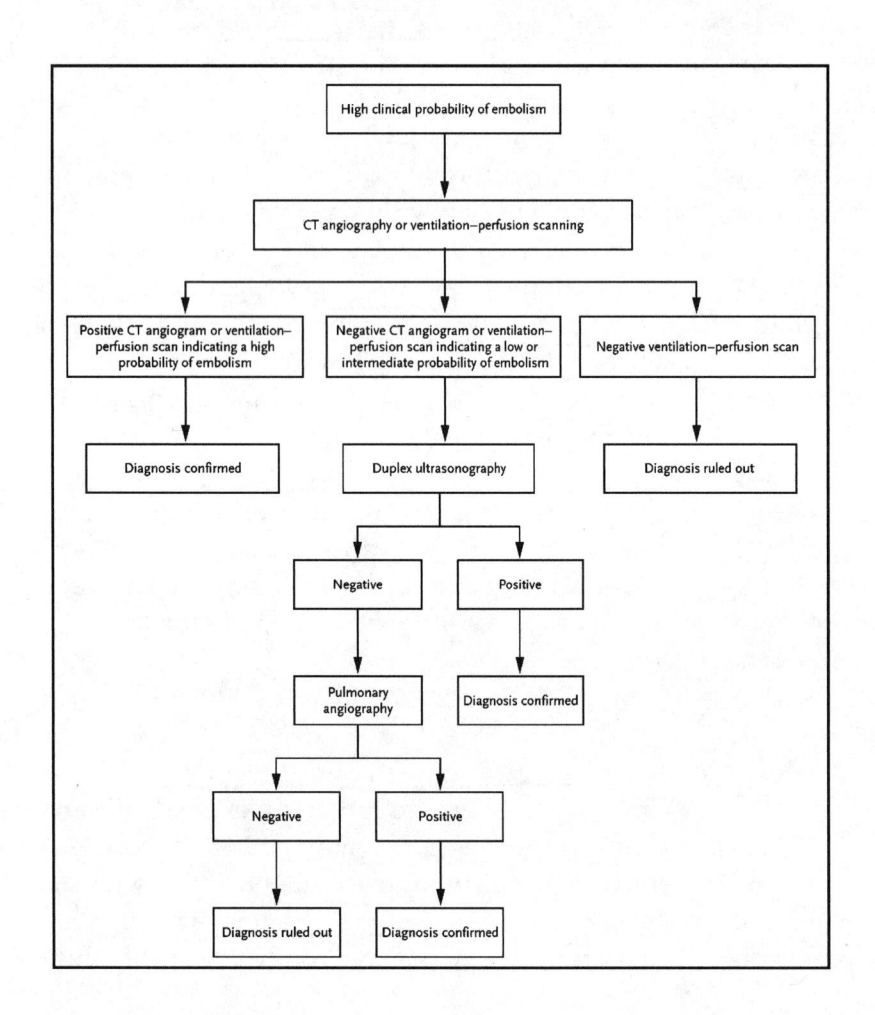

Figure 1. With permission from N Engl J Med 2003; 349:1247–1256.

Although subtherapeutic aPTT is strongly correlated with thromboembolic recurrence, a supratherapeutic aPTT does not appear to correlate with important bleeding complications. Instead, bleeding complications correlate with concurrent illness such as renal disease, heavy ethanol consumption, aspirin use, and peptic ulcer disease.

Based on this information, targeting an aPTT of 2.0 normal rather than 1.5 normal may be ideal. Adequate heparinization prevents additional clot formation, but the body's own fibrinolytic system must clear the clot that is already present so that patients who are hemodynamically unstable or who have poor cardiopulmonary reserve may remain at risk during early anticoagulation therapy. In patients without a contraindication for anticoagulation, heparin therapy should be instituted as soon as thromboembolic disease is considered. A loading dose of 5,000 to 10,000 units of heparin is indicated for PE (Table 1).

Failure to achieve adequate heparinization in the first 24 hours of treatment has been demonstrated to increase the risk of recurrent emboli.

Table 1. *Weight-Based Heparin Dosing for Pulmonary Embolism**

- Make calculations using total body weight in kilograms.
- Administer heparin, 80 U/kg, as an IV bolus.
- IV heparin infusion, 18 U/kg/h (20,000 U heparin in 500 mL of D5W = 40 U/mL).
- *Stat* aPTT 6 h after heparin bolus.
- Adjust heparin infusion based on sliding scale below:
  − aPTT (s)   Dose Change
    + aPTT <35   80-U/kg bolus, increase infusion rate by 4 U/kg/h
    + aPTT 35 to 45   40-U/kg bolus, increase infusion rate by 2 U/kg/h
    + aPTT 46 to 70   No change
    + aPTT 71 to 90   Reduce infusion rate by 2U/kg/h
    + aPTT >90   Hold heparin for 1 hr, reduce infusion rate by 3 U/kg/h
- Order aPTT 6 h after dosage change, adjusting heparin infusion by the sliding scale until aPTT is therapeutic (46 to 70 s).
- When two consecutive aPTTs are therapeutic, order aPTT (and readjust heparin drip) as needed every 24 h.
- Make changes as promptly as possible and round off doses to the nearest mL/hr (nearest 40 U/h).

*Adapted with permission from Raschke RA, Reilly BM, Guidry JR et al. The weight-based heparin dosing nomogram compared with a "standard care" nomogram: a randomized controlled trial. Ann Intern Med 1993; 119:874

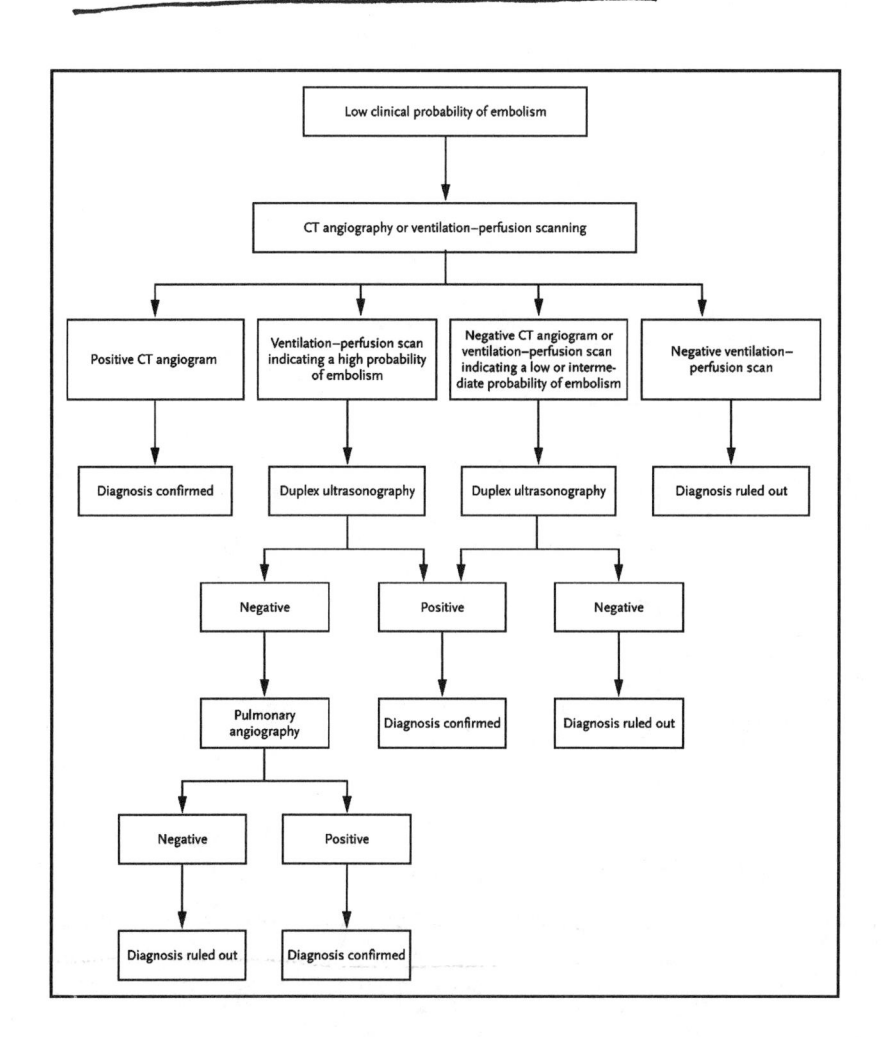

Figure 2. With permission from N Engl J Med 2003; 349:1247–1256.

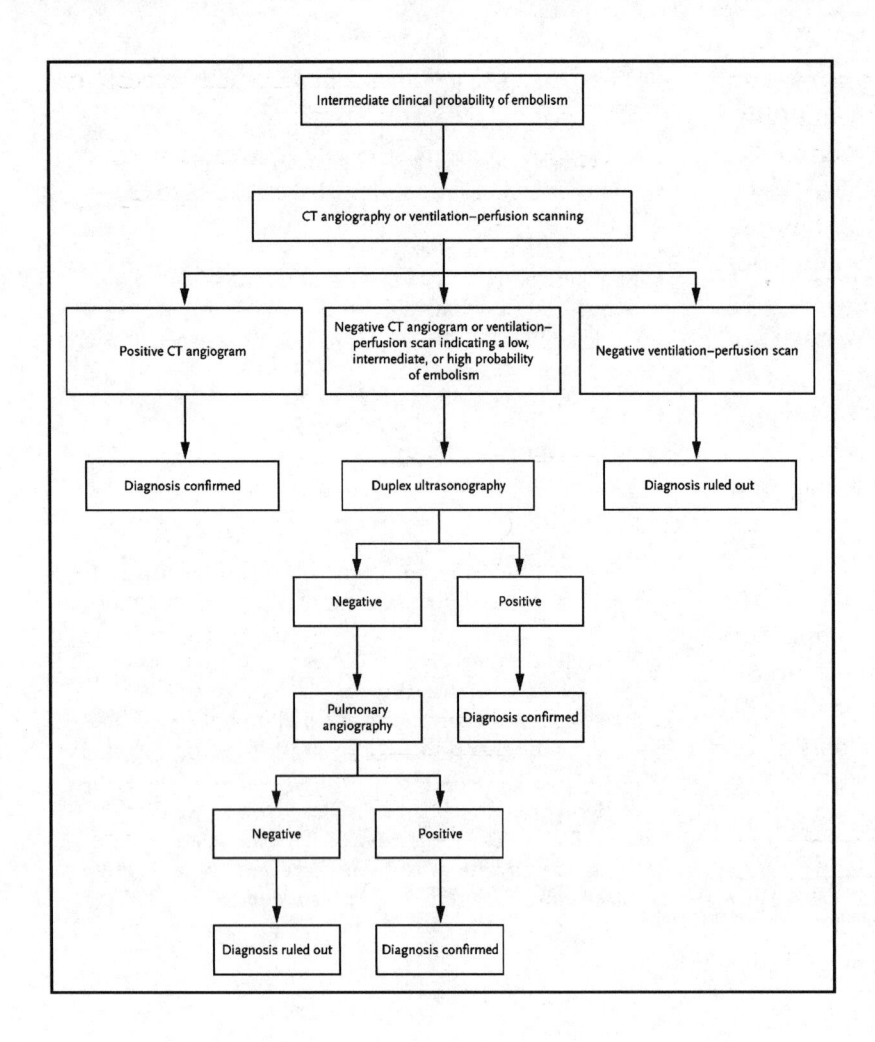

Figure 3. With permission from N Engl J Med 2003; 349:1247–1256.

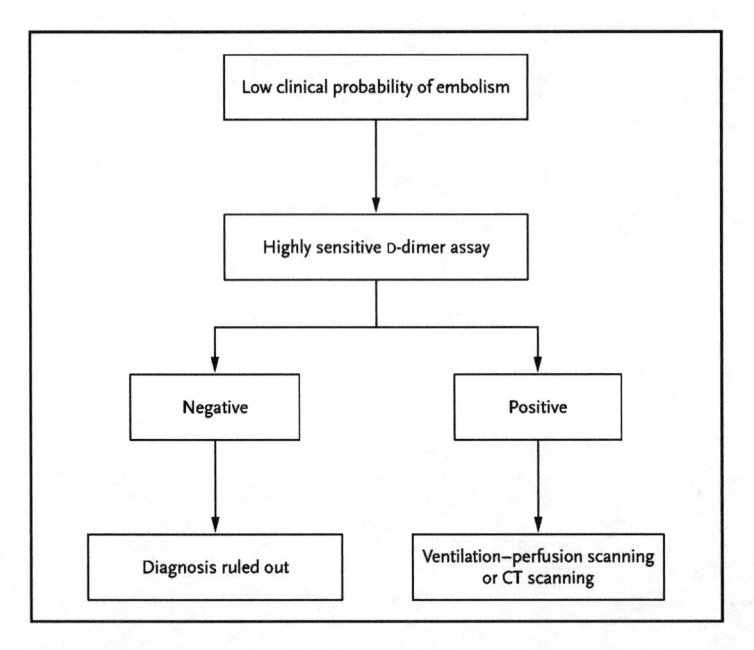

Figure 4. With permission from N Engl J Med 2003; 349:1247–1256.

Additionally, less heparin is typically required to maintain adequate anticoagulation after the first 48 hours of therapy.

Low-molecular-weight heparin (LMWH) is an effective subcutaneous therapy for DVT. It is at least as effective as standard heparin therapy in inpatient nonmassive PE and may be cost efficacious. An advantage of LMWH over unfractionated heparin is a decreased incidence of heparin-induced thrombocytopenia. A disadvantage in the critically ill patient, where the invasive procedures may be required, is that the longer half-life may be problematic. Decreased administration costs and no need for monitoring coagulation in most patients may make LMWH cost efficacious in the appropriate patient group. Thrombocytopenia is uncommon enough that no more than one platelet count is recommended during a treatment period of 5 to 7 days. If therapy is prolonged >7 days, subsequent platelet counts should be done. LMWH does not prolong the aPTT. Anti-factor Xa levels reflect LMWH activity but are not routinely necessary in most treated patients. LMWH dose adjustment is required in patients with renal insufficiency (creatinine clearance of <30 mL/min). In very large persons (>150 kg) or very small persons (<50 kg) appropriate dosing is difficult to ascertain and anti-factor Xa levels are needed to optimize dosing if LMWH is used. When bleeding occurs after recent administration of LMWH, protamine is recommended for reversal, but degree of effectiveness in this circumstance is somewhat cloudy.

It is important to remember that warfarin therapy is contraindicated in pregnancy and anticoagulation should be maintained with heparin. In addition, heparin dosage requirements are increased in pregnancy. Decreases in platelet count (heparin-induced thrombocytopenia or HIT) may occur with heparin therapy. A nonimmunologically mediated decrease in heparin (HIT-1) may occur, and is usually mild without dramatic drops in platelet count, occurs early in treatment, and does not usually require discontinuation of heparin. A more dramatic and clinically significant decrease in platelet count (HIT-2) may rarely occur in heparin therapy (days 3 to 4 or earlier with previous heparin exposure), is immunologically mediated, and does require immediate discontinuation of heparin therapy. Arterial thrombosis (white clot) may be a part of this more severe syndrome. When the platelet count falls precipitously or in a sustained fashion, heparin therapy should be stopped. When the platelet count falls to <100,000/mm³, heparin therapy should be stopped. There is a chance for cross-reactivity with LMWH and that is not advisable as a therapeutic option. Therefore, although LMWH might be chosen as a better option than unfractionated heparin in patients with thrombocytopenia at baseline, once thrombocytopenia occurs on unfractionated heparin, switching to LMWH is not a good option. With HIT-2, warfarin should not be instituted for 2 days because of the possibility of increased clot formation. Since 4 to 5 days may be required to achieve anticoagulation with warfarin in that circumstance, hirudin or heparinoid therapy is recommended to protect in the interim.

Thrombolytic Therapy

Indications for thrombolytic therapy are controversial since thrombolytic therapy has not been proven to alter clinical end points, such as mortality rates. Thrombolytic therapy followed by heparin has, however, been shown to provide more rapid improvement in RV function than heparin alone; therefore, its utility in the face of hemodynamic instability is its primary potential utilization. Severe hypoxemia despite maximum oxygen supplementation is also an accepted indication that rarely occurs.

All other uses are controversial (see discussion to follow). Streptokinase and recombinant plasminogen activator (rTPA) are both thrombolytic agents for consideration of treatment of PE. Traditional contraindications for thrombolytic therapy are active internal bleeding, recent acute cerebrovascular event (2 months), or recent cerebrovascular procedure (2 months). One report noted, however, the successful use of urokinase thrombolytic therapy of PE in 9 neurosurgical patients (mean 19 days after surgery) with no intracranial hemorrhage (1 subgaleal hematoma). Intracranial bleeding, a primary concern, occurs in 1 to 2% of patients with PE who are treated with thrombolytic therapy. Retroperitoneal hemorrhage can also be life-threatening, and most frequently occurs as a sequela of previous femoral vein access for pulmonary angiography or other associated femoral lines. Relative contraindications to thrombolytic therapy include any history of cerebrovascular event, a <10-day postpartum period, recent organ biopsy or puncture of a noncompressible vessel, recent serious internal trauma, surgery within the last 7 days, uncontrolled coagulation defects, pregnancy, cardiopulmonary resuscitation with rib fracture, thoracentesis, paracentesis, lumbar puncture, and any other conditions which place the patient at risk for bleeding. In general, angiographic documentation of PE should be obtained before thrombolytic therapy. Spiral CT diagnosis is sufficient. Occasionally, thrombolytic therapy may be considered in hemodynamically unstable patients with a high-probability perfusion scan who cannot be moved to receive pulmonary angiography. Bedside echocardiography, if immediately available, is also a consideration to offer additional support for diagnosis. When neither angiography nor perfusion scanning is possible, the patient is at risk for death, and the clinical scenario is strongly suggestive, echocardiography supporting PE may be adequate for diagnosis. No coagulation tests are typically necessary during thrombolysis. Blood samples should be limited during the thrombolytic-agent infusion period. Heparin should not be administered during thrombolysis, but heparin therapy should be resumed without a bolus when the aPTT is 1.5 to 2 times control. If bleeding should occur during thrombolytic therapy, this therapy should be discontinued to control hemorrhage due to the short half-life of the thrombolytic agent. If bleeding should persist, cryoprecipitate infusion or fresh-frozen plasma should be considered.

Although no study has demonstrated thrombolytic therapy-induced improvement in survival or decrease in recurrent thromboembolic events, its use is advocated by some in the presence of large clot burden or especially with echocardiographic evidence of acute RV dilation. This latter argument is based on the fact that RV dysfunction strongly correlates with mortality in patients with PE. Those who argue against thrombolytic use in this circumstance point to the low mortality rate once PE is diagnosed (8 to 9%), the absence of studies demonstrating clinical outcome benefit in this group, and the low but potentially catastrophic incidence of intracranial hemorrhage with thrombolytic therapy. One study evaluated 200 consecutive patients with documented PE (diagnosis made by high-probability $\dot{V}/\dot{Q}$, spiral CT, or angiography) who had echocardiography to document the presence or absence of acute RV dysfunction. Of the 65 normotensive patients with acute RV dysfunction (31% of patients), 6 developed PE-related shock after admission and 3 died. A contrasting study comes to an opposite opinion. Using a retrospective cohort analysis of two matched groups of 64 patients, the study concluded that although thrombolytic therapy improved lung scan more rapidly, there were no differences in recurrences or death rate from PE except increased death rate from bleeding. One study showed that although thrombolytic therapy of acute right ventricular dysfunction in the absence of hemodynamic instability did not decrease mortality, it did decrease escalation of therapy (institution of vasopressor therapy, intubation/mechanical ventilation, and secondary thrombolysis).

The management of free-floating RV thrombi remains controversial. Echocardiography usually demonstrates evidence of right ventricular overload (>90%), paradoxical interventricular septal motion (75%), and pulmonary hypertension (86%). The clots are usually worm-like, mortality is high (45%), and thrombolytic therapy, if not contraindicated, is recommended as the treatment of choice by some investigators. Infusion of a thrombolytic agent directly onto a pulmonary thrombus via the pulmonary artery has never been convincingly shown to be superior to infusion of the agent through a peripheral vein. There are some data in the radiology literature to suggest this may be useful for deep vein thrombus. The use of thrombolytic agents in PE remains controversial. The American College of Chest Physicians (ACCP) consensus statement of thromboembolism states that the use of thrombolytic agents continues to be highly individualized and clinicians should have latitude in their use. They are, however, recommended in general for hemodynamic instability and massive ileofemoral thrombosis.

In the United States, the most frequently used thrombolytic agent for the treatment of PE is rTPA. FDA-approved dosing is 100 mg over 2 h. In the patient with massive PE in whom death appears imminent without thrombolytic intervention, more rapid administration may be appropriate. One proposed alternative that seems reasonable in that circumstance is 40 mg over minutes followed by 60 mg over the remainder of the 2-h period. One study of PE as the cause of arrest noted a clinical diagnosis of PE made in 70% of patients (30% were not suspected until autopsy). In 21 of these 24 patients, r-TPA was administered; 2 of these patients survived to hospital discharge.

Inferior Vena Cava Filter

Traditional indications for inferior vena cava (IVC) filter placement include contraindication to anticoagulation, onset of bleeding with anticoagulation, and failure of anticoagulation to abate thromboembolic events. Other indications for filter placement include hemodynamically unstable patients who will not be given thrombolytic therapy, and patients with HIT as a bridge to warfarin therapy. Direct thrombin inhibitors, if available, are less invasive and more appropriate alternatives in this situation. The empiric use of IVC filter in patients with a large clot burden or poor cardiopulmonary reserve is more controversial. Filter placement may also be considered in patients with high risk for DVT and relative or absolute contraindications for anticoagulation prophylaxis of DVT. The decision to anticoagulate patients who have had an IVC filter placed is controversial, but the use of anticoagulation may prevent further clot formation and increase the patency rate of the filter over time and, therefore, facilitate venous drainage. Patency can be maintained, however, without concomitant heparin therapy. Documentation of deep venous thrombotic disease is usually required before placement of an IVC filter. A filter may also benefit patients at high risk for chronic anticoagulation, such as poorly compliant patients or patients at risk for falls. Complications of filter placement include vessel injury at the time of insertion, subsequent venous thrombosis at the insertion site, filter migration and embolization into the heart, filter erosion through the IVC, and IVC obstruction.

Pulmonary Embolism-Induced Hypoperfusion

The right ventricle cannot increase stroke volume in response to sudden increases in afterload. Instead, the RV dilates as ejection fraction decreases. Failure of the RV to compensate for the increased afterload produces hypotension and, if severe, syncope. Studies of hemodynamic profiles in patients with acute PE have demonstrated mean pulmonary artery pressures >40 mm Hg only in patients with preexisting cardiopulmonary disease, suggesting that the normal RV is incapable of generating pressures >40 mm Hg in the setting of acute pulmonary vascular bed obstruction.

Pulmonary artery catheterization may be useful to optimize therapy in the hypotensive patient but the catheters may be difficult to pass due to high pulmonary artery resistance and low-flow state. A right atrial pressure (RAP) of ~15 to 20 mm Hg is probably optimal. Overdistention of the RV (more likely when mean RAP is >20 mm Hg) may be problematic for several reasons. First, the RV may be made ischemic due to decreased coronary perfusion related to the high RV pressure since perfusion pressure of the right ventricle is approximated by aortic diastolic pressure minus mean RV pressure. With high right-sided pressures, left ventricular compliance may also be decreased as the interventricular septum shifts into the LV.

Based on the above, volume therapy is typically ineffective and may be deleterious with resultant overdistension of the RV. RV ischemia may be a primary cause or a major contributing factor to hypotension. Therapy should be targeted toward reducing RV afterload (RV work) by reducing pulmonary clot burden, avoiding volume-induced RV overdistension (RAP >20 mm Hg), and maintaining adequate aortic diastolic pressure (upstream filling pressure for the LV).

RV contractility may be improved by the use of inotropic drugs. Dopamine at doses beginning at 5 μg/kg/min is the recommended inotrope in the presence of hypotension. Dobutamine may be preferred in the presence of hypoperfusion but absence of hypotension. Isoproterenol alone should be avoided.

Vasopressors may also be beneficial by increasing aortic diastolic pressure when it is critically low. Combination inotrope/vasoconstrictor norepinephrine is recommended in the hypotensive patient. Vasoconstriction of systemic vascular bed with selective vasodilation of pulmonary vascular bed would be ideal. Inhaled nitric oxide has anecdotally been demonstrated to improve hemodynamics in PE by this mechanism. Benefit could only occur through vasodilation of PE-released humorally mediated vasoconstriction.

Surgical thrombectomy may be considered in situations of severe hemodynamic instability with a contraindication to thrombolytic therapy and close proximity to the operating room. Bypass capability is necessary and the clinical scenario should indicate a certain or almost certain clinical diagnosis of massive PE. It should also be considered when hemodynamic instability persists despite thrombolytic therapy.

Prevention of Pulmonary Embolism

The most powerful statement that can be made for prophylaxis is that, of the patients who die of pulmonary emboli, most patients survive <30 min after the event, which is not long for most forms of treatment to be effective. Without prophylaxis, the frequency of fatal PE is ~7% for emergency hip surgery, 2% after elective hip surgery, and 1% after elective surgery. Length of surgery, age, and type of surgery (hip, pelvis, knee, prostate) are important considerations for risk of emboli. Autopsy findings demonstrate that PE causes 5% of deaths in mechanically ventilated patients. The frequency of PE after myocardial infarction in the absence of prophylaxis may be ≤5%. The great majority of patients in the ICU should receive heparin prophylaxis for thromboembolic disease. The dose for general surgical patients or in medical patients is typically 5000 units of unfractionated heparin subcutaneously three times daily or LMWH once daily. Hemorrhagic side effects of low-dose heparin are rare (<2%) in patients without hemorrhagic diathesis. High-risk patients or those who have contraindications for heparin should receive intermittent pneumatic venous compression (IPVC), additively or as a replacement, respectively. Low-dose LMWH is the heparin of choice in knee surgery patients, hip surgery patients, and central nervous system trauma patients.

Recent reports of epidural hematoma after LMWH use in patients who have had epidural puncture should alert the physician to this potential complication with any anticoagulation in place, independent of type. IPVC is a nonpharmacologic prophylaxis alternative for knee surgery. IPVC is contraindicated in the face of arterial compromise of extremity. IPVC can be added to heparin prophylaxis in patients with additive risk factors. In high-risk patients such as those undergoing elective hip surgery, the use of either LMWH, adjusted-dose unfractionated heparin targeting heparin to prolong mid-dosing PTT measurement by 4 to 5 s, or low-dose warfarin is recommended. Low-dose warfarin can be instituted at 1 mg/day beginning 21 days before elective surgery and continuing through the postoperative hospitalization. For hip fracture surgery, LMWH or full-dose warfarin (INR 2.0 to 3.0) is recommended.

Clinically significant DVT develops in many trauma cases. Risk factors include advanced age, prolonged immobilization, severe head trauma, paralysis, pelvic and lower extremity fractures, direct venous trauma, shock, and multiple transfusions. Low-dose heparin or IPVC may not be effective in the highest-risk patient. In trauma patients at high risk for bleeding and those at high risk for pulmonary emboli, prophylactic IVC filter placement has been recommended by some investigators, especially if leg injury prevents application of pneumatic compression devices. Similar rationale has been offered when PE is diagnosed in advanced malignancy. Neither of these uses has been validated.

One study demonstrated that 52% of patients who had documented PE had received prophylactic therapy. Obviously, better prophylactic alternatives are needed.

Summary

PE is a treatable condition with a nonspecific clinical presentation that makes diagnosis difficult. CT scanning has become the primary diagnostic test. Predictive capability of negative CT studies in higher-risk patients is enhanced by additional studies (non-elevated D-dimer, negative leg ultrasound and low-probability $\dot{V}/\dot{Q}$ scan), occasionally pulmonary angiography is necessary. Thrombolytic therapy is indicated in patients with hemodynamic instability and no contraindications.

Annotated Bibliography

ACCP Consensus Committee on Pulmonary Embolism. Opinions regarding the diagnosis and management of venous thromboembolic disease. Chest 1998; 113:499–504
Question and answer format for controversial areas of VTE management.
Baile EM, King GG, Müller NL, et al. Spiral computed tomography is comparable to angiography for the

diagnosis of pulmonary embolism. Am J Respir Crit Care Med 2000; 161:1010–1015
Pig model using colored methacrylate beads and postmortem methacrylate casting showing no difference in diagnosis of subsegmental clot between angiography and spiral CT.

Bode FR, Dellinger RP. Deep vein thrombosis, pulmonary embolism. In: Gallagher TJ, ed. Postoperative care of the critically ill patient. Baltimore: Williams & Wilkins Co., 1995; 445–472.
Although this review is targeted toward the surgery patient, the basic principles are applicable to evaluation and management of thromboembolic disease in general in the critically ill patient.

Bounameaux H, de Moerloose P, Perrier A, et al. D-dimer testing in suspected venous thromboembolism: an update. QJM 1997; 90:437–442
Discusses potential use of D-dimer thresholds for refining diagnostic acumen in pulmonary embolism and the potential to use D-dimer to decrease invasive testing.

Chartier L, Béra J, Delomez M, et al. Free-floating thrombi in the right heart: Diagnosis, management, and prognostic indexes in 38 consecutive patients. Circulation 1999; 99:2779–2783
Argues that thrombolytic therapy is faster and more readily available for free-floating thrombi in the right heart and can be used as only therapy or as bridge to surgery.

Dalen JE, Banas JS, Brooks HL, et al. Resolution rate of acute pulmonary embolism in man. N Engl J Med 1969; 280:1194–1199
No resolution of PE by angiogram before day 14.

Dellinger RP. Prophylaxis of venous thromboembolism. In: Critical care symposium—1997. Anaheim, CA: Society of Critical Care Medicine, 1997; 51–76
An in-depth view of specific risk factors for development of deep vein thrombosis as well as recommended prophylactic regimens; significant literature review on surgical prophylaxis studies.

Dellinger RP. Pulmonary embolism. In: Parrillo JE, ed. Current therapy in critical care medicine. 3rd ed. Philadelphia: Mosby, 1997; 216–223
General review targeted toward diagnosis and treatment.

Dellinger RP: Pulmonary embolism. In: Vincent J-L, ed. Yearbook of intensive care and emergency medicine. Berlin: Springer-Verlag, 1997; 317–326
General review targeted toward diagnosis and treatment.

Elliott CG, Goldhaber SZ, Visani L, et al. Chest radiographs in acute pulmonary embolism. Chest 2000; 118:33–38
Review of chest radiographs in 2,454 patients with diagnosis of PE. Cardiomegaly (27%) was most common abnormal finding, as well as the most common finding.; Twenty-four percent were normal.

Fedullo PF, Tapson VF. The evaluation of suspected pulmonary embolism. N Engl J Med 2003; 349:1247–1256
General review on diagnosis with algorithms.

Fennerty T. The diagnosis of pulmonary embolism. BMJ 1997; 314:425–429
Concise, general review article on pulmonary embolism diagnosis.

Firdose R, Elamin EM. Recent advances in pulmonary embolism diagnosis and management. Compr Ther 2001; 27:156–162
General review.

Giordano A, Angiolillo DJ. Current role of lung scintigraphy in pulmonary embolism. Q J Nucl Med 2001; 45:294–301
A view on utility of $\dot{V}/\dot{Q}$ lung scanning from the nuclear medicine side.

Goldhaber SZ. Pulmonary embolism. N Engl J Med 1998; 339:93–104
Medical intelligence review article of pulmonary embolism management.

Goldhaber SZ. Unsolved issues in the treatment of pulmonary embolism. Thromb Res 2001; 103:V245–V255
Highlights areas of ongoing uncertainty.

Goodman LR, Lipchik RJ, Kuzo RS et al. Subsequent pulmonary embolism: risk after a negative helical CT pulmonary angiogram – prospective comparison with scintigraphy. Radiology 2000; 215:535–542

Goodman LR. Venous thromboembolic disease: CT evaluation. Q J Nucl Med 2001; 45:302–310
Points to improving ability to use CT results in decision making.

Gould MK, Dembitzer AD, Sanders GD, et al. Low-molecular-weight heparins compared with unfractionated heparin for treatment of acute deep venous thrombosis. a cost-effectiveness analysis. Ann Intern Med 1999; 130:789–799

Greco F, Bisignani G, Serafini O, et al. Successful treatment of right heart thromboemboli with IV recombinant tissue-type plasminogen activator during continuous echocardiographic monitoring. Chest 1999; 116:78–82
Study demonstrated complete resolution of all right heart clots studied when continuous echocardiography was employed after r-TPA.

Grifoni S, Olivotto I, Cecchini P, et al. Short-term clinical outcome of patients with acute pulmonary embolism, normal blood pressure, and echocardiographic right ventricular dysfunction. JAMA 2000; 101:2817–2822

Demonstrated significant morbidity and mortality developing in patients with PE, acute RV dysfunction, and initial hemodynamic stability.

Hamel E, Pacouret G, Vincentelli D, et al. Thrombolysis or heparin therapy in massive pulmonary embolism with right ventricular dilation: results from a 128-patient monocenter registry. Chest 2001; 120:6–8

Two retrospective cohort massive PE groups were matched with the exception of thrombolytic therapy. Although lung scan improved more rapidly in the thrombolytic group, there were no differences in recurrent PE with increased bleeding deaths in the thrombolytic group.

Hyers TM, Agnelli G, Hull RD, et al. Antithrombotic therapy for venous thromboembolic disease. Chest 2001; 119:176S–193S

Most recent ACCP consensus statement on therapy of PE.

Hyers TM. Venous thromboembolism. Am J Respir Crit Care Med 1999; 159:1–14

Concise general review of diagnosis and prevention of pulmonary embolism.

Jerges-Sanchez C, Ramirez-Rivera A, Garcia M, et al. Streptokinase and heparin versus heparin alone in massive pulmonary embolism: a randomized control trial. J Thromb Thrombolysis 1995; 2:227–229

Paper occasionally used to justify utility of thrombolytic therapy in massive PE and value of streptokinase in particular; however, only 4 patients in each group. Furthermore, all 4 patients in thrombolytic therapy group diagnosed in ED of hospital performing study while all 4 patients in heparin-only group transferred to that institution from other hospitals with recurrent PE on heparin.

Johnson MS. Current strategies for the diagnosis of pulmonary embolus. J Vasc Interv Radiol 2002; 13:13–23

General review of diagnostic modalities available for diagnoses and their severity and specificity.

Konstantinides S, Geibel A, Heuset G, et al. Heparin plus alteplace compared with heparin alone in patients with submassive pulmonary embolism N Engl J Med 2002; 347:1143–1150

Primary thrombolytic therapy decreased subsequent death and use of vasopressors/mechanical ventilation/secondary thrombolysis as a combined endpoint but no difference in mortality.

Kürkciyan I, Meron G, Sterz F, et al. Pulmonary embolism as cause of cardiac arrest: presentation and outcome. Arch Intern Med 2000; 160:1529–1535

10% salvage rate when r-TPA is given to patients with either confirmed PE or those highly likely to have PE.

Lorut C, Ghossains M, Horellou MH, et al. A noninvasive diagnostic strategy including spiral computed tomography in patients with suspected pulmonary embolism. Am J Respir Crit Care Med 2000; 162:1413–1418

A protocol was used for evaluation and decision as to presence or absence of PE using CT, Q scan, and D-dimer. Ultrasound was used in middle-ground situation as a final decision maker. Only 1.7% of untreated patients had PE over next 3 months.

Lund O, Nielsen TT, Schifter S, et al. Treatment of pulmonary embolism with full-dose heparin, streptokinase, or embolectomy. Thorac Cardiovasc Surg 1986; 32:240–246

Compared thrombolytic therapy with embolectomy for massive PE. Hospital mortality equal (21% and 22%), but 5-year survival better in embolectomy group. Nonrandomized study of 28 and 25 patients, respectively, but severity of illness score greater in embolectomy group at baseline.

McConnell MV, Solomon SD, Fayan ME, et al. Regional right ventricular dysfunction detected by echocardiography in acute pulmonary embolism. Am J Cardiol 1996; 78:469–473

The finding of abnormal wall motion in RV mid-free wall and normal motion in apex was very predictive of PE among patients with acute symptoms and evidence of pulmonary artery hypertension.

Miniati M, Pistolesi M, Maseri C, et al. Value of perfusion lung scan in the diagnosis of pulmonary embolism: results of the Prospective Investigative Study of Adult Pulmonary Embolism Diagnosis (PISA-PED). Am J Respir Crit Care Med 1996; 154:1387–1393

Studied the use of perfusion scanning/chest radiograph analysis without ventilation scanning in 890 consecutive patients with suspected pulmonary embolism. Abnormal scans were considered PE+ if scans demonstrated one or more wedge-shaped perfusion defect and PE− if they did not. Sensitivity was 92% (most patients with angiographically proven PE had PE+ scans) and specificity was 87% (most patients without angiographically proven PE had PE− scans). The addition of pretest clinical probability further heightened predictive capability.

Molina JE, Hunter DW, Yedlicka JW, et al. Thrombolytic therapy for post-operative pulmonary embolism. Am J Surg 1992; 163:375–380

Thirteen patients within 2 weeks of surgery (mean 9.6 days). Used modified urokinase regimen to demonstrate complete lysis of PE with no bleeding complications.

Musset D, Parent F, Meyer G, et al. Diagnostic strategy for patients with suspected pulmonary emobolism: a prospective multicentre outcome study. Lancet 2002; 360:1914–1920

Pandey AS, Rakowski H, Mickleborough LL, et al. Right heart pulmonary embolism in transit: A review of therapeutic considerations. Can J Cardiol 1997; 13:397–402

This article presents the challenges of reacting to the presence of right-heart clot on ultrasound as it is pertinent to decision-making in patients with pulmonary embolism. This finding is particularly problematic in the unstable patient and the patient with contraindication to thrombolytic therapy.

Perrier A, Howarth N, Didier D, et al. Performance of helical computed tomography in unselected outpatients with suspected pulmonary embolism. Ann Intern Med 2001; 135:88–97

Quinlan DJ, McQuillan A, Eikelboom JW. Low-molecular-weight heparin compared with intravenous unfractionated heparin for treatment of pulmonary embolism. Ann Intern Med 2004; 140:175–183

Quinn DA, Fogel RB, Smith CD, et al. D-dimers in the diagnosis of pulmonary embolism. Am J Respir Crit Care Med 1999; 159:1445–1449

Non-elevated D-dimers make PE very unlikely, while elevated D-dimers were not useful.

Raschke RA, Reilly BM, Guidry JR, et al. The weight-based heparin dosing nomogram compared with a "standard care" nomogram: a randomized controlled trial. Ann Intern Med 1993; 119:874–881

Valuable discussion and helpful summary of weight-based heparin anticoagulation therapy.

Rathbun SW, Raskob GE, Whitwett TL. Sensitivity and specificity of helical computed tomography in the diagnosis of pulmonary embolism: a systematic review. Ann Intern Med 2000; 132:227–232

A review of the 15 prospective English-language studies of use of helical (spiral) CT in the diagnosis of PE. Found that only two studies had consecutive patients, 8 studies had independently interpreted angiogram and CT, and only one study included a broad spectrum of patients. Concluded that there is not currently enough data to support withholding of heparin after negative spiral CT without additional testing. Large prospective trials are needed.

Ryu JH, Swensen SJ, Olson EJ, et al. Diagnosis of pulmonary embolism with use of computed tomographic angiography. Mayo Clin 2001; 76:59–65

This one would reflect critical care board timing for question writing.

Severi P, LoPinto G, Doggio R, et al. Urokinase thrombolytic therapy of pulmonary embolism in neurosurgical patients. Surg Neurol 1994; 42:469–470

Nine neurosurgery patients (mean 19 days following surgery) received urokinase. All survived, no intracranial hemorrhage, one subgaleal hemorrhage.

Stein PD, Afzal A, Henry JW, et al. Fever in pulmonary embolism. Chest 2000; 117:39–42

Demonstrated no source of fever (temp >100.0°F) other than PE in 14% of patients with angiographically documented PE. Fever correlated with DVT but not with infarction. Only 2 of 268 patients had temperatures > 103.0°F.

Stein PD, Athanasoulis C, Alavi A, et al. Complications and validity of pulmonary angiography in acute pulmonary embolism. Circulation 1992; 85:462–468

Interobserver radiologist agreement on angiographic diagnosis of pulmonary embolism: lobar 98%, segmental 90%, subsegmental 66%.

Stein PD, Huang H, Afzal A, Noor HA. Incidence of acute pulmonary embolism in a general hospital. Chest 1999; 116:909–913

Women >50 years old, but not women <50 years old, have greater incidence of PE than men.

Tapson VF, Carroll BA, Davidson BL, et al. The diagnostic approach to acute venous thromboembolism — clinical practice guidelines. Am J Respir Crit Care Med 1999; 160:1043–1066

Comprehensive clinical practice guideline for the diagnosis and treatment of DVT and PE. Extensive discussion of DVT diagnostic strategy. Also very good review on utility and risk of pulmonary angiogram.

The PIOPED Investigators. Value of the ventilation/perfusion scan in acute pulmonary embolism: results of the prospective investigation of pulmonary embolism diagnosis (PIOPED). JAMA 1990; 263:2753–2759

The article includes a discussion of the use of Bayes theorem, as well as the role of the previous cardiopulmonary disease and previous pulmonary embolism in reliability of scanning.

Turkstra F, Koopman MM, Buller HR. The treatment of deep vein thrombosis and pulmonary embolism. Thromb Haemost 1997; 78:489–496

Concise, general review article on treatment of deep-vein thrombosis and pulmonary embolism.

van Strijen MJL, de Monye W, Schiereck J, et al. Single-detector helical computed tomography as the primary diagnostic test in suspected pulmonary embolism: a multicenter clinical management study of 510 patients. Ann Intern Med 2003; 138:307–314

Verstraete M, Miller GAH, Bounameaus H, et al. Intravenous and intrapulmonary recombinant tissue-type plasminogen activator in the treatment of acute massive pulmonary embolism. Circulation 1988; 77:353–360

Demonstrated no beneficial effect of thrombolytic therapy infused into pulmonary artery versus peripheral administration.

Wiegand UKH, Kurowski V, Giannitsis E, et al. Effectiveness of end-tidal carbon dioxide tension for monitoring of thrombolytic therapy in acute pulmonary embolism. Crit Care Med 2000; 28: 3588–3592

End-tidal CO_2 decreases as thrombolytic therapy improves hemodynamics as indicator of decreased dead space.

Wood KE. Major pulmonary embolism – review of a pathophysiologic approach to the golden hour of hemodynamically significant pulmonary embolism. Chest 2002; 121:877–905

Excellent general review devoted to massive pulmonary embolism.

Notes

Notes

Endocrine Emergencies

James A. Kruse, MD

Objectives:

- To recognize the etiologies and clinical manifestations of endocrine crises involving the pancreas, thyroid, adrenal, and pituitary glands
- To review the optimal confirmatory laboratory tests for these disorders in the acute care setting
- To delineate the initial treatment for each specific endocrine emergency
- To cover important pearls and selected caveats related to the diagnosis and management of endocrine emergencies

Key words: adrenal insufficiency; diabetes insipidus; diabetic ketoacidosis; hyperosmolar-nonketotic dehydration syndrome; hypoglycemia; myxedema coma; pheochromocytoma; thyroid storm

Hypoglycemia

Hypoglycemia has numerous etiologies. Common causes in the ICU setting include sepsis, severe hepatic dysfunction, renal failure, and adrenal insufficiency. Administration of excessive therapeutic insulin is also common. Parenteral nutrition formulas contain high concentrations of dextrose, which can result in high circulating insulin levels in nondiabetic patients. Abruptly stopping such infusions can therefore induce hypoglycemia. Uncommon causes include pancreatic islet cell tumors, various nonpancreatic neoplasms (*eg*, hepatoma, sarcoma, lymphoma, leukemia, and carcinoid tumors) that secrete insulin-like factors, hereditary fructose intolerance, and glycogen storage disease. Certain drugs (*eg*, ethanol, sulfonylurea agents, β–adrenergic receptor blockers, pentamidine, quinidine, and disopyramide) can potentially cause hypoglycemia.

The classic diagnostic criteria for hypoglycemia are exemplified by Whipple's triad, which consists of hypoglycemia (blood glucose concentration <50 mg/dL) accompanied by classic symptoms of hypoglycemia, with resolution of these symptoms following administration of dextrose. The clinical findings of hypoglycemia are mainly either manifestations of the resulting hyperadrenergic state or the effects of neuroglycopenia. The latter include headache, visual disturbances, confusion, behavioral changes, delirium, stupor, coma, or seizures. Among the hyperadrenergic manifestations are tremulousness, anxiety, diaphoresis, palpitations, tachycardia, nausea, vomiting, and weakness. These signs and symptoms can be absent or blunted in patients taking β–adrenergic receptor blockers. In most cases the etiology is apparent or the episode represents an isolated event. Less commonly, repetitive unexplained episodes of hypoglycemia necessitate exclusion of obscure causes using assays for insulin and C-peptide levels, provocative testing, and in some cases drug testing.

If severe and prolonged, hypoglycemia can potentially result in devastating and permanent neurologic injury. For this reason it should be considered a medical emergency requiring acute treatment. Initial treatment consists of IV injection of concentrated dextrose (usually 50 mL of 50% dextrose solution). Blood can first be sampled for glucose analysis, if it does not delay dextrose administration for more than about a minute. If rapid assay, point of care testing is not used, dextrose should then be administered without waiting for the glucose assay result. IV administration of 25 g of dextrose is safe, even if the patient is subsequently found to not have hypoglycemia, or found to have hyperglycemia. This treatment is temporizing. Whatever mechanism caused the hypoglycemia is likely to still be present and the hypoglycemia is expected to recur once the 25 g of administered dextrose has been metabolized. Therefore, a continuous IV infusion of dextrose should be started. The final aspect of acute management is to provide for serial blood or serum glucose testing to detect possible recurrences and tailor the rate of ongoing dextrose administration. Serial glucose monitoring is especially critical in patients who are sedated or otherwise already have altered mentation or a depressed sensorium that can interfere with clinical detection of neuroglycopenic manifestations.

Diabetic Ketoacidosis

Diabetic ketoacidosis (DKA) occurs when there is a complete or near-complete lack of insulin. It is uncommon in older adults but is seen commonly in children and young adults with new onset or previously diagnosed type I diabetes mellitus. The two most common precipitating factors are noncompliance with insulin therapy and intercurrent medical illnesses, especially infection. Subjective manifestations include malaise, fatigue, polyuria, thirst, polydipsia, nausea, vomiting, and abdominal pain. Physical examination may reveal Kussmaul respirations, tachycardia, orthostatic or frank hypotension, acetone breath odor, abdominal tenderness, and alterations in the sensorium.

Laboratory findings include hyperglycemia, metabolic acidosis, ketonemia, ketonuria, and an elevation of the serum anion gap. The metabolic acidosis is due to production of excessive amounts of acetoacetic and β–hydroxybutyric acid. The former can be semiquantitatively assayed in the laboratory colorimetrically by reaction of serum or urine with nitroprusside. Acetone, a metabolic end-product of these two organic acids, also reacts with nitroprusside. Dissociation of loosely bound hydrogen ions on these acids forms β–hydroxybutyrate and acetoacetate, anions that are responsible for the elevated anion gap observed in the majority of patients with DKA. Glycosuria produces an osmotic diuresis and leads to depletion of water and potassium from the body. However, serum potassium levels are usually high in DKA at presentation, due to shifting of potassium from the intracellular compartment to the extracellular space as a result of the insulin deficiency. This hyperkalemia usually abates shortly after insulin treatment is initiated and can lead to rapid development of marked hypokalemia. Therefore, close monitoring of serum potassium is necessary with the expectation that potassium supplementation will be necessary soon after insulin therapy is under way. Hypophosphatemia can occur, either at presentation or more commonly during insulin administration. Specific diagnostic studies are utilized to rule out suspected precipitating factors, such as infection or myocardial infarction.

Treatment is initiated with vigorous isotonic IV fluid administration using normal saline initially. Hypotonic saline is substituted once intravascular volume is adequately replenished. Regular insulin is given first as an IV bolus at 0.15 U/kg, followed by a continuous IV infusion at 0.1 U/kg per hour, which is titrated against serial blood glucose measurements obtained at 1- to 2-h intervals. This monitoring is needed to minimize the risk of hypoglycemia, and to allow its prompt detection should it occur. Potassium supplementation is typically begun as soon as the serum potassium concentration falls to within the normal range. Phosphate is administered if hypophosphatemia is present. There are no systematic clinical trials showing that sodium bicarbonate therapy has a positive effect on outcome.

When blood glucose concentration falls below ~250 mg/dL, 5% dextrose is added to the IV fluid prescription but the IV insulin infusion is continued until the ketoacidosis resolves. Resolution of ketoacidosis is demonstrated by normalization of the serum anion gap and near-normalization of serum total CO_2 content. Once the ketoacidosis has resolved, the IV insulin infusion can be stopped and subcutaneously administered insulin substituted. Parenteral dextrose administration is then stopped and an appropriate oral diet prescribed.

Hyperosmolar-Nonketotic Dehydration Syndrome

Hyperosmolar-nonketotic dehydration syndrome (HONK) occurs in patients that have insulin deficiency that results in hyperglycemia, but still secrete enough insulin to prevent ketoacidosis from developing. Unlike DKA, it occurs more frequently in the elderly. Like DKA and other endocrine crises, an intercurrent illness frequently precipitates this disorder. Among the more common precipitating factors are sepsis, myocardial infarction, and stroke. Common subjective manifestations include polyuria and polydipsia, but marked sensorial depression can occur due to hyperosmolality caused by severe hyperglycemia.

Whereas in DKA the blood glucose concentration is typically between 400 and 800 mg/dL, HONK is characterized by blood glucose levels exceeding 800 mg/dL by definition, often well over 1,000 mg/dL, and on rare occasions over 2,000 mg/dL. Ketoacidosis is not present in classic cases of HONK, but mild degrees of ketosis or ketoacidosis are not uncommon. Pure HONK and pure DKA can be thought of as poles of a spectrum, with many patients represented in the overlap region of the spectrum such that some cases of DKA are associated with higher than typical blood glucose levels, and some cases of HONK have a degree of ketoacidosis.

As with DKA, glycosuria results in an osmotic diuresis, depleting extracellular water and potassium. In HONK, the marked elevations in blood glucose result in hyperosmolality and cause osmotic shifting of water from the intracellular space to the extracellular compartment. This can result in severe intracellular dehydration. In the brain, this intracellular dehydration is responsible for the sensorial depression or coma. The resulting brain shrinkage can lead to stretching of blood vessels between the skull and the cortical surface, potentially leading to parenchymal hemorrhage.

Renal losses of hypotonic fluid can lead to associated hypernatremia. On the other hand, the osmotic shifting of water from the cells to the extracellular space tends to lower plasma sodium by dilution. Although this latter effect by itself would tend to expand intravascular volume, the associated osmotic diuresis more than countervails and leads to intravascular volume depletion. The net effect of these forces determines actual plasma sodium concentration. The degree of hypernatremia is commonly used by clinicians as a means of estimating electrolyte-free water deficits in acutely ill patients, but its use for this purpose can be misleading in patients with HONK. Free water deficits are proportional to effective plasma osmolality, which in the absence of hyperglycemia is normally proportional to changes in plasma sodium concentration. In HONK, however, the sodium concentration may be normal or decreased (as described above) even though the plasma is hyperosmolar due to hyperglycemia. Even if the patient is hypernatremic, the degree of hypernatremia will under-represent the free-water deficit in so far as hyperglycemia tends to temper the plasma sodium concentration.

One way to estimate free-water deficits in this situation is to consider the adjusted serum concentration, after accounting for the expected effect of hyperglycemia on serum sodium concentration. This is conventionally done by adjusting the serum sodium concentration downward by 1.6 mmol/L for every 100-mg/dL elevation in glucose concentration. Applying this factor to the patient's reported serum sodium concentration allows the clinician to abstractly consider what the patient's sodium level would be if the same free-water deficit were present but in the absence of hyperglycemia.

Treatment of HONK is similar to that of DKA. Because the degree of dehydration is often much more severe than in DKA, more vigorous fluid replacement is usually required. Administering insulin before beginning fluid resuscitation can precipitate or worsen circulatory shock by driving glucose into cells, thereby lowering plasma osmolality and causing osmotic shifting of water from the intravascular compartment to the intracellular space, worsening hypovolemia. The choice of IV fluid composition initially is always normal saline. Even though hypotonic IV fluids can ameliorate the hyperosmolar state more rapidly, they are less effective at expanding intravascular volume. Treatment priority is given to correcting hypovolemia because the associated hypoperfusion represents a greater immediate threat to life than does hyperosmolality.

Myxedema Coma

Myxedema coma is the most severe expression of hypothyroidism. Etiologies of hypothyroidism include autoimmune thyroiditis, certain drugs (*eg*, propylthiouracil [PTU], amiodarone, lithium), thyroidectomy or radioactive iodine ablation with inadequate thyroid replacement therapy, and iodine deficiency. An intercurrent acute illness or injury (*eg*, infection, trauma, or surgery) frequently provokes the transition from a compensated to life-threatening state. Subjective manifestations of hypothyroidism can include fatigue, daytime somnolence, difficulty concentrating, cold intolerance, constipation, and myalgias. Objective findings may include goiter, an apathetic affect, lethargy or depressed sensorium, bradycardia or cardiac conduction disturbances, hypothermia, alopecia, dry skin, puffy facies, motor weakness, hoarseness, distant heart sounds, and absent or hypoactive deep tendon reflexes. For the hypothyroidism to be considered severe enough to be categorized as myxedema coma, a depressed level of consciousness is necessary. Hypoventilation is common in myxedema coma and a high proportion of patients progress, sometimes rapidly, to frank respiratory failure.

Arterial blood gas analysis demonstrates hypercapnia and hypoxemia in many patients with this disorder. Other nonspecific blood tests include hyponatremia, hypoglycemia, hyperlipidemia, and elevated creatine phosphokinase activity. Marked elevation of circulating thyroid-stimulating hormone (TSH) levels and depression of circulating free thyroxine (T_4) levels are diagnostic.

Patients who are severely ill often have abnormal thyroid function test results but no physical manifestations of hypothyroidism. Differentiating these false positive laboratory findings, also referred to as the sick euthyroid syndrome, from true hypothyroidism can therefore be difficult in critically ill patients. Most critically ill patients have low levels of free T_4 and tri-iodothyronine (T_3). T_3 is usually low early in the course of acute illness, but T_4 levels can also fall if the illness becomes more severe. Although less common, free T_4 levels are elevated in some patients with this syndrome. TSH is usually unaffected in sick euthyroid syndrome, but mild elevations are not uncommon. The syndrome is characterized by high circulating levels of reverse T_3, the inactive stereoisomer of the physiologically active form of T_3. Most authorities advise against therapeutic thyroid hormone administration to patients with euthyroid sick syndrome.

Specific treatment of myxedema coma consists of hormone replacement. This can be accomplished using a loading dose of thyroxine (eg, 300 to 500 µg IV), followed by daily doses of 50 to 200 µg. Stress doses of hydrocortisone are recommended to cover the possibility of coexistent adrenal insufficiency. For hypothermic patients, passive rewarming is preferred over active methods to avoid hypotension precipitation by cutaneous vasodilation. Endotracheal intubation and mechanical ventilation are frequently required, either for overt respiratory failure or airway protection due to deep coma.

Thyroid Storm

Thyroid storm is life-threatening thyrotoxicosis due to supraphysiologic circulating concentrations of free T_4 or T_3. This is an uncommon medical emergency. The cause is usually Graves' disease, an autoimmune disorder that represents the most common etiology of hyperthyroidism. The second most common etiology is toxic nodular goiter. Thyroid storm is rarely due to other etiologies of hyperthyroidism, although it can result from intentional overdose of thyroid replacement pharmaceuticals.

The distinction between thyrotoxicosis and thyroid storm is that the former can exist in a compensated state with mild to moderate symptoms, while the latter implies life-threatening effects consisting of either cardiac or central nervous system manifestations. Decompensation of thyrotoxicosis to thyroid storm is often triggered by an acute illness or injury. Subjective findings reported in thyrotoxicosis include nervousness, palpitations, fatigue, heat intolerance, dyspnea, anorexia, diarrhea, and weight-loss. Physical examination may reveal a goiter, supraventricular tachydysrhythmias (particularly atrial fibrillation or flutter), systolic hypertension with a widened pulse pressure, signs of congestive heart failure, tremors, hyperreflexia, and changes in mentation. Proptosis and pretibial myxedema may be present if the underlying etiology is Graves' disease. Signs of congestive heart failure or the presence of tachydysrhythmias, respiratory failure, or sensorial changes are common prominent features of thyroid storm.

TSH levels are low in nearly all cases of thyrotoxicosis due to feedback suppression of hypothalamic TSH secretion by high circulating levels of free T_4. Older TSH assays were unable to detect abnormally low TSH levels and could only be used for the diagnosis of hypothyroidism, but more sensitive assays are now routinely available and allow TSH measurement to extremely low concentrations. Plasma free T_4 levels are elevated in thyrotoxicosis, although there is a rare form of hyperthyroidism in which free T_4 levels can be within normal range but plasma T_3 concentrations are abnormally high. While there are no specific threshold biochemical levels that serve to demarcate thyroid storm from compensated thyrotoxicosis, thyroid function test results tend to be more severely abnormal in patients with storm. Other laboratory abnormalities sometimes observed in patients with hyperthyroidism are hypercalcemia and hyperbilirubinemia.

Because this condition can be rapidly progressive and life-threatening, patients with thyroid storm are treated in an ICU. This allows close cardiac and neurologic monitoring and early recognition of dehydration, cardiac dysrhythmias, heart failure, and respiratory failure. Thyroid ablation using radioactive iodine or thyroidectomy are options for treating thyrotoxicosis, but are not used in treating thyroid storm. The use of pharmacologic agents to inhibit thyroid hormone synthesis is another long-term therapeutic option in hyperthyroidism, but it represents the primary specific treatment of thyroid storm. PTU and methimazole are available for this purpose. These drugs stop ongoing synthesis of thyroid hormones; however, there can be enough preformed hormone stored within the thyroid gland to allow continued release into the circulation for days or weeks.

Lugol's iodine solution is traditionally administered as adjunctive therapy to block release of this stored hormone. Other iodine-containing agents, such as the oral radiocontrast agent sodium ipodate, oral potassium iodide solution, or IV sodium iodide, can also be used for this purpose. It is important not to administer any of these iodine-containing preparations until at least 1 h after PTU has been started. If iodine is given first it will augment thyroid hormone synthesis.

β–adrenergic receptor blocking drugs are routinely administered to patients with thyroid storm. Their primary purpose is to blunt the cardiovascular effects of thyrotoxicosis, including tachycardia and hypertension. Propranolol is traditionally used for this purpose, given initially in incremental doses by slow IV injection. High doses are often required to control atrial tachydysrhythmias. If there are relative contraindications to propranolol, a cardioselective β–blocker (eg, metoprolol) may be employed. Another alternative is the use of esmolol, which is given by continuous IV infusion. Since the drug has a short half-life, it has the advantage of rapid resolution of β–blockade after discontinuation of the infusion. Propranolol, sodium ipodate, and corticosteroids are known to inhibit conversion of T_4 to T_3 in peripheral tissues. Because T_3 is the more active thyroid hormone, inhibition of this peripheral conversion may have an adjunctive therapeutic role. Routine hydrocortisone administration has been recommended in thyroid storm because of the possibility of coexisting adrenal insufficiency.

Diabetes Insipidus

Diabetes insipidus (DI) occurs when water reabsorption at the distal renal tubules and collecting ducts is curtailed, resulting in polyuria and loss of urinary concentrating ability. In central DI the mechanism is lack of antidiuretic hormone (ADH) secretion by the posterior pituitary (ADH normally acts on the distal nephron to increase its permeability to water, resulting in reabsorption of water and production of concentrated urine). In nephrogenic DI the mechanism is intrinsic unresponsiveness of the distal nephron to the action of ADH. Both forms of the disorder can lead to dehydration. Otherwise normal subjects will eventually experience intense thirst and, if they have access to water, will exhibit polydipsia, preventing clinical dehydration. Patients with DI who also have sensorial changes that blunt thirst or the ability to act on it will develop dehydration unless it is provided therapeutically in adequate volumes. Other manifestations of DI are a reflection either of the underlying cause or the ensuing dehydration.

Central DI can be idiopathic or acquired. Acquired forms can be caused by head trauma, hypophysectomy, brain tumors, intracranial hemorrhage, anoxic encephalopathy, meningitis, encephalitis, granulomatous diseases of the brain, cerebrovascular aneurysm, and cerebral thromboembolic disease. Nephrogenic DI is associated with polycystic kidney disease, sickle-cell disease, medullary sponge disease, sarcoidosis, hypercalcemia, and prolonged hypokalemia. The drugs lithium, amphotericin B, demeclocycline, and vinblastine can also cause nephrogenic DI. There are congenital forms of both types of DI.

Polyuria occurs in DI but it is not specific for DI. Other causes of polyuria include excess fluid administration, diuretic use, hyperglycemia, and the polyuria that can occur after acute renal failure or relief of obstructive uropathy. Another cause is loss of the normal solute concentration gradient between the renal medulla and cortex (so-called "medullary washout"), which can occur after prolonged polyuria of any cause.

Although it is not specific for DI, hypernatremia is a common manifestation in hospitalized patients with DI, particularly in the ICU setting. On the other hand, hypernatremia is usually absent in patients with DI who are not acutely ill, since they will simply drink sufficient water to prevent the development of hypernatremia. Critically ill patients often have impaired thirst mechanisms or a globally diminished sensorium due to sedation or encephalopathy. These factors lead to dehydration and hypernatremia even in the absence of DI, with more rapid development of dehydration and hypernatremia in patients with DI.

The diagnosis of DI is classically made by depriving the patient of water to provoke mild dehydration and hypernatremia, and then examining the effect on urine output and concentrating ability. However, water deprivation testing should not be utilized in patients requiring intensive care because there is a risk of provoking hypovolemia in acutely ill or unstable patients. In addition, many critically ill patients with DI develop hypernatremia spontaneously making provocative testing unnecessary. The diagnosis can be made in these patients simply by demonstrating inappropriately low urine osmolality in the face of hypernatremia.

Water deprivation normally results in hypernatremia and elaboration of hyperosmolar urine with a total solute concentration exceeding 800 millimoles (mosm)/kg H_2O. In complete central DI the urine osmolality is below 300 mosm/kg H_2O, whereas in partial central DI it ranges between 300 and 800 mosm/kg H_2O. In the face of water deprivation, plasma ADH concentration is normally >2 pg/mL; however, in complete central DI, ADH is undetectable. In partial central DI, ADH levels may reach 1.5 pg/mL. Plasma ADH levels can exceed 5 pg/mL in nephrogenic DI. Discrimination of central from nephrogenic DI can be accomplished more simply by assaying urine osmolality before and after subcutaneous administration of 2 µg of desmopressin, an ADH analog. Normally this results in no more than a 5% increase in urine osmolality, but in complete central DI an increase of at least 50% is observed. An intermediate rise (ie, between 10% and 50%) is consistent with partial central DI. In nephrogenic DI, no change is expected because the nephron is refractory to both ADH and desmopressin.

Severe polyuria can occur in DI, in some cases exceeding 20 L/d. Careful monitoring of fluid intake and output, frequent measurement of serum sodium concentration, and judicious titration of IV fluids are important to prevent severe volume depletion. IV normal saline should be administered to patients who have or develop hypovolemia or signs of circulatory embarrassment, even though the patient is hypernatremic, because it will expand intravascular volume more effectively than hypotonic fluids, and because correction of hypovolemia takes priority over correction of hyperosmolality. Once intravascular volume is normalized, hypotonic fluids can be substituted, targeting correction of half of the free-water deficit during the first 24 h of therapy, and the remaining deficit over the next 48 h or so. It is imperative to take ongoing urinary fluid losses into account. Overhydration should be avoided because it can induce a water diuresis that increases the risk of medullary washout, potentially leading to sustained polyuria even if ADH replacement therapy is given or the DI otherwise resolves. Frequent monitoring of serum electrolytes is necessary because hypokalemia, hypomagnesemia, and hypophosphatemia can develop rapidly in some polyuric patients.

IV fluid administration and close monitoring may be adequate treatment for mild cases of DI in the ICU. For patients with central DI and marked polyuria, ADH replacement therapy is indicated to limit the polyuria and decrease the risk of dehydration. Aqueous vasopressin has a short duration of action that allows close titration. However, it can have potent vasoconstricting effects, particularly in critically ill patients and those with sepsis. If given subcutaneously or intramuscularly to these patients it can result in soft tissue necrosis. It can also provoke coronary ischemia in susceptible patients. Desmopressin is a safer alternative because it acts only on V_2 receptors in the nephron, and not on V_1 receptors located on vascular smooth muscle, and therefore lacks the vasoconstrictive effect of vasopressin. Desmopressin is typically dosed as 2 to 4 µg/d subcutaneously or IV in 2 divided doses. For stable patients, it is also available in an intranasal formulation, which is typically dosed at 10 to 40 µg/d in 2 to 3 divided doses.

As with central DI, the treatment of nephrogenic DI requires the same careful attention to fluid and electrolyte balance. However, ADH analogs are generally of no benefit in nephrogenic DI. Treatment for this variant otherwise consists of stopping any drugs that could be implicated as causative, and controlling polyuria with hydrochlorothiazide. Thiazide diuretics limit polyuria in nephrogenic DI by inducing mild volume contraction, stimulating sodium and water reabsorption in the proximal renal tubule and thereby diminishing water delivery to the distal nephron.

Adrenal Failure

Adrenal failure is the relative or absolute lack of adrenal corticosteroid production due to primary adrenal gland failure or secondary to insufficient adrenocorticotropic hormone (ACTH) elaboration by the anterior pituitary. Primary adrenal failure is most commonly due to autoimmune destruction of the adrenal glands, but is also caused by various infiltrative diseases involving the glands (*eg*, sarcoidosis, amyloidosis, or malignancy), including infectious diseases (*eg*, meningococcemia, pseudomonal infection, tuberculosis, or viral infections). Relative primary adrenal insufficiency is also observed in some patients with sepsis regardless of the specific micro-organism. An association between adrenal insufficiency and AIDS has been documented. Other causes include drug-induced adrenal impairment (*eg*, etomidate and ketoconazole), and hemorrhage or infarction affecting the glands. The most common cause of secondary failure is sudden withdrawal of chronic corticosteroid therapy. Other secondary causes include head trauma, brain tumors, stroke, pituitary surgery, infiltrative brain diseases, anoxic encephalopathy, and cranial radiation therapy.

Subjective manifestations of the disorder include anorexia, fatigue, nausea, vomiting, abdominal pain, diarrhea, myalgia, arthralgia, orthostatic lightheadedness, and salt craving. Physical examination may reveal orthostatic or frank hypotension, tachycardia, weight loss, abdominal tenderness, confusion, and hyper- or hypopigmented skin. An intercurrent illness or surgery can provoke adrenal crisis in patients with otherwise compensated adrenal insufficiency.

A variety of nonspecific laboratory abnormalities can be seen in adrenal insufficiency, including hyponatremia, hyperkalemia, hypercalcemia, hypoglycemia, prerenal azotemia, and a normal anion gap metabolic acidosis. Anemia, neutropenia, lymphocytosis, and eosinophilia can also be seen. Plasma cortisol levels <15 μg/dL are clearly abnormal in a severely stressed patient. In the acute setting, the diagnosis is conventionally confirmed by stimulation testing using a synthetic ACTH analog. Blood is first sampled for baseline plasma cortisol assay, and then re-sampled 30 and 60 min after giving 250 μg of cosyntropin IV. If warranted, treatment can be started after the poststimulation samples are obtained, without waiting for the assay results. Starting treatment with hydrocortisone before obtaining the poststimulation blood samples will result in falsely elevated plasma cortisol results. In highly unstable patients in whom a 1-h or so delay in therapy could be compromising, treatment can be initiated with one dose of dexamethasone at the time stimulation testing is begun. Unlike hydrocortisone, dexamethasone does not cross-react with laboratory cortisol assays. Adrenal failure is likely if the highest poststimulation cortisol level is <15 μg/dL. Levels >18 μg/dL are conventionally accepted as excluding most cases of adrenal insufficiency, but levels up to 25 mg/dL may represent an inadequate response in patients who are profoundly stressed.

Patients with adrenal crisis are fluid resuscitated and admitted to the ICU. Rapid initiation of fluid resuscitation is critical because most patients are severely volume-depleted. The preferred IV solution is 5% dextrose in isotonic saline, which expands intravascular volume and corrects or prevents hypoglycemia. The definitive treatment for adrenal crisis is IV hydrocortisone. The initial dose is 200 mg, followed by 300 mg/d given as either 100 mg IV every 8 h or 12.5 mg/h by continuous IV infusion.

Pheochromocytoma

Pheochromocytoma is an uncommon disorder caused by a usually benign tumor arising from the adrenal medulla and consisting of catecholamine-producing chromaffin cells. The tumor less commonly arises from extra-adrenal sites, particularly the organs of Zuckerkandl adjacent to the aortic bifurcation. The disorder is also associated with von Recklinghausen's disease as well as with types IIa and IIb multiple endocrine neoplasia syndrome. Manifestations are usually paroxysmal, typically lasting about 30 min, and most commonly consist of anxiety, headache, cutaneous flushing, tremors, and palpitations associated with hypertension. In some cases the hypertension is severe enough to be classified as a hypertensive emergency; ie, it can be accompanied by end-organ derangements such as acute left ventricular dysfunction and pulmonary edema. Diaphoresis, chest pain, nausea, vomiting, abdominal pain, tachydysrhythmias, and orthostatic hypo- or hypertension can also occur. Sustained hypertension occurs in some cases.

The manifestations of pheochromocytoma are the result of acute release of excessive amounts of catecholamines. Thus, the diagnosis is made by demonstrating increased production or circulating levels of these hormones. This is conventionally performed by assaying 24-h urinary excretion of the catecholamines epinephrine and norepinephrine, as well as their metabolic byproducts, the metanephrines and vanillylmandelic acid, and by assaying plasma catecholamine levels. However, the finding of normal plasma catecholamine and urinary metanephrine levels does not reliably exclude pheochromocytoma. More recent investigations have shown that the single best biochemical screening test is the plasma metanephrine assay. Normal plasma metanephrine results effectively exclude the diagnosis of pheochromocytoma.

Definitive diagnostic testing is problematic in the ICU setting because many acute physiologic derangements that are common among critically ill patients interfere with the relevant biochemical assays. Examples of these physiologic derangements include congestive heart failure, myocardial infarction, respiratory failure, renal failure, sepsis, hypoglycemia, hypothyroidism, anemia, peptic ulcer disease, neurologic abnormalities, dehydration, and a variety of drugs (eg, catecholamines, adrenergic receptor blocking agents, vasodilators, and diuretics). Thus, biochemical confirmation is best deferred until after the patient is stabilized and transferred out of the ICU. After the diagnosis of pheochromocytoma has been biochemically confirmed, the tumor is then localized using noninvasive imaging studies. These can include MRI, CT, and radiolabeled m-iodobenzylguanidine scintigraphy.

Surgical removal of the tumor is usually curative, but it entails considerable risk due to the prospect of provoking hypertensive crisis. To minimize this complication, surgery is delayed until the patient is stabilized, blood pressure is controlled, volume status is optimized, and any accompanying acute medical conditions are treated. In an acute episode of hypertensive crisis, the conventional pharmacologic agent of choice is phentolamine mesylate. This drug is a short-acting α-adrenergic receptor blocking agent that is initiated as sequential IV bolus doses (typically 2 to 5 mg) at intervals of 5 min or more until the desired blood pressure is reached. An alternative agent is sodium nitroprusside. Neither of these agents can be given chronically. For chronic α–adrenergic blockade, phenoxybenzamine can be used. β–adrenergic receptor blocking drugs are usually not necessary, but may be used adjunctively to control tachydysrhythmias. However, β–adrenergic blockers are contraindicated in patients who have not already received adequate α–adrenergic blockade because unopposed α–adrenergic stimulation can precipitate a hypertensive emergency.

The chapter, Endocrine Emergencies, is jointly held by the Society of Critical Care Medicine and the ACCP.

Annotated Bibliography

Annane D, Sebille V, Charpentier C, et al. Effect of treatment with low doses of hydrocortisone and fludrocortisone on mortality in patients with septic shock. JAMA 2002; 288:862-871

A clinical trial showing improved outcome in patients with septic shock, including those with relative adrenal insufficiency treated with 7 days of low-dose hydrocortisone and fludrocortisone.

Bichet DG. Nephrogenic diabetes insipidus. Am J Med 1998; 105:431-432

Supplemented by excellent illustrations, this review details the pathophysiology of nephrogenic DI.

Blevins LS, Wand GS. Diabetes insipidus. Crit Care Med 1992; 20:69-79

Another review that provides a good general overview of DI.

Genuth SM. Diabetic ketoacidosis and hyperglycemic hyperosmolar coma. Curr Ther Endocrinol Metab 1997; 6:438-447

A good tutorial review.

Kannan CR, Seshadri KG. Thyrotoxicosis. Disease-A-Month 1997; 43:601-677

An extensive review of the topic, with 144 references.

Kruse JA, Fink MP, Carlson RW, eds. Saunders Manual of Critical Care. Philadelphia, PA: WB Saunders, 2003; 164–193

Contains nine succinct chapters providing practical information on the clinical management of endocrine emergencies.

Lamberts SWJ, Bruining HA, de Jong FH. Corticosteroid therapy in severe illness. N Engl J Med 1997; 337:1285-1292

An excellent review of hypoadrenalism, focusing on the problems of diagnosis and management in the setting of critical illness. Discusses the concept of occult relative adrenal insufficiency.

Lenders JWM, Keiser HR, Goldstein DS, et al. Plasma metanephrines in the diagnosis of pheochromocytoma. Ann Intern Med 1995; 123:101-109

A study comparing the diagnostic sensitivity of plasma metanephrine measurement to measurement of plasma catecholamines and urinary metanephrines.

Oelkers W. Adrenal insufficiency. N Engl J Med 1996; 335:1206-1212

This report includes a good overview of various hormonal functional assessments, including provocative evaluations that are more complex than the rapid cosyntropin test.

Pacak K, Linehan WM, Eisenhofer G, et al. Recent advances in genetics, diagnosis, localization, and treatment of pheochromocytoma. Ann Intern Med 2001; 134:315-329

An update on neurochemical diagnostics, localization imaging, and surgical management.

Roberge RJ, Martin TG, Delbridge TR. Intentional massive insulin overdose: recognition and management. Ann Emerg Med 1993; 22:228-234

This review covers diagnostic and treatment considerations for managing hypoglycemia due to insulin overdose. The presentation includes a case report followed by a question and answer discussion.

Service FJ. Classification of hypoglycemic disorders. Endocrinol Metab Clin North Am 1999; 28(3):519-532

This entire issue is devoted to hypoglycemia. In addition to the article cited, the issue contains articles on the physiology of glucose counterregulation to hypoglycemia, drug-induced causes, diagnostic approaches, and others.

Singer I, Oster JR, Fishman LM. The management of diabetes insipidus in adults. Arch Intern Med 1997; 157:1293-1301

A comprehensive, practical review of short- and long-term management of patients with central and nephrogenic DI.

Smallridge RC. Metabolic and anatomic thyroid emergencies: a review. Crit Care Med 1992; 20:276-291

Provides a detailed review of the pathophysiology, diagnosis, and management of thyroid storm and myxedema coma. Contains 154 references.

Umpierrez GE, Khajavi M, Kitabchi AE. Review: diabetic ketoacidosis and hyper-glycemic hyperosmolar nonketotic syndrome. Am J Med Sci 1996; 311:225-233

A detailed review of hyperglycemic emergencies.

Viallon A, Zeni F, Lafond P, et al. Does bicarbonate therapy improve the management of severe diabetic ketoacidosis? Crit Care Med 1999; 27:2690-2693

A descriptive study and review of literature on the treatment of DKA with sodium bicarbonate.

Yamamoto T, Fukuyama J, Fujiyoshi A. Factors associated with mortality of myxedema coma: report of eight cases and literature survey. Thyroid 1999; 9:1167-1174

Examines the issue of high-dose versus low-dose thyroid replacement therapy for myxedema coma.

Zaloga GP, Marik PE, eds. Endocrine and metabolic dysfunction syndromes in the critically ill. Crit Care Clin 2001; 17:1-252

This entire bound issue is devoted to endocrine and metabolic disturbances pertinent to the ICU setting. Includes individual articles on thyroid, adrenal, pituitary, and glycemic crises.

Notes

Obesity and Critical Illness

Brian K. Gehlbach, MD

Objectives:

- Describe the cardiovascular effects of obesity.
- Describe the effects of morbid obesity on the respiratory system.
- Discuss the management of respiratory failure in the morbidly obese patient.

Key words: body mass index; obesity; obesity hypoventilation syndrome; obstructive sleep apnea

The Clinical Problem

The following definitions are customarily employed: overweight is defined as a body mass index (BMI) >25 kg/m², obesity is defined as a BMI >30 kg/m², and morbid obesity is defined as a BMI >40 kg/m². Some authorities extend the definition of morbid obesity to include individuals who have serious comorbidities and a BMI >35 kg/m².

Data from the 1999–2000 National Health and Nutrition Examination Survey[1] indicate that the prevalence of overweight, obese, and morbidly obese individuals continues to rise (64.5, 30.5, and 4.7%, respectively). It is therefore important for the intensivist to recognize the physiologic consequences of obesity in the critically ill patient as well as be aware of potential pitfalls in the management of such patients. This chapter will concentrate principally on the patient with morbid obesity.

Cardiovascular Effects of Morbid Obesity

Obesity is capable of promoting cardiovascular disease through a number of potential mechanisms including insulin resistance, hypertension, dyslipidemia, and coagulation abnormalities.[2,3] Furthermore, the hearts of such patients are exposed to chronic volume and pressure overload. Cardiac output increases in obesity as extracellular volume rises. This results in cardiac dilatation with subsequent eccentric left ventricular hypertrophy. Increased left ventricular afterload from chronic hypertension may further promote the development of left ventricular hypertrophy and diastolic heart failure. Systolic failure may be caused by ischemic heart disease, longstanding hypertension, or from obesity itself.

Certain obese patients present with pulmonary hypertension. It is important to recognize the many potential causes of this disorder and that obstructive sleep apnea (OSA), by itself, typically causes only mild pulmonary hypertension. When OSA is combined with obstructive lung disease or another chronic lung disease, however, severe pulmonary hypertension and cor pulmonale may result. The obesity hypoventilation syndrome (OHS), characterized by obesity and daytime hypercapnea and hypoxemia, is also associated with pulmonary hypertension that may be severe, and usually—although not always—with OSA as well. Diastolic heart failure is an important and often-overlooked cause of pulmonary hypertension in this population, while chronic thromboembolic disease should be given consideration given the increased risk of venous thromboembolism in obesity.

Implications for the Intensivist

A high index of suspicion for the presence of heart disease is merited in the morbidly obese patient, even in the absence of traditional risk factors such as tobacco use or diabetes. The difficulty of examining the morbidly obese patient sometimes frustrates the diagnosis of congestive heart failure, increasing the clinician's reliance on echocardiography to confirm the presence of systolic or diastolic dysfunction when congestive heart failure is suspected. Limitations of echocardiography in this setting include poor visualization of cardiac structures (particularly of the right ventricle) and an imperfect sensitivity for the diagnosis of diastolic dysfunction in this population. Selected patients may benefit from transesophageal echocardiography or invasive monitoring.

Pathophysiology of Respiratory Failure in Morbid Obesity

The effects of obesity on pulmonary function are highly variable, with physiologic impairment correlating only loosely with BMI and being influenced by the distribution of body fat (central vs peripheral) as well as the strength of the respiratory muscle pump.[4,5] The earliest change evident on pulmonary function tests is a decline in the expiratory reserve volume. Morbidly obese individuals and those with the OHS frequently exhibit a restrictive pattern, with reductions in total lung capacity, FVC, and FEV_1. An increase in airway resistance and a reduction in mid to late expiratory flows have been reported in some patients.[6] The compliance of the respiratory system is reduced, mostly because of reduced chest wall compliance. Small airway closure in the dependent regions of the lung causes mismatching of ventilation and perfusion with resulting arterial hypoxemia, typically worse in the supine position.[7] Ventilation near the closing volume of the lung predisposes the obese patient to atelectasis, particularly in the postoperative period. Respiratory drive is typically normal except in patients with the OHS, in whom it is reduced.

Implications for the Intensivist

The major consequence of these alterations is that morbidly obese patients may be particularly susceptible to respiratory failure. Typically, <5% of the total oxygen consumption is attributable to the work of breathing. Chronic lung diseases such as emphysema place an increased load on the respiratory system, with a corresponding increase in the oxygen consumed by the respiratory muscles (Vo_2RESP). In such cases, the neuromuscular competence of the respiratory system may just be sufficient to meet the increased load placed on it. Similar to emphysema, morbid obesity is associated with an increased baseline Vo_2RESP (up to 16% in a cohort of patients scheduled for bariatric surgery[8]) as well as a disproportionate rise in Vo_2RESP with increases in minute ventilation. This decrease in pulmonary reserve predisposes the morbidly obese patient to respiratory failure from seemingly trivial insults such as postoperative atelectasis or viral respiratory infection.

Evaluation of Respiratory Failure

The evaluation of morbidly obese patients with respiratory failure is challenging, in large part because of limitations in our usual diagnostic tools when used in this population. The chest radiograph is often difficult or even impossible to interpret, although sometimes changes seen over time are useful. CT is often unavailable due to the size of the patient. Frequently, the clinician is required to make diagnoses based on the data available: for example, congestive heart failure in the patient with frothy secretions from the endotracheal tube, hypoxemia refractory to high-flow oxygen, evidence of diastolic dysfunction on echocardiography, and an absence of signs of systemic inflammation. In such a patient, a response to empiric diuretic therapy may be diagnostic. Pneumonia may be suggested by fever, cough, sputum production, leukocytosis, and hypoxemia. Pulmonary embolism may be particularly difficult either to diagnose or exclude due to the inability to obtain a CT scan and the frequent nondiagnostic results of ventilation-perfusion scanning. While echocardiography may suggest the diagnosis by showing evidence of right-heart dilatation, this finding is not specific given other potential explanations for this finding such as cor pulmonale from the OHS or from the combination of severe OSA and obstructive lung disease. Still, at our institution, we frequently administer anticoagulates to the patient empirically when we encounter this finding, unless the history and physical findings clearly support an alternative diagnosis such as OHS and pulmonary embolism is deemed very unlikely. We also order serial leg studies to exclude the presence of a lower extremity deep venous thrombosis. D-dimer is rarely useful in this setting because of the low frequency of normal values obtained in this population.

Management of Respiratory Failure

The patient presenting with cardiopulmonary failure from sleep-disordered breathing and/or the OHS is best treated with noninvasive positive pressure ventilation, when possible. This therapy typically abolishes obstructive respiratory events, promotes sleep, unloads the respiratory muscles, decreases atelectasis, and avoids the risks associated with endotracheal intubation and sedation.

Cardiac function frequently improves as well through a variety of potential mechanisms including but not limited to improved right ventricular ejection due to decreased pulmonary vascular resistance. Severely volume overloaded patients with the OHS previously found to be resistant to diuretic therapy may undergo a "spontaneous" diuresis once adequate ventilation and oxygenation is achieved.

Intubation of the morbidly obese patient may be difficult, particularly in those patients with high Mallampati scores and large neck circumferences.[9,10] The morbidly obese patient is more likely to experience desaturation during attempted intubation because of a reduced functional residual capacity with attendant decreased oxygen stores. The risk of aspiration of gastric contents may be increased, so a "full stomach" should be assumed. An experienced operator should be present for the intubation, if possible.

Morbidly obese patients frequently require the provision of positive end-expiratory pressure of 8 to 15 cm H_2O in order to prevent atelectasis and improve gas exchange. The supine position places the diaphragm at a considerable disadvantage in such patients. It is therefore unreasonable to expect patients with marginal respiratory function to undergo spontaneous breathing trials without first placing them in the reverse Trendelenburg position.

Lung protective strategies are difficult to apply to the morbidly obese patient because of the inherent difficulty in detecting alveolar overdistension in this population. An elevated plateau pressure does not necessarily indicate alveolar overdistension because of the contribution of increased chest wall elastance to this value in the morbidly obese patient. When acute lung injury is present, the initial tidal volume should be 6 mL/kg of ideal body weight. If this results in an elevated plateau pressure (>30 cm H_2O), the need to reduce the tidal volume to prevent further lung injury is uncertain. A first step is to remeasure lung mechanics in the reverse Trendelenburg position. If the plateau pressure is still elevated, consideration should be given to reducing the tidal volume if this can be readily achieved. If not, plateau pressures up to 35 to 40 cm H_2O may still be acceptable in the extremely obese patient, although this is not known.

Selected patients are appropriate for early tracheostomy. This group includes patients with severe OSA refractory to medical therapy, when long-term nocturnal ventilation for the OHS is planned, and when the course of critical care and subsequent rehabilitation is expected to be prolonged.

Other Problems

Drug Dosing

While the volume of distribution for drugs with greater lipophilicity is generally increased, there are notable exceptions to this rule, indicating the importance of other typically unmeasured clinical variables such as plasma protein binding. Also problematic is the finding of significant intersubject variability in pharmacokinetics. It is therefore difficult to make generalizations regarding the dosing of drugs, and reference to published guidelines for individual drugs is recommended.[11,12] Close monitoring of clinically available serum drug levels is also advisable.

Nutritional Support

Lipolysis and fat oxidation is reduced in critically ill obese patients relative to nonobese subjects. This increases protein breakdown with the potential for adverse effects on immune function, wound healing, and lean muscle mass. Thus, while carefully controlled hypocaloric nutritional support that ensures adequate provision of protein may be safe, an effort to accelerate a program of weight loss while the patient is in the ICU should be avoided.[13] Because conventional equations for the provision of nutritional support are unreliable in this setting, indirect calorimetry should be used.

Establishing Vascular Access

Establishing central access can be particularly challenging in the critically ill patient. The femoral site should be avoided because of the increased risk of infection and thrombosis at this site; this site is often difficult to access as well because of intertrigo. While the subclavian vein is an attractive site for central access, the sharp angle required to enter the blood vessel can make passage of the dilator under the clavicle difficult. On occasion, the needle and the introducer may actually be too short for this site. As a result, the internal jugular vein is often the preferred site in the morbidly obese patient, even with the increased difficulty posed by a thick (and sometimes "short") neck. Ultrasound guidance may be useful when there is experience with this modality.

Venous Thromboembolism

The risk of venous thromboembolism is increased in obesity, meriting an aggressive approach to prophylaxis in such patients. While conclusive data to support this practice are lacking, the joint use of pneumatic compression boots and increased-dose subcutaneous heparin (7,500 U bid to tid) is appropriate.

Annotated References

1. Flegal KM, Carroll MD, Ogden CL, Johnson CL. Prevalence and trends in obesity among US adults, 1999–2000. JAMA 2002; 288:1723–1727
   Recent data from the National Health and Nutrition Examination Survey describing the prevalence of obesity and overweight in the United States.

2. Schunkert H. Obesity and target organ damage: the heart. Int J Obesity 2002; 26(suppl 4):S15–S20
   A review of the mechanisms of obesity-related cardiovascular disease.

3. Hall JE, Crook ED, Jones DW, et al. Mechanisms of obesity-associated cardiovascular and renal disease. Am J Med Sci 2002; 324:127–137
   A review of the mechanisms of obesity-related cardiovascular and renal disease.

4. Koenig SM. Pulmonary complications of obesity. Am J Med Sci 2001; 321:249–279
   Comprehensive review of the pulmonary complications of obesity, including a review of the effects of obesity on pulmonary function.

5. Unterborn J. Pulmonary function testing in obesity, pregnancy, and extremes of body habitus. Clin Chest Med 2001; 22:759–767
   A review of pulmonary function testing in obesity, pregnancy, and extremes of body habitus.

6. Rubinstein I, Zamel N, DuBarry L, et al. Airflow limitation in morbidly obese, nonsmoking men. Annals Intern Med 1990; 112:828–832
   Descriptive study of 103 obese, lifelong nonsmokers without cardiopulmonary disease compared with 190 healthy, nonobese nonsmoking control subjects.

7. Douglas FG, Chong PY. Influence of obesity on peripheral airways patency. J Appl Physiol 1972; 33:559–563
   The investigators demonstrated that "reduction in expiratory reserve volume due to obesity results in a tendency to closure of small peripheral airways in dependent lung zones," leading to impaired gas exchange.

8. Kress JP, Pohlman AS, Alverdy J, Hall JB. The impact of morbid obesity on oxygen cost of breathing at rest. Am J Respir Crit Care Med 1999; 160:883–886
   Describes the oxygen cost of breathing at rest in a cohort of morbidly obese patients scheduled for bariatric surgery.

9. Ogunnaike BO, Jones SB, Jones DB, et al. Anesthetic considerations for bariatric surgery. Anesth Analg 2002; 95:1793–1805
   A review of anesthetic considerations in the patient being evaluated for bariatric surgery.

10. Brodsky JB, Lemmens HJM, Brock-Utne JG, et al. Morbid obesity and tracheal intubation. Anesth Analg 2002; 94:732–736
    Analyzed risk factors for a difficult intubation in 100 consecutive morbidly obese patients undergoing elective surgery.

11. Marik P, Varon J. The obese patient in the ICU. Chest 1998; 113:492–498
    While not a recent review, there is very little new information since this was published. It includes a brief but readable discussion of drug dosing in obese patients.

12. Blouin RA, Warren GW. Pharmacokinetic considerations in obesity. J Pharm Sci 1999; 88:1–7
    A review of pharmacokinetic considerations in obesity.

13. Mechanick JI, Brett EM. Nutrition support of the chronically critically ill patient. Crit Care Clin 2002; 18:597–618
    Reviews nutrition support of the chronically critically ill patient, including the management of the obese patient.

Notes

Notes

Nervous System Infections and Catheter Infections

George H. Karam, MD, FCCP

Objectives:

- To review clinical presentations of nervous system infections that may present as serious or life-threatening processes
- To outline principles influencing diagnosis and management of nervous system infections
- To present an approach to infections related to catheters placed in the vasculature, urinary bladder, or peritoneum
- To summarize existing opinions and data about management of catheter-related infections

Key words: botulism; brain abscess; catheter-related infections; cavernous sinus thrombosis; encephalitis; meningitis; rabies; spinal epidural abscess

Introduction

Infection affecting various parts of the nervous system has the potential to be life-threatening or to result in severe sequelae if the infection is not appropriately diagnosed and treated. Although infections such as meningitis, encephalitis, and brain abscess are the most frequently encountered, processes such as spinal epidural abscess, septic intracranial thrombophlebitis, rabies, and botulism may present as emergent problems that require a high level of clinical suspicion for prompt diagnoses to be made. Infections associated with catheters placed in the vasculature, urinary bladder, or peritoneum can also result in morbidity and create diagnostic or therapeutic dilemmas for the clinician. This review will attempt to summarize these infections as they relate to the critical care setting.

Nervous System Infections

Meningitis

From 1986 to 1995, the median age of persons with bacterial meningitis increased from 15 months to 25 years, making meningitis in the United States predominantly a disease of adults rather than of infants and young children.[1]

The basic diagnostic tool in the diagnosis of meningitis is examination of cerebrospinal fluid (CSF). When such fluid is obtained, important clinical studies include (1) stains and cultures, (2) glucose, (3) protein, and (4) cell count with differential. Gram stain and culture of CSF are highly specific but may have a median sensitivity of about 75%. Helpful in understanding the pathogenesis of meningitis due to varied processes is the CSF glucose level. Glucose enters the CSF by facilitated transport across choroid plexuses and capillaries lining the CSF space.[2] Normally, the CSF-to-blood glucose ratio is 0.6. Although consumption of glucose by white blood cells and organisms may contribute to low CSF glucose levels (which is referred to as *hypoglycorrhachia*), the major mechanism for low glucose is impaired transport into the CSF; this classically occurs because of acute inflammation or with infiltration of the meninges by granulomas or malignant cells. Protein is usually excluded from the CSF but levels rise after disruption of the blood-brain barrier. Levels are lower in cisternal and ventricular CSF than in lumbar CSF. Usual elevations in patients with meningitis are in the 100 to 500 mg/dL range. Extreme elevations (*ie*, >1,000 mg/dL) are often indicative of subarachnoid block. When protein levels exceed 150 mg/dL, the fluid may appear xanthochromic.

The diagnosis of meningitis is made by the finding of a CSF pleocytosis and may occur on the basis of both infectious and noninfectious processes. In the absence of a positive stain on the CSF, the most helpful study in the initial approach to the patient with meningitis is a cell count with differential on the CSF. As summarized in Table 1, an approach for diagnosing the etiology of meningitis based on the CSF analysis would include three common categories: (1) polymorphonuclear meningitis, (2) lymphocytic meningitis with a normal glucose, and (3) lymphocytic meningitis with a low glucose. In addition, on rare occasions patients may have a predominance of eosinophils in the CSF, but eosinophilic meningitis is uncommon.

Polymorphonuclear Meningitis: Because of the acute inflammation, this process is usually associated with a low CSF glucose owing to impaired transport across the meninges. This is most notable with bacterial meningitis. In the differential diagnosis of polymorphonuclear meningitis, there are four major groups of disease: (1) bacterial infection, (2) the early meningeal response to any type of infection or inflammation, (3) parameningeal foci, and (4) persistent neutrophilic meningitis. Because of the sequelae that may be associated with a delay in therapy, the single most important cause of a polymorphonuclear meningitis is bacterial infection. Discussion in this syllabus will be limited to this topic.

Likely etiologic agents for bacterial meningitis are summarized in Table 2 from the perspectives of (1) the age of the patient and (2) underlying predispositions to meningitis. Presented in a different manner, rates of meningitis per 100,000 population in 22 counties in four states revealed the following: *Streptococcus pneumoniae*, 1.1; *Neisseria meningitidis*, 0.6; group B streptococci, 0.3; *Listeria monocytogenes*, 0.2; and *Haemophilus influenzae*, 0.2.[1] The most notable change in etiologic agents over the past decade has been the dramatic decrease in the incidence of *H influenzae* meningitis, which has occurred as a result of vaccination against this pathogen.

Although pneumococci are the most common pathogens in bacterial meningitis, the problematic strains of *S pneumoniae* are those that are penicillin-resistant. Strains with relative, or intermediate, resistance will have a penicillin minimal inhibitory concentration (MIC) of 0.12 to 1.0 µg/mL. High-level resistance to penicillin is defined as an MIC ≥2 µg/mL.[3] Compounding this problem is the inability of certain antibiotics to cross the blood-brain barrier effectively enough to yield CSF levels significantly above the MIC for the infecting organism. For pneumococcal meningitis caused by penicillin-susceptible strains, penicillin G and ampicillin are equally effective. Although high-dose penicillin (150,000 to 250,000 U/kg/d) has been useful in patients with pneumonia caused by strains of pneumococci with intermediate resistance, such high doses do not predictably lead to CSF levels of

Table 1. *An Approach to CSF Pleocytosis**

Polymorphonuclear	Lymphocytic With Normal Glucose	Lymphocytic With Low Glucose
Bacterial (see Table 2)	Viral meningitis	Fungal
Early meningitis	Enteroviruses, including poliovirus	Tuberculous
Tuberculosis	Herpes simplex virus (usually type 2)	Certain forms of meningoencephalitis (*eg*, herpes simplex) or viral meningitis
Fungal	HIV	Partially treated bacterial meningitis
Viral	Adenovirus	Carcinomatous meningitis
Drug-induced	Tick-borne viruses	Subarachnoid hemorrhage
Parameningeal foci	Meningoencephalitis, including viral causes	Chemical meningitis
Brain abscess	Parameningeal foci	
Subdural empyema	Partially treated bacterial meningitis	
Epidural abscess	Listeria meningitis	
Sinusitis	Spirochetal infections	
Mastoiditis	Syphilis	
Osteomyelitis	Leptospirosis	
Persistent neutrophilic meningitis	Lyme disease	
	Rickettsial infections	
	Rocky Mountain spotted fever	
	Ehrlichiosis	
	Infective endocarditis	
	Immune-mediated diseases	
	Sarcoidosis	
	Drug-induced	

*Although not clinically common in the United States, eosinophilic meningitis can occur, and the characteristic pathogens causing such a process are *Angiostrongylus cantonesis, Trichinella spiralis, Taenia solium, Toxocara canis, Gnathostoma spinigerum, Paragonimus westwermani,* and *Baylisascaris procyonis.*

Table 2. *Likely Pathogens in Bacterial Meningitis Based on Patient's Age or Underlying Conditions*

Neonates	Enterobacteriaceae Group B streptococci *Listeria monocytogenes*
<6 yr	*Neisseria meningitidis, Streptococcus pneumoniae Haemophilus influenzae*
6 yr to young adult	*N meningitidis, S pneumoniae*
Adults < 50 yr	*S pneumoniae, N meningitidis*
Alcoholic and elderly	*S pneumoniae, N meningitidis* Enterobacteriaceae *L monocytogenes*
Closed skull fracture	*S pneumoniae, H influenzae* *Staphylococcus aureus* Coagulase-negative staphylococci Gram-negative bacilli
Open skull fracture	Gram-negative bacilli, including *Klebsiella pneumoniae* and *Acinetobacter calcoaceticus* (when meningitis develops from a contiguous postoperative traumatic wound infection) *S aureus*
Penetrating trauma; Postneurosurgery	*S aureus* Coagulase-negative staphylococci Aerobic Gram-negative bacilli (including *Pseudomonas aeruginosa*)
CSF leak	*S pneumoniae, H influenzae* Gram-negative bacilli Staphylococci
CSF shunt–associated	Coagulase-negative staphylococci *S aureus* Aerobic Gram-negative bacilli (including *P aeruginosa*) *Propionibacterium acnes*
Diabetes	*S pneumoniae* Gram-negative bacilli *S aureus*
Defects in cell-mediated immunity	*L monocytogenes*
Concern of bioterrorism	*Bacillus anthracis*

penicillin that exceed the MIC of intermediately resistant strains.[4]

In 2002, the National Committee for Clinical Laboratory Standards began offering differing cephalosporin breakpoints for pneumococcal susceptibility based on the site of infections.[5] For *S pneumoniae* from a meningeal source, the ceftriaxone and cefotaxime breakpoints were listed as follows: susceptible, 0.5 μg/mL; intermediate susceptibility, 1 μg/mL; and resistant, 2 μg/mL. This was in contrast to nonmeningeal breakpoints, which were stated as follows: susceptible, 1 μg/mL; intermediate susceptibility, 2 μg/mL; and resistant, 4 μg/mL.[5] These recommendations have been repeated in subsequent National Committee for Clinical Laboratory Standards reports.[3] To assess the effect of these new criteria on reporting of nonsusceptible *S pneumoniae* isolates, the Centers for Disease Control and Prevention (CDC) analyzed cefotaxime MIC data from the Active Bacterial Core Surveillance of the Emerging Infections Program Network from 1998 to 2001.[6] This analysis indicated that after the new criteria were applied, the number of isolates defined as nonsusceptible to cefotaxime decreased 52.1 to 61.2% each year. Even though cefotaxime or ceftriaxone has been recommended for pneumococci with intermediate susceptibility to penicillin, clinical failures have been reported when these agents have been used for such strains. For isolates with high-level resistance, vancomycin is the drug of choice. The less-than-optimal penetration of vancomycin into CSF has an impact on this therapeutic option. Steroids given concomitantly for meningitis may further decrease vancomycin's penetration.

In December 2004, the Infectious Diseases Society of America (IDSA) published recommendations for the management of bacterial meningitis[7] to update recommendations that have been available since 1997.[8] A summary of the empiric therapy recommendations from those guidelines is included in Table 3. Because of the importance of *S pneumoniae*, including those strains demonstrating antibiotic resistance, the guidelines provided an approach to therapy of proven pneumococcal meningitis based on *in vitro* susceptibility. For penicillin-susceptible isolates, penicillin or ampicillin was suggested. With intermediate susceptibility to penicillin (MIC, 0.1 to 1.0 μg/mL), a third-generation cephalosporin was recommended. It was suggested that the regimen of a broad-spectrum cephalosporin plus vancomycin be used if the *S pneumoniae* isolate is resistant to penicillin (MIC ≥ 2 μg/mL) and to ceftriaxone and cefotaxime (MIC ≥ 1 μg/mL). Clinical data on the efficacy of rifampin in patients with bacterial

Table 3. *CSF Recommendations for Empiric Therapy of Meningitis When Lumbar Puncture Is Delayed or in Patients With a Nondiagnostic CSF Gram Stain**

Patient Group	Recommended Drugs
Age 2 to 50 yr	Vancomycin plus a third-generation cephalosporin
Age > 50 yr	Vancomycin plus ampicillin plus a third-generation cephalosporin
Penetrating head trauma, or postneurosurgery, or CSF shunt	Vancomycin plus ceftazidime or vancomycin plus cefepime[†], or vancomycin plus meropenem[‡]

*Adapted from Tunkel and colleagues.[7]
[†]Not approved by the Food and Drug Administration (FDA) for meningitis.
[‡]FDA-approved for bacterial meningitis in pediatric patients ≥3 mo old.

meningitis are lacking, but some authorities would use this agent in combination with a third-generation cephalosporin, with or without vancomycin, in patients with pneumococcal meningitis caused by highly penicillin- or cephalosporin-resistant strains.[7] This statement was qualified in the IDSA guidelines for treatment of bacterial meningitis with the comment that rifampin should be added only if the organism is shown to be susceptible and there is a delay in the expected clinical or bacteriologic response. The usual duration of therapy for pneumococcal meningitis is generally stated to be 10 to 14 days.[7]

The role of steroids in adults with meningitis has not been definitively established. An early opinion by experts in the field suggested that adult patients who might be candidates for steroid therapy in meningitis are those with a high CSF concentration of bacteria (*ie*, demonstrable bacteria on Gram stain of CSF), especially if there is increased intracranial pressure.[9] A prospective, randomized, double-blind, multicenter trial assessed the value of adjuvant treatment with dexamethasone compared with placebo in adults 17 years of age or older with suspected meningitis who had cloudy CSF, bacteria in CSF on Gram staining, or a CSF leukocyte count of >1,000/mm^3.[10] Early treatment with dexamethasone was shown to improve the outcome and did not increase the risk of GI bleed. The dose of dexamethasone used in this study was 10 mg IV q6h for 4 days. In the 2004 IDSA guidelines for the treatment of bacterial meningitis in adults, it was recommended that dexamethasone (0.15 mg/kg q6h for 2 to 4 days, with the first dose administered 10 to 20 min before, or at least concomitant with, the first dose of antimicrobial therapy) be given in adults with suspected or proven pneumococcal meningitis.[7] It was stated that adjunctive dexamethasone should not be given to adult patients who have already received antimicrobial therapy, because administration of dexamethasone in this circumstance is unlikely to improve patient outcome. Even though the data are inadequate to recommend adjunctive dexamethasone in adults with meningitis caused by bacterial pathogens other than *S pneumoniae*, it was acknowledged that some authorities would initiate dexamethasone in all adults because the etiology of meningitis is not always ascertained at initial evaluation.[7]

The infectious syndromes caused by *N meningitidis* are somewhat broad and include meningococcal meningitis, meningococcal bacteremia, meningococcemia (purpura fulminans and the Waterhouse-Friderichsen syndrome), respiratory tract infections (pneumonia, epiglottitis, otitis media), focal infection (conjunctivitis, septic arthritis, urethritis, purulent pericarditis), and chronic meningococcemia.[11] Important in the pathogenesis of the clinical illnesses caused by the meningococcus is the organism's natural reservoir in the nasopharynx. It is this site from which disease may develop. The epidemiology of meningococcal meningitis is evolving. The traditional groups of patients at risk have included children and young adults, especially college students or military recruits who live in relatively confined quarters. A report from Argentina described epidemic meningococcal disease in the northeastern part of that country associated with disco patronage, supporting the pathogenetic point that close confinement allows aerosolization and spread of the organism from the nasopharynx.[12] An additional observation from this study, which has been raised in previous studies, is the association with passive or active cigarette smoking. This report, which was titled "Disco Fever," expanded the closed settings in which meningococcal meningitis originates to include dance clubs and discos. Air travel–associated meningococcal disease has also been described and is defined as a patient who meets the case definition of meningococcal disease within 14 days of travel on a flight of at least 8-h duration.[13] Pneumonia, sinusitis, and tracheobronchitis are important sources of bacteremic meningococcal disease. Although meningitis is the characteristic infection caused by N meningitidis, a report from Atlanta noted that only 14 (32%) of the 44 adult patients with meningococcal infection had meningitis.[14] When it occurs, meningococcal meningitis is usually acute and often associated with purpuric skin lesions (although the Atlanta report noted that only 10 of the 14 adults with meningitis [71%] had a generalized rash). During the very early stages of infection, the CSF analysis may be relatively normal even though the clinical course is hyperacute with fever, nuchal rigidity, and coma. Although variably reported through the years, the potential for N meningitidis to cause purulent pericarditis should be noted. The illness may progress to acidosis, tissue hypoxia, shock, disseminated intravascular coagulopathy, and hemorrhagic adrenal infarction. The potential for β-lactamase-producing strains remains a concern, as does the existence of relatively resistant strains, presumably caused by alterations in the penicillin-binding proteins; however, active surveillance among a large, diverse population in the United States has failed to identify any such strains.[15] Penicillin or ampicillin, therefore, remains a drug of choice for treating meningitis caused by this pathogen. The usual duration of therapy is generally 7 days.[7]

With meningococcemia, a fulminant complication is acute, massive adrenal hemorrhage with the resultant clinical entity of the Waterhouse-Friderichsen syndrome. However, not all patients who die of meningococcemia have evidence of adrenal hemorrhage at autopsy, and many steroid-treated patients succumb despite therapy, implying that adrenal insufficiency may not be the primary cause of circulatory collapse. Because of the implications of such a complication, it would be helpful to have definitive recommendations about the role, if any, of steroids in management of patients with meningococcal meningitis. There are anecdotal reports in the literature of improved outcome in such patients treated with corticosteroids. In some patients with meningococcal infection, cortisol levels may be elevated. In contrast, other reports have noted that not all patients with severe meningococcal infection who have been given adrenocorticotropic hormone have responded to adrenocorticotropic hormone stimulation of cortisol production, and this raises the issues of whether adrenal reserves may be decreased in certain patients and whether steroids may have a role. In 1992, IDSA published a review of the role of steroids in patients with infectious diseases.[16] There were 10 infections for which steroids were strongly supported or suggested as having a role, and meningococcemia was not one of those listed. At the present time, the role of steroids in meningococcemia is unresolved. Because fulminant meningococcal septicemia represents an extreme form of endotoxin-induced sepsis and coagulopathy, with clinical consequences that include amputations and organ failure, investigators have addressed other potential therapeutic modalities that may be beneficial in patients with overwhelming meningococcal infection. The dual function of protein C as an anticoagulant and as a modulator of the inflammatory response was recently reviewed in the context of experimental data showing that activated protein C replacement therapy reduces the mortality rate for fulminant meningococcemia.[17] Such data become especially noteworthy given the efficacy and safety data about recombinant human activated protein C in patients with severe sepsis.[18]

In patients treated with penicillin for meningococcal meningitis, posttreatment with rifampin, ciprofloxacin, or ceftriaxone has been recommended to eradicate the nasal carrier state, as penicillin will not eliminate organisms at this site.[19] These recommendations are similar to those for chemoprophylaxis for individuals exposed to a person with known meningococcal disease. Those recommendations are summarized in Table 4. Prophylaxis is recommended for close contacts, which include household members, day-care center contacts, and anyone directly exposed to the patient's oral secretions (*eg*, kissing, mouth-to-mouth resuscitation, endotracheal intubation, endotracheal tube management). Because the rate of secondary disease for close contacts is highest during the first few days after the onset of disease in the primary patient, antimicrobial chemoprophylaxis should be administered as soon as possible (ideally within 24 h after the case is identified). Chemoprophylaxis administered >14 days has been stated to be of limited or no value.[13]

Since 1991, there have been increased numbers of outbreaks of serogroup C meningococcal disease in the United States. Meningococcal polysaccharide vaccine has been shown to be effective against serogroup C meningococcal disease in a community outbreak, with a vaccine efficacy among 2- to 29-year-olds of 85%.[20] Based on this observation, it has been recommended that emphasis be placed on achieving high vaccination coverage in future outbreaks, with special efforts to vaccinate young adults. The Advisory Committee on Immunization Practices and the American Academy of Pediatrics have recommended that health-care providers and colleges educate freshmen college students—especially those who live in dormitories—and their parents about the increased risk of meningococcal diseases and the potential benefits of immunization so that informed decisions about vaccination can be made.[21] A predisposing factor for neisserial infections is deficiency in the late complement components (*ie*, C5 to C8). Because previous studies have demonstrated an incidence as high as 39% in populations of patients with meningococcal infections, at a minimum, a screening test for complement function (CH_{50}) has been suggested for all patients who have invasive meningococcal infections[22]; it was also noted that direct assessment of complement (C5, C6, C7, C8, and C9) and properdin proteins should be considered.

Like the meningococcus, *H influenzae* may be isolated from the nasopharynx, and this may be the immediate source of invading pathogens. Rates of infection caused by this pathogen have decreased because of vaccination against *H influenzae*. In patients with meningitis due to this organism, a contiguous focus of infection such as sinusitis or otitis media should be investigated. In adults without these underlying processes, a search for a CSF leak, which may be the basis for the meningitis, is necessary. Because about one third of *H influenzae* isolates are β-lactamase producers, agents that are stable in the presence of these enzymes and that cross the blood-brain barrier should be used. The third-generation cephalosporins cefotaxime and ceftriaxone have had the most successful record of use in this regard. Even though the second-generation cephalosporin

Table 4. *Schedule for Administering Chemoprophylaxis Against Meningococcal Disease**

Drug	Age Group	Dosage	Duration/Route of Administration†
Rifampin‡	Children < 1 mo	5 mg/kg q12h	2 d
	Children ≥ 1 mo	10 mg/kg q12h	2 d
	Adults	600 mg q12h	2 d
Ciprofloxacin§	Adults	500 mg	Single dose
Ceftriaxone	Children <15 yr	125 mg	Single IM dose
	Adults	250 mg	Single IM dose

*Reprinted from the Centers for Disease Control and Prevention. MMWR Recomm Rep 2000; 49(RR-7):1-10.
†Oral administration unless indicated otherwise.
‡ Rifampin is not recommended for pregnant women because the drug is teratogenic in laboratory animals. Because the reliability of oral contraceptives may be affected by rifampin therapy, consideration should be given to using alternative contraceptive measures while rifampin is being administered.
§ Ciprofloxacin generally is not recommended for persons aged <18 yr or for pregnant and lactating women, because the drug causes cartilage damage in immature laboratory animals. However, ciprofloxacin can be used for chemoprophylaxis in children when no acceptable alternative is available.

cefuroxime is active against *H influenzae*, it has been shown to result in delayed sterilization of the CSF when compared with ceftriaxone.[23] A lower incidence of sensorineural hearing loss was demonstrated in children who adjunctively received dexamethasone (3.3%) vs those who did not receive steroids (15.5%). Similar findings have not been corroborated in adults. The usual duration of therapy for *H influenzae* meningitis is generally 7 days.[7]

Meningitis due to Gram-negative bacilli occurs most characteristically after neurosurgical procedures, with head trauma being a less likely predisposition. Medical conditions, including urosepsis, account for about 20% of episodes of this infection. In certain patient populations in which Gram-negative meningitis develops in the setting of impaired cell-mediated immunity, one should exclude *Strongyloides stercoralis* infection as the underlying predisposing cause. Of note, hyperinfection with the resultant predisposition to Gram-negative meningitis is uncommon in two groups of patients with defects in cell-mediated immunity: (1) transplant recipients who receive cyclosporine, because of the anthelminthic properties of this rejection agent; and (2) HIV-infected patients, unless the CD4$^+$ cell count is ≤200 cells/mm^3 and the patient is concomitantly receiving corticosteroids.[24] Parenterally administered aminoglycosides do not cross the blood-brain barrier after the 28th day of life. For these antibiotics to be useful beyond the neonatal period, they need to be administered intrathecally or intraventricularly. Chloramphenicol has activity against some Gram-negative bacilli, and it crosses the blood-brain barrier. Concern about toxicity issues such as aplastic anemia has decreased the use of this agent over the years, although it still plays an important role in persons with meningitis and type I (IgE-mediated) hypersensitivity to penicillins. Third-generation cephalosporins have become the mainstay of therapy for Gram-negative meningitis because of their spectrum and their penetration into the CSF. All of the presently available third-generation agents except for cefoperazone have an indication for meningitis due to susceptible pathogens. For meningitis due to *Pseudomonas aeruginosa*, ceftazidime is an efficacious agent. It is usually administered with a parenteral aminoglycoside, recognizing that this latter agent will not cross the blood-brain barrier in adults but that it might help to eradicate the site of infection outside the CNS that served as the focus for the meningitis. According to the recent IDSA guidelines for the management of bacterial meningitis, cefepime has greater *in vitro* activity than the third-generation cephalosporins against *Enterobacter* spp and *P aeruginosa*, and it has been used successfully in some patients with meningitis caused by these bacteria.[7] The guidelines summarized these observations by stating that they support cefepime as a useful agent in the treatment of patients with bacterial meningitis. This should be taken within the context that as of 2005, cefepime does not have an FDA-approved indication for the treatment of bacterial meningitis.[25] For meningitis due to Gram-negative pathogens, the IDSA guidelines list 21 days as the duration of therapy.[7]

Pharmacologic and microbiologic issues are important for two important pathogens that cause meningitis. *L monocytogenes* is an intracellular Gram-positive rod that characteristically infects persons with defects in cell-mediated immunity. It may also cause disease in diabetics and elderly persons, and about 30% of infected adults have no apparent risk. Acquisition has been associated with consumption of contaminated coleslaw, milk, and cheese. Although the CSF cellular response is usually polymorphonuclear, some patients present either with lymphocytes or with a normal glucose. Like fungal and tuberculous meningitis, Listeria meningitis has a predilection for involving the meninges at the base of the brain. This may lead to hydrocephalus. Ampicillin or penicillin is the drug of choice, and there is no significant activity by third-generation cephalosporins against this pathogen.[26] Some experts suggest the addition of an aminoglycoside given parenterally because of *in vitro* synergy. For those patients who are allergic to penicillin, trimethoprim-sulfamethoxazole is the agent of choice. Because of the intracellular location of this pathogen, 21 days of therapy has been recommended.[7] A review of *Staphylococcus aureus* meningitis divided this disease entity into two categories: (1) hospital-acquired and (2) community-acquired.[27] It was noted that hospital-acquired infection occurred as an occasional complication of neurosurgical procedures, with the presence of medical devices, or with certain skin infections; it generally had a favorable prognosis and a relatively low mortality rate. In contrast, community-acquired *S aureus* meningitis was associated with valvular heart disease, diabetes mellitus, or drug or alcohol abuse, and the mortality rate was significantly higher than for nosocomial infection. In this review of 28 patients with community-acquired *S aureus* meningitis, 8 had negative or no CSF culture. Of these 8 patients, 4 had received antibiotics prior to lumbar puncture. This finding is consistent with the observation that an important presentation of *S aureus* is in patients with addict-associated infective endocarditis. For *S aureus*, nafcillin or oxacillin has better activity against methicillin-sensitive strains than does vancomycin. In addition, the penetration of vancomycin into CSF may be variable, even in the setting of meningeal inflammation.

Beginning with the September 11, 2001, episode of terrorism in the United States, anthrax is an important consideration in the differential diagnosis of patients with a life-threatening illness that includes a meningeal component. Inhalational anthrax is a biphasic clinical syndrome with initial nonspecific flu-like symptoms (fatigue, malaise, myalgia, headache, nonproductive cough, and nausea/vomiting) followed by a second phase with hemodynamic collapse, septic shock/multi-organ dysfunction syndrome, and rapid death with overwhelming bacterial spread. It is during the stage of bacteremia that there is a strong likelihood of meningitis, which some sources cite as occurring in 50% of cases. The index case of bioterrorism anthrax in Florida presented with hemorrhagic meningitis,[28] which is characteristic of disseminated anthrax; however, meningitis without hemorrhage can occur with anthrax. In patients in whom infection with *Bacillus anthracis* is suspected to be the cause of meningitis, some have suggested adding either penicillin or chloramphenicol to the multidrug regimen that would be given for inhalational anthrax.[29]

Empiric therapy for meningitis has changed in recent years. In previously healthy, nonallergic individuals with acute pyogenic community-acquired meningitis in whom little information is available, ampicillin was suggested in a 1993 review as a reasonable empiric agent.[30] For patients with a type I (IgE-mediated) penicillin allergy, chloramphenicol was offered in that review as appropriate therapy. In 1997, recommendations suggested a broad-spectrum cephalosporin (*eg*, cefotaxime or ceftriaxone) as empiric therapy for individuals aged 18 to 50 years who have a nondiagnostic Gram stain.[8] As summarized in Table 3, the 2004 IDSA guidelines suggested vancomycin plus a third-generation cephalosporin as empiric therapy of meningitis when lumbar puncture is delayed or in patients with a nondiagnostic CSF Gram stain.[7] This evolution from 1993 to 2004 in the recommendations for empiric therapy of meningitis is influenced by penicillin resistance in pneumococci. The addition of ampicillin to a broad-spectrum cephalosporin plus vancomycin is reasonable empiric therapy for polymorphonuclear meningitis undiagnosed by Gram stain in patient populations with the following underlying conditions: (1) advanced age; (2) alcoholism; and (3) immunocompromised states. The activity by ampicillin against Listeria is an important component of the coverage in this regimen.

Certain epidemiologic situations may exist that influence the acquisition of specific pathogens, which may then cause meningitis. Those conditions (including skull fractures and shunt-associated infections), and the pathogens likely to occur in their setting, are summarized in Table 2.

Lymphocytic Meningitis With Normal Glucose: The meningeal response to infection or inflammation may be less marked in certain conditions, and the response may therefore be less associated with the inability to transport glucose across the meninges. Those conditions associated with the findings of lymphocytes and normal glucose in the CSF are listed in Table 1. The classic consideration in this differential has been viral meningitis. Enteroviruses, which are recognized causes of pleurodynia and pericarditis, are the most common cause of aseptic meningitis and characteristically cause a self-limited form of meningitis that presents with fever, headache, and lymphocytic pleocytosis, most often in the late summer or early fall. Recently, however, two other viruses have gained importance in the differential diagnosis of viral meningitis. With initial episodes or flares of genital herpes simplex virus infection, patients may develop meningitis as a systemic manifestation of their herpes infection. This process is distinctly different from the life-threatening entity of herpes encephalitis in that it is self-limited and does not require therapy. Because of the propensity for herpes genitalis to recur, this form of meningitis may similarly present as a recurrent form of lymphocytic meningitis. HIV has a predilection for neural tissue, and patients, including those with the acute retroviral syndrome, may present with viral meningitis that may resolve spontaneously. In those individuals who have risk factors for HIV and present with an illness consistent with viral meningitis, HIV infection is an important consideration.

Encephalitis may occur on the basis of both infectious and noninfectious causes. When these conditions are associated with WBCs in the CSF, the diagnosis of meningoencephalitis may be made. The traditional teaching has been that meningoencephalitis, like viral encephalitis, will give a normal glucose level in association with lymphocytes. As outlined in Table 1, herpes encephalitis may result in a low glucose level.

Spirochetal infections are an important cause of lymphocytic meningitis with normal glucose level. *Treponema pallidum*, the etiologic agent of syphilis, is a recognized cause of asymptomatic infection of the CNS in nonimmunocompromised hosts. Meningovascular syphilis has been increasingly diagnosed in the era of HIV infection; it may take the form of syphilitic meningitis or a stroke syndrome. In December 2004, new guidelines were published for the management of infections in HIV-infected persons.[31] Several important points were made regarding neurosyphilis. Because CNS disease can occur during any stage of syphilis, a patient who has clinical evidence of neurologic involvement with syphilis (eg, cognitive dysfunction, motor or sensory deficits, ophthalmic or auditory symptoms, cranial nerve palsies, and symptoms or signs of meningitis) should undergo a CSF examination. Because it is highly specific (although insensitive), the VDRL test in CSF (VDRL-CSF) is the standard serologic test for CSF. When reactive in the absence of substantial contamination of CSF with blood, it is considered diagnostic of neurosyphilis. However, with syphilitic meningitis, patients may present without symptoms of nervous system disease and analysis of their CSF may reveal only a few lymphocytes and a negative VDRL-CSF. The fluorescent treponemal antibody absorption test on CSF is less specific for neurosyphilis than the VDRL-CSF, but the high sensitivity of the study has led some experts to believe that a negative CSF fluorescent treponemal antibody absorption test excludes neurosyphilis.[31] The guidelines now state that a reactive CSF-VDRL and a CSF WBC count ≥10 cells/mm^3 support the diagnosis of neurosyphilis. An analysis of laboratory measures after treatment for neurosyphilis revealed that HIV-infected patients were less likely than non-HIV-infected patients to normalize their CSF-VDRL reactivity with higher baseline titers, even though the CSF WBC count and serum rapid plasma reagin reactivity in both populations were likely to normalize.[32] Neurosyphilis can present as cerebrovascular insufficiency, often in young patients with a stroke syndrome caused by an endarteritis, which most characteristically involves the middle cerebral artery.

According to guidelines,[31] the recommended regimen for patients with neurosyphilis is 18 to 24 million U/d of aqueous crystalline penicillin G, administered as 3 to 4 million U IV q4h or continuous infusion, for 10 to 14 days. If compliance with therapy can be ensured, patients may be treated with procaine penicillin (2.4 million U IM once daily) plus probenecid (500 mg orally 4 times a day), both for 10 to 14 days. Because these durations are shorter than the regimen used for late syphilis in the absence of neurosyphilis, some specialists administer benzathine penicillin (2.4 million U IM once per week for up to 3 weeks after completion of these neurosyphilis treatment regimens) to provide a comparable total duration of therapy. The CSF leukocyte count has been stated to be a sensitive measure of the effectiveness of therapy.

The classic presentation of neurologic Lyme disease, which is caused by *Borrelia burgdorferi*, is seventh nerve palsy (which may be bilateral) in association with a lymphocytic meningitis.

Leptospirosis, caused by *Leptospira interrogans*, is epidemiologically linked to such factors as infected rat urine or exposure to infected dogs. It presents as two distinct clinical syndromes.[33] Anicteric leptospirosis is a self-limiting illness, which progresses through two well-defined stages: a septicemic stage and an immune stage. The septicemic stage occurs after a 7- to 12-day incubation period and is primarily manifested as fever, chills, nausea, vomiting, and headache. The most characteristic physical finding during this stage is conjunctival suffusion. The causative organism can be isolated from blood or CSF at this point. Following a 1- to 3-day asymptomatic period, the immune stage develops; it is characterized by aseptic meningitis. Leptospira are present in the urine during this stage and may persist for up to 3 weeks. Icteric leptospirosis, or Weil syndrome, is a less common but potentially fatal syndrome that occurs in 5 to 10% of cases. Jaundice, renal involvement, hypotension, and hemorrhage are the hallmarks of this form of leptospirosis; however, the severity of these manifestations can vary greatly, and renal involvement is not universal. In icteric leptospirosis, the biphasic nature of the disease is somewhat obscured by the persistence of jaundice and azotemia throughout the illness, but septicemic and immune stages do occur. Leptospires can be isolated from blood or CSF during the first week and from the urine during the second week of illness. Additionally, the diagnosis can be made by demonstrating rising antibody titers. Treatment of leptospirosis involves intense supportive care as well as antibiotic coverage. The use of IV penicillin (1.5 million U every 6 h) has been shown to shorten the duration of fever, renal dysfunction, and hospital stay. In a prospective, open-label, randomized trial, ceftriaxone and penicillin G were shown to be equally effective for the treatment of severe leptospirosis.[34]

Over the years, Rocky Mountain spotted fever, which is caused by *Rickettsia rickettsii*, has been considered the classic rickettsial infection in the United States. Results of CSF analysis are usually normal unless patients have stupor or coma, in which case there may be a lymphocytic pleocytosis with normal glucose and elevated protein levels. An important emerging infection in the United States is ehrlichiosis. The clinical illness attributable to this infection is discussed in this syllabus in the section on encephalitis. The characteristic CSF abnormalities in patients with ehrlichiosis have been a lymphocytic pleocytosis with elevated protein. In a recent review of the subject, the CSF glucose level was normal in the majority of patients, with 24% of the patients having borderline low CSF glucose concentrations.[35] In this review, morulae were seen in CSF white cells in only a small minority of the patients. Clinical features supporting the diagnosis of ehrlichiosis are leukopenia (because of the intracellular location of the organism), thrombocytopenia, and elevated liver enzymes. From the limited clinical data available, it appears that chloramphenicol or tetracycline is the agent most frequently used for this infection.

Certain infectious diseases, such as infective endocarditis, may cause a lymphocytic pleocytosis with normal glucose that is the result of a vasculitis, which the infectious process causes in the CNS. A review of a 12-year experience at the Cleveland Clinic included the results of lumbar punctures done on 23 of 175 patients with endocarditis.[36] There was a CSF pleocytosis in 14 and no CSF WBCs in 9. Of the 14 patients who had a pleocytosis, the etiology was attributed to a stroke in 8 and to encephalopathy in 5; the remaining patient only had isolated headaches. No positive CSF cultures were reported in any of these 14 patients. Such information underscores a dilemma for the clinician managing a patient with endocarditis who has a CSF pleocytosis: Is the pleocytosis due to secondary bacterial seeding of the meninges, or is it due to other events associated with endocarditis that lead to a CNS response that is associated with a secondary cellular response?

A group of noninfectious causes of lymphocytic meningitis with a normal glucose level are described in Table 1.

Lymphocytic Meningitis With Low Glucose: With chronic processes, it is not surprising that the cellular CSF response would be lymphocytes. Low CSF glucose has been described in this syllabus as occurring due to impaired transport based on acute inflammation of the meninges. In certain conditions, glucose transport may be associated with infiltration of the meninges by either granulomatous processes or malignant cells. Such is the situation for several of the conditions summarized in Table 1 that cause lymphocytic meningitis with a low glucose level.

Viral meningitis due to mumps and lymphocytic choriomeningitis has characteristically been associated with a low CSF glucose. As previously discussed, certain forms of meningoencephalitis, including that due to herpes simplex virus, may present in this manner. Partially treated bacterial meningitis and certain chemical-induced meningitides may have similar findings. Four other groups of conditions are important in this setting are tuberculous meningitis, fungal meningitis, carcinomatous meningitis, and subarachnoid hemorrhage.

A review of 48 adult patients with tuberculous meningitis who were admitted to an ICU demonstrates the potential for this infectious process to cause serious disease.[37] It also emphasizes the difficulty often encountered in establishing the diagnosis. Repeated large volumes (10 to 20 mL) of CSF have a higher yield for acid-fast bacilli.[38] When four CSF smears for acid-fast bacilli are obtained, positive findings may occur in up to 90% of patients with tuberculous meningitis. Some studies have shown that elevated CSF titers of adenosine deaminase[39] or CSF chloride levels <110 mEq/L in the absence of bacterial infection support the diagnosis of tuberculous meningitis. Enzyme-linked immunosorbent assays (ELISAs) are felt by some to be helpful with this diagnosis. Polymerase chain reaction (PCR) for *Mycobacterium tuberculosis* may be helpful when performed on CSF, but false-negative results have been reported. Because of a predilection for tuberculous meningitis to involve the base of the brain, imaging studies of the CNS may reveal an obstructing hydrocephalus. In addition to antituberculous therapy with agents such as isoniazid, rifampin, pyrazinamide, and ethambutol, corticosteroids may play a role, especially in situations of increased intracranial pressure or obstruction resulting from the infection. The most recent guidelines of the American Thoracic Society give steroids in the treatment of tuberculous meningitis an A-1 recommendation.[40] A randomized, double-blind, placebo-controlled trial in Vietnam in patients >14 years of age with tuberculous meningitis showed that adjunctive treatment with dexamethasone improved survival but probably did not prevent severe disability.[41] From the series of patients with tuberculous meningitis admitted to an ICU, several important clinical points can be extracted[37]: (1) Ischemic lesions with signs of localization may be present. (2) Extrameningeal tuberculous infection may support the diagnosis. (Overall, the rate has been stated to be 40 to 45%, but in this review it was 66%.) (3) Clinical features and CSF profiles did not appear to be modified in the HIV-infected patients. (4) Delay to onset of treatment and the neurologic status at admission were identified as the main clinical prognostic factors. In low-incidence geographic areas, clinicians should suspect tuberculous meningitis in members of immigrant groups from high-incidence areas, as well as in patients who abuse alcohol or drugs and those with immunosuppression from any cause.[42]

Although fungal meningitis may be due to several etiologic agents, the two most common ones are *Cryptococcus neoformans* and *Coccidioides immitis*. Although both of these pathogens have been increasingly diagnosed as a cause of meningitis because of HIV infection, both caused meningitis in normal hosts prior to the AIDS era. Both organisms gain access to the body via the lungs. In HIV-infected persons with cryptococcal meningitis, there may be a lack of inflammation in the CSF, and therefore findings may include <20 CSF WBCs/mm^3 and a normal glucose level. The India ink stain, latex agglutination test, and fungal culture of the CSF are, therefore, important in the diagnosis. Potentially helpful in establishing the diagnosis are other sites of involvement, including lung, skin, and blood. Based on data from the Mycoses Study Group of the National Institutes of Health (NIH), it appears that therapy for cryptococcal meningitis in HIV-infected patients should begin with amphotericin B (0.7 mg/kg/d) in combination with flucytosine (100 mg/kg/d in persons with normal renal function) for the initial 2 weeks of therapy followed by fluconazole (400 mg/d orally) for an additional 8 to 10 weeks.[43] In the 381 patients with cryptococcal meningitis treated in this double-blind, multicenter trial, 13 of 14 early deaths and 40% of deaths during weeks 3 through 10 were associated with elevated intracranial pressure. Based on the association of elevated intracranial pressure and mortality in patients with cryptococcal meningitis, it was suggested that measurement of intracranial pressure be included in the management of such patients. Included in the recommendations were daily lumbar punctures, use of acetazolamide, and ventriculoperitoneal shunts for asymptomatic patients with intracranial CSF pressure >320 mm H$_2$O and for symptomatic patients with pressure >180 mm H$_2$O. More recently, it was recommended that in the absence of focal lesions, opening pressures ≥250 mm H$_2$O should be treated with large-volume CSF drainage (defined in this report as allowing CSF to drain until a satisfactory closing pressure had been achieved, commonly <200 mm H$_2$O).[44] The IDSA guidelines for the management of cryptococcal meningitis in

HIV-infected persons with opening CSF pressure of >250 mm H$_2$O recommended lumbar drainage sufficient to achieve a closing pressure ≤200 mm H$_2$O or 50% of initial opening pressure.[45] Maintenance therapy is required after completion of primary therapy, and studies have defined fluconazole (200 mg/d orally) as the agent of choice.

Meningitis due to *C immitis* commonly presents with headache, vomiting, and altered mental status. Although the CSF formula is usually one of lymphocytes with a low glucose level, eosinophils are occasionally present. In addition to direct examination and culture of CSF, complement-fixing antibodies in the CSF may be an especially important aid to the diagnosis of coccidioidal meningitis. As with cryptococcal meningitis, the epidemiologic history and the other body sites of involvement (including lung, skin, joints, and bone) are important in making the diagnosis. In contrast to cryptococcal meningitis, management strategies for coccidioidal meningitis may vary from patient to patient. Recent IDSA guidelines noted that oral fluconazole is currently the preferred therapy, with itraconazole being listed as having comparable efficacy.[46] It was acknowledged that some physicians initiate therapy with intrathecal amphotericin B in addition to an azole on the basis of their belief that responses may be more prompt with this approach. Because Coccidioides has a predilection for the basilar meninges, hydrocephalus may occur. Regardless of the regimen being used, this potential complication nearly always requires a shunt for decompression.

Other fungi have the capability of causing meningitis, but they are less likely to do so. Because CNS involvement may be clinically recognized in 5 to 10% of cases of progressive disseminated histoplasmosis, the diagnosis and management of CNS histoplasmosis has been recently reviewed.[47] As a general rule, fungal meningitis, like tuberculous meningitis, may involve the base of the brain and cause obstruction of CSF flow with resulting hydrocephalus.

Eosinophilic Meningitis: The subject of eosinophilic meningitis has been recently reviewed.[48]

Angiostrongylus cantonensis is a nematode that can infect humans who ingest poorly cooked or raw intermediate mollusk hosts, such as snails, slugs, and prawns. Infection can also occur when fresh vegetables contaminated with infective larvae are eaten. Once ingested, the infective larvae penetrate the gut wall and migrate to the small vessels of the meninges to cause a clinical picture of fever, meningismus, and headache. CSF analysis reveals an eosinophilic pleocytosis; larvae are usually not found. Such a process has been most characteristically described in Asia and the South Pacific. A recent report described an outbreak of meningitis due to *A cantonensis* that developed in 12 travelers who traveled to the Caribbean and whose clinical illness was strongly associated with the consumption of a Caesar salad at a meal.[49] From this outbreak, it was suggested that *A cantonensis* infection should be suspected among travelers at risk who present with headache, elevated intracranial pressure, and pleocytosis, with or without eosinophilia, particularly in association with paresthesias or hyperesthesias.

Less classic infectious causes of eosinophilic meningitis include *Trichinella spiralis*, *Taenia solium*, *Toxocara canis*, *Gnathostoma spinigerum*, *Paragonimus westermani*, and *Baylisascaris procyonis*. Important noninfectious causes include malignancy (*eg*, Hodgkin disease, non-Hodgkin lymphoma, and eosinophilic leukemia), medications (*eg*, ciprofloxacin, ibuprofen), and intraventricular medications or shunts.

Meningitis Caused by Protozoa or Helminth: Of the causes, five deserve special comment. The most common is due to *Toxoplasma gondii* and presents most often as multiple ring-enhancing lesions in HIV-infected patients. These lesions may be associated with a CSF pleocytosis, but meningitis is not the most likely presentation of CNS toxoplasmosis. Because this infection usually represents reactivation disease, the IgG antibody to Toxoplasma is positive in about 95% of these individuals. Therapy is with sulfadiazine and pyrimethamine.

Naegleria fowleri is a free-living amoeba that enters the CNS by invading the nasal mucosa at the level of the cribriform plate. The classic presentation is of an acute pyogenic meningitis in a person who recently swam in fresh water.[50] The CSF analysis shows a polymorphonuclear pleocytosis, many RBCs, and hypoglycorrhachia. The diagnosis is confirmed by identifying the organism on CSF wet mount as motile amoeba, or it can be made by biopsy of brain tissue. Amphotericin B administered systemically and intraventricularly is the drug of choice. Another amoebic pathogen infecting the nervous system is Acanthamoeba, which may infect individuals with defects in cell-mediated immunity (including patients with AIDS or after organ transplantation) and result in a granulomatous amoebic encephalitis. Clinical manifestations include mental status abnormalities, seizures, fever, headache, focal neurologic deficits, meningismus, visual disturbances, and ataxia. An important clinical clue may be preexisting skin lesions that have been present for months before CNS disease and may take the form of ulcerative, nodular, or subcutaneous abscesses. Pneumonitis may also be a part of the clinical presentation.

Neurocysticercosis, which is caused by the pork tapeworm *T solium*, is the most common cause of acquired epilepsy in the world and is highly endemic in all parts of the developing world where pigs are raised, especially Latin America, most of Asia, sub-Saharan Africa, and parts of Oceania.[24] Even though seizures are the most common manifestation of neurocysticercosis, other symptoms include headache, hemiparesis, and ataxia. Symptoms typically begin years after the initial infection, when a host inflammatory response develops against *T solium* antigens released after the death of the parasite. Although not the most classic presentation of neurocysticercosis, eosinophilic meningitis may be part of the clinical presentation. Brain imaging studies may reveal intracranial lesions, which may be cystic or calcified; because of chronic inflammation at the base of the brain, hydrocephalus may be present. The epidemiologic history, combined with brain imaging studies and serologies (serum enzyme-linked immunoelectrotransfer blot or CSF ELISA), helps make the diagnosis. The drug treatment of choice for neurocysticercosis includes albendazole or praziquantel; steroids should be given concomitantly to reduce edema produced by medical treatment, especially for meningeal infection.[24] Most experts agree that the inflammatory response produced by the death of the cyst produces symptomatic neurocysticercosis and that inactive infection (*ie*, presence of calcified or ring-enhancing lesions) does not require anthelminthics.[24]

As previously noted, *A cantonensis* may be a cause of eosinophilic meningitis.

Miscellaneous Issues in the Diagnosis and Management of Meningitis: The timing of diagnostic studies in patients with meningitis is of critical importance. An important issue is focality. Over the last several decades, many have limited the designation of focality to such processes as hemiparesis, isolated abnormalities on an imaging study of the brain, or an abnormal focus on an EEG. More recently, it has been stated that altered mental status indicates bilateral hemispheric or brainstem dysfunction and severely compromises the ability to determine whether the patient's neurologic assessment is nonfocal.

Because of the potential for severe neurologic sequelae in individuals with bacterial meningitis who are treated in a suboptimal manner, attention has been focused in recent years on the appropriate sequencing of diagnostic studies. A prospective study of 301 adults with suspected meningitis was conducted to determine whether clinical characteristics present before CT of the head was performed could be used to identify patients who were unlikely to have abnormalities on CT.[51] Thirteen baseline clinical characteristics were used to predict abnormal findings on head CT: age ≥ 60 years; immunocompromised state; history of CNS disease; seizure within 1 week before presentation; abnormal level of consciousness; inability to answer two questions correctly; inability to follow two commands correctly; gaze palsy; abnormal visual fields; facial palsy; arm drift; leg drift; and abnormal language (*ie*, aphasia, dysarthria, and extinction). From the results of the study, the authors concluded that adults with suspected meningitis who have none of the noted baseline features are good candidates for immediate lumbar puncture since they have a low risk of brain herniation as a result of lumbar puncture. It was acknowledged that such an approach would have resulted in a 41% decrease in the frequency of CT scans performed in the study cohort. When imaging is indicated, the following sequence of evaluation and management has been suggested: (1) obtain blood cultures; (2) institute empiric antibiotic therapy; and (3) perform lumbar puncture immediately after the imaging study if no intracranial mass lesion is present.[8]

Supporting the importance of the timing of antibiotics in patients with meningitis are the findings of a retrospective, observational cohort study of patients with community-acquired bacterial meningitis.[52] In this study, patients with microbiologically proven, community-acquired bacterial meningitis were stratified into three groups based on the clinical findings of hypotension, altered mental status, and seizures. Patients with none of these three predictor variables were in stage I; those with one predictor variable, stage II; and those with two or more predictor variables, stage III. Delay in therapy after arrival in the emergency department was associated with adverse clinical outcome when the patient's condition advanced from stage I or II to stage III before the initial antibiotic dose was given, a finding that underscores the need for prompt administration of antibiotics in patients with bacterial meningitis. This study was further interpreted as suggesting that the risk for adverse outcome is influenced more by the severity of illness than the timing of initial antibiotic therapy for patients who arrive in the emergency department at stage III.

A recent analysis of the causes of death in adults hospitalized with community-acquired bacterial meningitis provides some important insights.[53] Although 50% of the 74 patients had meningitis as the underlying and immediate cause of death, 18% of patients had meningitis as the underlying but not immediate cause of death, and 23% had meningitis as neither the underlying nor immediate cause of death. A 14-day survival end point discriminated between deaths attributable to meningitis and those with another cause. It was concluded that such an end point will facilitate greater accuracy of epidemiologic statistics and will assist investigations of the impact of new therapeutic interventions.

For many years, clinicians have relied on a CSF pleocytosis for diagnosing meningitis. Because of implications in both therapy and prophylaxis of meningitis, rapid and accurate diagnostic tests for bacterial meningitis are important. A recent report describes the potential role for broad-range bacterial PCR in excluding the diagnosis of meningitis and in influencing the decision to initiate or discontinue antimicrobial therapy.[54]

In the *Medical Knowledge Self-Assessment Program IX* of the American College of Physicians, it was acknowledged that there are at least four clinical entities in which patients may have fever, coma, and nuchal ridigity but a normal CSF analysis: (1) early bacterial meningitis; (2) cryptococcal meningitis with concomitant HIV infection; (3) parameningeal foci; and (4) herpes simplex encephalitis.[55]

Encephalitis

Characteristic of processes involving cortical brain matter are alterations of consciousness and/or cognitive dysfunction. A representative clinical entity with such findings is acute viral encephalitis, which occurs on the basis of direct infection of neural cells with associated perivascular inflammation, neuronal destruction, and tissue necrosis.[56] Pathologically, the involvement in acute viral encephalitis is in the gray matter. This may be associated with evidence of meningeal irritation and CSF mononuclear pleocytosis, in which the process is referred to as meningoencephalitis. In addition to infectious agents, which may cause direct brain injury, there are indirect mechanisms including induction of autoimmune diseases. This process is referred to as postinfectious encephalomyelitis and is characterized by widespread perivenular inflammation with demyelination localized to the white matter of the brain. The list of infectious and noninfectious processes causing encephalitis is lengthy and is partially summarized in Table 5. An additional process, which represents the sequelae of an infection, is production of neurotoxins as occurs with shigellosis, melioidosis, and cat-scratch disease.

Of all the mechanisms by which an infectious process leads to involvement of the brain, direct viral invasion of neural cells is the most classic. Although the most common cause of acute viral meningitis is enteroviral infection (notably coxsackie A and B viruses and echoviruses), it has been stated that <3% of the CNS complications from such infections would be classified as encephalitis. Diagnostic studies should include viral pharyngeal, rectal, and urine cultures, but confirmation using acute- and convalescent-phase serology is important because viral shedding from the sites of culture may occur without clinical disease. No specific therapy is available for enteroviral encephalitis.

From the clinical perspective, the most emergent encephalitis to diagnose is that due to herpes simplex virus (HSV).[57] This infection is characteristically caused by HSV type 1 and results in inflammation or necrosis localized to the medial-temporal and orbital-frontal lobes. Although it may have an insidious onset, in its most classic form HSV encephalitis presents as an acute, febrile, focal illness. Because of the temporal lobe localization, personality change may be prominent for a few days to as long as a week before other manifestations. Headache is also a prominent early symptom. Patients may progress rapidly from a nonspecific prodrome of fever and malaise, to findings such as behavioral abnormalities and seizures, to coma. A hallmark of the diagnosis is focality, which may be demonstrated with history (eg, changes in personality or in olfaction), physical examination, imaging studies of the brain, or EEG. These findings most characteristically involve the temporal lobes. Subtle clues to focality may include abnormalities such as changes in olfaction, which may be influenced by the fact that HSV might access the brain via the olfactory tract. CSF analysis may initially be unrevealing even in some acutely ill patients who have fever, nuchal rigidity, and coma. Characteristic features with lumbar puncture include increased intracranial pressure, CSF lymphocytosis, and the presence of RBCs in the CSF. Although CSF glucose is characteristically normal, patients may have hypoglycorrhachia. For many years, brain biopsy with viral culture was considered the gold-standard diagnostic study. In suspected cases, such pathologic examination of brain tissue often yielded another treatable diagnosis. Because of the invasiveness of the procedure and because neurosurgical services are not available at all

Table 5. Encephalitis*

Infectious	Postinfectious Encephalomyelitis	Noninfectious Diseases Simulating Viral Encephalitis
Viral	Vaccinia virus	Systemic lupus erythematosus
Rabies	Measles virus	Granulomatous angiitis
Herpes viruses: HSV 1 and 2, varicella-zoster, herpes B (simian herpes), Epstein-Barr, CMV, human herpes 6	Varicella-zoster virus	Behçet disease
Arthropod-borne (Table 6)	Rubella virus carcinomatous meningitis	Neoplastic diseases, including
Mumps	Epstein-Barr virus	Sarcoid
Lymphocytic choriomeningitis	Mumps virus	Reye syndrome
Enteroviruses: coxsackievirus, echovirus, hepatitis A	Influenza virus	Adrenal leukodystrophy
HIV	Nonspecific respiratory disease	Metabolic encephalopathies
Bacterial (including Brucella, Listeria, Nocardia, Actinomyces, relapsing fever, cat scratch disease, Whipple disease, infective endocarditis, parameningeal foci)	…	Cerebrovascular disease
M tuberculosis	…	Subdural hematoma
Mycoplasma pneumoniae	…	Subarachnoid hemorrhage
Spirochetes: syphilis, Lyme disease, leptospirosis		Acute multiple sclerosis
Fungal: including Cryptococcus, Coccidioides, Histoplasma, Blastomyces, Candida		Toxic encephalopathy, including cocaine-induced
Rickettsial: RMSF, typhus, Ehrlichia, Q fever	…	Drug reactions
Parasites: Toxoplasma, Naegleria, Acanthamoeba, Plasmodium falciparum, Trichinella, Echinococcus, Cysticercus, Trypanosoma cruzi	…	

*CMV = cytomegalovirus; RMSF = Rocky Mountain spotted fever.

hospitals, there has been attention to noninvasive diagnostic procedures. PCR analysis of CSF (when performed with optimal techniques in an experienced laboratory) has been reported to be 100% specific and 75 to 98% sensitive. In a decision model comparing a PCR-based approach with empiric therapy, the PCR-based approach yielded better outcomes with reduced acyclovir use.[58] Prompt initiation of IV therapy with acyclovir is critical in management of patients in whom this infection is suspected because prognosis is influenced by the level of consciousness at the time therapy is begun. It has been stated that one cannot anticipate an accuracy of >50% in the diagnosis of HSV encephalitis in the early course of the infection, even when one uses physical examination, spinal fluid analysis without PCR, and neuroimaging studies. Relapse of HSV encephalitis has been stated to occur in some patients 1 week to 3 months after initial improvement and completion of a full course of acyclovir therapy. Retreatment may be indicated in these patients.

The arthropod-borne encephalitides are a group of CNS infections in which the viral pathogen is transmitted to humans via a mosquito or tick vector. Of those described in Table 6, all are mosquito-borne except for Powassan encephalitis, which is transmitted by the tick *Ixodes cookei*. The distinguishing features of these illnesses are summarized in this table. Of these, Eastern equine encephalitis is associated with the highest mortality rate (30 to 70%), and this fulminant process results in neurologic sequelae in >80% of survivors. St. Louis encephalitis (SLE) is caused by a flavivirus, which induces clinical disease in about 1% of those infected. Following a nonspecific prodrome, patients may experience the abrupt onset of headache, nausea, vomiting, disorientation, and stupor. Common laboratory findings include inappropriate secretion of antidiuretic hormone and pyuria. In contrast to Eastern equine encephalitis, the overall mortality related to SLE is about 2%, with the highest mortality rate occurring in elderly persons. Emotional disturbances are the most common sequelae.

The outbreak of arboviral encephalitis described in metropolitan New York City in the late summer and fall of 1999 was caused by West Nile virus (WNV), a flavivirus that is serologically closely related to SLE virus and that was responsible for 61 human cases, including 7 deaths.[59] In 2002, the virus became much more widespread in its prevalence across the United States, making WNV an important diagnostic consideration in patients with an acute viral illness. In the summary of pertinent information on this virus,[60] several important points were made. It was noted that 1 in 5 infected persons had developed a mild febrile illness, with 1 in 150 developing meningitis, encephalitis, or both. Advanced age was the greatest risk factor for severe neurologic disease, long-term morbidity, and death. The most efficient diagnostic method noted in that review was IgM antibody-capture ELISA for IgM antibody to WNV in serum or CSF. Important bases for using this diagnostic study are that IgM antibody does not cross the blood-brain barrier and that 90% of serum samples obtained within 8 days of symptom onset had been positive for IgM antibody. A feature clinicians need to be familiar with is that related flaviviruses—such as those causing SLE or dengue—may produce a false-positive assay for WNV. The cited review presents a concise summary of the criteria for making possible, probable, and confirmed diagnoses of WNV based on the US national case definitions for WNV encephalitis. Recently reported is the experience with WNV infection in 28 patients, 54% of whom had a focal neurologic deficit at presentation.[61] In 47% of these patients with focal deficits, a meningitis or encephalitis syndrome was absent. During the outbreak of WNV in the summer of 2002, several

Table 6. *Arthropod-Borne Encephalitis*

Encephalitis	Mortality	Neurologic Sequelae
Eastern equine encephalitis	30–70%	80%
St. Louis encephalitis	2–20%	20%
California encephalitis	*	*
West Nile encephalitis	11%[†]	[‡]
Western equine encephalitis	5–15%	30%
Venezuelan equine encephalitis	1%	Rare
Powassan encephalitis	15%	...

*Uneventful recovery in most patients; abnormal EEGs in 75%, with seizures in 6 to 10%.
[†]Based on the 1999 outbreak in metropolitan New York, NY (MMWR Morb Mortal Wkly Rep 2000; 49:25–28).[59]
[‡]The limited data available suggest that many patients have substantial morbidity (Ann Intern Med 2002; 137:173–179).[60]

patients were described who presented with acute flaccid paralysis syndrome.[62] Noteworthy features in these patients included an asymmetrical weakness without pain or sensory loss in association with a CSF pleocytosis. Although some of these patients were initially thought to have Guillain-Barré syndrome, they did not have the symmetric pattern with sensory changes, paresthesias, and CSF protein elevation in the absence of CSF pleocytosis that are typical of Guillain-Barré syndrome. Preliminary interpretation of the findings of acute flaccid paralysis in WNV-infected patients is that the pattern is a polio-like syndrome with involvement of the anterior horn cells of the spinal cord and motor axons. Treatment for WNV encephalitis is supportive. Several approaches, including interferon-α2b and immunoglobulin with high titer against WNV, offer promise based on animal models and limited clinical experience.[63] Like SLE virus, WNV is transmitted principally by Culex mosquitoes.

Health-care providers should consider arboviruses in the differential diagnosis of aseptic meningitis and encephalitis cases during the summer months. According to recommendations by the CDC, serum (acute and convalescent) and CSF samples should be obtained for serologic testing, and cases should be reported promptly to state health departments.[64] Diagnosis of arbovirus encephalitis may be rapidly facilitated by testing acute serum or spinal fluid for virus-specific IgM antibody. Unfortunately, no effective specific therapy is available for any of these infections. Supportive measures should focus on cerebral edema, seizures, or ventilation if problems related to any of these occur.

HIV has tropism for neural tissue, and a significant number of patients will develop involvement of the CNS. As a part of the acute retroviral syndrome that follows initial infection with HIV, patients may develop an acute encephalitis that can include seizures and delirium and from which patients may spontaneously recover with few, if any, neurologic sequelae. On a chronic basis and occurring later in the course of HIV infection, patients may develop an encephalopathy associated with cerebral atrophy and widened sulci on CT studies of the brain. Clinical features may initially include forgetfulness and impaired cognitive function; these may progress to include weakness, ataxia, spasticity, and myoclonus.

The DNA polyoma virus JC is the etiologic agent in progressive multifocal leukoencephalopathy (PML). In this primary demyelinating process involving white matter of the cerebral hemispheres, patients present subacutely with confusion, disorientation, and visual disturbances, which may progress to cortical blindness or ataxia. CSF is characteristically acellular. A feature on neuroradiology imaging studies is lack of mass effect. No definitive therapy is presently available for this infection, and clinical efforts have recently focused on the role of immune reconstitution in modifying the clinical course of the illness. In a multicenter analysis of 57 consecutive HIV-positive patients with PML, neurologic improvement or stability at 2 months after therapy was demonstrated in 26% of patients who received highly active antiretroviral therapy, in contrast to improvement in only 4% of patients who did not receive this therapy (p = 0.03).[65] In this study, decreases in JC virus DNA to undetectable levels predicted a longer survival. In the context that untreated PML may be fatal within 3 to 6 months, the potential for preventing neurologic progression and improving survival by controlling JC virus replication becomes clinically relevant.

In recent months, there have been increasing reports of human rabies in the United States. Although this infection does not occur very often, it raises some important points about epidemiology, transmission, clinical presentation, and prevention. Rabies is probably best considered to be an encephalomyelopathy. After inoculation, the virus replicates in myocytes and then enters the nervous system via unmyelinated sensory and motor nerves. It spreads until the spinal cord is reached, and it is at this point in the clinical course that paresthesias may begin at the wound site. The virus then moves from the CNS along peripheral nerves to skin and intestine as well as into salivary glands, where it is released into saliva.[66] Knowledge of these factors allows an understanding of both clinical presentation and prevention. A review of the topic by the CDC stated that "…this infection should be considered in the differential diagnosis of persons presenting with unexplained rapidly progressive encephalitis."[67] A recent report acknowledges the potential for rabies to be spread through organ transplantation[68] and provides further support for the contention that rabies should be considered in any patient with unexplained encephalitis. It is the CNS involvement that leads to the cognitive dysfunction characteristic in encephalitis. Because the rabies virus may in the early stages localize to limbic structures, changes in behavior may result. Although an ascending paralysis simulating the Guillain-Barré syndrome has been described, the most classic presentation is of encephalitis associated with hypertonicity and hypersalivation. Noteworthy in Table 7 is that 13 of the 15 patients had pain and/or weakness, explainable since rabies is a myelopathic infection.[67-77]

Of the cases of bat-related rabies reported in the United States since 1980, the minority is definitively related to an animal bite. Only 3 of the 15 cases reported in the recent *Morbidity and Mortality Weekly Reports* cited in Table 7 were bite-related.

When the management of rabies in humans was reviewed in 2003,[78] it was acknowledged that the only survivors of the disease had received rabies vaccine before the onset of illness. In 2004, a previously healthy 15-year-old girl developed rabies after being bitten by a bat approximately 1 month before symptom onset. Her case represented the sixth known occurrence of human recovery after rabies infection; however, the case was unique because the patient received no rabies prophylaxis either before or after illness onset.[77] Despite this very rare occurrence, there is still a strong impetus for postexposure prophylaxis, which is discussed in the following paragraph. The cited review notes that the normal management of patients with rabies should be palliative. In those individuals who might be candidates for aggressive management, a combination of specific therapies was listed for consideration, including rabies vaccine, rabies immunoglobulin, monoclonal antibodies, ribavirin, interferon-α, and ketamine. A summary of the potential role of each of these agents was included. Because severe brain edema with herniation has been rare in patients with rabies and because corticosteroids have been associated with increased mortality and shortened incubation period in mouse models of rabies, the review stated that corticosteroids should not be used.

Rabies prophylaxis has been recently reviewed.[79] In individuals who were not previously vaccinated against rabies but have an indication for rabies postexposure prophylaxis, the treatment regimen includes local wound cleansing, human rabies immune globulin, and vaccine.

Table 7. *Clinical Presentation of Rabies**

Clinical Feature	Encephalitis Symptoms	Pain and Weakness	Findings of CI	Myoclonus	Paralysis	Autonomic Instability
Case 1[67]	Hallucinations	Left arm	Yes	Yes	Total body	No
Case 2[67]	Hypersalivation	Left arm	Yes	Yes	No	Yes
Case 3[69]	Confusion	Left face, ear	Yes	Yes	Vocal cord, ocular	No
Case 4[70]	Hallucinations	Right shoulder	Yes	No	No	Yes
Case 5[71]	Confusion	Right wrist	No	Yes	No	Yes
Case 6[71]	Confusion; hypersalivation	Right arm	No	Yes	Dysphagia	Yes
Case 7[71]	Disorientation; hypersalivation	No	No	No	No	Yes
Case 8[71]	No	Right arm	Yes	No	Flaccid paralysis	No
Case 9[71]	Delirium	Left arm	Yes	Yes	Dysphagia	Yes
Case 10[72]	Agitation	Both legs	Yes	No	No	Yes
Case 11[73]	Agitation; hypersalivation	Right arm	Yes	No	Dysphagia	Yes
Case 12[74]	Hallucinations; intractable seizures	Abdominal	No	No	Respiratory dysfunction	No
Case 13[75]	Ataxia; confusion	No	Yes	Yes	No	No
Case 14[76]	Confusion	Right arm	Yes	No	No	No
Case 15[77]	Hypersalivation	Left arm	Yes	Yes	Sixth nerve palsy	Yes

*CI = cerebrovascular insufficiency.

The doses of human rabies immune globulin and vaccine have been summarized.[79] The administration of rabies immune globulin has been modified, and recommendations now are that as much as anatomically feasible of the 20 IU/kg body weight dose should be infiltrated into and around the wound(s), with the remainder administered IM in the deltoid or quadriceps at a location other than that used for vaccine inoculation, to minimize potential interference. An important consideration is the prevention of rabies infection after exposure of family members or health-care providers to an index case. Possible percutaneous or mucous membrane exposure to a patient's saliva or CSF is an indication for postexposure prophylaxis. In the reports of the 15 patients summarized in Table 7, the following numbers of persons received postexposure prophylaxis: case 1, 46; case 2, 50; case 3, 60; case 4, 53; case 5, 48; case 6, 37; case 7, 71; case 8, 20; case 9, 27; case 10, 23; case 11, 46; case 12, 53; case 13, 8; case 14, 6; and case 15, 5. For persons in whom preexposure prophylaxis is indicated, only vaccine is recommended.[79]

A group of viruses, including dengue virus, enteroviruses, adenoviruses, and cytomegalovirus, may cause direct infection that results in encephalitis. In addition to viruses producing direct infection of the brain, certain viruses may cause a postinfectious encephalomyelitis. At one time, this form of CNS pathology accounted for about one third of fatal cases of encephalitis (with acute viral encephalitis being the major cause of infectious mortality in this category). With the elimination of vaccinia virus by vaccination for smallpox, the mortality attributable to postinfectious encephalomyelitis is now estimated to be 10 to 15% of cases of acute encephalitis in the United States. The pathogenesis of this process has not been definitively elucidated. The pathologic changes have been compared with those occurring in persons in whom acute encephalomyelitis developed following rabies immunization using vaccine prepared in CNS tissue. It has been suggested that certain viral infections may cause a disruption of normal immune regulation, with resultant release of autoimmune responses. The viruses that have been associated with postinfectious encephalomyelitis are summarized in Table 4. Treatment of patients with such problems is limited to supportive care.

Two common infections that usually have benign courses in adolescents and young adults may progress to serious disease, which may include involvement of the CNS. Mononucleosis due to Epstein-Barr virus may, on rare occasions, cause direct infection of the brain and an encephalitic process, which is the most common cause of death resulting from this infection. CNS infection is the most significant extrarespiratory manifestation of infection caused by *Mycoplasma pneumoniae*. Even though this organism has been isolated from the CSF, the mechanism by which it causes encephalitis is thought to be an autoimmune one.

Rickettsiae have the ability to produce infection of the CNS. Of these, the most characteristic is Rocky Mountain spotted fever (RMSF), caused by *R rickettsii*. After being transmitted to humans via a tick bite, this intracellular pathogen can produce a constellation of symptoms and signs that includes fever, petechial skin lesions (involving the palms, soles, wrists, and ankles), and a meningoencephalitis. Because of the skin lesions and neurologic involvement, acute forms of this infection may mimic disease caused by *N meningitidis*. Chloramphenicol is effective against both of these pathogens, but tetracycline is considered the usual first-line drug when only RMSF is suspected. In contrast to the distal skin lesions that progress centrally in RMSF, epidemic typhus caused by *Rickettsia prowazekii* is characterized by central lesions that move distally. This infection is more likely to occur during the winter months than is RMSF, which usually occurs during the late summer and early fall. The emerging rickettsial pathogen identified as a cause of nervous system involvement is Ehrlichia. Pathogens within the genus Ehrlichia have the propensity to parasitize either mononuclear or granulocytic leukocytes, with the resultant infections referred to as human monocytic ehrlichiosis or human granulocytic ehrlichiosis, respectively. The epidemiology of ehrlichiosis, including outdoor activity and exposure to ticks, is similar to that of RMSF, but in contrast to RMSF, ehrlichiosis is associated with rash in only about 20% of cases. In addition to causing the characteristic findings of fever, leukopenia, thrombocytopenia, and abnormal liver enzymes, nervous system involvement in ehrlichiosis may include severe headache, confusion, lethargy, broad-based gait, hyperreflexia, clonus, photophobia, cranial nerve palsy, seizures, blurred vision, nuchal rigidity, and ataxia. The characteristic CSF abnormalities have been a lymphocytic pleocytosis with an elevated protein level. In a recent review of the subject, the CSF glucose level was normal in the majority of patients, with 24% of the patients having borderline low CSF glucose concentrations. In this review, morulae were seen in CSF white cells in only a small minority of the patients. Radiographic and encephalographic studies did not reveal any lesions that supported a specific diagnosis. Although the definitive agent for treating this infection has not been established by clinical trials, it appears that chloramphenicol or tetracycline is the agent most frequently used. The clinical experience with this process has been limited, and the outcome in patients with nervous system involvement is not well established.

As summarized in Table 5, certain noninfectious diseases may mimic viral encephalitis.

Brain Abscess

Among bacterial infections of the CNS, brain abscess is the second most common. On a pathogenetic basis, this infection may develop after hematogenous dissemination of organisms during systemic infection (which often occurs in the context of such conditions as infective endocarditis, cyanotic congenital heart disease, and lung abscess), with extension from infected cranial structures (*eg*, sinuses or middle ear) along emissary veins, or as a consequence of trauma or neurosurgery. The classic presentation may include recent onset of severe headache, new focal or generalized seizures, and clinical evidence of an intracranial mass. In the nonimmunocompromised host, brain abscess represents a deviation from the classic tenet that *Bacteroides fragilis* is not a significant pathogen above the diaphragm. In the patient without predisposing factors, streptococci (including the *Streptococcus intermedius* [*milleri*] group) along with anaerobes (including *B fragilis*) are the predominant pathogens.[80] Excision or stereotactic aspiration of the abscess is used to identify the etiologic agents and has been recommended for lesions >2.5 cm.[81] Some experts have advocated using empiric antimicrobial therapy without aspiration of the abscess in patients who are neurologically stable and have an abscess <3 cm in diameter that is not encroaching on the ventricular system; however, if such a decision is made, they have advised that the patient must be followed meticulously with a brain imaging study such as CT or MRI, and enlargement of the abscess during therapy mandates surgery. Because of the lack of consistent efficacy of metronidazole against streptococci and upper airway anaerobic cocci, penicillin or a third-generation cephalosporin (*eg*, cefotaxime or ceftriaxone) is usually combined with this agent. An alternative to metronidazole in this regimen would be chloramphenicol. In the settings of penetrating head trauma, following neurosurgical procedures, or with acute bacterial endocarditis, therapy for *S aureus* should be included. Those patients with a presumed otic or sinus origin for their abscess should have coverage against enterobacteriaceae and *H influenzae* using a third-generation cephalosporin.

In HIV-infected persons, *T gondii* classically presents as fever, headache, altered mental status, and focal neurologic deficits, especially in individuals whose $CD4^+$ count falls below 100 cells/mm^3. Because the disease is due to reactivation of latent infection in about 95% of cases, IgG antibody to Toxoplasma is generally present. A review of neuroimaging studies in patients with AIDS is summarized in Table 8, with a key point being whether or not mass effect is present.[82] Imaging studies of the brain in AIDS patients with Toxoplasma brain abscess show multiple (usually ≥3) nodular contrast-enhancing lesions with mass effect found most commonly in the basal ganglia and at the gray-white matter junction. In the classic setting

Table 8. *Approach to Mass Lesions In HIV-Infected Persons**

Focal Lesions With Mass Effect in HIV-Infected Persons	Focal Lesion Without Mass Effect in HIV-Infected Persons
Toxoplasmosis Primary lymphoma of the CNS Cerebral cryptococcosis† Neurotuberculosis† Syphilitic gumma‡	Progressive multifocal leukoencephalopathy

*CNS = central nervous system. Adapted from Clin Infect Dis 1996;22:906–919.[82]

† Rarely present as abscesses.

‡ Rare presentation of neurosyphilis.

described above, empiric therapy with sulfadiazine and pyrimethamine is recommended. Clindamycin-containing regimens may be considered in sulfa-allergic patients. Brain biopsy is reserved for atypical presentations and for patients who do not respond to initial therapy. After acute therapy for toxoplasmic encephalitis, prophylaxis to prevent recurrence has been recommended with a regimen like sulfadiazine plus pyrimethamine plus leucovorin, but may be discontinued once CD4+ cells are >200/μL for ≥6 months.[83] The lesions of toxoplasmosis may be confused with primary CNS lymphoma, which also causes a mass effect due to surrounding edema and which may undergo central necrosis and present as ring-enhancing masses.

Spinal Epidural Abscess and Subdural Empyema

A review of spinal epidural abscess provides the basis for understanding two common threads included in literature published about this infection: reports of poor prognosis and appeals for rapid treatment.[84] Spinal epidural abscess represents a neurosurgical emergency because neurologic deficits may become irreversible when there is a delay in evacuating the purulent material. Although the basis for this irreversibility has not been definitively established, mechanisms for the associated spinal cord necrosis include a decrease in arterial blood flow, venous thrombosis, or direct compression of the spinal cord. The triad of findings that supports the diagnosis is fever, point tenderness over the spine, and focal neurologic deficits. The predisposing factors to this infection shed light on the likely pathogens. Skin and soft tissue are the most probable source of infection and provide an understanding of why S aureus is the most common pathogen in this infection. Spinal epidural abscess has been reported to follow surgery, trauma, urinary tract infections, and respiratory diseases. Of increasing importance are the reports of this infection occurring as a complication of lumbar puncture and epidural anesthesia. In 16% of cases, the source of infection may be unknown. Usual pathogens include S aureus, streptococci (both aerobic and anaerobic), and Gram-negative bacilli.

Gadolinium-enhanced MRI has replaced myelography as the diagnostic study of choice because it identifies not only mass lesions, but also signal abnormalities that are consistent with acute transverse myelopathy and spinal cord ischemia.[85]

Subdural empyema is an infection that occurs between the dura and arachnoid and that results as organisms are spread via emissary veins or by extension of osteomyelitis of the skull. The paranasal sinuses are the source in over half the cases, with otitis another likely predisposing condition. In young children, it is usually a complication of meningitis. The clinical features include fever, headache, vomiting, signs of meningeal irritation, alteration in mental status, and focal neurologic deficits that progress to focal seizures. The usual pathogens are aerobic streptococci (including S pneumoniae), staphylococci, H influenzae, Gram-negative bacilli, and anaerobes (including B fragilis). The diagnosis is often made using MRI, but CT scan with contrast enhancement may offer the advantage of imaging bone. Antibiotics directed against the likely pathogens and surgical interventions are mainstays of therapy.

Septic Intracranial Thrombophlebitis

Thrombosis of the cortical vein may occur as a complication of meningitis and is associated with progressive neurologic deficits, including hemiparesis, bilateral weakness, or aphasia. Thrombosis of the intracranial venous sinuses classically follows infections of the paranasal sinuses, middle ear, mastoid, face, or oropharynx, although the process may be metastatic from lungs or other sites. The most frequent pathogens are S aureus, coagulase-negative staphylococci, streptococci, Gram-negative bacilli, and anaerobes. Five anatomic sites may be involved with varying clinical presentations.[86] Superior sagittal sinus thrombosis results in bilateral leg weakness or in communicating hydrocephalus. Lateral sinus thrombosis produces pain over the ear and mastoid, with possible edema over the mastoid. Superior petrosal sinus thrombosis causes ipsilateral pain, sensory deficit, or temporal lobe seizures. Inferior petrosal sinus thrombosis may produce the syndrome of ipsilateral facial pain and lateral rectus weakness that is referred to as Gradenigo's syndrome.

Of the forms of venous sinus thrombosis, cavernous sinus thrombosis is the most frequently discussed. Within this sinus lie the internal carotid artery with its sympathetic plexus and the sixth cranial nerve. In the lateral wall of the sinus are the third and fourth cranial nerves, along with the ophthalmic and sometimes maxillary divisions of the trigeminal nerve. The clinical presentation is influenced by these anatomic considerations. The process, which is considered life-threatening, begins unilaterally but usually becomes bilateral within hours. High fever, headaches, malaise, nausea, and vomiting are the predominant findings. Patients progress to develop proptosis, chemosis, periorbital edema, and cyanosis of the ipsilateral forehead, eyelids, and root of the nose. Ophthalmoplegia may develop, with the sixth cranial nerve usually involved first. Trigeminal nerve involvement may manifest itself as decreased sensation about the eye. Ophthalmic nerve involvement may present as photophobia and persistent eye pain. Papilledema, diminished pupillary reactivity, and diminished corneal reflexes may also develop. The disease may be relentless in its progression to alteration in level of consciousness, meningitis, and seizures. The mainstays of therapy include broad-spectrum antibiotics and surgical drainage with removal of infected bone or abscess. The issue of anticoagulation in patients with suppurative intracranial thrombophlebitis is controversial. It is the opinion of some experts in the field that heparin followed by warfarin may be beneficial,[87] but heparin-induced thrombocytopenia has been noted as a potential complication. Steroids may be necessary if involvement of the pituitary gland leads to adrenal insufficiency and circulatory collapse.

Neuritis

Infection of nervous tissue outside of the CNS can take place on the basis of several pathogenetic mechanisms. Certain pathogens, such as *Borrelia burgdorferi* (the etiologic agent of Lyme disease), HIV, cytomegalovirus, HSV type 2, and varicella-zoster virus, can produce peripheral neuropathy. Direct infection of nerves may occur with *Mycobacterium leprae* and *Trypanosoma* spp. *Corynebacterium diphtheriae*, *Clostridium tetani*, and *Clostridium botulinum* can produce toxins that can injure peripheral nerves.

C diphtheriae produces a toxin that directly involves nerves to cause a noninflammatory demyelination. Clinical sequelae of such a process initially include local paralysis of the soft palate and posterior pharyngeal wall, followed by cranial nerve involvement, and culminating in involvement of peripheral nerves. Myocarditis occurs in as many as two thirds of patients, but <25% develop clinical evidence of cardiac dysfunction. Antitoxin is indicated in infected patients, along with antibacterial therapy. Both penicillin and erythromycin have been recommended as treatment of diphtheria by the World Health Organization. In a study in Vietnamese children with diphtheria that compared IM benzylpenicillin with erythromycin, both antibiotics were efficacious, but slower fever clearance and a higher incidence of GI side effects were associated with erythromycin.[88] Erythromycin resistance was noted in some of the isolates tested, but all were susceptible to penicillin. Both *C tetani* and *C botulinum* cause indirect nerve involvement on the basis of toxin production. The epidemiology of tetanus has changed somewhat in recent years. Joining elderly patients as a patient population at risk for tetanus are injection drug users who inject drugs subcutaneously (ie, "skin pop"). The toxin of *C tetani* is transported up axons and binds to presynaptic endings on motor neurons in anterior horn cells of the spinal cord. This blocks inhibitory input and results in uncontrolled motor input to skeletal muscle and tetanic spasm. Antitoxin is not available for this disorder, but tetanus immune globulin and tetanus toxoid are given for clinical disease. Prevention plays a pivotal role in controlling the number of cases of tetanus. A population-based serologic survey of immunity to tetanus in the United States revealed protective levels of tetanus antibodies ranging from 87.7% among those 6 to 11 years of age to 27.8% among those 70 years of age or older.[89] Although there is an excellent correlation between vaccination rates (96%) and immunity (96%) among 6-year-olds, antibody levels decline over time such that one fifth of older children (10 to 16 years of age) do not have protective antibody levels. Such data argue strongly for ongoing tetanus immunization throughout a person's life in an attempt to prevent this potentially fatal disease.

The toxin of *C botulinum* binds to the presynaptic axon terminal of the neuromuscular junction with inhibition of acetylcholine release. This results in a symmetric, descending, flaccid paralysis of motor and autonomic nerves, usually beginning with the cranial nerves. Recent reports of botulism have noted not only foodborne outbreaks associated with consumption of contaminated fish, commercial cheese sauce, and baked potatoes held in aluminum foil for several days at room temperature, but also wound botulism in injection drug users who injected Mexican black tar heroin subcutaneously. The classic presentation includes neurologic and GI findings. Nausea and vomiting may be followed by diminished salivation and extreme dryness of the mouth, and by difficulty in focusing the eyes that occurs due to interruption of cholinergic autonomic transmission. Patients progress to cranial nerve palsies (with common presentations being diplopia, dysarthria, or dysphagia) and then to a symmetrical descending flaccid voluntary muscle weakness that may progress to respiratory compromise. Normal body temperature and normal sensory nerve examination findings are typical, as is an intact mental status despite a groggy appearance. A large outbreak occurred in 1994 in El Paso, TX, and was traced to a dip prepared in a restaurant from potatoes that had been baked in aluminum foil and then left at room temperature for several days.[90] In that report, the following criteria were used for making the diagnosis of botulism: (1) an electromyographic (EMG) study showing an increase of ≥50% in the evoked train of compound muscle action potentials with rapid repetitive stimulation (20 to 50 Hz); (2) stool culture positive for *C botulinum*; and (3) blurred vision, dysphagia, or dysarthria in a person who did not have EMG findings indicating botulism and who did not have *C botulinum* detected in stool (findings consistent with the diagnosis of "suspected case"). In addition, the mouse inoculation test for toxin using serum, stool, or food may be positive. In a recent review of laboratory findings in foodborne botulism, the following were listed: normal CSF values; specific EMG findings (normal motor conduction velocities; normal sensory nerve amplitudes and latencies; decreased evoked muscle action potential; facilitation following rapid repetitive nerve stimulation); and standard mouse bioassay positive for toxin from clinical specimens and/or suspect food.[91] Researchers from the CDC and the Republic of Georgia's National Center for Disease Control studied 706 cases of botulism in Georgia, which has the highest reported rate of foodborne botulism of any country.[92] They discovered that the patients at highest risk of dying were those who reported to the hospital with shortness of breath and impaired gag reflex but no diarrhea. This constellation of symptoms, if validated in the United States and other countries as predictors of death, would allow doctors to give first consideration to patients who are at highest risk of dying in a botulism outbreak.[92]

Intestinal botulism, which occurs most commonly in infants and is rare in children and adults, is the most common form of human botulism in the United States.[93] Along with the traditional forms of botulism, there are two additional forms of importance. Since 1978, the CDC has recorded cases of botulism in which extensive investigation failed to implicate a specific food as the cause. These have been referred to as cases of "undetermined origin." Investigation has shown that some of these cases were caused by colonization of the GI tract by *C botulinum* or *Clostridium baratii* with *in vivo* production of toxin, analogous to the pathogenesis of infant botulism. In some cases of botulism strongly suspected to represent intestinal colonization, the patients had a history of GI surgery or illnesses such as inflammatory bowel disease, which might have predisposed them to enteric colonization. This form of botulism has been referred to as intestinal colonization botulism (also termed by some as adult-type infant botulism). Of more recent interest is inhalational botulism, which could occur as a component of bioterrorism with intentional release of aerosolized botulinum toxin.

As summarized in Table 9, antitoxin is indicated for adult botulism, which occurs on the

Table 9. *Toxin-Mediated Peripheral Neuritis*

Direct toxin injury
  Corynebacterium diphtheriae*
Indirect toxin injury
  Clostridium tetani
  Clostridium botulinum
    Traditional categories
      Adult botulism*
      Infant (intestinal) botulism†
      Wound botulism*
      Intestinal colonization botulism‡
  New category
    Inhalational botulism‡

*Antitoxin indicated.
†Role for botulism immune globulin IV (human) [BIG-IV].
‡See text.

basis of ingestion of preformed toxin, and for wound botulism, in which toxin is produced locally at the infected wound. A review of botulism has noted that antitoxin is released from the CDC for cases of intestinal colonization botulism.[94] With inhalational botulism, it has been suggested that antitoxin be given as early as possible based on clinical suspicion and should not be delayed while awaiting microbiologic testing.[95] It has been noted with this form of botulism that antitoxin might only prevent progression of disease but not reverse paralysis once it has occurred. It is important to be aware that skin testing should be performed to assess for sensitivity to serum or antitoxin prior to administration of antitoxin. In contrast, infant botulism, which occurs when the ingested organism produces toxin within the GI tract, does not respond to antitoxin. A human-derived human botulism immune globulin has been administered to infants with botulism and has been shown to reduce length of stay with this pattern of disease. Although this product is not yet commercially available, it may be obtained for the treatment of infant botulism under a Treatment Investigational New Drug protocol by contacting the California Department of Health Services (telephone (510) 540-2646). The acute, simultaneous onset of neurologic symptoms in multiple individuals should suggest a common source for the problem and increase the suspicion of botulism.

Certain toxins produced by fish and shellfish have been associated with neurologic involvement. Ciguatera fish poisoning follows consumption of marine fish (most characteristically grouper, red snapper, and barracuda) that have been contaminated with toxins produced by microalgae known as dinoflagellates. The classic constellation of findings involves GI, cardiovascular, and neurologic systems. The characteristic neurologic findings include paresthesias (which may be chronic) periorally and in distal extremities, often associated with a debilitating hot-to-cold reversal dysesthesia. Taste sensation is often altered. Implicated toxins include ciguatoxin (which induces membrane depolarization by opening voltage-dependent sodium channels), maitotoxin (which opens calcium channels), and palytoxin (which causes muscle injury). Therapy is primarily symptomatic and supportive. Paralytic shellfish poisoning is caused by consumption of shellfish (most characteristically butter clams, mussels, cockles, steamer clams, sea snails, or razor clams) or broth from cooked shellfish that contain either concentrated saxitoxin (a heat-stable alkaloid neurotoxin) or related compounds, with resultant sensory, cerebellar, and motor dysfunction. Characteristic neurologic findings include paresthesias of the mouth and extremities, ataxia, dysphagia, muscle paralysis, coma, and total muscular paralysis. Treatment is supportive.

The ascending paralysis that comprises the Guillain-Barré syndrome characteristically follows respiratory infection, GI infection (notably, Campylobacter infection), or immunization. The pathology is segmental inflammation with perivascular mononuclear cells and demyelination. An exact etiology for this process has not been elucidated.

Catheter-Related Infections

Urinary Bladder Catheters

A clinical situation frequently associated with injudicious use of antibiotics in the critical care setting is asymptomatic bacteriuria. In March 2005, the IDSA published guidelines for the diagnosis and treatment of asymptomatic bacteriuria in adults.[96] In that document, the diagnosis of asymptomatic bacteruria was based on results of a culture of a urine specimen collected in a manner that minimizes contamination. For asymptomatic women, *bacteriuria* was defined as two consecutive voided urine specimens with isolation of the same bacterial strain in quantitative counts $\geq 10^5$ cfu/mL. *Asymptomatic bacteriuria* was defined as (1) a single, clean-catch voided urine specimen with one bacterial species isolated in a quantitative count $\geq 10^5$ cfu/mL in men, or (2) a single catheterized urine specimen with one bacterial species isolated in a quantitative count $\geq 10^2$ cfu/mL in women or men. Of note is that pyuria accompanying asymptomatic bacteriuria was not considered to be an indication for antimicrobial therapy. In adults, two A-1 recommendations were made regarding treatment of asymptomatic bacteriuria in adults: (1) pregnant women, and (2) men scheduled to undergo transurethral resection of the prostate. An A-III recommendation was given for treatment of asymptomatic bacteriuria before urologic procedures (other than transurethral resection of the prostate) for which mucosal bleeding is anticipated. The guidelines stated that antimicrobial treatment of asymptomatic women with catheter-acquired bacteriuria that persists 48 h after indwelling catheter removal may be considered for treatment. Table 10 summarizes those situations where therapy for asymptomatic bacteriuria was not recommended and reviews situations where the data are evolving but not conclusive.[96-107]

A clinically important area, but one in which there are no definitive data, relates to renal transplant recipients. It has been acknowledged that urine culture surveillance and periodic renal scan or ultrasound examinations are recommended by some authors, at least during the first months after transplantation. Based on cited references that treatment of asymptomatic urinary tract infections in renal transplant recipients are largely unsuccessful and that such therapy may not have an observable effect on graft function, it was noted that asymptomatic urinary tract infections in this immunocompromised patient population may be left untreated.[101] Frequent or inappropriate use of antibiotics exerts selective pressures that are responsible for the increasing prevalence of bacterial resistance. Because of this, it is important to use antibiotics in situations where the clinical benefits exceed risks such as adverse effects and the selection of resistant organisms. A recent report of the NIH-sponsored Mycoses Study Group evaluated the issue of treatment for candiduria that was asymptomatic or minimally symptomatic.[108] Patients were randomly assigned to receive fluconazole (200 mg/d) or placebo for 14 days. In 50% of cases, the isolate was *Candida albicans*. At the end of treatment, urine was cleared in 50% of patients given fluconazole vs 29% of those given placebo. However, cure rate was about 70% in both groups at 2 weeks posttreatment. Although these data represented short-term eradication of candiduria (especially following catheter removal), the long-term eradication rates were not associated with clinical benefit. Notable in this study were the observations in the placebo group that candiduria resolved in about 20% of chronically catheterized patients when their catheter was only changed and in 41% of untreated patients when the catheter was removed.

Peritoneal Dialysis Catheters

Abdominal pain and/or fever and/or cloudy peritoneal fluid are the clinical features usually found in patients who are undergoing either continuous ambulatory peritoneal dialysis or automated peritoneal dialysis and who develop peritonitis. The organisms most frequently isolated

Table 10. *Treatment of Asymptomatic Bacteriuria in Adults*

Adults in Whom Therapy Is Recommended

Pregnant women[97-99]
Men about to undergo transurethral resection of the prostate or other urologic procedures for which mucosal bleeding is anticipated[96,100]

Adults in Whom Therapy May Be Considered

Women with catheter-acquired bacteriuria that persists 48 h after indwelling catheter removal

Persons in Whom Definitive Recommendations Are Not Available but for Whom Some Provide Therapy

Certain immunocompromised patients, especially those who are neutropenic or who have undergone renal transplantation (see comments in text about renal transplant patients[101])
Elderly persons with obstructive uropathy[102-105]
Patients with diabetes mellitus[106]
Persons with positive urine cultures both at the time of catheter removal and then again 1–2 wk after catheter removal[107]
Those undergoing certain types of surgery, particularly when prostheses or foreign bodies (notably vascular grafts) may be left in place
Some patients with struvite stones
Persons with spinal cord injury[96]
Catheterized patients while the catheter remains *in situ*[96]

in such processes have been coagulase-negative staphylococci (*eg*, *Staphylococcus epidermidis*) or *S aureus*, but the incidence of Gram-negative pathogens has increased in patients utilizing disconnect systems. When caused by *S aureus*, a toxic shock–like syndrome has been occasionally noted. The finding of >100 WBCs/mm^3, of which at least 50% are polymorphonuclear neutrophils, is supportive of the diagnosis of peritonitis. Recent trends in the management of this infection have been affected by the emergence of vancomycin resistance, both in enterococci as well as in *S aureus*. Vancomycin use has influenced this resistance. In a review of vancomycin-intermediate *S aureus*, it was noted that of the first 6 patients reported in the United States with this pathogen, all but 1 had had exposure to dialysis for renal insufficiency, with the resultant potential for recurrent vancomycin use.[109] In recognition of the contribution of injudicious use of vancomycin to the development of vancomycin resistance in Gram-positive organisms, the Advisory Committee on Peritonitis Management of the International Society for Peritoneal Dialysis recommended that traditional empiric therapy of catheter-associated peritonitis be changed from the regimen of vancomycin and gentamicin to a first-generation cephalosporin (*eg*, cefazolin or cephalothin in a loading dose of 500 mg/L and a maintenance dose of 125 mg/L) in combination with an aminoglycoside.[110] The committee stated further that modifications to this regimen could be made based on the organism isolated or on sensitivity patterns. In its more recent iteration of recommendations for treatment of adult peritoneal dialysis-related peritonitis,[111] the International Society for Peritoneal Dialysis suggested the substitution of ceftazidime for the aminoglycoside. Residual renal function is an independent predictor of patient survival. It is especially noteworthy that use of any aminoglycoside,[112] even when given for short periods, and the rate of peritonitis[113] are independent risk factors for the decline of residual renal function in patients using continuous ambulatory peritoneal dialysis. A concern about ceftazidime is its risk of selecting resistant Gram-negative organisms, including those that produce type I β-lactamases or extended-spectrum β-lactamases.[114] The role of empiric therapy with cefazolin has also been reported in potentially infected hemodialysis patients,[115] with vancomycin being reserved for confirmed resistant organisms.[116] Many episodes of catheter-associated peritonitis may be managed without removal of the catheter, but peritonitis that does not respond to antibiotic therapy and peritonitis associated with tunnel infections may be indications for catheter removal. Infection with Pseudomonas, a fungal pathogen, or mycobacteria often requires catheter removal for cure.[117] Another entity that influences the decision for catheter removal is relapsing peritonitis, defined as an episode of peritonitis caused by the same genus/species that caused the immediately preceding episode, occurring within 4 weeks of completion of the antibiotic course. If no clinical response is noted after 96 h of therapy for relapsing peritonitis, catheter removal is indicated; if the patient responds clinically, but subsequently relapses an additional time, catheter removal and replacement are recommended.[111]

Vascular Catheters

Of the 200,000 nosocomial bloodstream infections that occur each year in the United States, most are related to different types of intravascular devices. The IDSA, the Society of Critical Care Medicine, and the Society for Healthcare Epidemiology of America have recently published guidelines for management of intravascular catheter–related infections.[118] In their review, the following recommendations were made regarding blood cultures in cases of suspected catheter-associated bacteremia: (1) two sets of blood samples for culture, with a least one drawn percutaneously, should be obtained with a new episode of suspected central venous catheter–related bloodstream infection; and (2) paired quantitative blood cultures or paired qualitative blood cultures with a continuously monitored differential time to positivity should be collected for the diagnosis of catheter-related infection, especially when the long-term catheter cannot be removed. The recommendation regarding blood cultures noted in the preceding statement is different from those recommended in a recent *New England Journal of Medicine* review,[119] in which it was stated that "Two cultures of blood from peripheral sites should be evaluated because it is difficult to determine whether a positive culture of blood from a central venous catheter indicates contamination of the hub, catheter colonization, or a catheter-related bloodstream infection." Quantitative blood cultures simultaneously obtained through a central venous catheter and a peripheral vein and demonstrating a five- to 10-fold increase in concentration of an organism in catheter blood compared with peripheral blood have been reported to correlate well with catheter-related infections; however, some studies have not supported such a correlation. For tunneled catheters, a quantitative culture of blood from the central venous catheter that yields at least 100 cfu/mL may be diagnostic without a companion culture of a peripheral blood sample.[120] A new diagnostic method has been made possible by continuous blood culture monitoring systems and compares the time to positive cultures of blood drawn from the catheter and from a peripheral vein. One study has shown a sensitivity of 91% and a specificity of 94% in determining catheter-related infection when a blood culture drawn from a central venous catheter became positive at least 2 h earlier than the culture drawn from a peripheral vein.[121] These data have most applicability to tunneled catheters.

Over the past two decades, the medical literature has proposed several predictors of sepsis from a catheter. Although Gram stain of material from the tip of a catheter may be helpful with diagnosis of local infection, it is significantly less sensitive than quantitative methods. The most traditionally quoted study regarding predictors of catheter-related infection suggests that the presence of ≥15 colonies on a semiquantitative roll culture of the tip of a catheter or needle is most useful.[122] Although such techniques are relied on at present to assist in the determination of an infected catheter, some data have suggested that the semiquantitative culture may not be predictive of clinical outcome. When compared with qualitative cultures, quantitative methods—which include either (1) flushing the segment with broth or (2) vortexing or sonicating the segment in broth, followed by serial dilutions and surface plating on blood agar—have greater specificity in the identification of catheter-related infections. In the recently published guidelines for management of intravascular catheter-related infections,[104] the sensitivities of these three methods were listed as follows: sonication, 80%; roll plate method, 60%; and flush culture, 40 to 50%.

A review of 51 English-language studies published from 1966 to July 2004 studied the eight diagnostic methods that are most frequently used in clinical practice and for which performance data have been published: qualitative catheter segment culture, semiquantitative catheter segment culture (roll-plate method), or quantitative catheter segment culture, each combined with demonstrated concordance with results of concomitant blood cultures; qualitative blood culture drawn through an intravascular device (IVD); paired quantitative peripheral and IVD-drawn blood cultures; acridine orange leukocyte cytospin testing of IVD-drawn blood; and differential time to positivity of concomitant qualitative IVD-drawn and peripheral blood cultures (>2 h).[123] In this analysis, paired quantitative blood culture was the most accurate test for diagnosis of IVD-related bloodstream infection. However, most other methods studied showed acceptable sensitivity and specificity (both >0.75) and negative predictive value.

In the IDSA guidelines for the management of catheter-related infections, alternative routes of antibiotic administration were also discussed.[118] An important consideration is whether the infection is intraluminal or extraluminal. Catheters that have been in place for <2 weeks are most often infected extraluminally, whereas catheters in place for a longer duration were more likely to have intraluminal infection. Antibiotic solutions that contain the desired antimicrobial agent in a concentration of 1 to 5 mg/mL are usually mixed with 50 to 100 U of heparin (or normal saline) and are installed or "locked" into the catheter lumen during periods when the catheter is not used (eg, for a 12-h period each night). The volume of installed antibiotic is removed before infusion of the next dose of an antibiotic or IV medication or solution, and the most often used duration of such therapy is 2 weeks. Summarized in this review are some reports of cure of patients with infected tunneled catheters who were treated with both parenteral and lock therapy.

Of the pathogens most characteristically isolated as a complication of indwelling vascular catheters, coagulase-negative staphylococci, *S aureus*, and *Candida* spp have been most frequently reported. In immunocompromised patients with long-term indwelling catheters, *Corynebacterium jeikeium* and Bacillus spp are important, and notably both have vancomycin as the drug of choice for therapy. Gram-negative bacilli and atypical mycobacteria are also included as possible pathogens in this setting.

An important and common clinical question is whether a catheter-related intravascular infection can be cured with a long-term indwelling catheter left in place. The medical literature suggests that catheter-related coagulase-negative staphylococcal bacteremia may be successfully treated without recurrence in up to 80% of patients whose catheters remained in place and who received antibiotics.[124] In the 20% of patients who remained bacteremic while taking antibiotics with their catheters in place, metastatic infection was not a significant problem. For patients with vascular catheter-associated coagulase-negative staphylococcal bacteremia, the following recommendations have been made:[118] (1) if a central venous catheter is removed, appropriate systemic antibiotic therapy is recommended for 5 to 7 days; (2) if a nontunneled central venous catheter is retained and intraluminal infection is suspected, systemic antibiotic therapy for 10 to 14 days and antibiotic lock therapy are recommended; and (3) if a tunneled central venous catheter or an IVD is retained in patients with uncomplicated, catheter-related, bloodstream infection, patients should be treated with systemic antibiotic therapy for 7 days and with antibiotic lock therapy for 14 days.

Although some authors have suggested that infections caused by *S aureus* in the setting of a vascular catheter may respond to treatment with the catheter left in place, there are increasing reports of metastatic sites of infection by this organism when the catheter is not removed. As a result, it seems most prudent to remove the catheter when *S aureus* is isolated from the bloodstream.[125] A scoring system based on the presence or absence of four risk factors (community acquisition, skin examination findings suggesting acute systemic infection, persistent fever at 72 h, and positive follow-up blood culture results at 48 to 96 h) has been suggested as a means of clinically identifying complicated *S aureus* bacteremia.[126] With this system, the strongest predictor was a positive follow-up blood culture at 48 to 96 h. Because of the potentially devastating complications that may occur when *S aureus* seeds heart valves or bone, the issue of duration of therapy for bacteremia due to this pathogen in catheter-associated bacteremia is exceedingly important. It is well accepted that individuals with endocarditis or osteomyelitis occurring as complications of metastatic *S aureus* infection should receive a prolonged course of parenteral antimicrobial therapy, with 6 weeks as the frequently stated duration in these settings. The duration of therapy for patients with *S aureus* bacteremia that is catheter-related may be similar to that for *S aureus* bacteremia due to a drainable focus. Discussed frequently in the medical literature, therapy for this clinical problem has not been definitively established by clinical trials.

Based on the available data, the most frequently noted minimum duration of parenteral therapy in such settings is 2 weeks. However, before one makes the decision to limit parenteral therapy to this short course, all four of the following criteria should probably be met: (1) there is removal of the intravascular catheter or drainage of the abscess that was presumed to be the source of the bacteremia; (2) the bacteremia is demonstrated to promptly resolve with the removal or drainage; (3) there is prompt clinical response, including resolution of fever; and (4) heart valves are demonstrated to be normal. Some have suggested that transesophageal echocardiography (TEE) may be a cost-effective means of stratifying patients with catheter-associated *S aureus* bacteremia to a specific duration of therapy.[127] With infectious disease consultation as one of the six components of the evaluation, it was suggested that a 7-day course of antibiotics may be appropriate for patients with what has been termed "simple bacteremia" with *S aureus* if all of the other criteria are met: (1) TEE on day 5 to 7 of therapy was negative for both vegetations and predisposing valvular abnormalities; (2) negative surveillance culture of blood obtained 2 to 4 days after beginning appropriate antibiotic therapy and removal of focus; (3) removable focus of infection; (4) clinical resolution (afebrile and no localizing complaints attributable to metastatic staphylococcal infections within 72 h of initiating therapy and removal of focus); and (5) no indwelling prosthetic devices.[128] Even in such settings, patients with diabetes mellitus may still be at an increased risk for developing *S aureus* endocarditis, and some experts have suggested 4 weeks of therapy in this patient population even if heart valves are normal. Removal is suggested in the following settings of *S aureus* bacteremia: (1) nontunneled central vascular catheters; and (2) tunneled central vascular catheters or IVDs when there is evidence of tunnel, pocket, or exit-site infection.[118] In the recommendations just cited, it was noted that tunneled central vascular catheters or IVDs with uncomplicated intraluminal infection and *S aureus* bacteremia should be removed or, in selected cases, retained and treated with appropriate systemic and antibiotic lock therapy for 14 days. For patients who remain febrile and/or have bacteremia for >3 days after catheter removal and/or initiation of antibiotic therapy, a longer course of therapy and an aggressive workup for septic thrombosis and infective endocarditis should be instituted. Because the sensitivity of transthoracic echocardiography is low, it is not recommended for excluding a diagnosis of catheter-related endocarditis if TEE can be done.[118] It is important to reiterate that not all of the recommendations listed in this discussion of *S aureus* bacteremia have been definitively validated by clinical trials.

In a retrospective review of 51 patients with prosthetic heart valves in whom *S aureus* bacteremia developed, 26 (51%) had definite endocarditis using the modified Duke criteria for the diagnosis of endocarditis.[129] The risk of endocarditis was independent of the type, location, or age of the prosthetic valve. Because of the high mortality of prosthetic valve endocarditis, it has been recommended that all patients with a prosthetic valve in whom *S aureus* bacteremia develops should be aggressively screened and followed for endocarditis.[129]

Like *S aureus* and enterococci, Candida spp have a predilection to cause metastatic infection on heart valves and in bone when these organisms are bloodborne. In addition to the complications of endocarditis and osteomyelitis, Candida may seed the retina of the eye to cause retinal abscesses that proliferate into the vitreous and result in the clinical entity of Candida endophthalmitis. Because of the significant complications associated with candidemia, there are now two basic recommendations for patients with a positive blood culture for Candida: (1) the patient should receive a course of antifungal therapy[130]; and (2) intravascular lines should be removed.[131]

Risk factors cited for candidemia vary by reports, but the following is a representative list from international experts in the field: antibiotics; indwelling catheters; hyperalimentation; cancer therapy; immunosuppressive therapy after organ transplantation; hospitalization in ICUs; candiduria; and colonization with Candida spp.[132]

A clinical trial conducted by the Mycoses Study Group of the NIH compared amphotericin B with fluconazole in the treatment of candidemia in nonneutropenic and nonimmunocompromised patients.[133] In the 194 patients who had a single species of Candida isolated, 69% of the organisms were *C albicans*. The study concluded that fluconazole and amphotericin B were not significantly different in their effectiveness in treating candidemia. Since that study was performed, there has been an increasing prevalence of non-*albicans* strains of Candida in the bloodborne isolates from certain hospitals, and some of these strains may not respond to traditional doses of fluconazole. In their guidelines for the treatment of candidemia, the IDSA presented options for the treatment of candidemia based on the presence or absence of neutropenia.[134] In nonneutropenic patients, fluconazole, amphotericin B, and caspofungin were offered as options for therapy. In neutropenic patients, amphotericin B, a lipid preparation of amphotericin B, or caspofungin were recommended, with the absence of fluconazole in this patient population acknowledging the role of azole exposure as a risk factor for non-*albicans* strains of Candida. In a trial comparing the echinocandin caspofungin to amphotericin B in patients with Candida infection involving blood or another sterile body site, caspofungin was shown to be superior with significantly fewer drug-related adverse events than in the amphotericin B group.[135] Because echinocandins are more likely to have activity against non-*albicans* strains of Candida, they are potentially useful in patients who have previously been exposed to azole therapy or in whom empiric therapy is needed for presumed life-threatening fungal infection.

Other clinical situations for which catheter removal is necessary for cure of a catheter-related infection include the following: (1) bacteremia due to *C jeikeium* and Bacillus spp; (2) bacteremia with Gram-negative bacilli; (3) fungemia; (4) persistence of fever or bacteremia during therapy; (5) evidence of tunnel infection; and (6) rapid relapse after treatment. Currently available data do not support the need for scheduled replacement of short-term central venous catheters, either by guidewire exchange or through insertion at a new site.[136]

References

1. Schuchat A, Robinson K, Wenger JD, et al. Bacterial meningitis in the United States in 1995. N Engl J Med 1997; 337:970–976
2. Greenlee JE. Approach to diagnosis of meningitis: cerebrospinal fluid evaluation. Infect Dis Clin North Am 1990; 4:583–598
3. National Committee for Clinical Laboratory Standards. Performance standards for antimicrobial susceptibility testing: 14th informational supplement (vol 24). Wayne, PA: National Committee for Clinical Laboratory Standards, January 2004; M100S14
4. Friedland IR, McCracken GH Jr. Management of infections caused by antibiotic-resistant Streptococcus pneumoniae. N Engl J Med 1994; 331:377–382
5. National Committee for Clinical Laboratory Standards. Performance standards for antimicrobial susceptibility testing: 12th informational supplement (vol 22, no 1). Wayne, PA: National Committee for Clinical Laboratory Standards, January 2002; M100-S12
6. Centers for Disease Control and Prevention (CDC). Effect of new susceptibility breakpoints on reporting of resistance in Streptococcus pneumoniae—United States, 2003. MMWR Morb Mortal Wkly Rep 2004; 53:152–154
7. Tunkel AR, Hartman BJ, Kaplan SL, et al. Practice guidelines for the management of bacterial meningitis. Clin Infect Dis 2004; 39:1267–1284
8. Quagliarello V, Scheld WM. Treatment of bacterial meningitis. N Engl J Med 1997; 336:708–716
9. Quagliarello VJ, Scheld WM. New perspectives on bacterial meningitis. Clin Infect Dis 1993; 17:603–610
10. de Gans J, van de Beek D; European Dexamethasone in Adulthood Bacterial Meningitis Study Investigators. Dexamethasone in adults with bacterial meningitis. N Engl J Med 2002; 347:1549–1556
11. Rosenstein NE, Perkins BA, Stephens DS et al. Meningococcal disease. N Engl J Med 2001; 344:1378–1388
12. Cookson ST, Corrales JL, Lotero JO, et al. Disco fever: epidemic meningococcal disease in northeastern Argentina associated with disco patronage. J Infect Dis 1998; 178:266–269
13. Centers for Disease Control and Prevention. Exposure to patients with meningococcal disease on aircrafts—United States, 1999–2001. MMWR Morb Mortal Wkly Rep 2001; 50:485-489
14. Stephens DS, Hajjeh RA, Baughman WS, et al. Sporadic meningococcal disease in adults: results of a 5-year population-based study. Ann Intern Med 1995; 123:937–940
15. Rosenstein NE, Stocker SA, Popovic T, et al. Antimicrobial resistance of Neisseria meningitidis in the United States, 1997. Clin Infect Dis 2000; 30:212–213
16. McGowan JE, Chesney PJ, Crossley KB, et al. Guidelines for the use of systemic glucocorticosteroids in the management of selected infections. J Infect Dis 1992; 165:1–13
17. Alberio L, Lämmle B, Esmon CT. Protein C replacement in severe meningococcemia: rationale and clinical experience. Clin Infect Dis 2001; 32:1338–1346
18. Bernard GR, Vincent JL, Laterre PF, et al. Efficacy and safety of recombinant human activated protein C for severe sepsis. N Engl J Med 2001; 344: 699–709
19. Centers for Disease Control and Prevention. Prevention and control of meningococcal disease: recommendations of the Advisory Committee on Immunization Practices (ACIP). MMWR Recomm Rep 2000; 49[RR-7]:1–10
20. Rosenstein N, Levine O, Taylor JP, et al. Efficacy of meningococcal vaccine and barriers to vaccination. JAMA 1998; 279:435–439
21. Centers for Disease Control and Prevention. Meningococcal disease and college students: recommendations of the advisory committee on immunization practices (ACIP). MMWR Recomm Rep 2000; 49[RR-7]:13–20
22. Overturf GD. Indications for the immunological evaluation of patients with meningitis. Clin Infect Dis 2003; 36:189–194
23. Schaad UB, Suter S, Gianella-Borradori, et al. A comparison of ceftriaxone and cefuroxime for the treatment of bacterial meningitis in children. N Engl J Med 1990; 322:141–147
24. Walker M, Zunt JR. Parasitic central nervous system infections in immunocompromised hosts. Clin Infect Dis 2005; 40:1005–1015

25. Maxipime (cefepime hydrocholoride), product labeling. In: Physicians' desk reference. 59th ed. Montvale, NJ: Thomson PDR, 2005; 1207–1212
26. Lorber B. Listeriosis. Clin Infect Dis 1997; 24:1–11
27. Lerche A, Rasmussen N, Wandall JH, et al. *Staphylococcus aureus* meningitis: a review of 28 consecutive community-acquired cases. Scand J Infect Dis 1995; 27:569–573
28. Bush LM, Abrams BH, Beall A, et al. Index case of fatal inhalational anthrax due to bioterrorism in the United States. N Engl J Med 2001; 345:1607–1610
29. Mayer TA, Bersoff-Matcha S, Murphy C, et al. Clinical presentation of inhalational anthrax following bioterrorism exposure: report of 2 surviving patients. JAMA 2001; 286:2549–2553
30. Durand ML, Calderwood SB, Weber DJ, et al. Acute bacterial meningitis in adults: a review of 493 episodes. N Engl J Med 1993; 328:21–28
31. Centers for Disease Control and Prevention, National Institutes of Health, HIV Medicine Association/Infections Diseases Society of America. Treating opportunistic infections among HIV-infected adults and adolescents. MMWR 2004; 53[RR-15]: 1-112
32. Marra CM, Maxwell CL, Tantalo L, et al. Normalization of cerebrospinal fluid abnormalities after neurosyphilis therapy: does HIV status matter? Clin Infect Dis 2004: 38:1001–1006
33. Farr RW. Leptospirosis. Clin Infect Dis 1995; 21:1–6
34. Panaphut T, Domrongkitchaiporn S, Vibhagool A, et al. Ceftriaxone compared with sodium penicillin G for treatment of severe leptospirosis. Clin Infect Dis 2003; 36:1507–1513
35. Ratnasamy N, Everett ED, Roland WE, et al. Central nervous system manifestations of human ehrlichiosis. Clin Infect Dis 1996; 23:314–319
36. Salgado AV, Furlan AJ, Keys TF, et al. Neurologic complications of endocarditis: a 12-year experience. Neurology 1989; 39:173–178
37. Verdon R, Chevret S, Laissy J-P, et al. Tuberculous meningitis in adults: review of 48 cases. Clin Infect Dis 1996; 22:982–988
38. Kent SJ, Crowe SM, Yung A, et al. Tuberculous meningitis: a 30-year review. Clin Infect Dis 1993; 17:987–994
39. Lopez-Cortes LF, Cruz-Ruiz M, Gomez-Mateos J, et al. Adenosine deaminase activity in the CSF of patients with aseptic meningitis: utility in the diagnosis of tuberculous meningitis or neurobrucellosis. Clin Infect Dis 1995; 20:525–530

40. American Thoracic Society/Centers for Disease Control and Prevention/Infectious Diseases Society of America. Treatment of tuberculosis. Am J Respir Crit Care Med 2003; 167:603–662
41. Thwaites GE, Bang ND, Dung NH, et al. Dexamethasone for the treatment of tuberculous meningitis in adolescents and adults. N Engl J Med 2004; 351:1741–1751
42. Donald PR, Schoeman JF. Tuberculous meningitis. N Engl J Med 2004; 351:1719–1720
43. van der Horst CM, Saag MS, Cloud CA, et al. Treatment of cryptococcal meningitis associated with the acquired immunodeficiency syndrome. N Engl J Med 1997; 337:15–21
44. Graybill JR, Sobel J, Saag M, et al. Diagnosis and management of increased intracranial pressure in patients with AIDS and cryptococcal meningitis. Clin Infect Dis 2000; 30:47–54
45. Saag MS, Graybill RJ, Larsen RA, et al. Practice guidelines for the management of cryptococcal disease. Clin Infect Dis 2000; 30:710–718
46. Galgiani JN, Ampel NM, Catanzaro A, et al. Practice guidelines for the treatment of coccidioidomycosis. Clin Infect Dis 2000; 30:658–661
47. Wheat LJ, Musial CE, Jenny-Avital EJ. Diagnosis and management of central nervous system histoplasmosis. Clin Infect Dis 2005; 40:844–852
48. Lo Re V 3rd, Gluckman SJ. Eosinophilic meningitis. Am J Med 2003; 114:217–223
49. Slom TJ, Cortese MM, Gerber SI, et al. An outbreak of eosinophilic meningitis caused by *Angiostrongylus cantonensis* in travelers returning from the Caribbean. N Engl J Med 2002; 346:668–675
50. Centers for Disease Control and Prevention. Primary amebic meningoencephalitis—Georgia, 2002. MMWR Morb Mortal Wkly Rep 2003; 52:962–964
51. Hasbun R, Abrahams J, Jekel J, et al. Computed tomography of the head before lumbar puncture in adults with suspected meningitis. N Engl J Med 2001; 345:1727–1733
52. Aronin SI, Peduzzi P, Quagliarello VJ. Community-acquired bacterial meningitis: risk stratification for adverse clinical outcome and effect of antibiotic timing. Ann Intern Med 1998; 129:862–869
53. McMillan DA, Lin CY, Aronin SI, et al. Community-acquired bacterial meningitis in adults: categorization of causes and timing of death. Clin Infect Dis 2001; 33:969–975
54. Saravolatz LD, Manzor O, VanderVelde N, et al. Broad-range bacterial polymerase chain reaction

for early detection of bacterial meningitis. Clin Infect Dis 2003; 36:40–45

55. Karchmer AW, Barza M, Drew WL, et al. Infectious disease medicine. In: American College of Physicians' Medical Knowledge Self-Assessment Program IX (MKSAP IX). 1991; 307–353

56. Johnson RT. Acute encephalitis. Clin Infect Dis 1996; 23:219–226

57. Whitley RJ, Lakeman F. Herpes simplex virus infections of the central nervous system: therapeutic and diagnostic considerations. Clin Infect Dis1995; 20:414–420

58. Tebas P, Nease RF, Storch GA. Use of the polymerase chain reaction in the diagnosis of herpes simplex encephalitis: a decision analysis model. Am J Med 1998; 105:287–295

59. Centers for Disease Control and Prevention. Guidelines for surveillance, prevention, and control of West Nile virus infection—United States. MMWR Morb Mortal Wkly Rep 2000; 49:25–28

60. Petersen LR, Marfin AA. West nile virus: a primer for the clinician. Ann Intern Med 2002; 137:173–179

61. Watson NK, Bartt RE, Houff SA, et al. Focal neurological deficits and West Nile virus infection. Clin Infect Dis 2005; e59–e62

62. Centers for Disease Control and Prevention. Acute flaccid paralysis syndrome associated with West Nile virus infection—Mississippi and Louisiana. MMWR Morb Mortal Wkly Rep 2002; 51:825–828

63. Gea-Banacloche J, Johnson RT, Bagic A, et al. West nile virus: pathogenesis and therapeutic options. Ann Intern Med 2004; 140:545–553

64. Centers for Disease Control and Prevention. Arboviral disease—United States, 1994. MMWR Morb Mortal Wkly Rep 1995; 44:641–644

65. De Luca A, Giancola ML, Ammassari A, et al. The effect of potent antiretroviral therapy and JC virus load in cerebrospinal fluid on clinical outcome of patients with AIDS-associated progressive multifocal leukoencephalopathy. J Infect Dis 2000; 182:1077–1083

66. Plotkin SA. Rabies. Clin Infect Dis 2000; 30:4–12

67. Centers for Disease Control and Prevention. Human rabies—Montana and Washington, 1997. MMWR Morb Mortal Wkly Rep 1997; 46:770–774

68. Srinivasin A, Burton EC, Kuehnert MJ, et al. Transmission of rabies virus from an organ donor to four transplant recipients. N Engl J Med 2005; 352:1103–1111

69. Centers for Disease Control and Prevention. Human rabies—Texas and New Jersey, 1997. MMWR Morb Mortal Wkly Rep 1998; 47:1–5

70. Centers for Disease Control and Prevention. Human rabies—Virginia, 1998. MMWR Morb Mortal Wkly Rep 1999; 48:95–97

71. Centers for Disease Control and Prevention. Human rabies—California, Georgia, Minnesota, New York, and Wisconsin, 2000. MMWR Morb Mortal Wkly Rep 2000; 49:1111–1115

72. Centers for Disease Control and Prevention. Human rabies—California, 2002. MMWR Morb Mortal Wkly Rep 2002; 51:686–688

73. Centers for Disease Control and Prevention. Human rabies—Tennessee, 2002. MMWR Morb Mortal Wkly Rep 2002; 51:828–829

74. Centers for Disease Control and Prevention. Human rabies—Iowa, 2002. MMWR Morb Mortal Wkly Rep 2003; 51:47–48

75. Centers for Disease Control and Prevention. First human death associated with raccoon rabies—Virginia, 2003. MMWR Morb Mortal Wkly Rep 2003; 52:1102–1103

76. Centers for Disease Control and Prevention. Human death associated with bat rabies—California, 2003. MMWR Morb Mortal Wkly Rep 2004; 53:33–35

77. Centers for Disease Control and Prevention. Recovery of a patient from clinical rabies—Wisconsin, 2004. MMWR Morb Mortal Wkly Rep 2004; 53:1171–1173

78. Jackson AC, Warrell MJ, Rupprecht CE, et al. Management of rabies in humans. Clin Infect Dis 2003; 36:60–63

79. Rupprecht CE, Gibbons RV. Prophylaxis against rabies. N Engl J Med 2004; 351:2626–2635

80. Tattevin P, Bruneel F, Clair B, et al. Bacterial brain abscesses: a retrospective study of 94 patients admitted to an intensive care unit (1980 to 1999). Am J Med 2003; 115:143–146

81. Tunkel AR, Wispelwey B, Scheld WM. Brain abscess. In: Mandell GL, Bennett JE, Dolin R, eds. Mandell, Douglas, Bennett's principles and practice of infectious diseases. 5th ed. Philadelphia, PA: Churchill Livingstone, 2000; 1016–1028

82. Walot I, Miller BL, Chang L, Mehringer CM. Neuroimaging findings in patients with AIDS. Clin Infect Dis 1996; 22:906–919

83. Centers for Disease Control and Prevention. Guidelines for preventing opportunistic infections among HIV-infected persons—2002: recommendations of

the U.S. Public Health Service and Infectious Diseases Society of America. MMWR Recomm Rep 2002; 51[RR-8]:1–52
84. Darouiche RO, Hamill RJ, Greenberg SB, et al. Bacterial spinal epidural abscess: review of 43 cases and literature survey. Medicine 1992; 71:369–385
85. Stabler A, Reiser MF. Imaging of spinal infection. Radiol Clin North Am 2001; 39:115–135
86. Southwick FS, Richardson EP, Swartz MN. Septic thrombosis of the dural venous sinuses. Medicine 1986; 65:82–106
87. Bleck TP, Greenlee JE. Suppurative intracranial phlebitis. In: Mandell GL, Bennett JE, Dolin R, eds. Mandell, Douglas, Bennett's principles and practice of infectious diseases. 5th ed. Philadelphia, PA: Churchill Livingstone, 2000; 1034–1036
88. Kneen R, Pham NG, Solomon T, et al. Penicillin vs erythromycin in the treatment of diphtheria. Clin Infect Dis 1998; 27:845–850
89. Gergen PJ, McQuillan GM, Kiely M, et al. A population-based serologic survey of immunity to tetanus in the United States. N Engl J Med 1995; 332:761–766
90. Angulo FJ, Getz J, Taylor JP, et al. A large outbreak of botulism: the hazardous baked potato. J Infect Dis 1998; 178:172–177
91. Centers for Disease Control and Prevention. Outbreak of botulism type E associated with eating a beached whale—Western Alaska, July 2002. MMWR Morb Mortal Wkly Rep 2003; 52:24–26
92. Varma JK, Katsitadze G, Moiscrafishvili M, et al. Signs and symptoms predictive of death in patients with foodborne botulism—Republic of Georgia, 1980–2002. Clin Infect Dis 2004; 39:357–362
93. Centers for Disease Control and Prevention. Infant botulism—New York City, 2001–2002. MMWR Morb Mortal Wkly Rep 2003; 52:21–24
94. Shapiro RL, Hatheway C, Swerdlow DL. Botulism in the United States: a clinical and epidemiologic review. Ann Intern Med 1998; 129:221–228
95. Arnon SS, Schechter R, Inglesby TV, et al. Botulism toxin as a biological weapon: medical and public health management. JAMA 2001; 285:1059–1070
96. Nicolle LE, Bradley S, Colgan R, et al. Infectious Diseases Society of America guidelines for the diagnosis and treatment of asymptomatic bacteriuria in adults. Clin Infect Dis 2005; 40:643–654
97. Kaitz AL, Hodder EW. Bacteriuria and pyelonephritis of pregnancy: a prospective study of 616 pregnant women. N Engl J Med 1961; 265:667–672
98. Mittendork R, Williams MA, Kas EH. Prevention of preterm delivery and low birth weight associated with asymptomatic bacteriuria. Clin Infect Dis 1992; 14:927–932
99. Gratacos E, Torres PJ, Vila J, et al. Screening and treatment of asymptomatic bacteriuria in pregnancy prevents pyelonephritis. J Infect Dis 1994; 169:1390–1392
100. Stamm WE, Stapleton AE. Approach to the patient with urinary tract infection: asymptomatic bacteriuria. In: Gorbach SL, Bartlett JG, Blacklow NR, eds. Infectious diseases. 3rd ed. Philadelphia, PA: Lippincott Williams & Wilkins, 2004; 868–869
101. Munoz P. Management of urinary tract infections and lymphocele in renal transplant recipients. Clin Infect Dis 2001; 33 [suppl 1]:S53–S57
102. Nordenstam GR, Brandberg CA, Oden AS, et al. Bacteriuria and mortality in an elderly population. N Engl J Med 1986; 314:1152–1156
103. Nicolle LE, Bjornson J, Harding GK, et al. Bacteriuria in elderly institutionalized men. N Engl J Med 1983; 309:1420–1425
104. Abrutyn E, Mossey J, Berlin JA, et al. Does asymptomatic bacteriuria predict mortality and does antimicrobial treatment reduce mortality in elderly ambulatory women? Ann Intern Med 1984; 120:827–833
105. Boscia JA, Abrutyn E, Kaye D. Asymptomatic bacteriuria in elderly persons: treat or do not treat? Ann Intern Med 1987; 106:764–766
106. Zhanel GG, Harding GK, Nicolle LE. Asymptomatic bacteriuria in patients with diabetes mellitus. Rev Infect Dis 1991; 13:150–154
107. Warren JW. Catheter-associated urinary tract infections. Infect Dis Clin North Am 1987; 1:823–824
108. Sobel JD, Kauffman CA, McKinsey D, et al. Candiduria: a randomized, double-blind study of treatment with fluconazole and placebo. Clin Infect Dis 2000; 30:19–24
109. Fridkin SK. Vancomycin-intermediate and -resistant *Staphylococcus aureus*: what the infectious disease specialist needs to know. Clin Infect Dis 2001; 32:108–115
110. Keane WF, Alexander SR, Bailie GR, et al. Peritoneal dialysis-related peritonitis treatment recommendations. Perit Dial Int 1996; 16:557–573
111. Keane WF, Bailie GR, Boeschoten E, et al. Adult peritoneal dialysis-related peritonitis treatment recommendations: 2000 update. Perit Dial Int 2000; 20:396–411

112. Shemin D, Maaz D, St Pierre D, et al. Effect of aminoglycoside use on residual renal function in peritoneal dialysis patients. Am J Kidney Dis 1999; 34:14–20

113. Shin SK, Noh H, Kang SW, et al. Risk factors influencing the decline of residual renal function in continuous ambulatory peritoneal dialysis patients. Perit Dial Int 1999; 19:138–142

114. Paterson DL, Ko WC, Von Gottberg A, et al. International prospective study of *Klebsiella pneumoniae* bacteremia: implications of extended-spectrum β-lactamase production in nosocomial infections. Ann Intern Med 2004; 140:26–32

115. Marx MA, Frye RF, Matzke GR, et al. Cefazolin as empiric therapy in hemodialysis-related infections: efficacy and blood concentrations. Am J Kidney Dis 1998; 32:410–414

116. Tokars JI. Vancomycin use and antimicrobial resistance in hemodialysis centers. Am J Kidney Dis 1998; 32:521–523

117. Johnson CC, Baldessarre J, Levison ME. Peritonitis: update on pathophysiology, clinical manifestations, and management. Clin Infect Dis 1997; 24:1035–1047

118. Mermel LA, Farr BM, Sherertz RJ, et al. Guidelines for the management of intravascular catheter-related infections. Clin Infect Dis 2001; 32:1249–1272

119. McGee DC, Gould MK. Preventing complications of central venous catheterization. N Engl J Med 2003; 348:1123–1133

120. Capdevila JA, Planes AM, Palomar M, et al. Value of differential quantitative blood cultures in the diagnosis of catheter-related sepsis. Eur J Microbiol Infect Dis 1992; 11:403–407

121. Blot F, Schmidt E, Nitenberg G, et al. Earlier positivity of central-venous- versus peripheral-blood cultures is highly predictive of catheter-related sepsis. J Clin Microbiol 1998; 36:105–109

122. Maki DG, Weise CE, Sarafin HW. A semiquantitative culture method for identifying intravenous-catheter-related infection. N Engl J Med 1977; 296:1305–1309

123. Safdar N, Fine JP, Maki DG. Meta-analysis: methods for diagnosing intravascular device-related bloodstream infection. Ann Intern Med 2005; 142:451–466

124. Raad I, Davis S, Khan A et al. Impact of central venous catheter removal on the recurrence of catheter-related coagulase-negative staphylococcal bacteremia. Infect Control Hosp Epidemiol 1992; 13:215–221

125. Raad I. Intravascular-catheter-related infections. Lancet 1998; 351:893–898

126. Fowler VG, Olsen MK, Corey R, et al. Clinical identifiers of complicated *Staphylcoccus aureus* bacteremia. Arch Intern Med 2003; 163:2066–2072

127. Rosen AB, Fowler VG, Corey R, et al. Cost-effectiveness of transesophageal echocardiography to determine the duration of therapy for intravascular catheter-associated *Staphylococcus aureus* bacteremia. Ann Intern Med 1999; 130:810–820

128. Fowler VG Jr, Sanders LL, Sexton DJ, et al. Outcome of *Staphylococcus aureus* bacteremia according to compliance with recommendations of infectious diseases specialists: experience with 244 patients. Clin Infect Dis 1998; 27:478–486

129. El-Ahdab F, Benjamin DK, Wang A, et al. Risk of endocarditis among patients with prosthetic valves and *Staphylococcus aureus* bacteremia. Am J Med 2005; 118:225–229

130. Edwards JE Jr, Filler SG. Current strategies for treating invasive candidiasis: emphasis on infections in nonneutropenic patients. Clin Infect Dis 1992; 14(suppl 1):S106–S113

131. Rex JH. Editorial response: catheters and candidemia. Clin Infect Dis 1996; 22:467–470

132. Edwards JE Jr, Bodey GP, Bowden RA, et al. International conference for the development of a consensus on the management and prevention of severe candidal infections. Clin Infect Dis 1997; 25:43–59

133. Rex JH, Bennett JE, Sugar AM et al. A randomized trial comparing fluconazole with amphotericin B for the treatment of candidemia in patients without neutropenia. N Engl J Med 1994; 331:1325–1330

134. Pappas PG, Rex JH, Sobel JD, et al. Guidelines for treatment of candidiasis. Clin Infect Dis 2004; 38:161–189

135. Mora-Duarte J, Betts R, Rotstein C, et al. Comparison of caspofungin and amphotericin B for invasive candidiasis. N Engl J Med 2002; 347:2020–2029

136. O'Grady NP, Alexander M, Dellinger EP, et al. Guidelines for the prevention of intravascular catheter-related infections. Clin Infect Dis 2002; 35:1281–1307

Notes

Notes

Upper Gastrointestinal Bleeding, Lower Gastrointestinal Bleeding, and Hepatic Failure

Gregory T. Everson, MD

Objectives:

- To use clinical clues to differentiate between upper and lower gastrointestinal (GI) hemorrhage
- To examine results of vital signs, blood tests, and nasogastric aspirate to assess severity of GI hemorrhage and define immediate resuscitative measures
- To define the common causes of GI hemorrhage in the intensive care unit (ICU)
- To develop a diagnostic strategy and plan of management
- To discuss the advantages and disadvantages of therapeutic options for treatment of GI hemorrhage
- To distinguish between acute hepatitis, acute liver failure, fulminant hepatitic failure, and an acute flare of chronic liver disease
- To assess the clinical features that define poor outcome and need for emergent transplantation
- To define the main causes of acute liver failure in patients presenting to the ICU
- To initiate an appropriate plan for diagnosis and management
- To understand the indications, complications, and utility of intracranial pressure monitoring
- To describe advantages, disadvantages, and outcome of a wide array of treatments, including hepatocyte transplantation, bioartificial liver support, and transplantation (conventional and living donor liver transplantation using the right lobe)

Key words: acetaminophen; acute hepatitis; angiography; bioartificial liver; cerebral edema; diverticulosis coli; encephalopathy; endoscopy; gastrointestinal hemorrhage; hematemesis; hematochezia; hepatic failure; hepatocyte transplantation; liver transplantation; living donor liver transplantation; melena; N-acetyl cysteine; non-steroidal antiinflammatory drugs (NSAIDs); peptic ulcer disease; resuscitation; varices

Upper Gastrointestinal Hemorrhage

Upper gastrointestinal (UGI) hemorrhage accounts for 0.1% of all admissions to the hospital, occurs twice as frequently in men, is more common in the elderly, and remains a significant cause of ICU morbidity and mortality. For unknown reasons, UGI bleeding from peptic ulcer disease is more common in winter months. Current mortality from transfusion-requiring hemorrhage ranges from 5% to 15%. Mortality increases with age, hemodynamic instability, volume of transfusion requirement ($\geq$ 6 U pRBCs), evidence of organ dysfunction, underlying cardiopulmonary disease, and underlying liver disease. Risk of death increases 3-fold if the patient is already hospitalized at the time of the initial bleed. Three principles underline management: volume and blood product resuscitation, emergent endoscopy for diagnosis, and prompt definition and institution of therapy targeted to the underlying etiology. Surgical consultation should be obtained in the early stages of resuscitation and evaluation.

Case Presentation 1

A 42-year-old woman experienced sudden hematemesis at work while performing her usual secretarial duties. She was noted by co-workers to be pale, diaphoretic, and faint. Emergency medical technicians started peripheral intravenous lines and administered saline. On arrival at the emergency room, she was alert and oriented, pale, with BP 95/55, P 120, RR 22, T 37°C. She passed a melenic stool and examination revealed only a few scattered spider telangiectasia with mild hepatosplenomegaly. Two units of pRBCs were infused, a nasogastric tube was placed revealing dark blood with clots in the stomach, and she was admitted to the medical ICU. She described recent use of ibuprofen for headaches but denied alcohol or any knowledge of underlying liver disease. Past medical history was unremarkable except for receipt of blood transfusion at age 23 for postpartum hemorrhage.

Resuscitation

Initial assessment of severity of bleeding requires critical evaluation of vital signs. Hematocrit is not a reliable indicator of the degree of hemorrhage because it does not decrease immediately with acute bleeding. The decrease in hematocrit that occurs with bleeding is due to re-equilibration of body fluid and may take 24 to 72 h to manifest. The patient who has sustained an UGI hemorrhage typically exhibits features of hypovolemia or hypovolemic shock. Immediate measures are focused at restoring intravascular volume and maintaining tissue oxygenation. Two large-bore indwelling intravenous catheters should be placed early in the resuscitation effort and blood pressure immediately corrected with bolus infusion of normal saline. The ideal hematocrit guiding transfusion of blood or packed-RBCs is somewhat controversial, although most recommend a target hematocrit of 25% to 30% (this latter hematocrit is recommended for elderly patients, age >60 yrs, or in those with underlying ischemic cardiovascular disease). Oxygen delivery to tissues is insured by volume replacement to restore blood pressure, maintenance of RBC volume to restore oxygen-carrying capacity, and administration of nasal oxygen to saturate the carrying capacity of blood. Coagulopathic patients may require platelets, fresh frozen plasma, or cryoprecipitate (to replace fibrinogen). Calcium infusion may be required in those receiving massive units of citrate-treated stored blood since citrate may chelate calcium and lower its plasma concentration.

During resuscitative efforts the patient should be evaluated for underlying organ dysfunction due to the hemorrhage and examined for the presence of chronic liver disease. Lactic acidosis, renal failure, myocardial ischemia and infarction, bowel ischemia, cerebral ischemia, and limb ischemia may all complicate hemorrhagic shock. UGI hemorrhage in the setting of chronic liver disease is related to portal hypertension in approximately 50% of cases (varices or portal hypertensive gastropathy). Management is influenced significantly by the presence of underlying chronic liver disease and its etiology.

Etiology

The causes of UGI bleeding are given in Table 1. Endoscopy or radiologic imaging is required to establish the cause of bleeding. The most common etiology is duodenal ulcer disease, representing 30% to 35% of all cases of UGI bleeding. Bleeding from gastric ulcer is the next most common diagnosis, followed by Mallory-Weiss lesions, portal hypertensive gastropathy, and varices. However, a wide array of conditions may present with UGI hemorrhage (Table 1).

NSAIDs and Risk of Bleeding

The risk of bleeding with use of nonselective NSAIDs is approximately 0.5% after 6 months of ongoing treatment. Risk increases with age, history of ulcer disease, history of cardiovascular disease, and is related to dose of NSAID. Risk is reduced, but not eliminated, by use of the more selective COX-2 inhibitors (celecoxib, rofecoxib). Co-administration of nonselective NSAIDs to patients taking steroids or anticoagulation therapy (heparin or warfarin) increases the relative risk of bleeding up to 12-fold. *Helicobacter pylori*, although proven to increase the risk for ulcer disease, is not an independent risk factor for UGI bleeding. A number of studies have demonstrated the effectiveness of proton pump inhibitors (PPI) for preventing gastroduodenal ulcers in patient taking NSAIDs.

Table 1. *Causes of Upper Gastrointestinal Hemorrhage*

Esophageal	As % of All UGI Bleeds
Varices	10%
Erosive Esophagitis	2%
Mallory-Weiss lesion	5% to 15%
Medication-induced ulceration	≤1%
Caustic ingestion	≤1%
Infectious Esophagitis	≤1%
Herpes	
CMV	
HIV	
Candida	
Carcinoma	≤1%
Gastric	
Peptic Lesions	15% to 20%
Gastric ulcer	
Gastritis	
NSAID ulcers	
Dieulafoy's lesion	≤1%
Varices	1% to 3%
Portal Hypertensive Gastropathy	10% to 15%
Vascular malformations	≤1%
Neoplastic Lesions	≤1%
Carcinoma	
Lymphoma	
Leiomyoma	
Duodenum	
Peptic ulcer	30% to 35%
Vascular malformation	≤1%
Aorto-enteric fistula	≤1%
Hemobilia	≤1%
Hemosuccus pancreatitis	≤1%

Diagnosis

Initial findings at physical examination may be useful in providing clues as to the location of the bleeding lesion in the gastrointestinal tract. Evaluation of vital signs, abdominal examination, and appearance of the bowel movement may localize the bleeding site. A patient passing bright red blood per rectum with stable vital signs and a benign abdomen is most likely bleeding from a lower, left-sided colonic lesion. A hemodynamically stable patient passing purplish clots and darker blood may be bleeding from the right colon or small bowel. Mild to moderate UGI bleeding is characterized by loose, black bowel movements (melena). Development of melena requires a minimum bleed of ≥100 mL and prolonged residence in the gut (≥12 h). Massive bleeding from varices or an artery in an ulcer base, is often charateized by hemodynamic instability or shock, and hematemesis. With brisk bleeding from an UGI source (≥1000 mL), one may observe passage of red blood per rectum; almost always mixed with darker blood or clots and characterized by hypotension. Approximately 5% to 15% of cases, initially thought to be bleeding from a lower GI source, are actually bleeding from an UGI source.

Nasogastric (NG) tubes can be helpful diagnostically in some cases, but hemoccult testing of aspirates is not useful and not recommended. If the aspirate lacks blood and contains bile, an UGI source for ongoing active bleeding is less likely. However, 16% of UGI bleeds from duodenal ulcer disease are associated with a clear NG aspirate. The major role for NG tubes is to allow lavage and clearance of blood from the stomach for the purpose of performing endoscopy or other diagnostic studies. Other clues to an UGI source are elevation of BUN, hyperactive bowel sounds, and physical findings (spider telangiectasia, jaundice, hepatosplenomegaly, acanthosis nigracans, pigmented lip lesions, palpable purpura). Some gastroenterologists use the NG tube also to assess the patient for activity of ongoing bleeding and to determine prognosis. A patient admitted for melena, who has a clear NG aspirate, has a predicted mortality of <5%. In contrast, a patient admitted with hematochezia, who has a red NG aspirate, has a predicted mortality of ~30%.

Emergent endoscopy, after resuscitation of the patient and clearance of blood and clots from the stomach, is indicated for nearly all acute UGI bleeders. Not only is endoscopy diagnostic in over 90% of cases, it can also be used to provide definitive therapy (variceal ligation or sclerotherapy, electocautery, alcohol or sclerosant injection, biopsy for *H pylori* in some cases may lead to antibiotic treatment). In addition, endoscopy is useful in identifying patients at high risk of rebleeding who may benefit from early surgical intervention (visible vessel failing endoscopic management, giant ulcer, diffuse hemorrhagic gastritis, miscellaneous lesions) (Table 2).

Case 1 (continued)

Our patient underwent endoscopy which revealed esophageal varices with stigmata of recent hemorrhage (cherry red spot over varix) and minimal erosive gastritis. She was treated with endoscopic ligation of varices, had no further bleeding, and was discharged from the hospital 72 h after admission. Subsequent evaluation revealed cirrhosis due to chronic hepatitis C. Varices were eradicated by repeated ligation treatments and she underwent evaluation for liver transplantation.

Imaging studies may also be useful in localizing a bleeding source. If endoscopic studies are nondiagnostic and bleeding persists, a nuclear medicine Tc99m-RBC scan may indicate the site of bleeding. This scan is more sensitive than angiography and when sequential scans are performed the bleeding site may be localized in 60% to 80% of cases. Although the scan can localize bleeding

Table 2. *Prediction of Outcome After Upper Gastrointestinal Bleed From Peptic Lesions*

Increased Risk of Mortality is Associated With
- Age >60 years
- Hemodynamic instability with initial bleed
- Onset of bleeding during hospitalization for unrelated co-morbid condition
- History of cancer
- Underlying co-morbid conditions
- Endoscopic finding of giant ulcer
- Endoscopic finding of visible vessel in base of ulcer

Endoscopic Features Predictive of Rebleeding
- Spurting artery (actively bleeding)
- Nonbleeding but elevated visible vessel
- Adherent clot
- Flat cherry red or black spot with oozing

to a site in the bowel, etiology is rarely, if ever, defined from this study. Angiography is used in patients with higher bleeding rates and may be therapeutic if embolization of the bleeding site is performed. Angiography can be diagnostic for vascular lesions of the bowel. Meckel's scan (Technetium pertechnetate) is usually performed only after all other studies have failed to provide a diagnosis. Barium studies are not recommended in the initial evaluation of UGI bleeding.

Specific Therapeutic Approaches

Peptic Lesions

Bleeding from peptic lesions of the UGI tract is treated by:

1. Gastric acid suppression (proton pump inhibitors [PPIs] are favored over H2-blockers, but are not effective in the setting of active bleeding): High dose antisecretory therapy (IV PPI) significantly decrease the risk of rebleeding in patients with bleeding ulcers.
2. Octreotide, 50 µg bolus followed by 50 µg/h infusion. Use of octreotide for this indication is controversial, but some studies suggest that rebleeding rate is reduced by 30% to 50%.
3. Correction of coagulopathy
4. Therapeutic endoscopy (electocautery, injection of sclerosant) Effectiveness of endoscopic therapy is limited by arterial size. Arterial bleeders with diameter ≥2 mm usually do not respond and require surgery. Rebleeding after initial control with endoscopic treatment is best managed by repeat endoscopic therapy or radiologic intervention. Surgery is only necessary in ~10% of rebleeds.
5. Surgery, for those who fail endoscopic management
6. After resolution of the acute bleed, all patients with duodenal ulcer should be considered for triple therapy against H pylori. After an acute bleed, H pylori status should be determined before initiating triple therapy. The incidence of non-H pylori related duodenal ulcer is increasing and these patients have significantly worse outcomes if treated empirically for H pylori. Other peptic lesions may also require this therapy if the patient is H pylori-positive.

Varices

Risk of bleeding from esophageal varices is directly related to portal pressure (≥12 mm Hg), variceal size and appearance on endoscopy, advanced Child-Pugh score (Table 3), and coincident gastric varices. Mortality from UGI hemorrhage from varices ranges from 30% to 50%. The treatment of bleeding from esophageal varices is aimed at control of portal hypertension using pharmacological agents and direct application of endoscopic treatment to the bleeding variceal channels. A number of pharmacologic agents can lower portal hypertension: beta-blockers, nitroglycerin, vasopressin, and somatostatin. We currently favor use of octreotide or vapreotide since they are effective, well-tolerated, and have few side effects. A loading dose of 50 µg is administered initially, and followed by continuous infusion at 50 µg/h. The majority of patients bleeding from esophageal varices can be controlled by endoscopic ligation, especially if done with co-administration of long-acting somatostatin analogue. Endoscopic ligation treatment ("banding") is associated with fewer complications than endoscopic sclerotherapy and is currently the preferred modality. Patients bleeding from gastric varices or who rebleed from esophageal varices despite endoscopic treatment may require placement of a Sengstaken-Blakemore tube and performance of either transjugular intrahepatic portal-systemic shunt (TIPS) or surgical shunt (Table 4). TIPS placement is successful in 90% to 95% of cases, but TIPS may thrombose or stenose and require repeated radiological interventions. In addition, TIPS is costly and 15% of 30% of patients undergoing TIPS suffer from post-TIPS

Table 3. *Child-Pugh Criteria*

	1 point	2 points	3 points
Bilirubin (mg/dL)	<2	2–3	>3
Albumin (g/dL)	>3.5	2.8–3.5	<2.8
PT (sec prolonged)	1–3	4–6	>6
Ascites	None	slight	moderate
Encephalopathy	None	1–2	3–4

Grades: A = 4–6 points; B = 7-9 points; C = 10–15 points
Pugh's modification of the Child-Turcotte prognostic classification (Pugh RN, Murray-Lyon IM, Dawson JL, et al. Transection of the esophagus for bleeding of esophageal varices. Br J Surg 1973; 60:646)

Table 4. *Indications for and Contraindications to Transjugular Intrahepatic Portal-Systemic Shunt (TIPS)*

Indications	Contraindications

Accepted:
Gastroesophageal variceal hemorrhage
  refractory acute variceal bleeding
  refractory recurrent variceal bleeding
  bleeding from intestinal varices
Cirrhotic Hydrothorax
 	
Promising:
Refractory Ascites
Hepatorenal Syndrome
Budd-Chiari Syndrome
	Absolute:
	Heart failure with elevated CVP
	Polycystic liver disease
	Severe hepatic failure
	
	Relative:
	Active intrahepatic or systemic infection
	Portal vein occlusion
	Hypervascular hepatic neoplasms
	Poorly controlled hepatic encephalopathy
	Stenosis of celiac trunk

Table 5. *Risk of Death From Variceal Hemorrhage According to Severity of Liver Disease*

Child-Pugh Class A	≤5%
Child-Pugh Class B	≤25%
Child-Pugh Class C	>50%

Table 6. *Causes of Significant Acute Lower Gastrointestinal (LGI) Bleeding*

Diverticulosis	30%
Post-polypectomy	7%
Ischemic colitis	6%
Colonic ulcerations	6%
Neoplasm (cancer and polyps)	5%
Angiodysplasia	4%
Radiation proctitis	2%
Inflammatory bowel disease	2%
Miscellaneous lesions	12%
Undiagnosed LGI bleeding	26%

encephalopathy. Mortality rates from bleeding varices are directly related to Child-Pugh score, ongoing alcohol use, and comorbid illness. Mortality is over 50% in Child-Pugh class C cirrhotics (Table 5).

Lower Gastrointestinal Hemorrhage

The principles of management for lower GI (LGI) bleeding are similar to those mentioned above for UGI bleeding: resuscitation, diagnosis, and planning for specific therapy. One initial consideration in evaluating the LGI bleeder is to exclude an UGI source. A negative NG lavage may obviate the need for upper endoscopy, but nearly 5% to 15% of patients thought to have LGI bleeding are actually diagnosed with an UGI source, and about 5% are from the small bowel. The average age of LGI bleeders is 65 years. Causes of LGI bleeding include: hemorrhoids, angiodysplasia, diverticular disease, neoplastic lesions, inflammatory bowel disease, and other vascular lesions or tumors of the LGI tract (Table 6).

Diagnosis

Colonoscopy: The primary diagnostic test in LGI bleeding is colonoscopy after purgation of the bowel by use of Colyte. Studies comparing colonoscopy to air-contrast barium enema (ACBE) indicate that colonoscopy is far superior, identifying the source in ~70% of cases compared to only ~30% for ACBE. Another advantage of colonoscopy is the ability to provide treatment (cautery, polypectomy, sclerotherapy). However, there is a 2% risk of perforation with endoscopic treatments when administered in the setting of acute bleeding. Sigmoidoscopy should be reserved for the evaluation of minor LGI bleeding in relatively young patients (≤40 years).

Angiography: Angiography can be diagnostic in up to 75% of cases if the rate of bleeding is ≥0.5 mL/min. This diagnostic and therapeutic modality is usually restricted to cases where endoscopy is not possible due to large amounts of blood in the gut lumen or when certain treatments are planned (vasopressin infusion, embolization). Angiography is particularly useful in the diagnosis and management of isolated vascular malformation.

Other Techniques: Technetium-labeled RBC scans are often ordered because of the ease of performance of the test and the perception that valuable information is gained. However, these scans rarely provide definitive information regarding cause or localization of bleeding and cannot provide therapy. The usefulness of RBC scans is quite limited.

Etiology

Diverticular Disease: Diverticuli are the cause of LGI bleeding in 30% of all cases and 50% of those with active hemorrhage undergoing angiography. However, diverticuli are very common and prevalence increases with advancing age. Overall, only 3% of patients with diverticulosis coli ever experience LGI bleeding. When bleeding occurs, it is usually sudden, painless, and often from the right colon (in up to 70% of cases). Acute bleeding stops spontaneously in 80% of cases, but 20% to 25% rebleed. Localization of the site of bleeding is essential to plan appropriately for treatment, which may include segmental colonic resection or even subtotal colectomy.

The list of other relatively common causes of LGI bleeding is given in Table 6. Additional rare causes of LGI bleeding include infectious colitis, NSAID ulcers, rectal varices, vasculitis, and juvenile polyps. As with other causes of GI bleeding, treatment is directed at the underlying etiology.

Acute Hepatic Failure

Definitions

Acute Hepatitis: The standard definition of acute hepatitis is the development of acute liver parenchymal injury from exposure to hepatotoxins or infectious agents, such as viral hepatitis, toxins, or medications. Typical patients with self-limited disease exhibit variable elevations in transaminases (AST and ALT 100 to 1000 IU/L), limited elevations in bilirubin (<5 mg/dL), have normal serum albumin, and no coagulopathy (prothrombin time or INR is normal). Most patients with acute hepatitis recover uneventfully, but approximately 1% will experience severe injury with evidence of liver failure. Patients with chronic liver disease, such as chronic hepatitis C, who experience intercurrent acute hepatitis, such as acute hepatitis A, may experience hepatic decompensation and signs of liver failure.

Acute Liver Failure: Acute liver failure is defined by the development of coagulopathy (prothrombin time >2 sec prolonged, INR >1.5) in a patient with acute hepatitis who lacks underlying chronic liver disease. Patients with acute liver failure usually have greater elevations of AST and ALT levels with the initial injury (1000 to 5000 IU/L), often are jaundiced, and exhibit more constitutional symptoms. These patients are at risk for fulminant hepatic failure (FHF), although most recover uneventfully.

Fulminant Hepatic Failure: The classification of fulminant liver failure requires evidence of hepatic encephalopathy within 8 weeks of the onset of jaundice related to acute liver injury. One criterion for this diagnosis is the absence of underlying chronic liver disease, the only exception being Wilson's disease. There are approximately 2000 cases of FHF in the US each year.

Case Presentation 2

A 38-yr-old businessman presented with a 3-day history of progressive malaise, myalgia, and anorexia. In the last 24 hours he has noted dark urine and jaundice. His wife reports that the patient has been mildly confused. He and his family deny a past history of underlying medical illness, intravenous drug use, or other exposure to blood or blood products. He described his usual alcohol intake as 2 to 4 mixed drinks each day. In the week prior to the onset of his illness he drank from 5 to 8 mixed drinks each day and frequently skipped meals. In addition, he described taking 8 to 10 50-mg tablets of acetaminophen per day for the last 10 days for headaches. Physical examination revealed jaundice, mild hepatomegaly with tenderness to palpation, with no other features of cirrhosis. He was an icteric man who was unaware of the date and had mild asterixis. Laboratory values were as follows: ALT 6250 IU/L, AST 9,765 IU/L, total bilirubin 6.5 mg/dL, albumin 3.8 g/dL, prothrombin time 21.5 sec (INR 2.3), creatinine 2.2 mg/dL, and arterial pH 7.25.

Etiology

The main causes of acute hepatitis are viral hepatitis, drug-induced liver injury, and alcoholic hepatitis. Fulminant liver failure, defined by severe hepatocellular injury, coagulopathy and hepatic encephalopathy, is most often due, in order, to acetaminophen, drug toxicity, hepatitis B, and hepatitis A. However, the second leading diagnostic category for FHF is cryptogenic, cause unknown (Table 7). Recent data, since 1998, indicate that over 50% of cases of FHF in the US are due to acetaminophen (38%) or other idiosyncratic drug reactions (~14%). Sporadic cases of FHF due to both cocaine and Ecstacy have recently been described. FHF from mushroom poisoning occasionally occurs among inexperienced amateur mushroom fanciers. Infiltration of the liver with rapid progression of tumor growth can lead to FHF and has been described for breast carcinoma, lymphoma, and melanoma. Biopsy of the liver is required to establish the latter diagnoses. FHF may also occur in the third trimester of pregnancy related to acute fatty liver of pregnancy, HELLP syndrome, or disseminated Herpes infection.

Acetaminophen-induced acute liver failure occurs in the setting of intentional overdose (majority of cases), but a substantial portion occur as a "therapeutic misadventure." In these cases injury occurs despite taking doses of acetaminophen within the recommended therapeutic range, as little as 4 gm/day for several days, in the setting of moderate alcohol intake and fasting. Enhanced toxicity is due to induction of metabolizing enzymes by alcohol which increase formation of the toxic intermediate of acetaminophen and lead to depletion of hepatic glutathione. Liver injury in this circumstance is associated with towering AST levels, often >5,000 IU/dL, and mortality may exceed 20%. This high mortality rate contrasts with mortality of <1% after acetaminophen overdose among non-alcoholics. Recognition of the association of alcohol use with higher risk of FHF and death after acetaminophen use has led to labeling changes of over-the-counter acetaminophen preparations (Table 8).

Prognosis

A major determinant of prognosis is the level of encephalopathy (Table 9). Patients with FHF who have progressed to higher stages of encephalopathy (Stage III or IV) have the worst prognosis. Additional clinical features that indicate a poor prognosis include: metabolic acidosis, renal failure, severe jaundice, or markedly prolonged prothrombin time. The likelihood of survival varies with the cause of acute liver injury. Patients with acetaminophen overdose have a relatively favorable outcome, over 50% survive. Patients with fulminant hepatitis-A virus and hepatitis-B virus infection have an intermediate prognosis in the range of 30% to 50%. In contrast, patients with a fulminant presentation of Wilson's disease or severe sporadic non-A, non-B, non-C hepatitis have a survival rate of less than 10%.

Clinical Management

Once recognized, patients with fulminant liver failure should be transferred to a center with expertise in managing FHF and which can offer liver transplantation.

Table 7. *Causes of Acute Liver Failure*

Acetaminophen	20%
Cryptogenic	15%
Non-acetaminophen drug toxicity	12%
Hepatitis B	10%
Hepatitis A	7%
Autoimmune hepatitis	6%
Wilson's disease	6%
Miscellaneous*	24%

* Budd-Chiari syndrome, herpes simplex, paramyxovirus, Epstein-Barr virus, amanita poisoning, ischemia, malignant infiltration
Adapted from Schiodt FV, Atillasoy E, Shakil O, et al. Etiologic factors and outcome for 295 patients with acute liver failure in the United States. Liver Transplant Surg 1999; 5:29–34

Table 8. *Labeling of Acetaminophen*

Alcohol Warning:
- If you drink 3 or more alcoholic beverages every day, ask your doctor if you should take TYLENOL® or other pain relievers. Chronic heavy alcohol users may be at increased risk of liver damage when taking more than the recommended dose (overdose) of TYLENOL.®

Directions:
- Adults and children 12 years of age and older: Take 2 geltabs (500 mg/geltab) every 4 to 6 h as needed. Do not take more than 8 geltabs in 24 h, or as directed by a doctor.
- Do not use:
  – with any other product containing acetaminophen
  – for more than 10 days for pain unless directed by a doctor
  – for more than 3 days for fever unless directed by a doctor

Table 9. *Grades of Encephalopathy in Patients With Fulminant Hepatic Failure*

Grade 0: No alteration of mental status
Grade I: Awake and responsive
  Mild confusion and disorientation
  Altered personality
  Asterixis may or may not be present
Grade II: Awake, but agitated
  Increasingly confused and disoriented
  Hallucinations
Grade III: Increasing suppression of mental status
  Stuporous but arousable to vocal or tactile stimuli
  May require endotracheal tube for airway protection
Grade IV: Unresponsive to vocal or tactile stimulation
  Essentially comatose but with intact pupillary reflexes
  Usually still withdraw to painful stimuli

Irreversible Brain Injury (guidelines only):
1. Cerebral edema on brain imaging (CT or MRI) with ischemic necrosis, hemorrhage, and compromised perfusion
2. Sustained elevation of intracranial pressure by intracranial pressure (ICP) monitoring with cerebral perfusion pressure (mean arterial pressure [MAP] – ICP) of < 40 mm Hg for more than 4 h
3. Lack of brainstem function on neurologic examination (absent pupillary response, corneal reflex, gag reflex, and lack of any physiologic response or withdrawal to painful stimuli)

Case 2 (continued)

The patient described above had acute liver failure with encephalopathy and was transferred to a liver transplantation center. After transfer, the patient's neurological status, coagulation profile, and liver chemistries were carefully monitored. He underwent evaluation for liver transplantation, including living donation, but concern was raised about his chronic excessive alcohol use. Over the next 48 hours, his mental status deteriorated, and his INR increased, despite a precipitous decline in aminotransferases. He was listed at status 1 and received a cadaveric liver transplant and his clinical state, including neurologic condition, completely resolved.

General Measures: Indications for hospitalization include nausea and vomiting severe enough to result in dehydration, or severe impairment of liver function resulting in encephalopathy, ascites, GI bleed, or rising prothrombin time. All admitted patients should be placed on needle (HB, NANB) and stool (HA) precautions but not in isolation. Gloves should be worn when handling biological specimens and specimens should be clearly labeled (Hepatitis patient). All used instruments should be autoclaved or appropriately disposed. No effective antiviral therapy exists for acute viral hepatitis or FHF; corticosteroids are contraindicated as they may increase the risk of developing chronic hepatitis. Removal of the offending drug, toxin, or alcohol is the mainstay of therapy of drug-induced and alcoholic hepatitis, respectively. N-acetyl cysteine is an effective primary intervention for hepatic injury related to acetaminophen and is currently under investigation in the treatment of FHF due to other etiologies (Table 10).

Upper Gastrointestinal Bleed: By definition, patients with FHF have acute liver disease and, therefore, lack manifestations of cirrhosis, such as esophageal varices. Upper GI bleeding in the setting of FHF is typically not due to varices or portal hypertension. Upper GI bleeding in this setting is usually mild, controlled by correction of coagulopathy, and is usually due to either erosive gastritis or peptic ulcer disease. Emergent endoscopy is indicated to identify the bleeding lesion, plan management, and possibly to apply therapy. The key management issue is prevention of UGI bleeding

Table 10. *Use of N-Acetyl Cysteine in Treatment of Acetaminophen Overdose*

Oral Dosing Schedule
1. Avoid use of activated charcoal since it will bind *N*-acetyl cysteine, reducing its efficacy
2. Place nasogastric (NG) tube for administration of *N*-acetyl cysteine. *N*-acetyl cysteine is highly unpalatable; most patients cannot tolerate its oral administration. The NG tube is necessary to insure dosing of the medication.
3. Dosage: 140 mg/kg initially, followed by 70 mg/kg q4h, to a total of 17 doses of *N*-acetyl cysteine.
4. Toxicity: nausea, vomiting

Intravenous Dosing Schedule (Limited Availability in Research Centers)
1. Intravenous access for administration
2. Obtain informed consent
3. Dosage: Dilute in crystalloid solution to final concentration of 3%. Doses are infused over one hour through a 0.22 micron filter. Loading dose is 140 mg/kg initially, followed by 70 mg/kg q4h, to a total of 12 doses of N-acetyl cysteine.
4. Adverse reactions occur in approximately 15%: flushing and transient skin rash (usually responds to diphenhydramine), wheezing, nausea, vomiting. Patient should be monitored for anaphlyaxis (Rx with epinephrine, H1 and H2 blockers, supportive care).

by acid suppression with either H2-blockers (intravenously or orally) or PPIs (orally) or by use of sucralfate via the NG tube in patients who cannot take oral medications and in whom an adverse effect of H2 blockers (thrombocytopenia) is to be avoided. Doses of the first two agents are adjusted to achieve maximum acid suppression and optimum prophylaxis by monitoring gastric pH (target is pH ≥ 5) via an NG tube. Sucralfate is dosed at 1 g q6h, irrespective of gastric pH.

Encephalopathy: Encephalopathy is a hallmark of FHF and is also observed in patients with underlying chronic liver disease who sustain a superimposed acute liver injury. The mechanisms of encephalopathy differ but share some common features. Encephalopathy in the setting of chronic liver disease is linked to ammonia production (and several other factors) and responds to measures that effectively reduce blood ammonia levels: protein restriction, lactulose, and nonabsorbable oral antibiotics, such as neomycin.

In contrast, the encephalopathy of acute hepatic failure is usually related to cerebral edema. The exact mechanisms causing cerebral edema are unknown, however experiments with animal models suggest a role for brain ammonia, production of glutamine, retention of glutamine in astrocytes, and astrocyte swelling. Progressively worsening encephalopathy in patients with acute liver failure is an ominous clincal feature; development of grade III or IV encephalopathy may herald the death of the patient due to central herniation of the brain. Efforts to control the encephalopathy of acute liver failure are directed at preventing or resolving cerebral edema (Table 11). Because emerging evidence suggests that ammonia may play a role in the development of cerebral edema, we recommend limited use of protein (<40 g/d) and lactulose to purge the bowel. However, one must exercise caution in using lactulose in the setting of FHF; dosing should be monitored carefully and adjusted to avoid alterations in electrolytes and volume depletion. If lactulose (PO) is given simultaneously with IV mannitol, marked loss of free water may occur, inducing severe hypernatremia. Rapid shifts in sodium concentration have been associated with central pontine myelinolysis.

Coagulopathy: In general, the coagulopathy of acute liver failure is due to depletion of clotting factors related to inadequate hepatic production. Some patients exhibit features of disseminated intravascular coagulation or primary fibrinolysis. Once the patient is diagnosed with severe acute liver failure or FHF, we recommend administration of mephyton (vitamin K) 10 mg/d SQ. Prophylactic infusions of clotting factors are not of proven benefit. Use of clotting factors, such as blood, fresh frozen plasma and fresh platelets, should be restricted to ongoing bleeding, such as GI hemorrhage.

Table 11. *Measures Used To Monitor and Control Cerebral Edema Due to Fulminant Hepatic Failure*

1. Correction of metabolic abnormalities
   - Electrolytes (Na, K, Cl, HCO$_3$)
   - Acid-Base (if patient is on mechanical ventilation, induce mild respiratory alkalosis)
   - Glucose (maintenance intravenous glucose infusion)
2. Avoid over-transfusion or over-hydration
   - Carefully match intake and output once patient is euvolemic
   - Daily weights
   - Avoid use of blood products unless indicated for ongoing bleeding and correction of coagulopathy or to maintain hemostasis when intracranial monitor has been placed. In the latter circumstance, you may need to diurese the patient to avoid an excess intravascular volume, especially from plasma.
3. Institute dialysis in patients in renal failure
   - Continuous arteriovenous or venovenous hemodialysis is preferred over standard hemodialysis
   - Avoid severe volume shifts, stabilize blood pressure, maintain euvolemia, correct electrolyte and acid-base abnormalities
4. Mechanical ventilation (worsening encephalopathy, > Grade II)
   - Main indication in liver failure is airway protection to prevent aspiration pneumonia
   - Induce mild respiratory alkalosis (pH 7.45 to 7.50, Pco$_2$ 20 to 30 mm Hg)
   - Elevate the head of the bed 15 to 30 degrees
   - Use sedation to avoid having the patient "fight the ET tube"
5. Consider placement of intracranial pressure (ICP) monitor in the epidural space
   - Should be considered when patients evolve from stage II (agitated confusion) to stage III (stuporous) encephalopathy.
   - Maintain adequate platelet count (> 60,000 cells/mm3) with platelet transfusions and INR < 1.5 with fresh frozen plasma, if necessary.
   - Mannitol is used to control ICP in patients with intact renal function or in those on dialysis. Mannitol is given in 0.5 to 1.0 g/kg doses. Serum electrolytes, glucose, and osmolarity should be checked every 4 to 6 h. If ICP elevated, osmolarity < 310 mOsm/L H$_2$O, and Na <145 mEq/L, then give mannitol. Mannitol should be held if the patient has excessive serum osmolarity or significant hypernatremia.

Sepsis: Prophylactic antibiotics are not recommended. Blood, urine and sputum should be cultured frequently (even in absence of fever or other signs of infection) and antibiotic therapy directed toward specific organisms. Development of fever usually signifies intercurrent infection and should not be attributed to the liver injury, *per se*. Febrile patients should be fully cultured and treated empirically with antibiotics. The most common sources of infection are respiratory, urinary, and line sepsis. Currently we use vancomycin with a fluroquinolone in initial treatment and then tailor antibiotic use once results of cultures are known.

Glucose: Glycogen in the liver represents a main storage supply of glucose during periods of stress or fasting. Hepatic failure impairs glycogenolysis, and depletes the liver of its glycogen stores, resulting in severe, potentially life-threatening hypoglycemia. It is imperative that all patients with acute liver failure or FHF be treated with glucose infusions and that blood glucose levels are checked every 4 to 6 hours.

Liver Support Systems: Several methods have been used in FHF: exchange blood transfusion, plasmapheresis, cross circulation with human and baboon donors, hemoperfusion through isolated human or animal liver, hemodialysis (conventional and polyacrylonitrate), and column hemoperfusion (microencapsulated charcoal, albumin-covered amberlite XAD 7 Resin). Only exchange transfusion and charcoal hemoperfusion have been evaluated by controlled trial, and the mortality was either similar or greater in the treated group. Since none of these techniques has been demonstrated to improve survival, their use in FHF is not currently recommended (unless under IRB-approved protocols in major liver centers).

Bioartificial Liver: Extracorporeal liver assist devices (ELAD) or bioartificial liver machines (BAL) have recently emerged as potential therapeutic interventions in the treatment of FHF. However, their use currently is experimental and none has yet been conclusively shown, in randomized controlled trials, to improve outcome for patients with FHF. The major principle behind these devices is the use of a "bioreactor" which contains liver cells in a dialysis cartridge, external to the capillary luminae through which blood or plasma flows. The liver cells used in these reactors vary from primary porcine hepatocytes to transformed cells (subclones of HepG2 cells). "Toxins" or metabolites diffuse across the capillary membrane where the liver cells can remove, metabolize, or inactivate them. Experimental models suggest that removal of toxins and metabolites may reduce the neurotoxicity of FHF by inhibiting the formation of cerebral edema. In clinical terms, the goal is stabilization of neurological function to allow for hepatic regeneration or to bridge the patient to liver transplantation. Randomized controlled trials in the US are currently examining the efficacy of two different bioartificial livers in treatment of FHF.

Stange and colleagues recently reported use of a bioartificial liver (MARS) in 26 patients with chronic liver disease who had either acute or chronic liver failure. The treatments lowered plasma bilirubin and bile acids but effect on clinical outcome was unclear: nine patients with advanced liver disease (equivalent to UNOS 2A) died within an average of 15 days but the remainder survived and were thought to have benefited. Further studies will be needed to define benefit and overall utility.

Hepatocyte Transplantation

The principles guiding use of hepatocyte transplantation are similar to those of the bioartificial liver: provide support during a period of critical need so that the patient can be bridged to recovery or transplantation. One potential advantage of hepatocyte transplantation is the ability of liver stem cells to regenerate, raising the potential for repopulation of a dying or dead liver by allogeneic donor hepatocytes. The latter theoretical consideration has not been proven. Experience with hepatocyte transplantation in FHF is limited. We have used this technique in six patients who were not candidates for liver transplantation due to active substance abuse or who had prohibitive underlying medical illness and one patient listed for transplantation who had disseminated herpes infection. Despite a suggestion of improvement in neurologic status after hepatocyte transplantation, all seven died. Difficulties with this approach include: inadequacy of the supply of human hepatocytes, need for arterial puncture in a coagulopathic patient to access either splenic artery for intrasplenic infusion of hepatocytes or hepatic artery for intrahepatic infusion, need for transjugular approach to portal vein if intraportal infusion of hepatocytes is to be performed, compromise of arterial circulation to spleen or liver during infusion, and use of immunosuppression to prevent hepatocyte rejection in setting of severe hepatic failure. Clearly, at this point hepatocyte transplantation for FHF should be viewed as unproven and experimental.

Liver Transplantation

Liver transplantation is the only treatment that has been proven to improve survival in patients with FHF and grade III or IV encephalopathy. Survival of this group of patients without transplantation is 10% to 20%. Survival increases to 60% to 80% with liver transplantation. Patients with FHF are listed at status 1 and given top priority for transplantation. The major limitation in performance of liver transplantation is inadequate availability of donor organs. As of May 1, 2001, there were greater than 18,000 patients on the US waiting list for liver transplantation. In the last 4 years, the number of liver transplants performed has ranged from 4,000 to 4,500 annually. Although most UNOS regions in the US currently "share" livers between organ procurement organizations (OPO) within each region for status 1 patients, this practice does not increase total donor organ availability. Available organs from patients with more stable chronic liver disease are simply shifted to those with acute liver failure and in greatest immediate need. Expansion of the donor pool is essential to resolve the donor-recipient mismatch.

Adult Living Donor Liver Transplantation Using the Right Lobe: There are currently two major approaches to expanding the donor pool: splitting cadaveric donor livers and use of living donors. Split livers are used primarily in the setting of an adult and pediatric recipient simultaneously in need of urgent transplantation. The left lateral segment is transplanted into the child and the remaining liver is used for the adult. Splitting livers into right and left hemi-livers for implantation into two adult recipients is under investigation.

Living donor liver transplantation (LDLT) has been performed successfully in approximately 1500 pediatric cases, typically from parent to child using the lateral segment of the left lobe, and in over 800 adults, typically using either full left lobe or, more recently the right lobe. Donor safety is a major concern in the performance of LDLT. Current statistics suggest that donor mortality is approximately 0.13% for adult-to-pediatric cases and 0.25% for adult-to-adult cases. Recent surveys indicate that donors have been satisfied with their decision to donate and in one survey from our institution all indicated a willingness to donate again, if they could.

In adults with FHF, survival is dependent upon an adequate functional hepatic mass. The left lateral segment is not thought to have sufficient hepatocellular mass to support an adult patient. For this reason, living-donation of the left lateral segment for adults with FHF has not been actively pursued. In contrast, an increasing number of liver transplant centers have begun to use the right lobe from living donors to perform hepatic transplantation. Experience with this approach in FHF, however, is limited. At a recent NIH-sponsored workshop (December 2000), outcome after LDLT for FHF was reviewed. Fourteen patients had undergone LDLT for FHF, of these all survived the surgical procedure and the 1-year survival rate was 90%. These favorable results are encouraging, since results with cadaveric transplantation have yielded 1-year survival rates of 60% to 80%.

Examination of a single case is instructive. We used LDLT in a young woman with fulminant hepatitis who was in coma, on mechanical ventilation and dialysis, with CT evidence of cerebral edema. There was no cadaveric donor available in our region and her brother inquired into the feasibility of performing living donor transplantation. It should be noted that our center was already experienced with adult-to-adult, right lobe, living donor transplantation in patients with chronic liver disease. The patient sustained complete clinical and neurological recovery following the living-donor transplant. The donor was discharged from the hospital within one week of surgery. Liver volume in both recipient and donor regenerates rapidly after resection and implantation; within 2 to 12 weeks liver volume normalized. Increasing availability of surgical expertise to perform this procedure may allow more widespread application and timely transplantation of patients with FHF.

Bibliography

Portal Hypertension

1. Cales P, Masliah C, Bernard B, et al. Early administration of vapreotide for variceal bleeding in patients with cirrhosis. N Engl J Med 2001; 344:23–28
2. Corley DA, Cello JP, Adkisson W, et al. Octeotide for acute esophageal variceal bleeding: a meta-analysis. Gastroenterology 2001; 120:946–954
3. Grace ND. Diagnosis and treatment of gastrointestinal bleeding secondary to portal hypertension. Am J Gastroenterol 1997; 92:1081–1091
4. Grace ND, Bhattacharya K. Pharmacologic therapy of portal hypertension and variceal hemorrhage. Clinics in Liver Disease 1997; 1:59–75
5. Pagliaro L, D'Amico G, Sorrenson TA, et al. Prevention of first bleeding in cirrhosis: A meta-analysis of randomized trials of non-surgical treatment. Ann Intern Med 1992; 117:59–70

Upper GI Bleed

6. Gostout CJ, Wang KK, Ahlquist DA. Acute gastrointestinal bleeding: Experience of a specialized management team. J Clin Gastroenterol 1992; 14:260–267
7. Lau JYW, Sung JJY, Lam YH, et al. Endoscopic retreatment compared with surgery in patients with recurrent bleeding after initial endoscopic control of bleeding ulcers. N Engl J Med 1999; 340:751–756
8. Rockall TA, Logan RF, Devlin HB, et al. Selection of patients for early discharge or outpatient care after acute upper gastrointestinal haemorrhage: National audit of acute upper gastrointestinal haemorrhage. Lancet 1996; 347:1138–1140
9. Rockall TA, Logan RFA, Devlin HB, et al. Incidence and mortality from acute gastrointestinal hemorrhage in the United Kingdom. Br Med J 1995; 311:222–226
10. Rockey DC, Koch J, Cello JP, et al. Relative frequency of upper gastrointestinal and colonic lesions in patients with positive fecal occult-blood tests. N Engl J Med 1998; 339:153–159
11. Zimmerman J, Siguencia J, Tsvang E. Predictors of mortality in patients admitted to hospital for acute gastrointestinal hemorrhage. Scand J Gastroenterol 1995; 30:327–331
12. Kaviani MJ, Hashemi MR, Kazemifar AR, et al. Effect of oral omeprazole in reducing re-bleeding in bleeding peptic ulcers: a prospective, double-blind, randomized, clinical trial. Aliment Pharmacol Ther 2003; 17:211–216
13. Lau JY, Sung JJ, Lee KK, et al. Effect of intravenous omeprazole on recurrent bleeding after endoscopic treatment of bleeding peptic ulcers. N Engl J Med 2000; 343:310–316
14. Graham DY, Agrawal NM, Campbell DR, et al. Ulcer prevention in long-term users of nonsteroidal anti-inflammatory drugs: results of a double-blind, randomized, multicenter, active- and placebo-controlled study of misoprostol vs lansoprazole. Arch Intern Med 2002; 162:169–175
15. Lai KC, Lam SK, Chu KM, et al. Lansoprazole for the prevention of recurrences of ulcer complications from long-term low-dose aspirin use. N Engl J Med 2002; 346:2033–2038
16. Ekstrom P, Carling L, Wetterhus S, et al. Prevention of peptic ulcer and dyspeptic symptoms with omeprazole in patients receiving continuous non-steroidal anti-inflammatory drug therapy: a Nordic multicentre study. Scand J Gastroenterol 1996; 31:753–758
17. Ciociola AA, McSorley DJ, Turner K, et al. Helicobacter pylori infection rates in duodenal ulcer patients in the United States may be lower than previously estimated. Am J Gastroenterol 1999; 94:1834–1840
18. Bytzer P, Teglbjaerg PS. Helicobacter pylori-negative duodenal ulcers: prevalence, clinical characteristics, and prognosis--results from a randomized trial with 2-year follow-up. Am J Gastroenterol 2001; 96:1409–1416

Lower GI Bleed

19. Bokhari M, Vernava AM, Ure T, Longo WE. Diverticular hemorrhage in the elderly – Is it well-tolerated? Dis Colon Rectum 1996; 39:191–195
20. Richter JM, Christensen MR, Kaplan LM, et al. Effectiveness of current technology in the diagnosis and management of lower gastrointestinal hemorrhage. Gastrointest Endosc 1994; 41:93–98

Acute Liver Failure

21. Belay ED, Bresee JS, Holman RC, et al. Reye's Syndrome in the United States from 1981 through 1997. N Engl J Med 1999; 340:1377–1382

22. Charlton M, Adjei P, Poterucha J, et al. TT-Virus infection in North American blood donors, patients with fulminant hepatic failure, and cryptogenic cirrhosis. Hepatology 1998; 28:839–842
23. Clemmesen JO, Larsen FS, Kondrup J, et al. Cerebral herniation in patients with acute liver failure is correlated with arterial ammonia concentration. Hepatology 1999; 29:648–653
24. Hoofnagle JH, Carithers RL, Shapiro C, et al. Fulminant hepatic failure: summary of a workshop. Hepatology 1995; 21:240–252
25. Lee WM. Medical progress: Acute liver failure. N Engl J Med 1993; 329:1862–1872
26. Lee WM. Acute liver failure. Clin Perspect Gastroenterol. 2001 March/April; 101–110
27. Lee WM, Williams R. Acute Liver Failure. Cambridge, UK: Cambridge University Press, 1997
28. Riordan SM, Williams R. Use and validation of selection criteria for liver transplantation in acute liver failure. Liver Transplantation 2000; 6:170–173
29. Schiodt FV, Atillasoy E, Shakil AO, et al. Etiology and outcome for 295 patients with acute liver failure in the United States. Liver Transplant Surg 1999; 5:29–34
30. Schiodt FV, Rochling FA, Casey DL, Lee WM. Acetaminophen toxicity in an urban county hospital. N Engl J Med 1997; 337:1112–1117
31. Shakil AO, Kramer D, Mazariegos GV, et al. Acute liver failure: Clinical features, outcome analysis, and applicability of prognostic criteria. Liver Transpl 2000; 6:163–169
32. Stange J, Mitzner SR, Klammt S, et al. Liver support by extracorporeal blood purification: a clinical observation. Liver Transpl 2000; 6:603–613
33. Strom SC, Chowdhury JR, Fox IJ. Hepatocyte transplantation for the treatment of human disease. Semin Liver Dis 1999; 19:39–48
34. Trotter J, Wachs M, Everson GT, et al. Adult-to-adult right hepatic lobe living donor liver transplantation. N Engl J Med 2002; 346:1074–1082
35. Tsiaoussis J, Newsome PN, Nelson LJ, et al. Which hepatocyte will it be? Hepatocyte choice for bioartificial liver support systems. Liver Transpl 2001; 7:2–10

Notes

Infections in AIDS Patients and Other Immunocompromised Hosts

George H. Karam, MD, FCCP

Objectives:

- To propose an approach to the immunocompromised patient based on identification of defects in three major host defense systems
- To review the likely pathogens, their clinical presentations, and therapeutic options in patients with neutropenia
- To summarize the various limbs in humoral immunity, with particular attention to the clinical situations of asplenia and splenic dysfunction
- To outline the categories and clinical presentations of pathogens likely to be encountered with deficits of cell-mediated immunity
- To focus on the broadening number of clinical issues in patients whose cell-mediated immunity defect is on the basis of HIV infection

Key words: asplenia; cell-mediated immunity; HIV; humoral immunity; neutropenia

---

In the clinical approach to patients with fever presumed to be infectious in etiology, a basic consideration is whether the patient is a normal host or one who is immunocompromised. A traditional method has been to consider host defense in immunocompromised patients as being in one of two categories: (1) mechanical factors, including barrier systems such as skin and mucous membranes (which are protective against infection) or foreign bodies such as intravascular and urinary catheters (which predispose to infection); and (2) cellular host defense, which includes the three major categories of primary neutrophil defense, humoral immunity, and cell-mediated immunity. Use of an approach that identifies the defective limb of host defense allows for directed therapeutic decisions that are based on likely pathogens for the involved site.

Recent attention has been focused on the concept of type 1 and type 2 immunity as they interrelate with humoral and cell-mediated immunity.[1] Subpopulations of CD4+ lymphocytes are important in both humoral immunity and cell-mediated immunity, with T helper type 1 (Th1) and T helper type 2 (Th2) cells being the most relevant. All T helper lymphocytes start out as naive Th0 cells, which, after being activated, are capable of "polarizing" or differentiating into either Th1 or Th2 effector cells. Although multiple factors are involved, the key to polarization of Th0 cells into the Th1 phenotype is interleukin (IL)-12, whereas IL-4 is needed for Th2 polarization. These events may not occur until an activated T cell arrives at the site of danger and samples the local cytokine milieu to determine if an inflammatory or antibody response is appropriate. In questionable circumstances, the Th2 outcome is favored over the Th1 differentiation because IL-4 dominates IL-12. Th1 cells, which are involved with type 1 immunity, secrete interferon-gamma (IFN-γ), IL-2, and lymphotoxin-α as the cytokines chiefly responsible for their proinflammatory effect. The Th1 cell is associated with strong cell-mediated immunity and weak humoral immunity. Th2 cells are involved with type 2 immunity, are influenced by IL-4, IL-10, and IL-13, stimulate high titers of antibody production, and are associated with suppression of cell-mediated immunity and with strong humoral immunity. When integrated into the traditional approach of cell-mediated immunity and humoral immunity, type 1 and type 2 immunity have important therapeutic implications in the care provided for immunocompromised patients.

Primary Neutrophil Function

The polymorphonuclear leukocyte is the major phagocyte for both primary neutrophil defense and humoral immunity. Once a pathogen is ingested by these cells and is intracellular, killing is generally an easy process. Pathogens that classically infect patients with primary neutrophil problems are those that may be ingested without opsonization. The system of neutrophil defense has been described as being responsible for defending against organisms that are easy to eat and easy to kill.[2]

An important pathophysiologic consideration is that polymorphonuclear leukocytes may have either an extravascular or intravascular location. After leaving the bloodstream, these phagocytes go to two major sites: the subepithelial area of skin and the submucosal area of the GI tract. Recognition of this fact allows for an understanding of the organisms that classically infect neutropenic patients.

As represented in Table 1, neutrophil dysfunction may occur on either a qualitative or quantitative basis. Qualitative defects characteristically occur in children and are associated with polymorphonuclear leukocytes that are normal in number but abnormal in function. Classic qualitative defects of polymorphonuclear leukocytes are related to dysfunction in one of the following processes: (1) diapedesis (the ability to leave the intravascular space via endothelial channels); (2) chemotaxis (movement to the site of infection); (3) ingestion (the process of attaching to the pathogen and then getting that pathogen within the cell, where killing takes place); and (4) intracellular killing (which may occur via either oxygen-dependent or oxygen-independent mechanisms).

Quantitative defects, which are the more characteristic neutrophil problems in adults, clinically present as the entity interchangeably referred to as either granulocytopenia or neutropenia. Characteristic conditions that may lead to neutropenia are listed in Table 1. Although eosinophils are classified as granulocytes, for most clinical purposes the granulocyte count is calculated by adding the percentage of polymorphonuclear leukocytes and band forms, and then multiplying the total WBC count by that percentage. In the guidelines of the Infectious Diseases Society of America (IDSA) for management of febrile, neutropenic patients, a calculated granulocyte count of <500 cells/mm^3 indicates absolute neutropenia; a granulocyte count <1,000 cells/mm^3 with a predicted decline to <500 cells/mm^3 should be considered neutropenia.[3] In the setting of neutropenia and fever, the clinician must assume that the patient has impaired natural defense against the pathogens defended against by this limb of host defense.

The clinical course of patients with neutropenia is variable and may be explained in part by the integrity of the gut mucosa. In conditions such as aplastic anemia or HIV-associated neutropenia, the gut mucosa is usually intact, and those patients have a lower incidence of bacteremia. In contrast, patients who receive chemotherapeutic agents that cause mucositis have loss of both the mechanical barrier of gut mucosa and submucosal polymorphonuclear leukocytes. These patients are more likely to experience Gram-negative bacteremia and fungemia.

Infections due to bacteria are classically encountered when the neutropenia is either rapid in development or profound (especially with counts <100 cells/mm^3). The pathogens most likely to infect neutropenic patients are listed in Table 2. The bacteria characteristically involved are skin and gut flora, as might be predicted from the loss of subepithelial and submucosal polymorphonuclear leukocytes. Although any of the enterobacteriaceae (*eg*, *Escherichia coli* or *Klebsiella*) may cause infection in this setting, the most life-threatening

Table 1. *Conditions Causing Neutrophil Dysfunction*

Qualitative Defects
    Impaired diapedesis
    Impaired chemotaxis
    Impaired ingestion
    Impaired intracellular killing
Quantitative Defects (Neutropenia)
    Acute leukemia
    Invasion of bone marrow by neoplasms
    Treatment with agents toxic to marrow
    Drug idiosyncrasy
    Splenic sequestration syndromes
    HIV-associated neutropenia
    Idiopathic chronic neutropenia

Table 2. *Important Pathogens Causing Infection in Neutropenic Patients*

Gram-positive organisms
    Staphylococcus aureus
    Coagulase-negative staphylococci
    Viridans streptococci
    Enterococci
    Corynebacterium jeikeium
Enterobacteriaceae
Pseudomonas aeruginosa
Anaerobes, including *Bacteroides fragilis*
Fungi
    Yeasts, most notably Candida spp
    Filamentous fungi, most notably Aspergillus spp

pathogen is *Pseudomonas aeruginosa*. Because of this (and despite the relative decline in the incidence of infection caused by this pathogen in neutropenic patients), a basic principle in empiric therapy of febrile neutropenic patients is coverage of *P aeruginosa*. The classic skin lesion that suggests such an infection is ecthyma gangrenosum. These lesions have a central area of hemorrhage surrounded by a halo of uninvolved skin with a narrow pink or purple rim. Histologically, the infection involves dermal veins, and clinically it may progress to bullae formation. Although other Gram-negative pathogens have been reported to cause such a process, the clinician should assume that ecthyma gangrenosum is caused by *P aeruginosa* until this pathogen has been excluded.

In recent years, infections caused by Gram-positive organisms have significantly increased in neutropenic patients. These pathogens, which are listed in Table 2, have increased in part because of the expanded use of invasive devices such as intravascular catheters, which breach the mechanical barrier of the skin. The important clinical finding of cavitary pulmonary infiltrates may be a clue to infection by either *Staphylococcus aureus* or *Corynebacterium jeikeium*. Notable among the Gram-positive pathogens is infection caused by viridans streptococci (eg, *Streptococcus mitis*), which may result in the viridans streptococcal shock syndrome. In a recent prospective study of 485 episodes of bacteremia in neutropenic patients with cancer,[4] viridans streptococci caused a total of 88 episodes (18%). Ten of these 88 cases (11%) were associated with serious complications, including ARDS plus septic shock (5 cases), ARDS (3 cases), and septic shock (2 cases). Of the patients with serious complications of their streptococcal bacteremia, 3 (30%) had a cutaneous rash, which in other reports has been associated on occasion with desquamation. Severe oral mucositis, high-dose chemotherapy with cyclophosphamide, and allogeneic bone marrow transplantation were the only variables found to be significantly associated with the development of complications. In patients with complications, 36% of these pathogens showed diminished susceptibility to penicillin, and approximately one half were resistant to ceftazidime. In a more recent review,[5] two additional risk factors for viridans streptococcal bacteremia in neutropenic patients were cytosine arabinoside and antimicrobial prophylaxis with either trimethoprim/sulfamethoxazole or a fluoroquinolone.

The experience with antibiotic prophylaxis during the neutropenic period after autologous peripheral blood stem cell transplantation provides an important insight into a potential problem regarding viridans streptococci.[6] Despite the use of levofloxacin prophylaxis, viridans group streptococcal bacteremia developed in 6 of 37 patients (16.2%) who underwent transplantation over a 2-month period in 2001. All 6 patients presented with fever and mucositis after a mean of 4.5 days of neutropenia, and septic shock developed in 3 days. All six viridans group streptococcal isolates from these patients exhibited distinct patterns on pulsed-field gel electrophoresis. A conclusion of this paper was that the use of levofloxacin may select viridans group streptococci with diminished susceptibility to levofloxacin and other quinolones with enhanced activity against Gram-positive organisms and, therefore, may not be optimal for preventing viridans group streptococcal bacteremia in neutropenic patients.

A life-threatening complication that may occur in patients who have received chemotherapy is neutropenic enterocolitis. Previously referred to as typhlitis because of the cecum as the predominant site in many cases, neutropenic enterocolitis may involve the terminal ileum, the cecum, and the colon (with the ascending portion the most frequently involved). Pathogenetically, the process may occur on several bases including destruction of GI mucosa by chemotherapy, intramural hemorrhage due to severe thrombocytopenia, and alterations in GI tract flora. Patients characteristically present with the triad of fever, abdominal pain, and diarrhea, but these findings may be seen with other conditions including *Clostridium difficile* toxin–induced colitis and ischemic colitis. Ultrasound findings include echogenic thickening of the mucosa and bowel wall. Although isodense cecal wall thickening is the most notable CT finding, the distal ileum and remaining colon are also frequently involved. Although optimal therapy has not been definitively established, conservative medical management appears to be effective for most patients.[7]

Although the level of temperature elevation that mandates antimicrobial therapy in neutropenic patients may be influenced by the degree of neutropenia, fever in neutropenic patients has been defined as a single oral temperature of >38.5°C (101°F) or as a temperature of ≥38.0°C (100.4°F) over at least 1 h. In such patients, empiric antibiotics should be started after appropriate cultures are obtained. Because the patients do not have adequate neutrophils to provide natural host defense, all antimicrobial agents administered should be bactericidal. The classic regimen has been an antipseudomonal β-lactam antibiotic (eg, piperacillin or ceftazidime) in combination with an aminoglycoside. Although some centers acknowledge a decreasing prevalence of infection caused by *P aeruginosa*, the recommendation for coverage against this pathogen in febrile neutropenic patients is prompted by the higher rates of mortality that may occur when this pathogen infects neutropenic patients. According to a review of 410 episodes of Pseudomonas bacteremia in patients with cancer from 1972 to 1981, outcome was related to the interval between the onset of the bacteremia and the institution of appropriate therapy.[8] Of the neutropenic patients in this study who had *P aeruginosa* bacteremia and in whom therapy was delayed, 26% died within 24 h and 70% died within 48 h. In an update of these data from 1991 to 1995 in the same institution, the incidence of *P aeruginosa* bacteremia decreased between the two study periods from 4.7 to 2.8 cases per 1,000 admissions.[9] *P aeruginosa* bacteremia remained the most common in acute leukemia, where the frequency did not change. Overall cure rate was 80% in the latter study period vs 62% in the earlier study. The outcome among 230 patients who received appropriate therapy was related to the duration of bacteremia, with cure rates similar among patients who had bacteremia from 1 to 3 days (85%) but greater among patients with >3 days of bacteremia (for which the cure rate was only 50%.) A conclusion of the latter paper was that antibiotic regimens for empiric therapy in neutropenic patients and especially patients with acute leukemia should still provide coverage against *P aeruginosa*.[9]

Influenced by multiple factors, including the potential for acute mortality in neutropenic patients who are bacteremic with *P aeruginosa*, in its most recent recommendations for management of febrile neutropenic patients the IDSA has offered suggestions for empiric antimicrobial therapy.[3] In these recommendations, it was noted that the initial evaluation should determine (1) whether the patient is at low risk for complications (with the specifics defined in these guidelines), and (2) whether vancomycin therapy is needed. For low-risk adults only, an oral regimen using ciprofloxacin plus amoxicillin-clavulanate was suggested. Options in patients for monotherapy with vancomycin not being needed included one of the following agents: cefepime or ceftazidime; or imipenem or meropenem. Options for combination therapy were an aminoglycoside plus an antipseudomonal penicillin, cephalosporin (cefepime or ceftazidime), or carbapenem. In those patients in whom vancomycin is indicated (discussed in the following paragraph), three options were presented: cefepime or ceftazidime plus vancomycin, with or without an aminoglycoside; carbapenem plus vancomycin, with or without an aminoglycoside; or an antipseudomonal penicillin plus an aminoglycoside and vancomycin. Prior to the publication of the 2002 IDSA guidelines, a prospective, multicenter, double-blind, randomized clinical trial showed piperacillin-tazobactam given as monotherapy to be as effective as the combination of piperacillin-tazobactam plus amikacin for the treatment for adults who were febrile and neutropenic.[10] Even though an antipseudomonal penicillin was offered as an option in the 2002 IDSA guidelines for combination therapy without vancomycin and for therapy in which vancomycin was indicated, it was not presented as an option for monotherapy when vancomycin was not indicated.

An ongoing controversy remains regarding whether an agent like vancomycin, which would cover such pathogens as methicillin-resistant *S aureus*, penicillin- and cephalosporin-resistant *Streptococcus pneumoniae*, and *C jeikeium*, should be included in the initial regimen. Because of the risk of selecting vancomycin-resistant enterococci or vancomycin-resistant staphylococci with injudicious use of vancomycin, the IDSA guidelines for management of febrile neutropenic patients discouraged vancomycin use in routine empiric therapy for a febrile neutropenic patient and recommended that this agent be used in the following settings: (1): clinically suspected serious catheter-related infections (eg, bacteremia, cellulitis); (2) known colonization with methicillin-resistant *S aureus* or penicillin- and cephalosporin-resistant *S pneumoniae*; (3) positive results of blood cultures for Gram-positive bacteria before final identification and susceptibility testing; and (4) hypotension or other evidence of cardiovascular impairment.[3]

The guidelines of the American Society of Clinical Oncology (ASCO) for colony-stimulating factors were published in the *Journal of Clinical Oncology*.[11] Clinical situations for which recommendations were made in adults include the following: (1) when the expected incidence of neutropenia is ≥40% (although there are some special circumstances detailed in the ASCO guidelines that might be a valid exception); (2) as adjuncts to progenitor-cell transplantation; (3) after completion of induction chemotherapy in patients ≥55 years of age who have acute myeloid leukemia; and (4) after completion of the first few days of chemotherapy of the initial induction or first postremission course in patients with acute lymphoblastic leukemia. In the 1996 ASCO guidelines, colony-stimulating factors were recommended after documented febrile neutropenia in a prior chemotherapy cycle to avoid infectious complications and maintain dose intensity in subsequent treatment cycles when chemotherapy dose reduction is not appropriate.[12] This was modified in the 2000 guidelines because there were no published regimens that have demonstrated disease-free or overall survival benefits when the dose of chemotherapy was maintained and secondary prophylaxis was instituted. Based on these data, it was recommended that, in the setting of many tumors but exclusive of curable tumors (*eg*, germ cell tumors), dose reduction after an episode of severe neutropenia should be considered as a primary therapeutic option. Colony-stimulating factors should be avoided in patients receiving concomitant chemotherapy and radiation therapy, particularly involving the mediastinum. Because no large-scale prospective, comparative trials evaluating the relative efficacy of granulocyte colony-stimulating factor vs granulocyte-macrophage colony-stimulating factor were available, guidelines about the equivalency of these preparations were not proposed. Certain patients with fever and neutropenia are at higher risk for infection-associated complications and have prognostic factors that are predictive of poor clinical outcome. The use of a colony-stimulating factor in such high-risk patients may be considered, but the benefits in these circumstances have not been proven. Potential clinical factors mentioned in the 2000 guidelines include profound neutropenia (absolute neutrophil count <100/µL), uncontrolled primary disease, pneumonia, hypotension, multiorgan dysfunction (sepsis syndrome), and invasive fungal infection. Age >65 years and posttreatment lymphopenia were mentioned as potentially being other high-risk factors, but it was acknowledged that these have not been consistently confirmed by multicenter trials.

Prolonged neutropenia is a major predisposition to fungal infection. Although the list of fungal organisms identified in neutropenic patients has increased significantly in recent years, the most important pathogens to consider are Candida spp and Aspergillus spp. On the basis of neutropenia, indwelling catheters, broad-spectrum antibiotics, and mucositis, neutropenic patients are at risk for candidemia. The clinical presentation may range from unexplained fever to a septic appearance. Autopsy series have suggested that as many as 50% of patients with evidence of metastatic candidal infections in visceral organs may have had negative antemortem blood cultures for Candida.[13] The characteristic clinical infection in this setting is chronic disseminated candidiasis, which has also been referred to as hepatosplenic candidiasis. This illness may present as unexplained fever, right upper quadrant tenderness, and elevated alkaline phosphatase. During the period of neutropenia, imaging studies may be negative, but as the granulocyte count improves, patients may demonstrate bull's-eye liver lesions on ultrasound and hypodense liver defects on abdominal CT scan.[14] In the 2004 guidelines of the IDSA for treatment of candidemia, the options for neutropenic patients included amphotericin B, liposomal amphotericin B, and caspofungin.[15] Noteworthy is that fluconazole, which was recommended in the treatment of candidemia in nonneutropenic patients, was not included as a treatment option in neutropenic patients. This recommendation is probably an acknowledgement of the evolving trend toward non-*albicans* species of Candida and of the potential role of azole therapy in selecting for such pathogens.

Aspergillus is a nosocomial pathogen that may be associated with vascular invasion and extensive tissue necrosis. The lungs are a prime site of infection, with a spectrum of disease that includes pulmonary infiltrates or cavitary lung lesions; infection of the paranasal sinuses and CNS may also occur.[16] Because of the nosocomial nature of this organism, it may be introduced into the skin with catheter insertion. With the lack of both intravascular and subepithelial polymorphonuclear leukocytes, and because of the vascular invasion, the skin lesions may be concentrically enlarging and necrotic. Blood cultures are not likely to reveal this pathogen. In a randomized trial comparing voriconazole with standard amphotericin B for primary treatment of invasive aspergillosis, voriconazole was demonstrated to be more effective than amphotericin B.[17] An evolving body of clinical data regarding this topic has led to the recent comment that voriconazole will likely become the drug of choice for treatment of invasive aspergillosis.[18]

There is not a consensus recommendation about when empiric antifungal therapy should be started for neutropenic patients who have persistent fever. The IDSA's clinical guidelines for treatment of infections caused by Candida suggest starting antifungal treatment when there is persistent unexplained fever despite 4 to 7 days of appropriate antibacterial therapy,[15] but the IDSA guidelines for therapy in febrile neutropenic patients suggest beginning empirical antifungal treatment when there is persistent fever for >3 days after antibacterial therapy is instituted in patients expected to have neutropenia for longer than 5 to 7 more days.[3] Because amphotericin B has activity against most Candida spp as well as Aspergillus, it has been the agent most often used. Liposomal amphotericin B has been shown to be as effective as conventional amphotericin B for empiric antifungal therapy in patients with fever and neutropenia, and it is associated with fewer breakthrough fungal infections, less infusion-related toxicity, and less nephrotoxicity.[19] More recently, a randomized, international, multicenter trial found that voriconazole (a new second-generation triazole with both Aspergillus and Candida activity) was comparable to liposomal amphotericin B for empiric antifungal therapy.[20] A statistically significant and noteworthy observation in this report was that patients receiving voriconazole had more episodes of transient visual changes (22%) than did those receiving liposomal amphotericin B (1%). In a blinded, randomized, international multicenter noninferiority study of caspofungin (50 mg daily; 70 mg on day 1) vs liposomal amphotericin B (3 mg/kg daily) for therapy of persistently febrile neutropenic patients, both agents were comparable in overall success; however, caspofungin was associated with more successful outcome in patients with baseline fungal infections ($p = 0.043$) and had fewer drug-related adverse events ($p < 0.001$).[21]

Humoral Immunity

To be ingested by polymorphonuclear leukocytes, there is a requirement that certain organisms undergo opsonization, a process in which those organisms are encased by a factor which then allows the phagocyte to attach. Once intracellular, these organisms are readily killed by the phagocyte. The humoral immune system provides for such opsonization through its major components of antibody and complement and may be summarized as providing protection against pathogens that are hard to eat but easy to kill.[2]

The antibody component of humoral immunity is dependent on the transformation of B lymphocytes into plasma cells, which produce as major opsonins IgG and IgM. A structural part of these antibodies is a component referred to as the Fc segment. Polymorphonuclear leukocytes have a receptor for this Fc segment. These Fc segments attach to the Fc receptor on the phagocyte, allowing the polymorphonuclear leukocyte to ingest the organism in a process that has been referred to as the "zipper" phenomenon of phagocytosis.

In addition to antibody, complement may serve as an opsonizer. Of the various complement components, the one most important for opsonization is C3b, which may be generated through two different pathways. In the classic complement pathway, the formation of antigen-antibody complexes turns on the complement cascade. Once C3 is activated, it is cleaved by C3 esterase to yield C3b. A limitation of the classic complement pathway is the requirement for antibody production, which may take hours to develop. In situations such as the acute development of pneumococcal infection, there is an immediate need for host defense that cannot wait for antibody production. It is in this setting that the alternative complement pathway (also known as the properdin system) becomes important. Instead of requiring an antigen-antibody complex to turn on the cascade, the alternative pathway is dependent on cell wall components such as teichoic acid and peptidoglycans found in Gram-positive organisms and lipopolysaccharides found in Gram-negative organisms. These lead to proteolytic cleavage of C3 to generate C3b, and this mechanism can lead to immediate opsonization. In addition to its opsonizing ability and its initiation of the membrane attack complex of complement, C3b can be joined by factors B and D to form a C3 convertase, which is highly labile. When bound by properdin, the C3 convertase is stabilized and can then cleave more C3 to generate more C3b, with a resultant amplification of the alternative complement pathway. Some clinical evidence exists that patients who have undergone splenectomy have a decrease in alternative pathway-mediated activation of C3.[22]

There are four clinically relevant situations within the category of defective humoral immunity: (1) disorders of immunoglobulin production; (2) asplenia or hyposplenic states; (3) hypocomplementemia; and (4) impaired neutralization of toxins.

The major clinical situations that result in disorders of immunoglobulin production are summarized in Table 3. Included in these processes is the lack of B-cell regulation, with its resultant production of abnormal immunoglobulins occurring on the basis of T-cell deficiency states in conditions such as HIV infection.

The characteristic pathogens infecting patients with impairment of immunoglobulin production are included in Table 4. Among the bacteria, the common feature is encapsulation, with the capsule essentially making them slippery and therefore dependent on opsonization for phagocyte attachment. Of the pathogens defended against by humoral immunity, the one that most frequently causes an acute life-threatening infection is *S pneumoniae*. In recent years, it has been noted that the severity of infection with *S pneumoniae* may be accentuated in patients with alcoholism or in those who are HIV-infected. In both patient groups, this pathogen may initially present as the etiologic agent of community-acquired pneumonia, which may be multilobar, with a high incidence of bacteremia and an increased risk of ARDS. An important consideration regarding infection with this pathogen is the increasing prevalence of penicillin resistance. Despite appropriate antibiotics and supportive care, the mortality in this setting remains high.

Also included among the pathogens that infect patients with defects in immunoglobulin production are certain viruses, including enteroviruses, influenza viruses, and arboviruses. Enteroviruses, particularly echovirus 24, have been associated with a clinical complex consisting of dermatomyositis-like skin lesions, edema, and neurologic problems. This has been referred to as chronic enteroviral meningoencephalitis.

Common variable immunodeficiency (CVI) is associated with functional abnormalities of both B and T cells but is usually classified as a primary antibody deficiency syndrome. Characterized by hypogammaglobulinemia and recurrent bacterial infections, CVI usually does not become clinically

Table 3. *Major Clinical Situations Resulting in Disorder of Immunoglobulin Production*

Congenital agammaglobulinemias
Common variable immunodeficiency (acquired hypogammaglobulinemia)
Heavy chain disease
Waldenström's macroglobulinemia
Multiple myeloma
B-cell lymphomas
Chronic lymphocytic leukemia
T-cell deficiency states
Hyposplenic states

Table 4. *Pathogens in Patients With Defective Humoral Immunity*

Disorders of Immunoglobulin Production
    Streptococcus pneumoniae
    Haemophilus influenzae
    Encapsulated strains of Gram-negative bacilli
    Enteroviruses, particularly echovirus 24
    Influenza viruses
    Arboviruses
    Pneumocystis jiroveci (formerly *P carinii*)
    Giardia lamblia
Asplenic State or Splenic Dysfunction
    Streptococcus pneumoniae
    Capnocytophaga canimorsus
    Babesia microti
    Plasmodium spp
    Haemophilus influenzae
    Neisseria spp

apparent until the second or third decade of life. Affected patients have an increased risk of autoimmune, granulomatous, and lymphoproliferative diseases. Even though recurrent bacterial infections of the respiratory tract are the most common, diarrhea due to *Giardia lamblia* is frequently encountered. This reflects the importance of local immunoglobulin production in the GI tract as a component of defense against *G lamblia*. Because some of the common pathogens infecting the respiratory or GI tracts are dependent on antibody production for host defense, concomitant infection of these two body sites should raise the suspicion of immunoglobulin deficiency states such as CVI. IV immunoglobulin may be efficacious in patients with this clinical entity, but anaphylaxis with such therapy has been reported.

Anatomic asplenia, as well as the hyposplenic states that occur in persons with sickle cell disease (due to autoinfarction of the spleen) and in patients with Hodgkin disease (especially after therapy), are also important predispositions to infection. The propensity for infection in these patients occurs on the basis of impairment of several immunologic functions: (1) relative to other lymphoid organs, the spleen has a greater percentage of B lymphocytes and is therefore involved in the production of antibody to polysaccharide antigens; (2) the spleen participates as a phagocytic organ, removing opsonin-coated organisms or damaged cells from the circulation; and (3) alternative complement-mediated activation of C3 may be decreased in patients after splenectomy. An important clinical clue to heighten awareness of both functional and anatomic asplenia is the presence of Howell-Jolly bodies on the peripheral blood smear.

The important pathogens involved in infections in patients without a spleen or with splenic dysfunction are summarized in Table 4.[23] Responsible for about 80% of overwhelming infections in asplenic patients, *S pneumoniae* should be given a particularly high index of suspicion because the clinical entity of post-splenectomy pneumococcal sepsis may initially present as only a flu-like illness with fever and myalgias.[24] Within the course of a few hours, untreated patients may develop a fulminant course that includes disseminated intravascular coagulation, purpura fulminans, symmetrical peripheral gangrene, shock, and ultimately death. Although *S pneumoniae* and *Haemophilus influenzae* are pathogens encountered in patients with either disorders of immunoglobulin production or splenic dysfunction, the pathogens infecting the asplenic or hyposplenic patient are otherwise different. Also included are two pathogens, *Babesia microti* and *Plasmodium* spp, that infect erythrocytes to cause hemolytic states and that require removal of parasitized RBCs by the spleen as a protective defense. *Capnocytophaga canimorsus* produces an acute illness with eschar formation following dog bites to asplenic individuals.[25]

Patients with deficiencies in the late complement components (C5 through C8) may present with recurrent *Neisseria* spp infections. The total hemolytic complement (CH_{50}) is the best screening test for this population. If the assay is normal, one can essentially exclude complement deficiency. In addition, an X-linked properdin deficiency associated with absence of the alternative complement pathway may produce a similar picture of severe meningococcal disease.

Completing the spectrum of clinical problems that may occur on the basis of defective humoral immunity is less-than-optimal neutralization of toxins produced in diphtheria, tetanus, and botulism.

IV gammaglobulin is a polyvalent antibody product containing the IgG antibodies that regularly occur in the donor population as well as traces of IgA and IgM and immunoglobulin fragments. Its half-life of 3 weeks allows for once-monthly dosing for prophylaxis in patients with primary humoral immunodeficiency. For bone marrow transplant patients ≥20 years of age, it has been shown to decrease the risk of septicemia and certain other infections, interstitial pneumonia of infectious or idiopathic etiology, and acute graft-vs-host disease in the first 100 days posttransplant.[26] In this patient population, dosing is more frequent than in prophylaxis for primary humoral immunodeficiency. Contraindications to its use include selective IgA deficiency and severe systemic reactions to human immune globulin.

Prevention of disease with vaccine is important in patients with defects in humoral immunity, although responses to vaccine may be attenuated. The 23-valent pneumococcal vaccine is recommended for adults with functional or anatomic asplenia, chronic cardiovascular disease, chronic pulmonary disease, diabetes mellitus, alcoholism, chronic liver disease, cerebrospinal fluid (CSF) leaks, and immunocompromised states including malignancy and HIV infection. In the review by the Centers for Disease Control and Prevention (CDC),[27] revaccination once was recommended for two groups: (1) persons aged ≥2 years who are at highest risk for serious pneumococcal infection and those who are likely to have a rapid decline in pneumococcal antibody levels (*eg*, functional or anatomic asplenia, HIV infection, leukemia, lymphoma, Hodgkin disease, multiple myeloma, generalized malignancy, chronic renal failure, nephrotic syndrome, other conditions associated with immunosuppression [including transplantation], and those receiving immunosuppressive chemotherapy [including steroids]), provided that 5 years has elapsed since receipt of the first dose of pneumococcal vaccine; and (2) persons aged ≥65 years if they received the vaccine 5 years previously and were <65 years old at the time of the primary vaccination. In an overall analysis not limited to immunocompromised patients, the effectiveness of pneumococcal conjugate vaccine has been demonstrated to prevent disease in young children for whom the vaccine is indicated and may be reducing the rate of disease in adults.[28] This report noted that the vaccine provides an effective tool for reducing disease caused by drug-resistant strains. Routine vaccination with the quadrivalent *Neisseria meningitidis* vaccine is recommended for certain high-risk groups, including persons who have terminal complement component deficiencies and those who have anatomic or functional asplenia.[29] Although the need for revaccination of adults has not been determined, antibody levels to *N meningitidis* rapidly decline over 2 to 3 years, and revaccination may be considered 3 to 5 years after receipt of the initial dose. Prophylaxis options against meningococcal infection based on the patient population being treated include rifampin (600 mg orally q12h for 2 days), ciprofloxacin (500 mg orally as single dose in nonpregnant adults), or ceftriaxone (250 mg IM as a single dose). *H influenzae* B vaccines are immunogenic in splenectomized adults and may be considered for this group.[30] When elective splenectomy is planned, pneumococcal, meningococcal, and *H influenzae* B vaccination should precede surgery by at least 2 weeks, if possible.

Cell-Mediated Immunity

The cell-mediated immune system is dependent on the interrelationship of T lymphocytes with macrophages. In contrast to primary neutrophil defense and humoral immunity, in which the polymorphonuclear leukocyte is the major phagocyte, the predominant phagocytic cell in cell-mediated immunity is the macrophage. On initial exposure to an antigen, T lymphocytes become sensitized. When restimulated, these sensitized T lymphocytes produce a group of lymphokines, including macrophage activation factor. It is this substance that stimulates macrophages to better ingest and kill pathogens. In contrast to polymorphonuclear leukocytes, macrophages can readily ingest microorganisms but have a difficult time with intracellular killing. This system may be summarized as providing protection against pathogens that are easy to eat but hard to kill.[2]

Some of the disorders and clinical situations associated with defects in cell-mediated immunity are listed in Table 5. With aging alone, patients have a decrease in cell-mediated immunity. Pregnant women in their third trimester have a transient loss of cell-mediated immunity, which spontaneously reconstitutes itself within about 3 months of delivery.[31] Immunosuppressive drugs (including corticosteroids and cyclosporine) and HIV infection are associated with defects in this limb of host defense. Both steroids and HIV infection decrease total T lymphocyte numbers, resulting in production of abnormal amounts of lymphokines like macrophage activation factor. In contrast, cyclosporine does not decrease lymphocyte numbers but decreases the functional capacity of lymphocytes to produce lymphokines. Irrespective of the mechanism, a

Table 5. *Important Clinical Situations Associated With Defects in Cell-Mediated Immunity*

Aging
During and following certain viral illnesses
Thymic dysplasia
Congenital situations associated with defects in cell-mediated immunity
Third trimester of pregnancy
Lymphatic malignancies of T-cell origin
Immunosuppressive therapy, especially corticosteroids and cyclosporine
AIDS and HIV-related disorders

Table 6. *Pathogens in Disorders of Cell-Mediated Immunity*

Bacteria	Fungi	Viruses	Parasites/Protozoa	Others
Mycobacteria	Cryptococcus	Herpes simplex	Pneumocystis	*Treponema pallidum*
Listeria	Histoplasma	Varicella-zoster	Toxoplasma	Chlamydiae
Nocardia	Coccidioides	Cytomegalovirus	Strongyloides	Rickettsiae
Rhodococcus	Blastomyces	Epstein-Barr virus	Giardia	
Salmonella	Candida	Polyoma viruses	Cryptosporidium	
Legionella	Aspergillus	Adenoviruses	Isospora	
Brucella		Measles virus	Trypanosoma	
Bartonella (formerly Rochalimaea)			Microsporidia	
			Leishmania	
			Amebae	

decrease in the production of macrophage activation factor decreases the stimulus for macrophages to optimally serve as the primary phagocytic cell in this host defense system.

The pathogens infecting patients with defects in cell-mediated immunity are summarized in Table 6 and can be divided into five categories: (1) bacteria (having as a common characteristic an intracellular location); (2) fungi (which often become clinically manifested in the setting of previous epidemiologic exposure); (3) viruses (most characteristically, DNA viruses); (4) parasites and protozoa; and (5) a miscellaneous group (some include spirochetes in this category).

Intracellular Bacteria

Mycobacterium tuberculosis

Although tuberculosis (TB) can be a problem in any patient with defective cell-mediated immunity, it has attracted recent attention because of the copathogenesis that may occur in individuals who are dually infected with the intracellular pathogens *M tuberculosis* and HIV-1. It has been suggested by some that mycobacteria and their products may enhance viral replication by inducing nuclear factor κ-B, the cellular factor that binds to promoter regions of HIV.[32] The presentation of TB in HIV-infected persons is variable and is influenced by the level of immunosuppression. With CD4+ counts >300 cells/μL, the pattern of typical reactivation TB with cavitary disease or upper lobe infiltrates is more common. When CD4+ cells fall to <200/μL, the pattern of disease is more typically middle to lower lobe disease with or without intrathoracic lymphadenopathy.[33] In patients with CD4+ counts at this level, extrapulmonary TB has been reported in at least 50%. Persons with serologic evidence of HIV infection and pulmonary TB fulfill the case definition for AIDS. These individuals with drug-susceptible strains tend to respond well to standard antituberculous therapy given as a short-course regimen for 6 months.[34] After initiation of antituberculosis therapy, some patients experience a paradoxical reaction, which is the temporary exacerbation of TB symptoms in the form of hectic fevers, lymphadenopathy, worsening of chest radiographic findings, and worsening of extrapulmonary lesions. These reactions are not associated with changes in *M tuberculosis* bacteriology, and patients generally feel well with no signs of toxicity. Such reactions have been attributed to recovery of delayed hypersensitivity response and an increase in exposure and reaction to mycobacterial antigens after bactericidal antituberculosis therapy is initiated. These reactions have been especially notable in individuals concurrently treated with antituberculosis and antiretroviral therapy. A noteworthy issue in HIV-infected patients is the interaction between antituberculosis drugs and antiretroviral therapy, including that with protease inhibitors. The rifamycins (*eg*, rifampin and rifabutin) accelerate the metabolism of protease inhibitors through induction of hepatic P_{450} cytochrome oxidases. Rifabutin has comparable antituberculous activity but with less hepatic P_{450} cytochrome enzyme-inducing effect than rifampin. The joint document of the American Thoracic Society, CDC, and IDSA on the treatment of tuberculosis includes recommendations for use of rifamycins in the treatment of tuberculosis.[34]

Two clinically relevant trends related to TB deserve comment. One is an apparent increase in TB reactivation associated with tumor necrosis factor-α inhibitors (eg, infliximab) used to treat rheumatoid arthritis and Crohn disease, with extrapulmonary TB being especially noted.[35] The other relates to the reports of liver failure and death after 2 months of therapy with rifampin and pyrazinamide.[36]

Some recent attention has focused on measures that foster type 1 immunity as a means of treating patients with TB, including those who may not have responded to initial therapy. Because IL-2 has a central role in regulating T-cell responses to *M tuberculosis*, a randomized, placebo-controlled, double-blinded trial in 110 HIV-negative, smear-positive, drug-susceptible pulmonary TB patients was conducted using adjunctive immunotherapy with recombinant IL-2.[37] In this trial, IL-2 did not enhance bacillary clearance or improvement in symptoms in HIV-seronegative adults with drug-susceptible TB.

A significant change has recently occurred regarding TB infection. For many decades, the terms "preventive therapy" and "chemoprophylaxis" were used to describe the status of persons with a positive tuberculin test but no symptoms or signs of active TB. The word *preventive* was inaccurate in that it referred to use of an agent such as isoniazid to prevent development of active TB in persons known or likely to be infected with *M tuberculosis*; it was not intended to imply prevention of true primary infection. To more accurately describe such therapy, in an official statement in 2000 the American Thoracic Society introduced the terminology "latent tuberculosis infection" (LTBI) as a substitute for "preventive therapy" and "chemoprophylaxis."[38] It acknowledged the role of LTBI as an important element in control of TB. It has been noted that HIV-infected persons with a positive tuberculin skin test have about a 7% chance per year of developing tuberculous disease, which exceeds the standard estimated lifetime risk of approximately 10% for the reactivation of LTBI in nonimmunocompromised persons with positive purified protein derivative tests.[39] In a prospective cohort study of persons with HIV infection in the United States, the annual risk of active TB among HIV-infected persons with a positive tuberculin test was 4.5 cases per 100 person-years of observation.[40] Based on such facts, it is recommended that HIV-infected persons with a tuberculin skin test with ≥5-mm induration be given treatment for latent tuberculosis. In the 2000 guidelines for treatment of LTBI, tuberculin positivity was also set at ≥5-mm induration for patients with organ transplants and other immunosuppressed patients receiving the equivalent of ≥15 mg/d of prednisone for 1 month or more. The risk of TB increases with a higher dose and longer duration of corticosteroids.

Mycobacterium avium *Complex*

Among individuals with defective cell-mediated immunity, *Mycobacterium avium* complex (MAC) classically infects HIV-infected persons when their CD4+ cells are <50/μL. In patients with AIDS, there are several lines of evidence suggesting that most patients with disseminated MAC have recently acquired the organisms, in contrast to the reactivation that is common with TB.[41] Adherence of the organisms to the gut wall is the initial event in invasion, followed by entry into the lamina propria and then phagocytosis by macrophages. Local replication of organisms leads to the endoscopically visible 2- to 4-mm punctate lesions that are the hallmark of MAC disease in the gut. The clinical presentation is that of a wasting syndrome marked by fever, night sweats, weight loss, diarrhea, anorexia, and malaise. Despite positive sputum cultures, serious pulmonary infection is not common in HIV-infected patients. The organism is most characteristically isolated from blood, stool, respiratory secretions, bone marrow, GI tract mucosa, and lymph nodes (although granuloma formation is minimal or absent). A unique pathophysiologic abnormality seen in about 5% of AIDS patients with MAC disease is marked elevations (20 to 40 times normal) in serum alkaline phosphatase with little elevation of transaminases, bilirubin, or other parameters of hepatic function. This is believed to occur on the basis of interference with enzyme metabolism rather than because of hepatic tissue destruction.

In those patients with symptomatic disease, a multidrug regimen is recommended that should include either clarithromycin or azithromycin in combination with ethambutol.[42] With advanced immunosuppression (CD4+ <50/μL), with high mycobacterial loads, or in the absence of effective antiretroviral therapy, the treatment guidelines recommend that adding a third drug be considered. Additional drugs that may be added to this regimen include rifabutin (as an A-1 recommended agent) or ciprofloxacin, levofloxacin, or amikacin (as C-III recommendations). The response to therapy is variable among patients, and the acquisition of drug resistance is common, especially with monotherapy. Although rifabutin was the initial agent approved for prophylaxis against MAC infection, more recent recommendations for the prevention of opportunistic infections in HIV-infected persons have listed azithromycin or clarithromycin as the agent of choice when the CD4+ count is <50/μL.[43]

Listeria monocytogenes

This intracellular Gram-positive rod characteristically infects persons with malignancy, diabetes mellitus, or renal transplantation followed by immunosuppressive therapy.[44] Neonates and pregnant women are also at risk, and the infection occurs with increased frequency with cirrhosis. About one third of patients in some series have no known risk factor, and Listeria has only recently been considered a cause of febrile GI illness in immunocompetent persons.[45] Listeria may be acquired via consumption of certain contaminated raw vegetables (with coleslaw as a source in some outbreaks), certain contaminated canned products (with sterile canned corn kernels as the source in one outbreak), raw food from animal sources (eg, beef, pork, or poultry), unpasteurized milk, or foods made from raw milk (notably, certain soft cheeses).

The most common clinical presentations are of CNS infection, sepsis, or a flu-like illness. When it causes acute meningitis, Listeria may be associated with a variable glucose level or with a CSF lymphocytosis or monocytosis. Gram stain of the CSF is positive in only about one fourth of patients. The infection has a predilection for the base of the brain with resultant focal neurologic signs, particularly cranial nerve involvement, in up to 40% of patients. Hydrocephalus may be a complication of this localization. Bacteremia is another common presentation, with cerebritis or brain abscess being less frequent.

Therapy is with high-dose IV ampicillin or penicillin.[46] Some favor the addition of a parenteral aminoglycoside with these agents even for treatment of meningitis, recognizing that the aminoglycosides administered parenterally in adults will not cross the blood-brain barrier but may help eradicate infectious sites outside the CNS.[47] For penicillin-allergic patients, trimethoprim-sulfamethoxazole is possibly effective. Extremely noteworthy is that cephalosporin therapy has no role in treating infection caused by Listeria. Because of the intracellular location of the organisms, 3 weeks of therapy is recommended for serious infections.

Nocardia asteroides

These filamentous aerobic Gram-positive rods are weakly acid-fast and characteristically produce disease in patients who have lymphoreticular neoplasms or have received long-term corticosteroid therapy. Because the organism most commonly infects humans through the respiratory tract, the classic pattern of infection is pulmonary disease, which may take the form of nodular infiltrates, cavitary lesions, or diffuse infiltrates with or without consolidation. Pustular skin lesions and neurologic disease in the form of encephalitis or brain abscess complete the triad of the most common presentations by this pathogen. The liver and kidneys are less likely to be involved. In the report from the Johns Hopkins Hospital of 59 patients diagnosed with nocardiosis over an 11-year time span, Nocardia was isolated most commonly from the respiratory tract (76%), followed by soft tissue (13%), blood (7%), and CNS (5%).[48] In this series, the infection was common in AIDS patients as well as in transplant recipients. In both groups of patients, disease developed in some despite prophylactic therapy against other pathogens with trimethoprim/sulfamethoxazole.

Standard therapy is with sulfonamides.[49] Trimethoprim-sulfamethoxazole is often used because of its convenient IV dosing; however, it has not been definitively proven that the combination is synergistic at the drug ratios that usually are achieved in serum or CSF.

Rhodococcus equi

Formerly called *Corynebacterium equi*, this partially acid-fast, aerobic, intracellular Gram-positive rod-coccus was first described in 1967 as the cause of disease in humans.[50] Even though the organism has been rarely reported to cause infection in immunocompetent patients, immunocompromised patients, especially those with HIV infection, are the ones most likely to develop clinical disease due to this pathogen. The most characteristic pattern of infection is described as a progressive pneumonia that may cavitate. Bacteremia is common in immunocompromised patients. Like Nocardia, it has also been associated with neurologic and skin lesions.

The intracellular location has made the organism difficult to treat, and principles of therapy include a prolonged duration of antibiotics, often in association with drainage. *In vitro*, *R equi* is usually susceptible to erythromycin, rifampin, fluoroquinolones, aminoglycosides, glycopeptides (*eg*, vancomycin), and imipenem; it has been suggested that immunocompromised patients and patients with serious infections receive IV therapy with two-drug or three-drug regimens that include vancomycin, imipenem, aminoglycosides, ciprofloxacin, rifampin, and/or erythromycin.[51] The choice of agents used and the duration of therapy are dependent on both the patient's host defense status and the site of infection. Oral antibiotics may be an option in certain immunocompetent patients with localized infection.

Salmonella spp

Patient populations with defective cell-mediated immunity that develop bacteremia with this intracellular Gram-negative rod include those with hematologic malignancies, systemic lupus erythematosus, and HIV infection. In those persons with HIV infection, a febrile typhoidal illness without diarrhea accounts for about 45% of the disease caused by this pathogen. More common is an illness associated with fever, severe diarrhea, and crampy abdominal pain. Compared with Shigella and Campylobacter, there is a lower incidence of bloody diarrhea and fecal leukocytes with Salmonella infection. Recurrent nontyphoidal bacteremia is considered an indication for secondary antibacterial prophylaxis in HIV-infected persons.[43]

Legionella spp

Legionella is a pathogen recognized to have the potential for causing acute mortality in patients with pulmonary infections, including even those who are not immunocompromised.[52] This pathogen causes more severe disease in transplant recipients, patients who receive corticosteroids, and HIV-infected persons. Immunocompromised patients with legionellosis may present with variable patterns of multisystem disease. Fever with a scanty productive cough is often described. In individuals receiving corticosteroids, cavitary lung lesions with abscess formation may occur. Dissemination seems to occur via bacteremic spread of the organism. In a review of Legionnaires disease, the most common extrapulmonary site was reported to be the heart (including myocarditis and pericarditis), and one would need to assume that such organ system involvement might be possible in immunocompromised patients.[53] Other patterns of extrapulmonary involvement by Legionella may take the form of sinusitis, cellulitis, pyelonephritis, and pancreatitis. Patients with hairy-cell leukemia, a disorder of monocyte deficiency and dysfunction, have an increased incidence of Legionella pneumonia. Legionella infection should be suspected in those individuals who do not respond to therapy with a β-lactam antibiotic. Useful in the acute diagnosis is the Legionella urinary antigen assay, which has been stated to be 70% sensitive and 100% specific in diagnosing infection caused by *Legionella pneumophila serogroup I*.

Erythromycin has traditionally been considered the agent of choice for treatment of this infection,[54] but recent reviews have suggested that the fluoroquinolones may be more efficacious.[53] Because of increased efficacy and the fact that macrolides such as erythromycin may have pharmacologic interactions with immunosuppressive agents used in transplant patients, some investigators feel that a fluoroquinolone should be added to the standard regimen for treating Legionnaires disease in transplant recipients with nosocomial pneumonia if the causative agent has not been identified. Some have suggested that rifampin be used as adjunctive therapy for severe Legionella infections, but this must be taken in context with the facts that (1) no prospective studies have evaluated such therapy, and (2) rifampin has the potential to induce the cytochrome P_{450} system and, therefore, cause a significant interaction with immunosuppressive therapy.

Brucella spp

Even though intracellular brucellae require cell-mediated immunity for eradication, the spectrum of brucellosis in immunocompromised hosts has not been frequently described. Because of the ability for splenic localization with the formation of suppurative lesions that might require splenectomy, this organism may cause further impairment of an otherwise compromised immune system.

Bartonella (Formerly Rochalimaea) spp

The small Gram-negative organisms in this genus may be demonstrated with Warthin-Starry staining or by electron microscopy. The patterns of infection in HIV-infected persons include the following: (1) bacteremia (in the absence of focal vascular proliferative response in tissue); (2) bacillary angiomatosis; and (3) peliosis hepatitis.[55] Bacillary angiomatosis presents in the later phases of HIV infection, usually with CD4+ counts <100 cells/μL. The condition is associated with a unique vascular lesion that may involve virtually every organ system, either alone or in association with other sites of involvement.[56] Of these, skin lesions are the most commonly recognized, with characteristic lesions being red and papular and therefore resembling Kaposi sarcoma. Lesions characteristically are associated with a long duration of symptoms or physical findings prior to diagnosis. Species causing such a process include *Bartonella henselae* and *Bartonella quintana*. Peliosis hepatitis refers to the blood-filled peliotic changes in the parenchyma of the liver or spleen that occur because of infection with these two species. Because these organisms are at present difficult to culture from blood or tissue, histopathology may be the study that directs further diagnostic evaluation. Erythromycin or doxycycline is considered the preferred agent.[42]

Fungi

Cryptococcus neoformans

Cryptococcal meningitis is an important infection in HIV-infected persons, particularly when CD4+ counts are <100 cells/μL, but may also occur in other populations, including elderly persons. The organism enters the body through the lungs, and the associated finding of pulmonary infiltrates in an HIV-infected person with meningitis should raise the suspicion of this diagnosis. The organism has a propensity to enter the bloodstream and may be detected in routine blood cultures. The resulting fungemia is often associated with multisegment pulmonary infiltrates and with skin lesions. Infection in the HIV population may present as a noninflammatory infection of the CNS, and the clinical features are therefore different from what one might expect in classic forms of meningitis caused by other pathogens. The history is frequently of a subacute or chronic illness associated mainly with headache. Physical examination may not reveal classic findings such as nuchal rigidity. Because of the lack of inflammation in the CNS, the CSF formula may include <20 WBC/mm³, normal glucose, and normal protein. These findings make CSF studies such as India ink stain, cryptococcal antigen, and fungal culture mainstays in the diagnosis.

The National Institute of Allergy and Infectious Diseases Mycoses Study Group and AIDS Clinical Trials Group reported their findings in 381 patients with cryptococcal meningitis treated in a double-blind multicenter trial.[57] Conclusions from this trial of AIDS-associated cryptococcal meningitis were that induction treatment for 2 weeks with the combination of amphotericin B (0.7 mg/kg/d) plus flucytosine (100 mg/kg/d in patients who were tolerant of this agent), followed by therapy with fluconazole (400 mg/d orally for 8 weeks) is safe and effective and should be considered the treatment of choice. The authors noted that high intracranial pressures have been associated with catastrophic neurologic deterioration and death in the absence of hydrocephalus. Of the patients in this study, 13 of 14 early deaths and 40% of deaths during weeks 3 through 10 were associated with elevated intracranial pressure. Based on the association between elevated intracranial pressure and mortality in patients with cryptococcal meningitis, it was suggested that measurement of intracranial pressure be included in the management of such patients. Included in the recommendations were daily lumbar punctures, use of acetazolamide, and ventriculoperitoneal shunts for asymptomatic patients with intracranial CSF pressure >320 mm H$_2$O and for symptomatic patients with pressures >180 mm H$_2$O. More recently, it was recommended that in the absence of focal lesions, opening pressures ≥250 mm H$_2$O should be treated with large-volume CSF drainage (defined in this report as allowing CSF to drain until a satisfactory closing pressure had been achieved, commonly <200 mm H$_2$O).[58] IDSA guidelines for the management of cryptococcal meningitis in HIV-infected persons with opening CSF pressure of >250 mm H$_2$O recommended lumbar drainage sufficient to achieve a closing pressure ≤200 mm H$_2$O or 50% of initial opening pressure.[59]

Maintenance therapy is required after completion of primary therapy, and studies have identified fluconazole as the agent of choice.[60,61] In an international observational study reported by the International Working Group on Cryptococcosis, discontinuation of maintenance therapy for cryptococcal meningitis was stated to be safe if the CD4+ cell count increases to >100 cells/μL while the patient is receiving highly active antiretroviral therapy (HAART).[62] These findings were consistent with previous recommendations by the US Public Health Service and the IDSA that discontinuation of secondary prophylaxis may be an option when CD4+ cells are >100 to 200 cells/μL for ≥6 months.[43] Recurrent cryptococcal infection should be suspected in patients whose serum cryptococcal antigen test results revert back to positive after discontinuation of maintenance therapy.[62]

Histoplasma capsulatum

The clinical entity of progressive disseminated histoplasmosis has become increasingly recognized because of HIV infection. The illness may occur on the basis of either reactivation or primary disease, making the epidemiologic history of travel to or residence in endemic areas crucial. Although patients may present with such nonspecific findings as fever, fatigue, weakness, and weight loss, a characteristic presentation in about half of patients is diffuse interstitial or miliary pulmonary infiltrates that are associated with hypoxemia and mimic *Pneumocystis jiroveci* (previously *Pneumocystis carinii*) pneumonia. These patients may concomitantly demonstrate reticuloendothelial involvement in the forms of hepatosplenomegaly, lymphadenopathy, and bone marrow involvement. A subgroup may present with a septic syndrome that can include disseminated intravascular coagulation. Small intracellular periodic acid-Schiff positive, yeast-like organisms are the characteristic morphologic form of the organism. Although the organism may be isolated from sputum, tissue, or blood, the *H capsulatum* polysaccharide antigen from blood, urine, or CSF may serve as a more rapid diagnostic study. In the IDSA guidelines for treating disseminated histoplasmosis, immunocompromised patients were divided into those with AIDS and those without AIDS.[63] In those without AIDS who were sufficiently ill to require hospitalization, amphotericin B (0.7 to 1.0 mg/kg/d) was recommended. It was noted that most patients respond quickly to amphotericin B and can then be treated with itraconazole (200 mg qd or bid) for 6 to 18 mo. For patients with AIDS, it was recommended that therapy be divided into an initial 12-week intensive phase to induce a remission in the clinical illness and then followed by a chronic maintenance phase to prevent relapse. Amphotericin B was recommended for patients sufficiently ill to require hospitalization, with replacement by itraconazole, 200 mg twice daily (when the patient no longer requires hospitalization for IV therapy), to complete a 12-week total course of induction therapy. Itraconazole (200 mg tid for 3 days and then bid for 12 weeks) was recommended for patients who have mild or moderately severe symptoms and do not require hospitalization. Maintenance therapy with itraconazole for life was included in the recommendations.

Coccidioides immitis

In HIV-infected persons as well as in transplant recipients, this fungal pathogen occurs most commonly in those individuals from endemic areas. The illness may resemble Pneumocystis pneumonia with diffuse reticulonodular infiltrates. The classic clinical pattern of disease, manifested as dissemination to sites such as meninges, skin, and joints, is not altered by HIV infection. In the IDSA guidelines for the treatment of coccidioidomycosis, it was noted that the presence of bilateral reticulonodular or miliary infiltrates produced by C immitis usually implies an underlying immunodeficiency state.[64] In such circumstances, therapy usually starts with amphotericin B. Several weeks of therapy is often required for improvement, at which point an oral azole may replace amphotericin. The IDSA guidelines for treatment of coccidioidomycosis offer recommendations for the management of meningitis, including a role for oral fluconazole in certain patients.

Candida spp

Host defense against Candida is provided by both neutrophils and cell-mediated immunity. In addition, the immunocompetent host may develop bloodborne infection with this pathogen, and notable risk factors for this include surgery (particularly of the GI tract), broad-spectrum antibiotics, hyperalimentation, and intravascular catheters.[15] With HIV infection, Candida may present in a hierarchical pattern. With CD4+ counts in the 400 to 600 cells/μL range, women may develop recurrent vulvovaginal candidiasis. At CD4+ levels of ~250 cells/μL, oral candidiasis is the expected clinical entity. The clinical presentation of odynophagia in a patient with oral candidiasis and a CD4+ count of <100 cells/μL strongly raises the diagnosis of Candida esophagitis. These candidal infections generally respond well to therapy, and because of this, primary prophylaxis is not generally recommended. A recent trend has been toward non-*albicans* strains of Candida[65] and toward strains of *Candida albicans* that are fluconazole-resistant.[66] Patterns of azole use have probably contributed to such problems. Recurrent use of fluconazole in HIV-infected patients has been associated with an increasing number of reports of Candida spp resistant to this agent. In a bone marrow transplant unit in which patients were given fluconazole (400 mg/d, oral or IV) for the first 75 days after transplantation, 5% of patients became colonized with fluconazole-resistant strains of *C albicans*, and 53% of patients had at least one mouthwashing sample that yielded non-*albicans* species of Candida during the course of their bone marrow transplantation.[67]

Aspergillus spp

As is the case with Candida, Aspergillus may cause infection in patients with defects in either neutrophil function or cell-mediated immunity. In addition to being a nosocomial pathogen, infection with this agent may represent reactivation disease. This may be especially notable in patients who have received a bone marrow transplant or solid organ transplant. In AIDS patients with the concomitant problems of neutropenia, corticosteroid therapy, or ethanol use, invasive pulmonary or disseminated aspergillosis may occur. This tends to present in the later stages of HIV infection, especially when CD4+ cells are <50/μL. Voriconazole is the preferred therapy for invasive aspergillosis in HIV-infected patients.[42]

Aspergillus infection and its treatment provide some important insights into the evolving clinical importance of type 1 immunity. Patients with chronic granulomatous disease have an increased incidence of infection with Aspergillus. Treatment of these patients with recombinant IFN-γ stimulates killing of this pathogen and reduces the frequency and severity of clinically apparent fungal infection.[1] This observation is important in that it conveys a treatment option for IFN-γ based on an understanding of the role of type 1 immunity in defending against certain fungal pathogens. The traditional treatment for Aspergillus has been amphotericin B given at maximum tolerated doses (*eg*, 1 to 1.5 mg/kg/d) and continued despite modest increases in serum creatinine.[68] Lipid formulations of amphotericin have noteworthy roles in two circumstances: (1) for the patient who has impaired renal function or develops nephrotoxicity while receiving amphotericin B deoxycholate[68] and (2) for patients who have undergone bone marrow transplantation.[69] The echinocandin caspofungin has been recently approved for patients in whom amphotericin fails. Itraconazole has been suggested as an alternative form of therapy in certain settings of Aspergillus infection. In a randomized trial comparing voriconazole with standard amphotericin B for primary treatment of invasive aspergillosis, voriconazole was demonstrated to be more effective than amphotericin B.[17] An evolving body of clinical data regarding this topic has led to the recent comment that voriconazole, which is available in both IV and oral formulations, will likely become the drug of choice for treatment of invasive aspergillosis.[18,42]

Viruses

Herpes Simplex Virus

The patterns of herpes simplex virus (HSV) infection vary according to the underlying immunosuppression status. Patients with hematologic or lymphoreticular neoplasms may develop disseminated mucocutaneous HSV lesions. In transplant patients, esophagitis, tracheobronchitis, pneumonitis, or hepatitis are characteristic presentations, with hepatitis caused by HSV presenting most classically as the triad of high fever, leukopenia, and markedly elevated aminotransferase levels.[70] HIV-infected persons can have a vast array of clinical conditions caused by HSV, including esophagitis, colitis, perianal ulcers (often associated with urinary retention), pneumonitis, and a spectrum of neurologic diseases. Acyclovir remains the drug of choice for these infections. However, acyclovir-resistant strains have emerged, for which foscarnet may be the alternative therapy.

Varicella-Zoster Virus

As is the case with HSV infection, varicella-zoster virus (VZV) may present differently according to the underlying type of immunosuppression. With both chickenpox and shingles in patients with solid and hematologic malignancies, cutaneous dissemination may occur and may be associated with such visceral involvement as pneumonitis, hepatitis, and meningoencephalitis. Herpes zoster may be multidermatomal in HIV-infected persons, and this may be the initial clue to the diagnosis of HIV infection. Treatment options for both varicella and zoster have been summarized.[71] Acyclovir, famciclovir, and valacyclovir are discussed according to the disease, the pattern of immunosuppression, and the requirement for IV vs oral therapy. With the depression of cell-mediated immunity that occurs during the third trimester of pregnancy,[31] there is increased risk of dissemination of VZV to the lungs during pregnancy. A recently published case-control analysis of 18 pregnant women with VZV pneumonia compared with 72 matched control subjects identified cigarette smoking and >100 skin lesions as markers for the development of varicella pneumonia in pregnancy.[72] In immunocompromised patients and pregnant women who are exposed to chickenpox and in whom there is no clinical or serologic evidence of immunity to VZV, administration of varicella-zoster immune globulin may prevent or significantly modify VZV infection.[71]

Cytomegalovirus

For perspective, it is important to recognize the three major consequences of cytomegalovirus (CMV) infection in solid organ transplantation recipients: (1) CMV disease, including a wide range of clinical illnesses; (2) superinfection with opportunistic pathogens; and (3) injury to the transplanted organ, possibly enhancing chronic rejection.[73] The virus may be present in the forms of latency (infection without signs of active viral replication), active infection (viral replication in blood or organs), and primary infection (active infection in a previously nonimmune seronegative person). A recent study addressed the impact of primary infection in bone marrow recipients who were CMV-seronegative and who received stem cells from CMV-seropositive recipients.[74] These patients died of invasive bacterial and fungal infections at a rate greater than that of patients who did not have primary infection, and it was hypothesized that primary CMV infection has immunomodulatory effects that predispose to such secondary infections.

The spectrum of clinically active CMV infection in immunocompromised patients is broad and may vary according to the immunosuppressive condition. In HIV-infected patients, the classic presentation has been chorioretinitis but may also include GI ulcerations, pneumonitis, hepatitis, encephalopathy, adrenalitis, and a painful myeloradiculopathy. Some immunosuppressed patients present with only a mononucleosis-like syndrome consisting of fever and lymphadenopathy.

New approaches in both hematopoietic stem cell or solid organ transplant recipients emphasize the use of prophylactic or preemptive therapy based on CMV monitoring.[75] Although serologic tests have previously been suggested to have a potential role in directing CMV therapy in bone marrow transplant patients and heart transplant patients, serologies are not the most reliable studies in predicting the presence of CMV infection or clinical disease. The appearance of CMV protein pp65 in peripheral blood leukocytes has proved to be superior to tests based on virus isolation[73] and has correlated with subsequent development of CMV disease. In addition to CMV antigenemia, DNA/RNAemia (especially quantitative polymerase chain reaction) is clinically useful, and detection tests for both are methods of choice for diagnosis and monitoring of active CMV infection after organ transplantation.

For the purpose of developing consistent reporting of CMV in clinical trials, definitions of CMV infection and disease were developed and published.[76] In addition, an approach to the management of CMV infection after solid organ transplantation has been recently published, and several clinically relevant messages provided it.[73] In managing CMV infection, the clinician needs to be aware of four types of treatment options: (1) therapeutic use (treatment based on the presence of established infection); (2) prophylactic use (use of antimicrobial therapy from the earliest possible moment); (3) preemptive use (antimicrobial therapy before clinical signs of infection); and (4) deferred therapy (initiation of therapy after onset of disease). In the therapeutic setting of CMV disease after solid organ transplantation, IV ganciclovir is the drug of choice, with anti-CMV hyperimmunoglobulin preparations being useful adjuncts in seronegative recipients of seropositive organs and with foscarnet (because of its inherent toxicity) being considered as rescue therapy. Although ganciclovir has for years been the mainstay of therapy for CMV retinitis in AIDS patients, valganciclovir (an oral prodrug of ganciclovir) has been approved as an effective treatment option. In addition, studies are ongoing using valganciclovir as both preemptive and definitive therapy of CMV infections in transplant patients. An immune reconstitution syndrome including visual blurring months after successful therapy of CMV retinitis has been described in AIDS patients who have started HAART.[77]

The role for prophylaxis against CMV was summarized based on the type of organ transplanted.[76] With detection of CMV antigenemia at a predefined level, IV ganciclovir may have a role in preventing CMV disease in certain patient populations. Secondary prophylaxis has been recommended but may be discontinued if the CD4+ cell count reaches >100 to 150 cells/μL and remains at this level for ≥6 months with no evidence of active CMV disease.[43]

Epstein-Barr Virus

The pathobiology of Epstein-Barr virus (EBV) is important in understanding the evolution of EBV-associated disease in immunocompromised patients. Although early studies indicated that EBV replicated in epithelial cells in the oropharynx, more recent studies suggest that B cells in the oropharynx may be the primary site of infection.[78] This has led to the thought that resting memory B cells are the site of persistence of EBV within the body, with the number of latently infected cells remaining stable for years.[79] What has not been definitively elucidated at the present time is the role of oral epithelial cells in the transmission and latency of EBV. Even though the finding of antibodies against EBV viral proteins and antigens is consistent with the fact that there is some degree of humoral immunity to the virus, it is the cellular immune response that is the more important for controlling EBV infection. Important among the proteins produced by EBV is latent membrane protein 1, which acts as an oncogene and whose expression in an animal model has resulted in B-cell lymphomas. In patients who have AIDS or have received organ or bone marrow transplants, an inability to control proliferation of latently EBV-infected cells may lead to EBV lymphoproliferative disease, which in tissue may take the form of plasmacytic hyperplasia, B-cell hyperplasia, B-cell lymphoma, or immunoblastic lymphoma.[78] It has been suggested that therapy for EBV lymphoproliferative disease should include reduction in the dose of immunosuppressive medication when possible. More specific, definitive recommendations for therapy are not available, but potential options have been reviewed.[78]

Completing the spectrum of EBV disease in immunocompromised patients is oral hairy leukoplakia, a common, nonmalignant hyperplastic lesion of epithelial cells seen most characteristically in HIV-infected patients. In its classic presentation, hairy leukoplakia presents as raised white lesions of the oral mucosa, especially on the lateral aspect of the tongue. Contributing to the ongoing attempts to elucidate the pathobiology of EBV, a study of serial tongue biopsy specimens from HIV-infected patients demonstrated EBV replication in normal tongue epithelial cells (in contrast to the lack of active viral replication in certain EBV-associated malignancies) and suggested that the tongue may be a source of EBV secretion into saliva.[80] In this clinical trial, valacyclovir treatment completely abrogated EBV replication, resulting in resolution of hairy leukoplakia when it was present, but EBV replication returned in normal tongue epithelial cells after valacyclovir treatment. These findings are consistent with clinical experience that the lesions of hairy leukoplakia respond to antiviral therapy but recur once therapy is stopped. Topics not evaluated in this study, but important in the understanding of EBV, are whether other oral epithelial cells support viral replication and whether oral epithelial cells participate with B cells in viral latency.

Polyoma Viruses
(Including JC Virus and BK Virus)

Clinically important members of this class of double-stranded DNA viruses include BK virus and JC virus. Primary infection with BK virus is generally asymptomatic and occurs in childhood. Following primary infection, the virus can remain latent in many sites, with the most notable being the kidney. With cellular immunodeficiency, the virus can reactivate and cause clinical disease. Although the kidney, lung, eye, liver, and brain are sites of both primary and reactivated BK virus-associated disease, the most characteristic disease entities are hemorrhagic and nonhemorrhagic cystitis, ureteric stenosis, and nephritis, and these occur most often in recipients of solid organ or bone marrow transplants.[81]

JC virus is the etiologic agent in progressive multifocal leukoencephalopathy (PML). In this primary demyelinating process involving the white matter of the cerebral hemispheres, patients present subacutely with confusion, disorientation, and visual disturbances, which may progress to cortical blindness or ataxia. CSF is characteristically acellular. A feature on neuroradiology imaging studies is lack of mass effect. No definitive therapy is presently available for this infection, and clinical efforts have recently focused on the role of immune reconstitution in modifying the clinical course of the illness. In a multicenter analysis of 57 consecutive HIV-positive patients with PML, neurologic improvement or stability at 2 months after therapy was demonstrated in 26% of patients who received HAART in contrast to improvement in only 4% of patients who did not receive HAART (p = 0.03).[82] In this study, decreases in JC virus DNA to undetectable levels predicted a longer survival. In the context that untreated PML may be fatal within 3 to 6 months, such potential for preventing neurologic progression and improving survival by controlling JC virus replication becomes clinically relevant.

Adenoviruses

In immunocompromised patients, these DNA viruses may produce generalized illness that classically involves the nervous system, respiratory system, GI tract, and liver. This class of viruses has recently emerged as a major problem in some bone marrow transplant units. The infections may have a fulminant course, which may result in death. No drug has been shown to be definitively beneficial in these patients, although IV ribavirin may be effective in some.

Measles Virus

Because individuals are protected against measles by cell-mediated immunity and since measles may cause severe illness in HIV-infected persons, protection via vaccine is an important consideration. A basic tenet in infectious diseases has been that live-virus vaccines should not be administered to immunocompromised patients. An exception has been use of measles vaccine, a live-virus vaccine, in asymptomatic HIV-infected individuals and potentially in those with symptomatic HIV infection. Fatal giant-cell pneumonitis has been described in a young male measles vaccine recipient with AIDS.[83] Even with the overwhelming success of measles immunization programs, this case has prompted reappraisal of recommendations and some have suggested that it may be prudent to withhold measles-containing vaccines from HIV-infected persons with evidence of severe immunosuppression.

Emerging Viral Pathogens in Persons With Defects in Cell-Mediated Immunity

There have been increasing reports of infections caused by respiratory syncytial virus or parainfluenza virus, particularly in persons who have received bone marrow or solid organ transplantation. The spectrum of disease caused by these pathogens is evolving, with the lung being an important target organ. These viruses should be considered to be among the pathogens that may cause pneumonia in patients with defects in cell-mediated immunity.

Parasites and Protozoa

P jiroveci (Previously P carinii)

In recognition of its genetic and functional distinctness, the organism that causes human Pneumocystis pneumonia has been recently renamed *P jiroveci*, but despite this change, the use of the acronym PCP is not precluded because it can be read Pneumocystis pneumonia.[84] The clinical setting in which *P jiroveci* pneumonia (PCP) develops continues to evolve. In the pre-AIDS era, this pathogen was described as a cause of rapidly progressive infection in patients with malignant diseases, especially during the time of steroid withdrawal. Following the onset of the AIDS epidemic in the early 1980s, PCP was most often diagnosed in HIV-infected persons. Following the widespread use of HAART in the mid-1990s, HIV-associated PCP has decreased, and it has been recently reported that PCP may in certain settings be diagnosed more often in non-HIV immunocompromised patients than in those with HIV infection.[85] Host defense against Pneumocystis includes humoral immunity; however, because of the overwhelming predominance of infection by this pathogen in HIV-infected persons, it has been included in this section of pathogens that infect patients with defective cell-mediated immunity.

Although diffuse interstitial infiltrates are the most characteristic pulmonary finding with PCP, patients may present with focal infiltrates, cavitary lesions, or nodular lung lesions. Findings that support, but do not prove, the diagnosis of PCP in an HIV-infected patient with pulmonary infiltrates include a CD4+ cell count <250 cells/μL, a WBC count <8,000 cells/mm³, and an elevated serum lactate dehydrogenase. PCP may occur as part of the presentation of the acute retroviral syndrome. In the review of PCP from the Clinical Center at the National Institutes of Health,[85] diagnostic studies for PCP were reviewed. It was noted that traditional stains on sputum or from BAL specimens for the cyst form of *P jiroveci* have been the mainstay of diagnosis in most settings. Direct immunofluorescent staining using monoclonal antibody 2G2 (which detects both cysts and trophozoites) has been used for many years in the algorithm of the National Institutes of Health Clinical Center for diagnosing PCP. This stain is performed first on induced sputum, and if that smear is negative, then a BAL specimen is obtained for the same study. Ongoing investigation has been focused on the development of a quantitative polymerase chain reaction assay that can be performed on oral washes or gargles and that might allow a clinician not only to diagnose PCP at an earlier stage than has traditionally been possible, but also to distinguish between colonization and disease with *P jiroveci*.

Trimethoprim-sulfamethoxazole is the current first-line therapeutic agent. As alternative therapy, pentamidine has been recommended for severe PCP.[42] Clindamycin/primaquine has been compared with trimethoprim-sulfamethoxazole in a clinical trial and found to be a reasonable alternative therapy for mild to moderate PCP.[42] Also listed as alternative therapy for mild to moderate disease are dapsone plus trimethoprim, atovaquone, or trimetrexate with leucovorin. Adjunctive corticosteroid therapy is recommended for patients with PCP whose room air Pao$_2$ is <70 mg Hg or whose arterial-alveolar oxygen gradient is >35 mm Hg.[86] It is important that steroids are started at the time antipneumocystis therapy is initiated in an attempt to prevent the lung injury that may occur when this pathogen is killed. The dramatic decrease in the number of cases of PCP relative to the number of patients with HIV infection has been attributable to prophylaxis, which is recommended for those patients with a CD4+ cell count <200 cells/μL,

CD4+ cells <14% of total lymphocyte count, constitutional symptoms such as thrush or unexplained fever >100°F for ≥2 weeks (regardless of the CD4+ count), or a previous history of PCP. Based on several clinical investigations, it seems that discontinuing prophylaxis in patients with adequate immune recovery is a useful strategy that should be widely considered.[43,87–89]

Toxoplasma gondii

Patient populations at higher risk for toxoplasmosis include those with hematologic malignancies (particularly patients with lymphoma), bone marrow transplant, solid organ transplant (including heart, lung, liver, or kidney), or AIDS.[90] In the vast majority of immunocompromised patients, toxoplasmosis results from reactivation of latent infection, but in heart transplant patients and in a small number of other immunocompromised patients, the highest risk of developing disease is in the setting of primary infection (ie, a seronegative recipient who acquires the parasite from a seropositive donor via a graft).[91]

Although pulmonary disease due to this pathogen is associated with nonspecific radiographic findings of which bilateral pulmonary interstitial infiltrates are most common, neurologic disease is the classic pattern. In HIV-infected persons, it classically presents as fever, headache, altered mental status, and focal neurologic deficits, especially in individuals whose CD4+ count falls below 100 cells/μL. Because the disease is due to reactivation of latent infection in about 95% of cases, IgG antibody to Toxoplasma is generally present. Imaging studies of the brain show multiple (usually ≥3) nodular contrast-enhancing lesions, found most commonly in the basal ganglia and at the gray-white matter junction. Mass effect is characteristic with these lesions.[92]

In the classic setting, empiric therapy with sulfadiazine and pyrimethamine is recommended; the total duration of acute therapy should be at least 6 weeks.[42] Clindamycin-containing regimens may have a role in sulfa-allergic patients. Brain biopsy should be considered in immunocompromised patients with presumed CNS toxoplasmosis if there is a single lesion on MRI, a negative IgG antibody test result, or inadequate clinical response to an optimal treatment regimen or to what the physician considers to be an effective prophylactic regimen against T gondii.[90] Trimethoprim-sulfamethoxazole given for PCP prophylaxis serves as primary prophylaxis for toxoplasmosis, but should not be used for therapy. After acute therapy for toxoplasmic encephalitis, maintenance therapy is recommended but may be discontinued when the CD4+ cell count is >200/μL for ≥6 months.[43]

Strongyloides stercoralis

Infection with this parasite has often been described in patients with COPD who have been receiving chronic steroid therapy and who present with Gram-negative bacteremia. Among patients with defects in cell-mediated immunity, bacteremia secondary to the hyperinfection is uncommon in two groups: (1) transplant recipients who receive cyclosporine (because of the anthelminthic properties of this rejection agent); and (2) HIV-infected patients, unless the CD4+ cell count is ≤200 cells/mm^3 and the patient is concomitantly receiving corticosteroids.[91] The bacteremia occurs because of this organism's hyperinfection cycle, during which filariform larvae penetrate the intestinal mucosa, pass to the lungs by way of the bloodstream, break into alveolar spaces, and ascend to the glottis where they are swallowed into the intestinal tract to continue their process of autoinfection. Infection with this pathogen should be suspected in a patient with a defect in cell-mediated immunity who presents with clinical features that include generalized abdominal pain, diffuse pulmonary infiltrates, ileus, shock, and meningitis. Eosinophilia is often absent in steroid-treated patients.

In recent years, recommendations for therapy have changed based on the recognition that thiabendazole may not be consistently efficacious and that albendazole may be superior. Ivermectin may also be more effective than thiabendazole.

Cryptosporidium parvum

Although self-limited diarrhea associated with waterborne outbreaks has been noted in normal hosts, the clinical presentation of watery diarrhea, cramping, epigastric pain, anorexia, flatulence, and malaise in an HIV-infected patient suggests the diagnosis of cryptosporidiosis. Four clinical syndromes have been identified[93]: chronic diarrhea (in 36% of patients); cholera-like disease (33%); transient diarrhea (15%); and relapsing illness (15%). Biliary tract symptoms similar to cholecystitis have been noted in 10% of cases. Diagnosis is confirmed by finding characteristic acid-fast oocysts on examination of feces.

No predictably effective antimicrobial therapy is available, and management consists largely of symptomatic treatment of diarrhea. Effective antiretroviral therapy (to increase CD4+ count to >100 cells/μL) has been noted to result in complete, sustained clinical, microbiologic, and histologic resolution of HIV-associated cryptosporidiosis.[42]

Isospora belli

Like cryptosporidiosis, this pathogen is acid-fast and can cause a very similar diarrheal illness. In contrast to cryptosporidiosis, the pathogen is larger, oval, and cystic, and very importantly, responds to therapy with trimethoprim-sulfamethoxazole.[42]

Microsporidia

These obligate intracellular protozoa are probably transmitted to humans through the ingestion of food contaminated with its spores, which are resistant to environmental extremes. *Enterocytozoon bienuesi* produces a protracted diarrheal illness accompanied by fever and weight loss similar to that caused by Cryptosporidium; it is reported to occur in 20 to 30% of patients with chronic diarrhea not attributable to other causes. *Enterocytozoon cuniculi* has been described as an etiologic agent for hepatitis, peritonitis, and keratoconjunctivitis.

Transmission electron microscopy with observation of the polar filament is considered the gold standard for diagnosis, but the Brown-Brenn stain and the Warthin-Starry silver stain are commonly used for detecting microsporidia in tissue culture. The modified trichrome stain has been used in clinical diagnostic laboratories to detect microsporidia in fluids.[94]

Treatment guidelines have recommended the initiation and optimization of antiretroviral therapy with immune reconstitution to a CD4+ count >100 cells/μL.[42] Albendazole may be the most effective drug to treat disseminated (not ocular) and intestinal infection attributed to microsporidia other than *E bienuesi*.[42] For GI infections caused by *E bienuesi*, fumagillin has been suggested as being effective. For ocular infection, fumidil in saline eye drops and albendazole for management of systemic infection have been recommended.

Amoebae

Naegleria and Acanthamoeba are free-living amoebae that have the potential to infect humans. Of thevse, Acanthamoeba spp may infect individuals with defects in cell-mediated immunity (including patients who have AIDS or have undergone organ transplantation) and result in granulomatous amebic encephalitis. Clinical manifestations include mental status abnormalities, seizures, fever, headache, focal neurologic deficits, meningismus, visual disturbances, and ataxia. An important clinical clue may be preexisting skin lesions that have been present for months before CNS disease is clinically manifested, lesions may take the form of ulcerative, nodular, or subcutaneous abscesses. Pneumonitis may also be a part of the clinical presentation.

There are few data regarding therapy for granulomatous amebic encephalitis, but it appears that the diamidine derivatives pentamidine, propamidine, and dibromopropamidine have the greatest activity against Acanthamoeba.

Leishmania spp

In endemic areas of the world, these pathogens infect patients with defective cell-mediated immunity and cause a febrile illness with visceral involvement, most notably hepatomegaly and splenomegaly. Recently, leishmaniasis has been increasingly described in HIV-infected persons from endemic regions and may take a chronic relapsing course. Pentavalent antimonials (with sodium stibogluconate as the representative agent) may be useful for this infection. Notable is that the drug may cause dose-related QT prolongation on ECG, with arrhythmias (atrial and ventricular) and sudden death occasionally. It is contraindicated in patients with myocarditis, hepatitis, or nephritis.

Antimony resistance has been noted in some HIV-infected patients; in such situations, liposomal amphotericin B has been shown to be potentially effective because it targets infected macrophages and reaches high levels in plasma and tissues.

Of the relevant disease models influencing the understanding of the clinical significance of type 1 and type 2 immunity, leishmaniasis is important. Biopsy specimens from patients with localized infection with *Leishmania braziliensis* were consistent with a protective type 1 immune response that included prominent messenger RNA coding for IL-2 and IFN-γ.[95] As the lesions in patients became more destructive, there was a switch to a marked increase in the level of IL-4 messenger RNA, which is consistent with a failed type 2 immune response. Such data have been interpreted as an eloquent demonstration of the facts that type 1 immunity is the key to protection against Leishmania infections in humans and that a high infectious burden suppresses the human immune system from mounting type 1 responses. This has implications for therapy, which has included the use of IFN-γ as an adjunctive agent for visceral leishmaniasis.

Trypanosoma cruzi

With immunosuppression including HIV infection, reactivation of this pathogen can occur. In both posttransplantation infection and HIV-associated infection, patients may present with headache, cognitive changes, seizures, and hemiparesis.[42] In addition to the characteristic lesions seen with Chagas disease, immunosuppressed patients have an increased incidence of neurologic disease, with neuroimaging studies showing large solitary or multiple ring-enhancing lesions with surrounding edema.[42]

Miscellaneous Pathogens

Chlamydiae

This group of intracellular pathogens has been listed in some recent reviews of pathogens defended against by cell-mediated immunity. Although patients with a defect in this host defense system may be at increased risk for chlamydial infections, such problems have not been classically described.

Rickettsiae

As with chlamydiae, rickettsiae are intracellular pathogens defended against by cell-mediated immunity. Recent reviews have not described immunocompromised patients as being at increased risk for infection by pathogens in this group.

Treponema pallidum

Defense against this pathogen may include a role for macrophages and other antigen-presenting cells, such as dendritic cells, that process and present treponemal antigens to helper T cells. HIV-infected patients can have abnormal serologic test results, including unusually high, unusually low, or fluctuating titers. However, aberrant serologic responses are uncommon, and most specialists believe that both treponemal and nontreponemal serologic tests for syphilis can be interpreted in the usual manner for patients who are infected with both HIV and *T pallidum*.[95] With HIV infection, treponemal infection is more likely to have an atypical clinical presentation, be aggressive, or invade sites, such as the CNS. A reactive CSF-VDRL and a CSF WBC count ≥10 cells/mm^3 support the diagnosis of neurosyphilis.[42] Although the VDRL test on CSF is the standard serologic test for neurosyphilis, it may be nonreactive when neurosyphilis is present. The CSF fluorescent treponemal antibody absorption test is less specific for neurosyphilis than the VDRL-CSF, but the high sensitivity of the study has led some experts to believe that a negative CSF fluorescent treponemal antibody absorption test excludes neurosyphilis.[96] Such considerations are important, since HIV-1 infection might be associated with mild mononuclear CSF pleocytosis (5–15 cells/mm^3), particularly among persons with peripheral blood CD4$^+$ counts >500 cells/mm^3.[42] In addition to meningitis, a characteristic clinical presentation of syphilis in the CNS is stroke in a young person.

The recommended regimen for the treatment of patients with neurosyphilis is aqueous penicillin G (18 to 24 million U/d, administered as 3 to 4 million U IV q4h or as continuous infusion) for

10 to 14 days.[42,95] If compliance with therapy can be insured, an alternative regimen is procaine penicillin (2.4 million U IM once daily) plus probenecid (500 mg orally 4 times a day), both for 10 to 14 days. Because the duration of treatment recommended for neurosyphilis is shorter than for latent syphilis, some experts recommend administering benzathine penicillin (2.4 million IM once weekly) for up to 3 weeks on completion of the neurosyphilis regimen to provide a comparable total duration of therapy. It is recommended that all HIV-infected persons be tested for syphilis and that all persons with syphilis be tested for HIV. Spinal fluid examination has been recommended for all HIV-infected persons with latent syphilis or with neurologic abnormalities. Some experts have recommended spinal fluid examination for any HIV-1-infected person with syphilis, regardless of stage.[42]

Summary

The identification of a defect in neutrophil function, humoral immunity, or cell-mediated immunity allows the clinician to better focus on the most likely pathogens involved in an infectious process. An approach to the immunocompromised patient based on pathogenesis of disease should result in more directed, cost-effective therapy and in improved patient outcome.

References

1. Spellberg B, Edwards JE Jr. Type 1/type 2 immunity in infectious diseases. Clin Infect Dis 2001; 32:76–102
2. Karam GH, Griffin FM. An approach to diagnosing and treating infections in immunocompromised patients. In: Parrillo JE, ed. Current therapy in critical care medicine. St Louis, MO: Mosby–Year Book, 1997; 281–288
3. Hughes WT, Armstrong D, Bodey GP, et al. 2002 guidelines for the use of antimicrobial agents in neutropenic patients with cancer. Clin Infect Dis 2002; 34:730–751
4. Marron A, Carratalà J, González-Barca E, et al. Serious complications of bacteremia caused by viridans streptococci in neutropenic patients with cancer. Clin Infect Dis 2000; 31:1126–1130
5. Tunkel AR, Sepkowitz KA. Infections caused by viridans streptococci in patients with neutropenia. Clin Infect Dis 2002; 34:1524–1529
6. Razonable RR, Litzow MR, Khaliq Y, et al. Bacteremia due to viridans group streptococci with diminished susceptibility to levofloxacin among neutropenic patients receiving levofloxacin prophylaxis. Clin Infect Dis 2002; 34:1469–1474
7. Gomez L, Martino R, Rolston KV. Neutropenic enterocolitis: spectrum of the disease and comparison of definite and possible cases. Clin Infect Dis 1998; 27:695–699
8. Bodey GP, Jadeja L, Elting L. Pseudomonas bacteremia. Arch Intern Med 1985; 145:1621–1629
9. Chatzinikolaou I, Abi-Said D, Bodey GP, et al. Recent experience with *Pseudomonas aeruginosa* bacteremia in patients with cancer: retrospective analysis of 245 episodes. Arch Intern Med 2000; 160:501–509
10. Del Favero A, Menichetti F, Martino P, et al. A multicenter, double-blind, placebo-controlled trial comparing piperacillin-tazobactam with and without amikacin as empiric therapy for febrile neutropenia. Clin Infect Dis 2001; 33:1295–1301
11. Ozer H, Armitage JO, Bennett CL, et al. 2000 update of recommendations for the use of hematopoietic colony-stimulating factors: evidence-based, clinical practice guidelines. J Clin Oncol 2000; 18:3558–3585
12. American Society of Clinical Oncology. Update of recommendations for the use of hematopoietic colony-stimulating factors: evidence-based clinical practice guidelines. J Clin Oncol 1996; 14:1957–1960
13. Armstrong D. Treatment of opportunistic fungal infections. Clin Infect Dis 1993; 16:1–9
14. Thaler M, Pastakia B, Shawker TH, et al. Hepatic candidiasis in cancer patients: the evolving picture of the syndrome. Ann Intern Med 1988; 108:88–100
15. Pappas PG, Rex JH, Sobel JD, et al. Guidelines for treatment of candidiasis. Clin Infect Dis 2004; 38:161–189
16. Patterson TF, Kirkpatrick WR, White M, et al. Invasive aspergillosis: disease spectrum, treatment practices, and outcomes. Medicine (Baltimore) 2000; 79:250–260
17. Herbrecht R, Denning DW, Patterson TF, et al. Voriconazole versus amphotericin B for primary therapy of invasive aspergillosis. N Engl J Med 2002; 347:408–415

18. Johnson LB, Kauffman CA. Voriconazole: a new triazole antifungal agent. Clin Infect Dis 2003; 36:630–637
19. Walsh TJ, Finberg RW, Arndt C, et al. Liposomal amphotericin B for empirical therapy in patient with persistent fever and neutropenia. N Engl J Med 1999; 340:764–771
20. Walsh RJ, Pappas P, Winston DJ, et al. Voriconazole compared with liposomal amphotericin B for empirical antifungal therapy in patients with neutropenia and persistent fever. N Engl J Med 2002; 346:225–234
21. Walsh T, Teppler H, Donowitz G, et al. Caspofungin versus liposomal amphotericin B for empirical antifungal therapy in patients with persistent fever and neutropenia. N Engl J Med 2004; 351:1391–1402
22. de Ciutiis A, Polley MJ, Metakis LJ, et al. Immunologic defect of the alternate pathway-of-complement activation postsplenectomy: a possible relation between splenectomy and infection. J Natl Med Assoc 1978; 70:667–670
23. Barza MJ, Schooley RT. Case records of the Massachusetts General Hospital (Case 29-1986). N Engl J Med 1986; 315:241–249
24. Norris RP, Vergis EN, Yu VL. Overwhelming postsplenectomy infection: a critical review of etiologic pathogens and management. Infect Med 1996; 13:779–783
25. Parsonnet J, Baluta A, Versalovic J. Case records of the Massachusetts General Hospital (Case 17-1999). N Engl J Med 1999; 340:1819–1826
26. Sullivan KM, Kopecky KJ, Jocom J, et al. Immunomodulatory and antimicrobial efficacy of intravenous immunoglobulin in bone marrow transplantation. N Engl J Med 1990; 323:705–712
27. Centers for Disease Control and Prevention. Prevention of pneumococcal disease: recommendations of the Advisory Committee on Immunization Practices (ACIP). MMWR Recomm Rep 1997; 46(RR-8):1–24
28. Whitney CG, Farley MM, Hadler J, et al. Decline in invasive pneumococcal disease after the introduction of protein-polysaccharide conjugate vaccine. N Engl J Med 2003; 348:1737–1746
29. Centers for Disease Control and Prevention. Prevention and control of meningococcal disease: recommendations of the Advisory Committee on Immunization Practices (ACIP). MMWR Recomm Rep 2000; 49(RR-7):1–20
30. Centers for Disease Control and Prevention. Recommendations of the Advisory Committee on Immunization Practices (ACIP): use of vaccines and immune globulins for persons with altered immunocompetence. MMWR Recomm Rep 1993; 42(RR-4):1–12
31. Weinberg ED. Pregnancy-associated depression of cell-mediated immunity. Rev Infect Dis 1984; 6:814–831
32. Havlir DV, Barnes PF. Tuberculosis in patients with human immunodeficiency virus infection. N Engl J Med 1999; 340:367–373
33. Haas DW, Des Prez RM. Tuberculosis and acquired immunodeficiency syndrome: a historical perspective on recent developments. Am J Med 1994; 96:439–450
34. American Thoracic Society/Centers for Disease Control and Prevention/Infectious Diseases Society of America. Treatment of tuberculosis. Am J Respir Crit Care Med 2003; 167:603–662
35. Keane J, Gershon S, Wise RP, et al. Tuberculosis associated with infliximab, a tumor necrosis factor α-neutralizing agent. N Engl J Med 2001; 345:1098–1104
36. Update: fatal and severe liver injuries associated with rifampin and pyrazinamide for latent tuberculosis infection, and revisions in American Thoracic Society/CDC recommendations—United States, 2001. MMWR Morb Mortal Wkly Rep 2001; 50:733–735
37. Johnson JL, Ssekasanvu E, Okwera A, et al. Randomized trial of adjunctive interleukin-2 in adults with pulmonary tuberculosis. Am J Respir Crit Care Med 2003; 168:185–191
38. American Thoracic Society. Targeted tuberculin testing and treatment of latent tuberculosis infection. Am J Respir Crit Care Med 2000; 161:S221–S247
39. Selwyn PA, Hartel D, Lewis VA, et al. A prospective study of the risk of tuberculosis among intravenous drug users with human immunodeficiency virus infection. N Engl J Med 1989; 320:545–550
40. Markowitz N, Hansen NI, Hopewell PC, et al. Incidence of tuberculosis in the United States among HIV-infected persons. Ann Intern Med 1997; 126:123–132
41. Horsburgh CR. The pathophysiology of disseminated *Mycobacterium avium* complex disease in AIDS. J Infect Dis 1999; 179(suppl 3):S461–S465
42. Centers for Disease Control and Prevention, National Institutes of Health, HIV Medicine

Association/Infectious Diseases Society of America. Treating opportunistic infections among HIV-infected adults and adolescents. MMWR Recomm Rep 2004;53(RR-15):1–112

43. Guidelines for preventing opportunistic infections among HIV-infected persons—2002: recommendations of the U.S. Public Health Service and the Infectious Diseases Society of America. MMWR Recomm Rep 2002; 52(RR-8):1–52

44. Wing EJ, Gregory SH. *Listeria monocytogenes*: clinical and experimental update. J Infect Dis 2002; 185(suppl 1):S18–S24

45. Aureli P, Fiorucci GC, Caroli D, et al. An outbreak of febrile gastroenteritis associated with corn contaminated by *Listeria monocytogenes*. N Engl J Med 2000; 342:1236–1241

46. Lorber B. Listeriosis. Clin Infect Dis 1997; 24:1–11

47. Tunkel AR, Hartman BJ, Kaplan SL, et al. Practice guidelines for the management of bacterial meningitis. Clin Infect Dis 2004; 39:1267–1284

48. Walensky RP, Moore RD. A case series of 59 patients with nocardiosis. Infect Dis Clin Pract 2001; 10:249–254

49. Lerner PI. Nocardiosis. Clin Infect Dis 1996; 22:891–905

50. Verville TD, Huycke MM, Greenfield RA, et al. *Rhodococcus equi* infections of humans: 12 cases and a review of the literature. Medicine 1994; 73:119–132

51. Weinstock DM, Brown AE. *Rhodococcus equi*: an emerging pathogen. Clin Infect Dis 2002; 34:1379–1385

52. Torres A, Serra-Batlles J, Ferrer A, et al. Severe community-acquired pneumonia: epidemiology and prognostic factors. Am Rev Respir Dis 1991; 144:312–318

53. Stout JE, Yu VL. Legionellosis. N Engl J Med 1997; 337:682–687

54. Edelstein PH. Antimicrobial chemotherapy for Legionnaires' disease: a review. Clin Infect Dis 1995; 21(suppl 3):S265–S276

55. Koehler JE, Sanchez MA, Garrido CS, et al. Molecular epidemiology of bartonella infections in patients with bacillary angiomatosis-peliosis. N Engl J Med 1997; 337:1876–1883

56. Koehler JE, Sanchez MA, Tye S, et al. Prevalence of *Bartonella* infection among human immunodeficiency virus-infected patients with fever. Clin Infect Dis 2003; 37:559–566

57. van der Horst CM, Saag MS, Cloud CA, et al. Treatment of cryptococcal meningitis associated with the acquired immunodeficiency syndrome. N Engl J Med 1997; 337:15–21

58. Graybill JR, Sobel J, Saag M, et al. Diagnosis and management of increased intracranial pressure in patients with AIDS and cryptococcal meningitis. Clin Infect Dis 2000; 30:47–54

59. Saag MS, Graybill RJ, Larsen RA, et al. Practice guidelines for the management of cryptococcal disease. Clin Infect Dis 2000; 30:710–718

60. Powderly WG, Saag MS, Cloud GA, et al. A controlled trial of fluconazole or amphotericin B to prevent relapse of cryptococcal meningitis in patients with acquired immunodeficiency syndrome. N Engl J Med 1992; 326:793–798

61. Saag MS, Cloud GA, Graybill JR, et al. A comparison of itraconazole versus fluconazole as maintenance therapy for AIDS-associated cryptococcal meningitis. Clin Infect Dis 1999; 28:291–296

62. Mussini C, Pezzotti P, Miro JM, et al. Discontinuation of maintenance therapy for cryptococcal meningitis in patients with AIDS treated with highly active antiretroviral therapy: an international observational study. Clin Infect Dis 2004; 38:565–571

63. Wheat J, Sarosi G, McKinsey D, et al. Practice guidelines for the management of patients with histoplasmosis. Clin Infect Dis 2000; 30:688–695

64. Galgiani JN, Ampel NM, Catanzaro A, et al. Practice guidelines for the treatment of coccidioidomycosis. Clin Infect Dis 2000; 30:658–661

65. Pfaller MA, Diekema DJ, Jones RN, et al. International surveillance of bloodstream infections due to Candida species: frequency of occurrence and in vitro susceptibilities to fluconazole, ravuconazole, and voriconazole of isolates collected from 1997 through 1999 in the SENTRY antimicrobial surveillance program. J Clin Microbiol 2001; 39: 3254–3259

66. Rex JH, Rinaldi MG, Pfaller MA. Resistance of Candida species to fluconazole. Antimicrob Agents Chemother 1995; 39:1–8

67. Marr KA, Seidel K, White TC, et al. Candidemia in allogeneic blood and marrow transplant recipients: evolution of risk factors after adoption of prophylactic fluconazole. J Infect Dis 2000; 181:309–316

68. Stevens DA, Kan VL, Judson MA, et al. Practice guidelines for diseases caused by Aspergillus. Clin Infect Dis 2000; 30:696–709

69. Wingard JR, Kubilis P, Lee L, et al. Clinical significance of nephrotoxicity in patients treated with amphotericin B for suspected or proven aspergillosis. Clin Infect Dis 1999; 29:1402–1407

70. Farr RW, Short S, Weissman D. Fulminant hepatitis during herpes simplex virus infection in apparently immunocompetent adults: report of two cases and review of the literature. Clin Infect Dis 1997;24:1191–1194
71. Cohen JI, Brunell PA, Staus SE, et al. Recent advances in varicella-zoster virus infection. Ann Intern Med 1999; 130:922–932
72. Harger JH, Ernest JM, Thurnau GR, et al. Risk factors and outcome of varicella-zoster virus pneumonia in pregnant women. J Infect Dis 2002; 185:422–427
73. van der Bij, Speich R. Management of cytomegalovirus infection and disease after solid-organ transplantation. Clin Infect Dis 2001; 33(suppl 1): S33–S37
74. Nichols WG, Corey L, Gooley T, et al. High risk of death due to bacterial and fungal infection among cytomegalovirus (CMV)-seronegative recipients of stem cell transplants from seropositive donors: evidence for indirect effects of primary CMV infection. J Infect Dis 2002; 185:273–282
75. Dykewicz CA. Summary of the guidelines for preventing opportunistic infections among hematopoietic stem cell transplant recipients. Clin Infect Dis 2001; 33:139–144
76. Ljungman P, Griffiths P, Paya C. Definitions of cytomegalovirus infection and disease in transplant recipients. Clin Infect Dis 2002; 34:1094–1097
77. Karavellas MP, Azen SP, MacDonald JC, et al. Immune recovery vitritis and uveitis in AIDS: clinical predictors, sequelae, and treatment outcomes. Retina 2001; 21:1–9
78. Cohen JI. Epstein-Barr virus infection. N Engl J Med 2000; 343:481–492
79. Babcock GJ, Decker LL, Volk M, et al. EBV persistence in memory B cells in vivo. Immunity 1998; 9: 395–404
80. Walling DM, Flaitz CM, Nichols CM, et al. Persistent productive Epstein-Barr virus replication in normal epithelial cells *in vivo*. J Infect Dis 2001; 184:1499–1507
81. Reploeg MD, Storch GA, Clifford DB. BK virus: a clinical review. Clin Infect Dis 2001; 33:191–202
82. De Luca A, Giancola ML, Ammassari A, et al. The effect of potent antiretroviral therapy and JC virus load in cerebrospinal fluid on clinical outcome of patients with AIDS-associated progressive multifocal leukoencephalopathy. J Infect Dis 2000; 182:1077–1083

83. Angel JB, Walpita P, Lerch RA, et al. Vaccine-associated measles pneumonitis in an adult with AIDS. Ann Intern Med 1998; 129:104–106
84. Stringer JR, Beard CB, Miller RF, et al. A new name (*Pneumocystis jiroveci*) for Pneumocystis from humans. Emerg Infect Dis 2002; 8:891–896
85. Kovacs JA, Gill VJ, Meshnick S, et al. New insights into transmission, diagnosis, and drug treatment of *Pneumocystis carinii* pneumonia. JAMA 2001; 286:2450–2460
86. Bozzette SA. The use of corticosteroids in *Pneumocystis carinii* pneumonia. J Infect Dis 1990; 162:1365–1369
87. de Quiros JCLB, Miro JM, Peña JM, et al. A randomized trial of the discontinuation of primary and secondary prophylaxis against *Pneumocystis carinii* pneumonia after highly active antiretroviral therapy in patients with HIV infection. N Engl J Med 2001; 344:159–167
88. Ledergerber B, Mocroft A, Reiss R, et al. Discontinuation of secondary prophylaxis against *Pneumocystis carinii* pneumonia in patients with HIV infection who have a response to antiretroviral therapy. N Engl J Med 2001; 344:168–174
89. Trikalinos TA, Ioannidis JPA. Discontinuation of *Pneumocystis carinii* prophylaxis in patients infected with human immunodeficiency virus: a meta-analysis and decision analysis. Clin Infect Dis 2001; 33:1901–1909
90. Montoya JG. Laboratory diagnosis of *Toxoplasma gondii* infection and toxoplasmosis. J Infect Dis 2002; 185(suppl 1):S73–S82
91. Walker M, Zunt JR. Parasitic central nervous system infections in immunocompromised hosts. Clin Infect Dis 2005; 40:1005–1015
92. Walot I, Miller BL, Chang L, et al. Neuroimaging findings in patients with AIDS. Clin Infect Dis 1996; 22:906–919
93. Manabe YC, Clark DP, Moore RD, et al. Cryptosporidiosis in patients with AIDS: correlates of disease and survival. Clin Infect Dis 1998; 27:536–542
94. Didier ES. Microsporidiosis. Clin Infect Dis 1998; 27:1–8
95. Pirmez C, Yamamura M, Uyemura K, et al. Cytokine patterns in the pathogenesis of human leishmaniasis. J Clin Invest 1993; 91:1390–1395
96. Centers for Disease Control and Prevention. Sexually transmitted diseases treatment guidelines 2002. MMWR Recomm Rep 2002; 51(RR-6): 1–8

Notes

Nutritional Support in the Critically Ill Patient

Gregory M. Susla, PharmD

Objectives:

- To provide an overview of the metabolic response to critical illness
- To discuss the indications and goals for nutritional support in critically ill patients
- To discuss the various route of administration for administering nutrition support
- To discuss the monitoring of a patient receiving nutritional support
- To discuss the complications associated with nutritional support

Key words: catheter-related sepsis; enteral nutrition; immune-enhancing nutrition; injury stress response; metabolic cart; nutritional assessment; nitrogen balance; total parenteral nutrition

---

Critical illness occurs through a variety of point events such as trauma, sepsis, burn injury, respiratory failure, etc. The metabolic response that occurs following the insult includes hypermetabolism, protein catabolism, hyperglycemia, hypoalbuminemia, and fluid overload. The degree and duration of the hypermetabolic response is individual specific. There is a rapid breakdown of endogenous proteins and depletion of glucose stores after injury to meet the increased metabolic demands of the body.

The first hours after injury are known as the ebb phase of injury, in which the emphasis is on support of cardiopulmonary and other vital functions with little or no importance given to nutrition. The flow phase, or the generalized catabolic response, begins after the restoration of perfusion, and may last for several days to weeks. During this phase, the wound has priority and the body mobilizes protein stores as an additional energy source. The body begins to shift emphasis from the wound back onto the body as a whole as the injury begins to repair and heal itself. This begins the anabolic phase, in which protein stores begin to be replenished. After the wound is healed, the focus returns to rebuilding the body to its premorbid state. However, there may be intercurrent illnesses during the primary illness. The patient may experience, sepsis, acute renal failure, or multiorgan system failure after the initial insult. The metabolic impact of these morbidities may be additive on the body and can reverse the anabolic phase of the illness.

Stress Hypermetabolism

Stress hypermetabolism is a generalized response in which energy and substrates are mobilized to support inflammation, immune function, and tissue repair. Stress hypermetabolism is characterized by increased oxygen consumption, which may exceed 180 mL/min/m^2; the cardiac index may exceed 4.5 L/min/m^2 and minute ventilation may exceed 15 L/min. Carbohydrate metabolism is altered, resulting in hyperglycemia secondary to insulin resistance. Glucose oxidation is increased but decreased overall as a fraction of total calories. Increased gluconeogenesis is poorly suppressed by glucose or insulin infusions. Gluconeogenesis produces glucose that is utilized by glucose-dependent tissues such as the brain, erythrocytes, inflammatory cells, and wound tissue. There is increased Cori cycle activity with the conversion of lactate to glucose.

Fat metabolism is increased with oxidation of all chain lengths. Plasma linoleic acid and arachidonic acids are decreased while oleic acid levels increase. Triglyceride clearance decreases with progression of multiorgan failure. There is usually an absence of ketonemia. Hyperinsulinemia in response to elevated blood glucose concentrations results in suppression of lipid mobilization from body stores, and in the absence of an exogenous source of essential fatty acids, clinical essential fatty acid deficiency may develop in as little as 10 days.

Increased protein catabolism occurs to provide energy and to support protein synthesis. With inadequate caloric intake, energy sources are derived from excessive protein breakdown and gluconeogenesis. Whole-body protein synthesis and protein catabolism is increased with an overall net increase in protein catabolism, resulting in a rapid decrease in lean body mass and an increase in ureagenesis and urinary nitrogen losses. In skeletal muscle, release is increased and amino acid uptake decreases. Amino acids are also mobilized from connective tissue and unstimulated gut. Amino acids undergo extrahepatic oxidation and are redistributed to viscera, wounds, and WBCs; they are used as a gluconeogenic substrate and for hepatic synthesis of acute-phase reactant proteins. Stress hypermetabolism is also characterized by the increased extra hepatic utilization of branched chain amino acids as an oxidative fuel source. Overall, weight loss usually exceeds that from bed rest or starvation. Intracellular electrolytes such as potassium, magnesium, and phosphate are depleted and there are increased urinary losses of copper and zinc. The respiratory quotient (RQ) during stress hypermetabolism typically ranges between 0.8 and 0.85. The consequences of long-term hypermetabolism include immune system deficiency, diaphragm atrophy, cardiac cachexia, renal dysfunction, multiple organ failure and death.

Hormonal Effects

The hormonal response to stress includes increased growth hormone production for energy and protein conservation, cachectin for energy utilization, and glucagon for gluconeogenesis stimulation and protein catabolism. Increased cortisol levels stimulate stress protein catabolism, ureagenesis, hepatic gluconeogenesis and fluid retention. Increased antidiuretic hormone secretion results in fluid retention. Catecholamine release stimulates the sympathetic nervous system, resulting in increases in heart rate and respiration, glycogenolysis, gluconeogenesis, lipolysis, and aldosterone secretion, producing alterations in electrolyte and water balance. Insulin stimulates glucose uptake and metabolism, protein synthesis, and lipogenesis.

Paracrine System

Tumor necrosis factor increases stress protein catabolism, increases energy expenditure, and inhibits lipoprotein lipase. Interleukin-1 stimulates adrenocorticotropic hormone, increases the release of cortisol and glucagon, and stimulates gluconeogenesis and protein catabolism. Interleukin-2 activates lipolysis and decreases α-adrenergic inhibition of hormone-sensitive lipase. Platelet activating factor also stimulates gluconeogenesis.

The typical metabolic response to injury based on level of stress is outlined in Table 1.

Table 1. *Metabolic Response to Injury*

Level of Stress	Insult	UUN,* g/d	Glucose, mg/dL
Mild	Elective surgery	5–10	150 ± 25
Moderate	Trauma	10–15	150 ± 25
Severe	Sepsis	>15	250 ± 25

*1 g nitrogen = 6.25 g protein = 1 oz muscle.

Goals of Nutritional Support

The goals of nutritional therapy are to provide support consistent with the patient's needs, nutritional state, and available routes of administration in order to limit protein catabolism, prevent or treat macro- and micronutrient deficiencies, provide nutrients consistent with existing metabolism, and avoid complications. Providing metabolic support during critical illness is different from providing nutrition in the setting of malnutrition. These differences are outlined in Table 2.

Indications for Nutritional Support

Any critically ill patient unable to eat normally should receive nutritional support to avoid the development of severe protein/calorie depletion and other nutritional deficiencies. Patients in whom malnutrition is likely to occur include hypermetabolic patients and all patients in whom a prolonged course of critical illness is anticipated. Routine surgical patients expected to eat within 5 to 7 days will probably not benefit from nutritional support. There is no data to support the idea that early nutritional support significantly alters outcome for acutely ill patients, but therapy should be started as soon as the need is recognized (usually within the first week of illness). Indicators of adverse outcomes include weight loss >10% of usual body weight within the

Table 2. *Nutrition vs Metabolic Support*

Setting	Nutritional Support	Metabolic Support
Basis	Starvation	Metabolic stress
REE	Decreased	Increased
RQ	Low (0.65)	High (0.85)
Focus	Emphasis on visceral proteins and lean body mass	Preservation of organ structure and function; no substrate limitation; support metabolism
Fuel	Glucose or ketones	Mixed
Nonprotein cal/g nitrogen	≥150:1	≤100:1
Protein, g/kg/d	1–1.5	1.5–2.0
Nonprotein calories as fat, %	0–80	25–30
Mediator activation	–	+++
Regulatory responsiveness	++++	+
Proteolysis	+	+++
Branch chain oxidation	+	+++
Hepatic protein synthesis	+	+++
Ureagenesis	+	+++
Urinary nitrogen loss	+	+++
Gluconeogenesis	+	+++
Ketone body formation	+++	+

preceding 3 to 4 weeks, serum albumin <2.8 g/dL, serum transferrin <170 mg/dL, skin test anergy, and starvation for >5 days. Current nutrition support can prevent specific nutritional deficiencies, minimize starvation effects, and modulate to some extent the metabolic process of disease, but it cannot abolish the ongoing protein catabolism and wasting of lean body mass associated with stress hypermetabolism. Early nutritional intervention is imperative: "One day of delay equals 3 to 5 days of catch-up."

Patient Evaluation

A general patient assessment must be completed before any form of nutritional support is begun. This assessment includes a review of the patient's medical, dietary, and medication history and a physical examination. Weight is an unreliable assessment parameter in the ICU setting because of the rapid and frequent fluid shifts and often the lack of knowledge of the premorbid weight. The measured weight may not reflect the real body cell mass. Anthropometric measurements have not been standardized for critically ill patients and their measure may not be accurate in the edematous patient. The creatinine-height index has not been validated in critically patients, and skin testing may be difficult to perform in critically ill patients, especially if they are being treated with steroids or other immunosuppressive therapies.

Table 3. *Visceral Protein Indices*

Protein	Nutritional Status
Albumin, g/dL	Normal: >3.5
	Mild depletion: 2.8–3.5
	Moderate, 2.2–2.8
	Severe, <2.2
Transferrin, mg/dL	Mild depletion, 150–200
	Moderate, 100–150
	Severe, <100
Prealbumin, mg/dL	Normal, >18
	Mild depletion, 10–18
	Moderate, 5–10
	Severe, <5

Hepatic secretory function can be assessed by measuring albumin and prealbumin. Albumin is not a good assessment tool because it will drop by 30 to 50% within the first 24 h of critical illness as a result of decreased hepatic synthesis, loss to the extravascular space because of capillary leak, and dilution from fluid resuscitation. Also, albumin's long half-life makes it better suited for monitoring nutritional status over the long term in the outpatient setting. The correlation between baseline levels of albumin, prealbumin, and transferrin and the level of malnutrition is presented in Table 3.

Assessing Energy Expenditure

One of the goals in providing nutritional support to critically ill patients is providing nutrients

Table 4. Factors Affecting REE

Increase REE	Decrease REE
Critical illness	Starvation
Excessive glucose infusion	Sleep
Increasing size	Female sex
Male sex	Increasing age
Fever	Hypoventilation
Hyperventilation	Flow phase of injury
Impending respiratory failure	Mechanical ventilation
Ebb phase of injury	Narcotics
Activity, movement, nursing care	Sedatives
Pain	Paralytics
Catecholamines	ß-Blockers
Steroids	

Table 5. General Caloric Recommendations

Stress Level	Caloric Recommendation, kcal/kg/d
Low	20
Moderate	25–30
High	35

Table 6. Harris-Benedict Equations With Modifying Factors

Male: REE = 66.47 + [13.75 (weight, kg)] + [5 (height, cm)] − [6.76 (age, yr)]
Female: REE = 655.2 + [9.56 (weight, kg)] + [1.7 (height, cm)] − [4.77 (age, yr)]

Activity Factor	Stress Factor
Confined to bed: 1.2	Surgery: 1.1–1.2
Ambulatory: 1.3	Infection: 1.2–1.6
Fever: 1.13 per degree above 37°C	Trauma: 1.1–1.8
	Sepsis: 1.4–1.8

consistent with their degree of metabolism. Thus, it is important to measure or estimate the caloric needs of the patient. The basal metabolic rate (BMR) is the amount of energy expended under basal conditions while at complete rest, shortly after awakening, and after a 12-h fast. BMR varies with age, sex, and body size and typically ranges from 1,000 to 2,000 calories/d. BMR is measured in healthy, ambulatory patients. Resting energy expenditure (REE) is usually measured in critically ill patients. REE is defined as the energy expenditure measured 2 h after a meal, in the postabsorptive state, under rest and thermal neutrality; REE is approximately 10% higher than BMR. REE accounts for 75 to 90% of total energy expenditure, the remainder of which is accounted for by thermogenesis resulting from nutrition intake, environmental factors, and physical activity. The kidney, brain, and liver account for approximately 70% of REE, with the brain accounting for 20% of total body oxygen consumption. The work of breathing accounts for about 3% of REE, but this figure increases to about 26% with impending respiratory failure. The REE can range from 10% below to 23% above the steady-state REE throughout a 24-h period in the ICU. The numerous factors that can affect REE are listed in Table 4.

General Recommendations: There are numerous methods for calculating or estimating energy expenditure in critically ill patients. General recommendations can be used based on the presumed level of stress. These recommendations are listed in Table 5.

Disease-Specific Recommendations: Disease-specific recommendations are available for most critical illnesses. These recommendations may have been prospectively or retrospectively determined, but are often determined in nonhomogeneous patient populations during an unknown point of illness. These equations offer no advantage over general recommendations and usually result in unnecessary complex calculations for determining energy expenditure.

Harris-Benedict Equation: The Harris-Benedict Equation is an equation commonly used to estimate energy expenditure in critically ill patients. The equation itself tends to under-predict energy expenditure in critically ill patients, so the results of the equation are usually adjusted based on the activity and stress factors of the patient. The Harris-Benedict equation with the activity and stress factors is given in Table 6. Energy expenditure will be predicted accurately in only about 33% of critically ill patients when the Harris-Benedict equation is used with its associated activity and stress factors. In general, multiplying the REE calculated by the Harris-Benedict equation by 1.2 gives a pretty good estimate of the caloric needs of a typical critically ill patient.

American College of Chest Physicians Consensus Guidelines: The American College of Chest Physicians (ACCP) Consensus Panel on Nutrition Support published its recommendations in the 1990s (Table 7). The goals of consensus process were as follows: (1) define the clinical ICU settings

Table 7. *ACCP Recommendations*

Substrate	Dose	Comment
Total calories	25 kcal/kg/d	Based on usual body weight
Glucose	30–70% of total calories	Maintain glucose <225 mg/dL
Fat	15–30% of total calories	Maintain triglyceride <500 mg/dL
Protein	1.2–1.5 g/kg	Maintain BUN <100 mg/dL

Table 8. *Respiratory Quotients*

RQ	Fuel Source	Condition
0.8–0.95	Mixed	Ideal
0.6–0.7	Fat	Starvation
1.0	Carbohydrate	Excess carbohydrate
>1.0	Fat synthesis	Overfeeding

where nutritional therapy benefits patient outcomes; (2) define the goals of nutrition therapy; and (3) identify the nutrition needs of ICU patients. These recommendations provide an acceptable approach for developing a nutritional regimen for a critically ill patient.

Hemodynamic Equation: A hemodynamic equation may be used to determine REE. The equation is based on the Fick equation and requires that a pulmonary catheter be in place in order to determine the cardiac output (CO), and arterial oxygen saturation (Sao_2), and venous oxygen saturation (Svo_2):

$$REE = 95.18 \times hemoglobin \times CO \times (Sao_2 - Svo_2)$$

The equation provides a reliable estimate of energy expenditure that can be measured in real time. The results of the equation are stable as long as the patient is stable. Use of the equation allows one to determine the patient's energy expenditure as the his condition changes and adjust the nutrition prescription accordingly.

Indirect Calorimetry: Indirect calorimetry determines REE and RQ by measuring oxygen consumption ($\dot{V}o_2$), carbon dioxide production ($\dot{V}co_2$), and minute ventilation by expired gas analysis. The metabolic rate or REE is calculated using the Weir equation:

$$REE = (3.9 \times \dot{V}o_2) + (1.1 \times \dot{V}co_2) - 2.8 \times UUN$$

where UUN is urinary urea nitrogen. When values for REE measured on one day are compared to values measured on subsequent days, an average daily variability of 15% occurs. RQ is calculated by the equation $RQ = \dot{V}co_2/\dot{V}o_2$. The RQ reflects the percent of substrate utilization of fat and carbohydrate by the body, which may or may not coincide with the percentage of substrates being administered by enteral or parenteral nutrition. The RQ values for the fuel sources used in providing nutritional support are listed in Table 8.

Fuel Sources

Glucose

The primary fuel sources for feeding critically ill patients are glucose, fat, and protein. A minimum of 100 g/d of glucose is needed to provide an optimal energy substrate for certain parts of the body such as the brain, blood elements, and wound sites and to obtain a maximal protein-sparing effect. Amounts greater than 500 to 600 g/d are not recommended because the normal rate of glucose oxidation is 0.4 to 1.2 mg/kg/min and can only increase to 2 to 4 mg/kg/min with glucose infusion, up to a maximum of 5 to 7 mg/kg/min with severe physiologic stress. Exogenous insulin will not increase glucose oxidation beyond this point, although it still may stimulate protein synthesis. Stress gluconeogenesis and protein catabolism are poorly suppressed by glucose administration. Glucose is used to provide up to 60 to 70% of calories or approximately 20 kcal/kg/d. Glucose provides 3.4 kcal/g. The RQ associated with glucose metabolism is 1.0. Excessive glucose infusion administration leads to hyperglycemia, excessive CO_2 production, hyperinsulinemia, suppressed lipolysis, and hepatic steatosis. The ACCP consensus guidelines on nutrition support in critically ill patients recommends maintaining the blood glucose at <225 mg/dL. However, given the current trend for intensive insulin therapy and tight glucose control, it is probably wise to keep the glucose <150 mg/dL.

Table 9. *Protein Doses*

Condition	Dose
Normal health	Mixed
Critical illness	1.5–2 g/kg/d
Acute renal failure	0.5 g/kg/d
Intermittent dialysis	1 g/kg/d
Continuous renal replacement therapy	1.5 g/kg/d
Hepatic failure	0.5 g/kg/d

*Maintain BUN <100 mg/dL.

Fat

Seriously ill patients have a decreased ability to utilize carbohydrates and it has been suggested that fat may be a preferable energy source in critically ill patients. Fat administration prevents essential fatty acid deficiency that can develop in an unfed critically ill patient or patients fed a glucose- and protein-only nutrition prescription. The amount of fat needed to avoid essential fatty acid deficiency is unknown, but as little as 3 g/d may be sufficient to avoid this complication. Fat administration provides up to 25 to 30% of calories during critical illness. Fat provides 9 kcal/g and the maximum administration rate is 1 g/kg/d, keeping the triglyceride level less than 500 mg/dL. The RQ associated with fat administration is approximately 0.7. Excess fat administration results in hyperlipidemia, impaired immune function, and hypoxemia. Several clinical situations in which the fat dose may need be increased are listed in Table 9.

Protein

Daily protein turnover is 200 to 300 g, with a nitrogen requirement of 0.4 g/kg/d in stable adults. There is a much greater loss of nitrogen in patients with severe illness, with protein requirements increasing up to 1.5 to 2 g/kg/d. The kcal-to-nitrogen ratio is decreased from 150:1 to 100:1 in critically ill patients compared with starved patients. Protein provides 4 kcal/g and has an RQ of 0.8. Protein is administered to support stress protein synthesis (such as hepatic synthesis of acute-phase reactant proteins), immune function, and the repair process. The recommended dose of protein is 1.5 to 2 g/kg/d, but needs to be adjusted for the presence of renal failure, hepatic failure, and intermittent or continuous renal replacement therapy. The goal is to maintain the BUN at <100 mg/dL. The dose adjustments for renal dysfunction are given in Table 10.

Table 10. *Indications for Increased Fat Administration*

Need to minimize CO_2 production to facilitate weaning from mechanical ventilation

Need to increase parenteral calories while giving minimal additional volume

Need to decrease glucose load because of severe hyperglycemia (diabetic patients, patients receiving steroids)

Electrolytes

The process of refeeding is associated with major changes in electrolyte balance. During malnutrition there is a loss of potassium, magnesium, and phosphorus, and a gain in sodium and water. It is necessary to supply additional electrolytes, especially potassium, magnesium, calcium, and phosphorus, during the initial states of feeding.

Micronutrients

Vitamins and trace elements are essential for the utilization of protein, carbohydrates, and fat. Vitamins are enzyme cofactors in many metabolic pathways and are important in normal food substrate utilization and host defenses. Multivitamins are usually given on a daily basis in doses based on the current recommended daily allowance.

Trace elements are added to parenteral nutrition solutions to maintain good nutritional status. There are seven essential trace elements in humans: iron, zinc, copper, chromium, selenium, and iodine.

Caution should be used when hospitals only supply standardized parenteral nutrition support solutions. These solutions are usually designed to replenish the typical malnourished patients and may not meet the needs of a critically ill hypermetabolic patient. The nutrition recommendations for critically ill patients are summarized in Table 11.

Route of Administration

The decision to feed the patient enterally vs parenterally depends on several factors. Enteral

Table 11. *Nutritional Support in the Hypermetabolic Patient**

Nutrient	Recommendation
Total calories	25–30 kcal/kg/d
	BEE × 1.2
Glucose	20 kcal/kg/d
	5 g/kg/d
	60–70% of calories
Fat	10 kcal/kg/d
	1 g/kg/d
	15–40% of calories
Protein	1.2–2.0 g/kg/d
	10–15% of calories
Trace elements/vitamins	Recommended daily allowance
Electrolytes	Maintain normal levels

*BEE = Basal energy expenditure.

nutrition is the preferred route of administration and enteral solutions may be infused into the stomach or small bowel. The gut is the major interface between the host and the environment. Undernutrition impairs the adaptation and barrier function. Enteral feeding may prevent small bowel villous atrophy, prevent mucosal thinning, and decrease intestinal permeability. Whether this reduces the risk of the gut as a driver for bacterial translocation and multisystem organ failure remains to be determined in humans. Enteral nutrition is less expensive and associated with fewer metabolic and infectious complications than parenteral nutrition. Figure 1 shows the decision-making algorithm for deciding on the route of administration for feeding a patient.

Enteral Nutrition

Enteral nutrition may be accomplished unless an absolute contraindication exists such as a perforated viscus, obstruction, vomiting, or impending abdominal surgery is present or suspected. Relative contraindications to enteral feeding include enterocutaneous fistula, severe diarrhea, inflammatory bowel disease, or other conditions requiring temporary bowel rest. Small bowel feedings are efficacious in the presence of mild or resolving pancreatitis and low-output enterocutaneous fistula (<500 mL/d). The presence of bowel sounds and the passage of flatus or stool are not necessary for the initiation of enteral feeding. Small bowel feeding may be accomplished even in the absence of bowel sounds, gastric atony, and colonic ileus.

Feeding into the stomach may be the preferred route because of the ease of tube placement, the fact that it is more physiologic, and the possible protection against stress-ulcer formation. Feeding into the small bowel is often associated with difficulty in tube placement and easier tube displacement. Continuous infusion is the preferred delivery method regardless of the site of feeding tube placement. There is no difference in aspiration rates for gastric vs small bowel feeding. Isotonic feeding solutions can be started at 10 to 20 mL/h and titrated up to the goal rate as the patient tolerates the infusion. The issue of residual volume is somewhat controversial when delivering feeding solutions into the stomach. Most patients can tolerate residual volume up to 150 to 200 mL/h. It important to consider the volume of gastric juices and the infusion rate of the enteral solution when determining the maximum allowable residual volume for a patient.

Several dietary characteristics should be considered when selecting the most appropriate nutrition solution: (1) nutrient completeness with reasonable fluid limitation; (2) digestibility and absorbability; (3) residue content; (4) lactose content; (5) osmolarity; (6) viscosity; (7) stability; (8) preparation requirements; (9) versatility; and (10) cost.

There are several classifications of enteral feeding available: polymeric, oligomeric, and modular. Polymeric formulas contain 100% of the recommended daily allowance for vitamins and minerals when a total daily prescription of approximately 2 L is administered. These formulas are semi-isotonic or hypertonic, have a relatively high carbohydrate-to-fat ratio, are low in residue, and are sodium and lactose free. The nitrogen source is natural protein (egg, soy, or lactalbumin) that may be intact or partially hydrolyzed. These formulas require the ability to digest protein, carbohydrate, and fat. A polymeric formula should be the initial choice for nutritional supplementation when the GI tract and absorption are intact.

Oligomeric formulas are composed of elemental or nearly elemental nutrients that require minimal digestion and are usually hyperosmolar. They are almost completely absorbed and leave little residue in the colon. Oligomeric diets contain either crystalline amino acids or oligopeptides and amino acids. The carbohydrate sources are

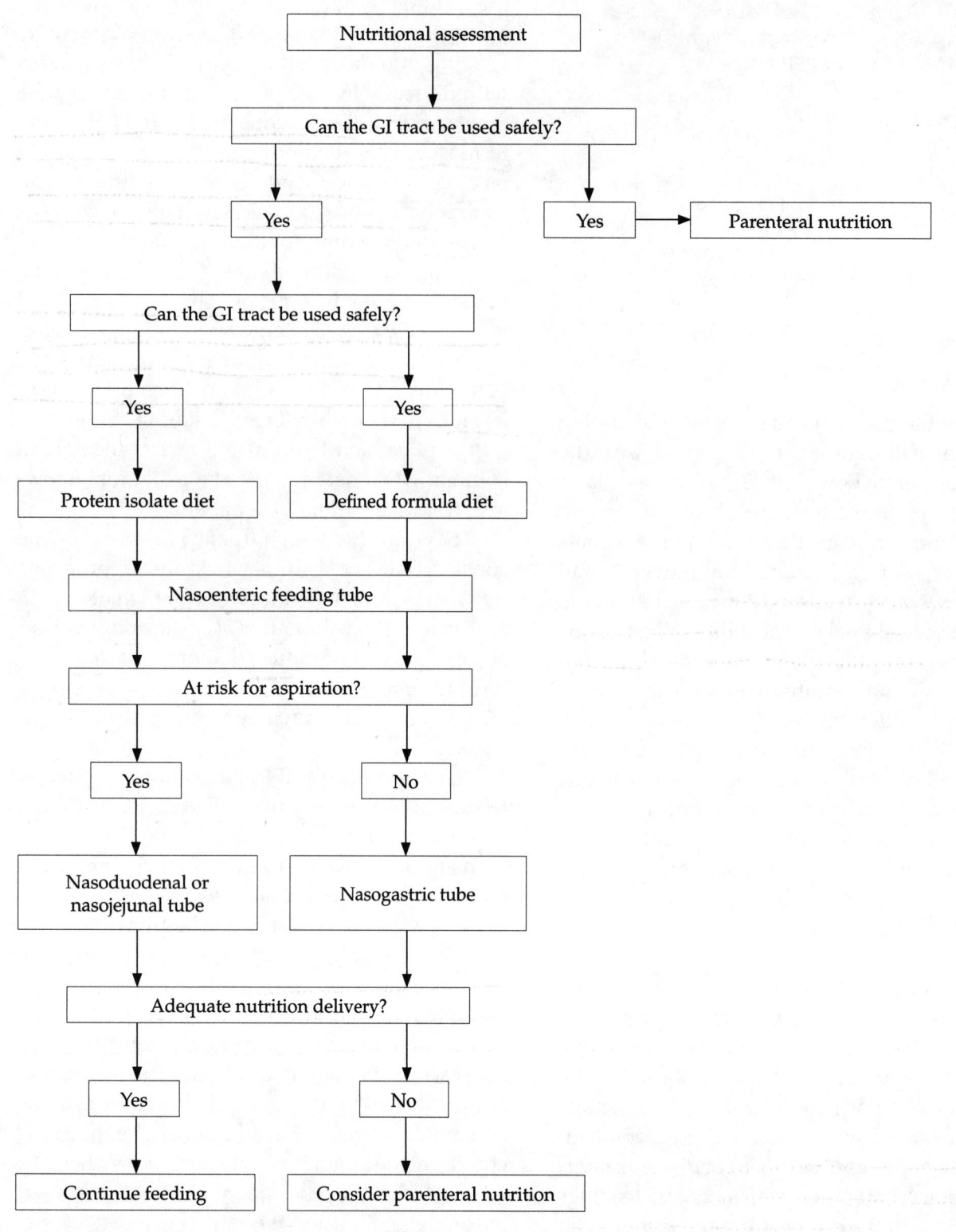

Figure 1.

oligosaccharides and disaccharides with variable amounts of fat. They contain all essential vitamins and minerals. These formulas require digestion of carbohydrates and fat, so pancreatic activity is required. Diarrhea may occur if these formulas are administered too fast because they are hyperosmolar. These formulas may be useful during periods of digestive or absorptive insufficiency, such as during the transition stage of gut recovery following peritonitis, prolonged ileus, or major surgery.

Modular diets consist of single or multiple nutrients that can be combined to produce a nutritionally complete diet for patients with unusual requirements that cannot be met with standard formulas. Dietary modules can be used to prepare custom-made feedings or to supplement fixed-ratio formulas. Single-entity modular products are available for protein, carbohydrate, and fat fuel sources.

There are specialized formulas for hepatic encephalopathy, renal failure, and respiratory failure. The benefit of these formulas over standard formulas remains controversial. The careful use of the standard formulas with appropriate monitoring may achieve the same nutritional end point while avoiding complications.

Parenteral Nutrition

The indications for parenteral nutrition are few. Parenteral nutrition should be considered when oral/enteral intake is not possible, is insufficient, or is contraindicated. Parenteral nutrition is indicated in the setting of a nonfunctioning GI tract, when bowel rest is required, in cases of intractable vomiting or diarrhea, in cases of severe malnutrition where the patient is unable to maintain adequate oral intake, and when patients are intolerant of enteral feeding. Parenteral nutrition is contraindicated when treatment is expected to last <5 days, the patient has a functioning GI tract, and the prognosis does not warrant aggressive nutritional support. Parenteral nutrition increases the risk of infectious and metabolic complications, depletes the liver of antioxidants, and promotes cholestasis.

Parenteral nutrition solution is composed of dextrose and amino acids mixed with lipids, or with lipids administered separately. Vitamins and trace elements are added to the dextrose/amino acid solution. Parenteral nutrition solutions are hyperosmolar and must be infused through a central vein. Parenteral nutrition solutions contain essential and nonessential amino acids. Special solutions for renal and hepatic failure are available and are similar in composition to enteral formulas. Again, the benefits of these solutions over traditional protein solutions remain controversial.

Specialized Formulations and Additives

A number of trials have evaluated the benefits of immune-enhancing formulas. However, not all trials have included critically ill patients, and the critically ill patient populations varied, including patients with trauma, those with burns, mixed-ICU patients, and septic ICU patients. Although some trials showed improved outcomes, several trials suffered from small sample sizes and the use of noncommercial control diets. Three meta-analyses concluded that there were improved patient outcomes with these diets. It is difficult to recommend the routine use of the specialized formulas until larger controlled studies using readily available commercial formulas are conducted.

Arginine

Arginine is a nonessential amino acid that has purported immune-enhancing and wound-healing properties, which may result from its role as a stimulant of growth hormone, glucagon, prolactin, and insulin release. Arginine is a precursor of nitric oxide, which is produced by a number of cells including vascular endothelial cells, macrophages, neutrophils, and neurons. The benefits of arginine-supplemented diets remain controversial. Whether arginine supplementation will result in improved outcomes in unknown.

Glutamine

Glutamine is a nonessential amino acid and the most abundant amino acid in the body. Glutamine is synthesized primarily in skeletal muscle and lungs and plays a role in maintaining acid-base balance in the kidney. It is a primary fuel source for enterocytes and colonocytes, a fuel source for lymphocytes and macrophages, and a precursor for nucleotide synthesis. Glutamine uptake by the small intestine and by immunologically active cells may exceed glutamine synthesis and release from skeletal muscle during catabolic illness, making glutamine essential during these conditions. Supplemental glutamine may increase protein synthesis to decrease protein breakdown and to improve nitrogen balance. Glutamine also has been shown to enhance intestinal adaptation after

Table 12. *Monitoring Nutritional Support*

Parameter	Frequency	Goal
Glucose	q6h initially, then daily	<150 mg/dL
Electrolytes	Daily and prn	Normal levels
Magnesium, phosphorus	Daily	Normal levels
Visceral protein	Twice weekly, then weekly	Normal levels
Triglyceride	Initially, then weekly	≤500 mg/dL
Liver function	Initially, then weekly	Normal levels
Prothrombin time	Initially, then weekly	Normal levels
Nitrogen balance	Initially, then weekly and prn	2–4 g positive
Indirect calorimetry	Initially, then weekly and prn	RQ, 0.8–0.9
Weight	Daily	Stable weight in the setting of static fluid balance
Fluid balance	Daily	Euvolemia

bowel resection, to attenuate intestinal and pancreatic atrophy associated with parenteral and elemental feeding. In critically ill patients, glutamine supplementation may enhance D-xylose absorption, reflecting increased small bowel absorptive capacity; in stable patients, it may attenuate villous atrophy and increased intestinal permeability associated with parenteral nutrition.

Monitoring

Baseline and follow-up monitoring parameters for patients receiving nutritional support are listed in Table 12.

Additional monitoring parameters specific to parenterally fed patients include checking the catheter insertion site to monitor for the development of a local site infection. Monitoring of enteral nutrition includes obtaining a chest radiograph before enteral nutrition solution is started to ensure that the feeding tube is placed properly in the stomach or small bowel. Gastric residual volumes should be measured on an hourly basis in patients receiving enteral nutrition in the stomach. In general, gastric residual volumes >200 mL may require modification of the infusion rate or the use of small bowel feedings. All enterally fed patients should be monitored for the development of diarrhea.

One of the difficulties associated with the use of enteral nutrition is ensuring that patients receive their total daily caloric requirement. A patient's actual caloric intake should be determined on a daily basis. Only 65% of patients are given an infusion rate sufficient to achieve their daily caloric goal, only 78% of ordered enteral solution may be delivered, and only 20 to 40% of patients may ever reach goal infusion rates. Additionally, up to 67% of patients may experience avoidable cessations in their enteral nutrition solution infusions.

One of the goals of nutrition support is to deliver enough nutrition to meet the metabolic demands of the patient. All patients must have the efficacy of the nutrition regimens assessed at least weekly. This typically includes the measurement of visceral protein levels and nitrogen balance. The most commonly monitored markers of visceral protein stores are albumin, transferrin, prealbumin, and retinal binding protein. The half-lives vary among the four parameters: albumin, 21 days; transferrin, 9 days; prealbumin, 2 days; and retinal binding protein, 12 h. The half-lives and time to steady state are too long for albumin and transferrin to make them clinically useful in monitoring therapy in a critically ill patient. The half-life of retinol binding protein is too short, often resulting is extreme variability between measurements. Prealbumin's half-life provides fairly good flexibility to assess the adequacy of a patient's nutrition regimen once to twice weekly. Prealbumin and nitrogen balance should stabilize once the patient's condition stabilizes and his caloric needs are being met. Prealbumin will increase and nitrogen balance will become less negative and eventually positive as the patient begins to heal. Declining prealbumin and worsening nitrogen balance indicates that the patient's caloric needs are not being met and the patient is continuing to break down endogenous protein stores as an energy source. Changes in a patient's illness that usually result in worsening nutritional indices include the onset of an intercurrent illness such as new-onset sepsis, renal failure, or respiratory failure. Other interventions that lead to an increase in energy expenditure and a reduction in nutritional

Table 13. *Nitrogen Balance Calculation*

Nitrogen in = Protein in (g)/6.25*
Nitrogen out = UUN (mg/dL) × urine volume (dL) × 1.2†
Nitrogen balance = Nitrogen in − Nitrogen out

*6.25 g protein contains 1 g nitrogen.
†Multiply UUN × 1.2 to account for nonmeasured, non-urea nitrogen in urine.

---

indices if the nutritional regimen is not adjusted accordingly include discontinuing narcotics, sedatives, or paralytic agents, as well as weaning from mechanical ventilation. The formula for calculating nitrogen balance is presented in Table 13. The nutritional-support regimen should be reassessed when there is a change in the patient's severity of illness, work of breathing, or drug therapy, and when the nutrition indices worsen.

Complications

Parenteral Nutrition

The complications associated with parenteral nutrition include metabolic, infectious, and mechanical problems. Metabolic complications include alterations in water and electrolyte balance. Excessive nutrient intake can result in hyperglycemia, excessive CO_2 production with an RQ >1, ventilator dependence, and fatty liver. Glucose given in excess of the caloric needs of the patient is stored as fat. This process of lipogenesis can result in RQ values as high as 8.0, causing increases in CO_2 production and resulting in increases in minute ventilation to maintain the $Paco_2$ within a stable clinically acceptable range. Central venous catheter complications have been reported in up to 15% of patients and include catheter misdirection, artery puncture, pneumothorax, hydrothorax, air embolism, cardiac injury with tamponade, arrhythmia, and stroke.

Hepatic steatosis, or fatty infiltration of the liver, can occur within the first 3 weeks of nutritional support with a dextrose-only-based parenteral nutrition regimen. This usually manifests as increases in transaminases. The etiology is excessive glucose administration, essential fatty acid deficiency, hyperinsulinemia, and carnitine deficiency. However, this condition is reversible after total parenteral nutrition is stopped. Intra- and extrahepatic cholestasis usually occurs after >3 weeks of parenteral therapy and results from periportal or pericentral canalicular bile plugging, bile staining, and lymphocytic triaditis. Elevated canalicular enzymes and bilirubin are the usual signs of cholestasis. Gallbladder sludge can develop after 4 to 6 weeks of parenteral therapy. Hepatobiliary complications usually result from stasis from a lack of enteral nutrition, taurine deficiency, and toxic bile production (lithocholate) by intestinal bacteria. The diagnosis is usually clinical and typically responds to changes in formula or route of nutritional therapy. Avoiding excess glucose administration or using enteral nutrition can prevent hepatobiliary complications. Progression to chronic liver disease rarely occurs in adults.

Enteral Nutrition

Although considered safer than parenteral nutrition, enteral nutrition can be associated with a number of mechanical, GI, or metabolic complications. Mechanical complications include knotting or clogging of the feeding tube and improper tube placement. Improper tube placement can be prevented by endoscopic visualization or fluoroscopic guidance. Tube placement should always be confirmed before starting tube-feeding infusions. Flushing may relieve clogged tubes; if not, the tube must be replaced. Other mechanical problems include epistaxis, nasopharyngeal erosions, sinusitis, otitis, gagging, esophageal reflux, esophagitis, tracheoesophageal fistulas, and ruptured esophageal varices. Nasoenteral tubes are not recommended for patients with known or suspected cribriform plate fracture because of the risk of inadvertent tube placement into the cranial vault.

GI complications include nausea and vomiting, diarrhea resulting from fast infusion rates, lactose intolerance, fat intolerance, hyperosmolarity, and delayed gastric emptying. Nausea and vomiting can occur in up to 20% of enterally fed patients. Careful formula selection and management can avoid most of these complications. Diarrhea is the most common GI complication to manage in enterally fed patients and develops in 10 to 25% of tube-fed patients. Common causes of diarrhea are multifactorial and include infectious, dietary, and drug-induced factors. In general, diarrhea is secretory and not an indication to stop enteral feeding. Many enteral solutions are hypertonic and can lead to osmotic diarrhea. The volume and rate of infusion can be common cause of diarrhea. Increasing abdominal distention necessitates stopping the feedings and conducting a medical evaluation. Many patients receiving enteral nutrition may be receiving liquid medications containing sorbitol through their feeding tube, which can cause osmotic-induced diarrhea. An evaluation is required if the volume of diarrhea exceeds 1,000 mL/d. Antidiarrheal agents may be used if a relevant medical or surgical cause is not found, including *Clostridium difficile* enterocolitis.

There are fewer metabolic complications with enteral nutrition than with parenteral nutrition. These complications include nutrient intolerance and fluid and electrolyte imbalance. Patients with preexisting glucose intolerance, such as diabetics or patients taking steroids, may experience hyperglycemia.

Aspiration may occur in up to 40% of patients who are fed enterally. Although gross aspiration can occur, proper patient positioning and frequent monitoring of gastric residual volumes can prevent much of this aspiration.

Selected Readings

Alexander E, Susla GM, Burstein A, et al. Retrospective evaluation of commonly used equations to predict energy expenditure in mechanically ventilated critically ill patients. Pharmacotherapy 2004; 24:1659–1967

American Society of Parenteral and Enteral Nutrition. Guidelines for the use of parenteral and enteral nutrition in adult and pediatric patients. JPEN J Parenter Enteral Nutr 2002; 17(suppl):1S–138S

Barton R. Nutrition support in critical illness. Nutr Clin Practice 1994; 9:127–139

Beale RJ, Bryg DJ, Bihari DJ. Immunonutrition in the critically ill: a systematic review of clinical outcomes. Crit Care Med 1999; 27:2799–2805

Cerra F, Hirsch J, Mullen K, et al. The effect of stress level, amino acid formula, and nitrogen dose on nitrogen retention in traumatic and septic stress. Ann Surg 1987; 205:282–287

Cerra F, Rios Benitez M, Blackburn G, et al. Applied nutrition in ICU patients. Chest 1997; 111:769–778

Heyland D, Cook DJ, Winder B, et al. Enteral nutrition in the critically ill: a prospective study. Crit Care Med 1995; 23:1055–1060

Heyland DK, Drover KW, McDonald S, et al. Effect of postpyloric feeding on gastroesophageal regurgitation and pulmonary microaspiration: results of a randomized controlled trial. Crit Care Med 2001; 29:1495–1501

Heyland DK, Dhaliwal R, Day, A, et al. Validation of the Canadian clinical: practice guidelines for nutrition support in mechanically ventilated, critically ill patients; results of a prospective observational study. Crit Care Med 2004; 32:2260–2266

Jeevanandam M, Shamos R, Peterson SR. Substrate utilization in early support of critically ill multiple trauma victims. JPEN J Parenter Enteral Nutr 1992; 16:511–520

Kudsk KA, Croce MA, Fabian TC, et al. Enteral versus parenteral feeding: effects on septic mortality after blunt and penetrating abdominal trauma. Ann Surg 1992; 215:503–513

Long CL, Schaffel N, Geiger JW, et al. Metabolic response to injury and illness: estimation of energy and protein needs for indirect calorimetry and nitrogen balance. JPEN J Parenter Enteral Nutr 1979; 3:452–456

Long CL, Nelson KM, Akin JM, et al. A physiologic basis for the provision of fuel mixtures in normal and stress patients. J Trauma 1990; 30:1077–1086

McClave SA, Sexton LK, Spain D, et al. Enteral tube feeding in the intensive care unit: factors impeding adequate delivery. Crit Care Med 1999; 27:1252–1256

McClave SA, Snider HL. Use of indirect calorimetry in clinical nutrition. Nutr Clin Pract 1992; 7:207–221

McClave SA, Lukan JK, Stefater JA, et al. Poor validity of residual volumes as a marker for risk of aspiration in critically ill patients. Crit Care Med 2005; 33:324–330

Mackenzie SL, Zygun DA, Whitmore BL, et al. Implementation of a nutrition support protocol increases the proportion of mechanically ventilated patients receiving enteral nutrition targets in the adult intensive care unit. J Parenter Enteral Nutr 2005; 29:74–80

Mizock BA. Alterations in carbohydrate metabolism during stress: a review of the literature. Am J Med 1995; 98:75–83

Novak F, Heyland DK, Avenell A, et al. Glutamine supplementation in serious illness: a systematic review of the evidence. Crit Care Med 2002; 30:2022–2029

Peter JV, Moran JL, Phillips-Hughes J. A metaanalysis of treatment outcomes of early enteral versus parenteral nutrition in hospitalized patients. Crit Care Med 2005; 33:213–220

Simpson F, Doig GS. Parenteral vs enteral nutrition in the critically ill patient: a meta-analysis of trials using the intention to treat principle. Intensive Care Med 2005; 31:12–23

Notes

Notes

Acute Renal Failure in the Critically Ill

Richard S. Muther, MD

Objectives:

- To develop a systematic approach to the differential diagnosis of acute renal failure
- To learn prevention techniques for critically ill patients at high risk for acute renal failure
- To learn specific and supportive treatment options for acute renal failure
- To review various dialysis options and their indications

Key words: glomerular hemodynamics; glomerulonephritis; interstitial nephritis; obstructive uropathy; prerenal azotemia; renal replacement therapies

---

Acute renal failure (ARF) is an abrupt decrease in glomerular filtration rate (GFR) resulting in the accumulation of waste products in the blood (acute azotemia). ARF comprises a spectrum of disorders but is usually due to an alteration in systemic or intrarenal hemodynamics or an acute renal parenchymal disease. While renal functional recovery (dialysis independence) is common in survivors of ARF, chronic azotemia may result in a significant percentage of patients. Subsequent progression to end stage renal disease (ESRD) may occur, particularly in those whose ARF complicates preexisting azotemia.

Acute azotemia may also be related to various nonrenal factors (pseudorenal failure), decreased renal perfusion (prerenal azotemia), or urinary tract obstruction (postrenal azotemia). *Pseudorenal failure* occurs when GI bleeding, corticosteroids, tetracyclines, severe catabolic states, or hyperalimentation alter urea metabolism, increasing the BUN without a change in GFR. Similarly, the serum creatinine may increase with creatine release from damaged muscles (rhabdomyolysis), blocked renal tubular creatinine secretion (trimethoprim and cimetidine), or interference with the creatinine assay (cefoxitin, acetone, alpha-methyldopa). Malnutrition and severe muscle wasting may spuriously decrease the plasma urea and creatinine concentrations, respectfully. One should always consider these nonrenal factors as a potential explanation for acute azotemia (Table 1).

Prerenal azotemia occurs when renal perfusion is compromised by an absolute decrease in extracellular fluid volume (ECV) (*eg*, hemorrhage, GI fluid losses, burns), a decrease in the "effective" circulating volume (heart failure, ascites), or the accumulation of fluid in a "third space" (*eg*, pancreatitis, acute abdomen, bowel surgery, muscle trauma). It may occasionally occur with high intra-abdominal pressures (>15 mm Hg bladder pressure) after trauma or surgery (abdominal compartment syndrome).[1] Correction of the intravascular volume defect or abdominal pressure should result in improved renal perfusion and resolution of azotemia. In most series, prerenal azotemia has a 90% survival rate, but if unrecognized or untreated, it can evolve into ARF and a significantly worse prognosis.

The diagnosis of prerenal azotemia is based on the physical examination demonstrating an alteration of ECV and on several urinary indexes (Table 2). Of these, the fractional excretion of sodium (FENa) is most reliable.[2] The FENa measures the ratio of the sodium excreted (urinary sodium × volume) to the sodium filtered (serum sodium × GFR) by the following formula:

$$FENa = (UNa/SNa) \div (Ucr/Scr) \times 100$$

where U indicates urine; Na, sodium; S, serum; cr, creatinine. The test can be done with a spot sample of urine and blood. The FENa is <1% when acute azotemia is prerenal but >1% with ARF. A few exceptions must be kept in mind. Rhabdomyolysis, contrast nephropathy, acute glomerulonephritis, and sepsis are all causes of ARF in which the FENa may be spuriously low, particularly early in the clinical course.[3] In addition, patients with severe heart failure or cirrhosis often have a FENa of <1% despite ARF.[4] Diuretics, glucosuria, or preexisting renal insufficiency will falsely elevate the FENa in a patient with prerenal azotemia. When diuretics elevate the FENa, a fractional excretion of urea of <35% accurately indicates prerenal azotemia.[5] The clinician must

Table 1. *Causes of Pseudorenal Failure*

Nonrenal causes of elevated urea
    Corticosteroids
    Hyperalimentation
    GI bleeding
Nonrenal causes of elevated creatinine
    Increased creatine release from skeletal muscle
        Rhabdomyolysis
    Interference with creatinine assay
        Acetone
        Cefoxitin
        Flucytosine
        Methyldopa
    Blocked tubular creatinine secretion
        Cimetidine
        Trimethoprim

Table 2. *Diagnostic Indices of Prerenal Azotemia and Acute Tubular Necrosis*

Variable	PRA*	ATN
BUN:creatinine ratio	20	10
Urine osmolality, mosm/L	>350	±300
Urine:plasma osmolality ratio	>1.5	1.0
Urine sodium, mEq/L	<20	>30
FENa	<1%	>1%
Fractional excretion of urea	<35%	>50%

*PRA = prerenal azotemia.

be alert to these potential pitfalls of the FENa when approaching the acutely azotemic patient.

In addition to a low FENa and fractional excretion of urea, prerenal azotemia usually causes a low urinary Na level (<20 mEq/L), high urine osmolality (>350 milliosmols (mosm)/L), and an elevated BUN:creatinine ratio (>20). The urine sediment may show granular casts but is usually devoid of cellular elements. Oliguria is virtually universal unless a diuretic or glucosuria is present. ARF, on the other hand, causes a high urine Na level (>30 mEq/L), isosthenuria (urine osmolality ~300 osm/L), and a BUN:creatinine ratio near 10. Prerenal azotemia is confirmed if the urinary output improves and the azotemia resolves with the administration of isotonic fluids, improvement in the underlying heart failure, or correction of the third-space defect.

An obstruction to urine flow may cause *postrenal azotemia*. Although anuria is expected, fluctuating or even high urine volumes may result if the blockage is partial. As long as the obstruction is relatively recent (days to weeks) and the serum creatinine level relatively low (<5 mg/dL), correcting the obstruction will usually resolve the azotemia. With urethral or prostatic obstruction, a Foley catheter will suffice. This and a renal ultrasound are required diagnostic steps in any patient with acute azotemia. For patients with one kidney, a CT scan (without contrast) or even a retrograde pyelogram may be necessary to positively exclude obstruction. Upper tract obstruction may require a ureteral stent or percutaneous nephrostomy.

After excluding pseudorenal, prerenal, and postrenal azotemia, one must consider the various renal parenchymal or hemodynamic derangements responsible for ARF. These include diseases that primarily affect the glomerulus (glomerulonephritis), interstitium (interstitial nephritis), blood vessels (vascular occlusion or vasculitis), or tubules (acute tubular necrosis [ATN]).

Differential Diagnosis of ARF in the ICU

Although ATN is the most common cause of ICU-acquired ARF,[6] important glomerular, interstitial, and vascular diseases must be considered (Table 3).

Glomerular Diseases

Fulminant *glomerulonephritis* due to bacterial endocarditis, lupus erythematosus, staphylococcal septicemia, visceral abscesses, hepatitis B antigenemia, Goodpasture's syndrome, or idiopathic rapidly progressive (crescentic) glomerulonephritis is not uncommon in a major ICU. Once considered, these diagnoses are not difficult to make. The urinalysis will show dysmorphic RBCs (those with multiple surface irregularities), RBC casts, and moderate to heavy proteinuria. Hypertension is variably present. Blood cultures, serologic testing (antinuclear antibody, antineutrophilic cytoplasmic antibodies, hepatitis B surface antigen, and antiglomerular basement membrane antibody), and a search for visceral abscess may be rewarding. An urgent renal biopsy should be strongly considered whenever acute glomerulonephritis is suspected, as aggressive specific therapy (eg, plasma exchange, corticosteroids, and/or cyclophosphamide) is often required.

Alterations in *glomerular hemodynamics* are increasingly recognized as a cause of ARF. These

Table 3. *Differential Diagnosis of ARF*

I. Glomerular
   A. Altered glomerular hemodynamics
      1. Hepatorenal syndrome
      2. Angiotensin-converting enzyme inhibitors/angiotensin receptor blockers
      3. Nifedipine/nitroprusside
      4. Cyclosporine/tacrolimus
      5. NSAIDs
      6. Hypercalcemia
   B. Glomerulonephritis
      1. Infectious
         a. Bacterial endocarditis
         b. "Shunt" nephritis
         c. Visceral abscess
         d. Hepatitis antigenemia
         e. Poststreptococcal glomerulonephritis
      2. Lupus erythematosus
      3. Rapidly progressive glomerulonephritis
      4. Goodpasture's syndrome

II. Vascular
   A. Hypertensive crisis
   B. Microangiopathy
      1. Thrombotic thrombocytopenic purpura
      2. Hemolytic uremic syndrome
   C. Renal artery thrombosis/thromboembolism
   D. Cholesterol emboli syndrome
   E. Vasculitis
      1. Wegener's granulomatosus
      2. Polyarteritis nodosa
      3. Microscopic polyarteritis
      4. Hypersensitivity vasculitis
      5. Henoch-Schönlein purpura
      6. Cryoglobulinemia

III. Interstitial
   A. Allergic interstitial nephritis
   B. Bacterial pyelonephritis
   C. Viral (cytomegalovirus, measles, mumps)
   D. Rickettsial disease
   E. Tumor lysis
   F. Urate/oxalate nephropathy
   G. Multiple myeloma
   H. Infiltrative (lymphoma, leukemia)
   I. Sarcoidosis
   J. Immune (SLE, Sjögren's, tubulointerstitial nephritis uveitis)

IV. Tubular (ATN)
   A. Toxic
      1. Aminoglycosides
      2. Platinum
      3. Radiographic contrast agents
      4. Amphotericin B
      5. Solvents (CCl4, ethylene glycol)
      6. Rhabdomyolysis/myoglobinuria
      7. Intravascular hemolysis
      8. Acetaminophen
   B. Ischemic
      1. Hypotension/shock
      2. Hemorrhage
      3. Sepsis

---

include afferent arteriolar vasoconstriction (hepatorenal syndrome) or efferent arteriolar vasodilatation (angiotensin-converting enzyme inhibitors). The latter is usually seen when severe cardiac failure, ECV depletion, or bilateral renal artery stenosis already compromises renal blood flow. In addition, less well-defined derangements in intrarenal hemodynamics likely contribute to the ARF of sepsis, potent vasodilators (nitroprusside and nifedipine),[7] and the nonsteroidal anti-inflammatory drugs (NSAIDs). In these cases, the urine sediment is usually bland, and results of the renal biopsy (if performed) are normal. Recovery of renal function is expected provided the offending drug is removed or the underlying condition is corrected.

Hepatorenal syndrome (HRS) refers to ARF that occurs in the setting of severe liver failure after other obvious causes are excluded. The patient demonstrates avid sodium retention (urinary sodium <10 mEq/L; FENa <1%) and oliguria not responding to ECV expansion. The urine sediment is usually benign. The onset may be insidious or abruptly precipitated by ECV depletion (GI bleeding, diuretics, paracentesis) or sepsis. Because the liver is critical to both urea and creatinine generation, patients with cirrhosis and ascites are at high risk despite normal serum values. In one study, the incidence of HRS was 18% at 1 year and 39% at 5 years in cirrhotic patients with ascites.[8]

HRS likely results from nitric oxide-induced splanchnic vasodilatation with consequent activation of the renin angiotensin and sympathetic nervous systems.[9] Thus, cardiac output is high and systemic vascular resistance is low ("septic physiology") despite elevated renal vascular resistance. Other theories of pathogenesis include an imbalance of vasoconstrictor/vasodilator prostaglandins (supported by elevated urinary 20-hydroxyeicosatetraenoic acid, a vasoconstrictor prostaglandin), endotoxemia, endothelin-induced renal vasoconstriction, release of false neurotransmitters, or an increase in sympathetic tone pursuant to elevated hepatic sinusoidal pressure.

The preferred treatment of HRS is liver transplantation. As a bridge to transplant, various medical therapies may be tried. Norepinephrine infusion should be tried, particularly in patients with a mean arterial pressure <60 mm Hg. The sympatholytic agent clonidine may transiently improve GFR. Data on misoprostol and *N*-acetylcysteine are conflicting. There are promising preliminary reports using both terlipressin (an antidiuretic hormone analog) given with albumin infusions[10] and the combination of midodrine and octreotide.[11] Peritoneovenous shunting and the transjugular intrahepatic portosystemic shunt have high complication rates and are generally reserved as a last resort in refractory patients.

Interstitial Diseases

Acute interstitial nephritis is usually due to allergy. Penicillins, cephalosporins, sulfonamides, diuretics, and NSAIDs are the most common offending agents, although the list of agents reported to cause acute interstitial nephritis is legion. Patients typically have fever, rash, arthralgias, and eosinophilia. Pyuria (sterile) dominates the urinary sediment, although hematuria and proteinuria are also common. Eosinophiluria (best evaluated by Hansel's stain) is demonstrated in many cases, often excepting NSAIDs. Other causes of eosinophilia and eosinophiluria associated with ARF (such as atheroemboli or rapidly progressive glomerulonephritis) are usually easily distinguished on clinical grounds.

Tumor lysis syndrome refers to a variety of metabolic complications associated with lymphoreticular or (rarely) solid malignancies. Hyperuricemia (usually >15 mg/dL) and hyperphosphatemia (usually >8 mg/dL) each may cause ARF; the latter usually follows lytic therapy while the former often precedes treatment of the primary malignancy. Hypocalcemia and hyperkalemia often complicate the early clinical course. Patients are usually oligoanuric and the urinary sediment frequently reveals amorphous urates or urate crystals. Urinary alkalinization is not routinely recommended as it may actually enhance renal parenchymal calcium phosphate deposition. ECV expansion with isotonic crystalloid or mannitol has prophylactic benefit. Although allopurinol has not completely eliminated the ARF of tumor lysis, it does help (at high dosages of 600 to 900 mg/d, if possible).

Other causes of ARF due to interstitial nephritis are less common but include viral or bacterial pyelonephritis, multiple myeloma, uric acid nephropathy, and occasionally infiltrative disorders such as lymphoma, leukemia, and sarcoidosis. Oxalate nephropathy may complicate acute ethylene glycol ingestion (with elevated anion and osmolar gap). The urine sediment in these cases is usually bland, but crystalluria, pyuria, and WBC casts can be seen, even in the absence of infection.

Vascular Diseases

Vascular disease is a frequently overlooked cause of ARF. *Malignant hypertension*, usually accompanied by retinopathy, thrombocytopenia, and microangiopathy, can cause ARF. Microangiopathy and thrombocytopenia also accompany *hemolytic uremic syndrome* or *thrombotic thrombocytopenic purpura*. Renal *infarction* due to trauma, thrombosis, or thromboembolism can cause ARF with fever, hematuria, acute flank pain, ileus, leukocytosis, and an elevated lactate dehydrogenase level, a syndrome that mimics an acute abdomen. Thromboembolism usually arises from the heart in patients with severe left ventricular failure or atrial fibrillation.

Cholesterol emboli syndrome (CES) refers to renal atherosclerotic or cholesterol microemboli that may occur following aortic manipulation (surgery or catheterization) or systemic anticoagulation. Besides ARF, GI bleeding (due to microinfarcts), livido reticularis of the lower extremities, patchy areas of ischemic necrosis in the toes, hypocomplementemia, and eosinophilia are common. It is important to distinguish CES from a thromboembolic event, as therapeutic anticoagulation is dangerous in patients with CES but necessary for those with the latter.

Renal *vasculitis* (Wegener's granulomatosis, polyarteritis nodosa, hypersensitivity vasculitis, and Henoch-Schönlein purpura) often causes ARF. These disorders are identified by their multisystem manifestations, very active urine sediment (hematuria, pyuria, RBC and WBC casts, and proteinuria), and, in the case of Wegener's granulomatosis and polyarteritis nodosa, the presence of antineutrophilic cytoplasmic antibodies in the serum.

Tubular Diseases

The most common cause of hospital- and ICU-acquired ARF is *ATN*,[6] which is broadly divided into toxic and ischemic causes. In fact,

ATN in the ICU setting is usually attributed to a conspiracy of factors including hypovolemia, poor cardiac output, nephrotoxins, and sepsis.

Among the more common toxins causing ATN are the aminoglycoside antibiotics. Risk factors for *aminoglycoside nephrotoxicity* include volume contraction, age, hypokalemia, concomitant use of other nephrotoxins, and a short dosing interval. After an initial loading dose (2 to 3 mg/kg), the maintenance dose (1 mg/kg) should be adjusted based on the patient's creatinine clearance (Ccr) (estimated by the formula Ccr = body weight (kg)/serum creatinine) or calculated GFR. The routine use of peak and trough serum levels does not decrease the likelihood of ATN.

Radiographic contrast agents may cause ARF in patients who have preexisting renal insufficiency, diabetes mellitus, and poor left ventricular function, or who undergo multiple studies in a 24-h period. The volume of contrast used (>1.5 mL/kg) appears directly related to nephrotoxicity. Nonionic and isosmolar contrast appears less nephrotoxic. The best prophylaxis appears to be isotonic sodium bicarbonate (150 mEq/L; 300 mL over 1 h precontrast then 100 mL/h postcontrast for 1 L)[12] and *N*-acetylcysteine (600 mg po q12h; two doses before and two doses after the procedure).[13] IV mannitol, furosemide (either before or after contrast), dopamine, calcium channel blockers and fenoldopam do not appear to lessen nephrotoxicity. Theophylline may decrease nephrotoxicity in patients at very high risk, particularly those in whom crystalloid is contraindicated.

Although most cases of contrast nephrotoxicity are nonoliguric and resolve within a few days, it significantly increases hospital mortality and cost. Patients may require acute dialysis, but permanent loss of renal function is not likely to occur. CES is potentially a more serious, although less common, renal complication for patients undergoing radiographic contrast studies.

Massive *intravascular hemolysis* or *rhabdomyolysis* may produce ARF. Common causes of rhabdomyolysis include drugs (*eg*, heroin, cocaine, statins), major crush injuries, alcohol, seizures, and muscle compression syndromes. All have the potential of producing myoglobinuria and ARF, particularly if ECV depletion or shock exists simultaneously. Hyperkalemia, hyperuricemia, hyperphosphatemia, and hypercreatinemia (low BUN:creatinine ratio) also result. Hypocalcemia often occurs early, but hypercalcemia (as high as 12 to 14 mg/dL) appears during recovery.[14] An elevated creatine phosphokinase level and dark heme-positive urine without RBCs are major diagnostic clues. Prophylaxis against ATN depends on aggressive IV crystalloid. The addition of mannitol and bicarbonate (1/2 normal saline solution with 12.5 g of mannitol per liter and 50 mEq of $NaHCO_3$ per liter at 250 to 500 mL/h) may be a useful adjunct.

Ischemic insults to the kidney occur with prolonged hypotension, suprarenal aortic or renal artery occlusion (either with clot or clamp), and sepsis. The renal tubular cells are particularly susceptible to ischemic insult because their baseline balance between oxygen supply and demand is tenuous.[15] Thus, whenever systemic or intrarenal blood flow decreases slightly, ischemic insult to the tubular cells may occur. This may help to explain the beneficial effects attributed to loop diuretics shown in some studies. By inhibiting active chloride and sodium transport in the ascending limb of the loop, these agents decrease metabolic work and therefore, oxygen requirements.[15] Figure 1 diagrams the factors affecting oxygen supply and demand in the tubular cells of the renal medulla.

Sepsis appears to cause >50% of all cases of hospital-acquired oliguric ARF, and it is particularly common in the critically ill patient. In addition, the prognosis of sepsis-induced ARF appears directly related to the severity of the sepsis. Sepsis causes a simultaneous decrease in systemic vascular resistance and increase in renal vascular

Oxygen Supply		Oxygen Demand	
Increase	**Decrease**	**Increase**	**Decrease**
Fenoldopam	CsA	Hypovolemia	Furosemide
Dopamine	NSAID	NSAID	CCBs
ANP	Myoglobin	Contrast	Dopamine
Hypervolemia	Contrast	Ampho B	
CCBs	Hypovolemia		

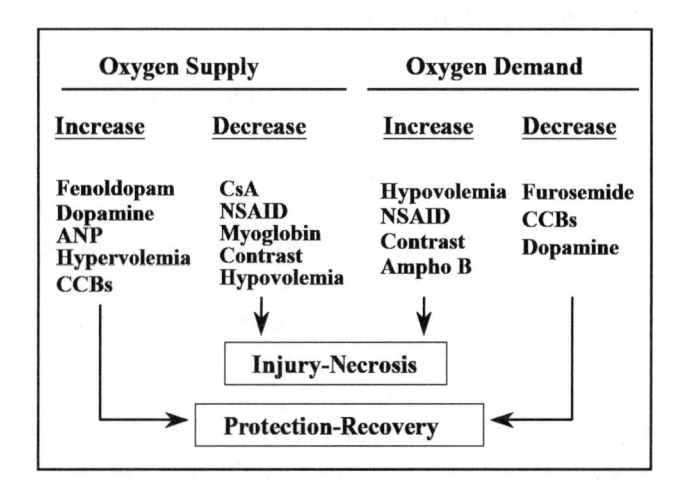

↓ ↓
Injury-Necrosis
Protection-Recovery

Figure 1. Factors which may affect renal tubular oxygen supply and demand.

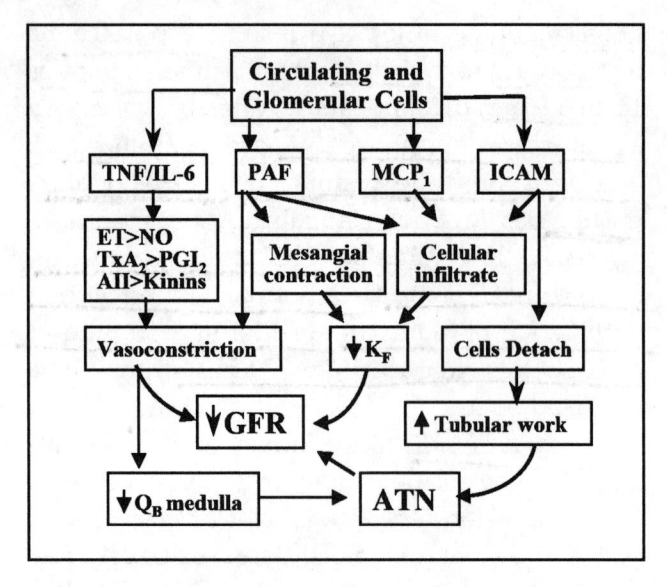

Figure 2. Factors contributing to acute renal failure in sepsis. (Abbreviations: TNF, tumor necrosis factor; IL, interleukin; PAF, platelet activating factor; MCP, monocyte chemoattractant protein; ICAM, intercellular adhesion molecule; ET, endothelin; NO, nitric oxide; TxA, thromboxane; PGI, prostacyclin; AII, angiotensin II; K_F, glomerular permeability; Q_B, blood flow.)

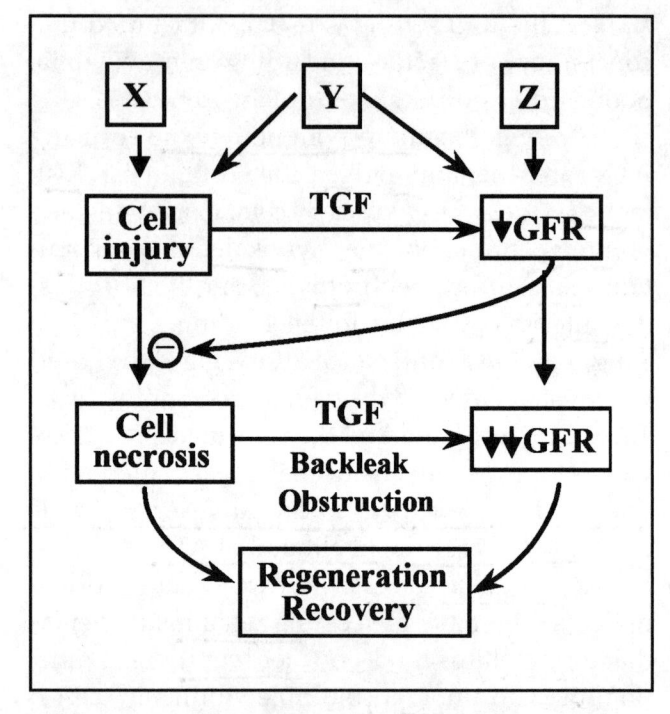

Figure 3. Pathophysiology of acute renal failure. A given insult (*eg*, X, Y or Z) may directly effect a renal tubular cell injury, a decrease in glomerular filtration rate (GFR) or both. Tubular glomerular feedback (TGF) ensures a decline in GFR if the tubules are primarily affected, which may retard the development of tubular necrosis. If acute tubular necrosis occurs, tubular obstruction and backleak of ultrafiltrate contribute to a more pronounced and prolonged decrease in GFR.

resistance, reducing renal plasma flow and GFR.[16] Both circulating and glomerular cells react to endotoxins by producing a variety of cytokines and autacoids, decreasing renal perfusion and increasing renal tubular cell work (Fig 2). ARF can occur even without systemic hypotension. Fever, leukocytosis, and other overt signs of sepsis may be absent. A mild alteration in mental status or respiratory alkalosis may be the only clinical clue. Oliguria and/or azotemia in this setting should be considered occult septicemia unless disproved.

Pathophysiology of ARF

Either a toxic or ischemic insult can initiate an intrarenal cascade that manifests as clinical ARF (Fig 3). The primary renal tubular cellular event appears to be decreased production and increased degradation of adenosine triphosphate, thus increasing local production of phospholipases, hypoxanthine, and adenosine. Phospholipases destabilize tubular cell membranes, causing redistribution of integrin receptors from the basolateral to the luminal surface, decreasing intercellular adhesion. Disruption and shedding of renal tubular cells may then result in intratubular obstruction and back-leak of tubular fluid.

The cells of the thick ascending limb of Henle and the S_3 segment of the proximal tubule appear uniquely susceptible to ischemic injury. Because of marginal medullary blood flow and the unique anatomy of the vasa rectae, these very metabolically active cells (responsible for the bulk of sodium transport) normally function in borderline hypoxia.[15] Seemingly minor decrements in perfusion may cause substantial injury to these cells. Here, oxygen free radicals (generated from hypoxanthine and by infiltrating neutrophils) may play a role. Platelet activating factor released during injury increases vascular permeability and contributes to the infiltration of neutrophils by upregulating adhesion molecules (intercellular adhesion molecule, or ICAM-1) on endothelial cells.

Injured renal tubular cells may also release vasoconstrictor prostaglandins, adenosine, endothelin, or other substances that affect intraglomerular hemodynamics (afferent arteriolar vasoconstriction or efferent arteriolar vasodilatation) or glomerular capillary permeability in such a way as to decrease GFR.[17] This phenomenon is known as *tubuloglomerular feedback*. The net result is a prolonged decrement in GFR with varying degrees of urine output. All of these events may occur without an alteration in systemic hemodynamics or even renal blood flow (RBF).

Simultaneous with these events causing renal functional decline, other factors appear to mediate a regenerative or repair process.[18] Release of various cytokines from injured cells appears to recruit and activate macrophages, which synthesize growth factors (such as epidermal and transforming growth factors), stimulating renal tubular cell regeneration and recovery. Production of vasodilator prostaglandins and nitric oxide may aid this renal recovery.

Clinically, these pathophysiologic mechanisms appear to produce a brief initial decrease in RBF and GFR, followed by a prolonged (days to weeks) maintenance phase in which GFR remains low but RBF returns to normal. Oliguria may occur during this maintenance period, and dialysis is often necessary. The recovery phase is marked first by increasing urinary volume and finally by return of GFR.

Treatment of ARF

Several therapies for ARF show promise *in vitro* and in animal studies, including diuretics, dopamine, natriuretic peptides, calcium channel blockers, endothelin antagonists, growth factors, and oxygen free-radical scavengers. Application of these therapies in human clinical trials proves disappointing. Therefore, in 2005, *the treatment for ARF remains largely preventive and supportive.*

Prevention

Because the risk and the mortality of ARF are high in critically ill patients, prevention is the best therapy. Table 4 lists several common risk factors for ARF and suggestions for prophylaxis. The most common risk factor is ECV depletion. Volume expansion can minimize the risk of ARF from radiographic contrast agents, cisplatin, and NSAIDs. *N*-acetylcysteine appears effective in preventing contrast and possibly cisplatin nephrotoxicity. Mannitol may at least partially abrogate

Table 4. *Prevention of Acute Renal Failure**

Risk Factor	Strategy for Prevention
Renal hypoperfusion	Avoid nephrotoxins
ECV depletion	Isotonic crystalloids
Hypotension	Replete ECV with crystalloid, colloid; inotropic agents if needed; vasopressors
Congestive heart failure	Inotropic agents; cautious use of ACEIs
Cirrhosis/ascites	Avoid NSAIDs. Colloid with paracenteses. Norepinephrine if hypotensive. Clonidine? Peritoneovenous shunt or TIPS?
Third-space ECV	Colloid, isotonic crystalloids
PEEP	Isotonic crystalloids
Renal artery stenosis	Avoid ACEIs with diuretics
Preexisting azotemia	Avoid ECV depletion; cautious use of nephrotoxins
Sepsis	Avoid ECV depletion; cautious use of nephrotoxins
Nephrotoxins	Avoid ECV depletion and other nephrotoxins
Aminoglycosides	Use alternative agent if possible; lengthen dosing interval; correct hypokalemia
Chemotherapy	Expand ECV; mannitol; N-acetylcysteine, possibly theophylline for platinum
Radiocontrast agents	Expand ECV with normal sodium bicarbonate; *N*-acetylcysteine; limit dose; use nonionic, isoosmolar contrast with preexisting azotemia
Cyclosporine	Calcium channel blockers
NSAIDs	Cautious use in congestive heart failure, cirrhosis, ECV depletion; avoid simultaneous triamterene
Rhabdomyolysis	Expand ECV. Mannitol? HCO_3?
Hyperuricemia	Expand ECV; alkalinize urine unless serum phosphorus elevated; allopurinol
Electrolyte disorders	
Hypokalemia	Correct
Hypophosphatemia	Correct
Hyperphosphatemia	Avoid calcium therapy; avoid alkalinization; expand ECV; short-term intestinal binders
Hypercalcemia	Avoid phosphorus therapy; expand ECV; furosemide

*ACEI = angiotensin-converting enzyme inhibitor; TIPS = transjugular intrahpatic portosystemic shunt.

the ARF caused by rhabdomyolysis and cisplatin, but not that caused by contrast agents. Limiting the dose and simultaneous exposure appears important in avoiding contrast, aminoglycoside, and cisplatin toxicity. Alkali may limit the nephrotoxicity of myoglobinuria and uric acid. Allopurinol should be used before chemotherapy whenever tumor lysis is anticipated. Adjusting the dosing interval for changes in Ccr is important to prevent aminoglycoside toxicity. Polyuria or an increasing creatinine level should prompt additional widening of the dosing interval. Correcting hypokalemia and expanding ECV are also helpful. Although the peak aminoglycoside level correlates with antibacterial effect, there is little evidence that monitoring trough levels minimizes or avoids nephrotoxicity.

Although some data support abdominal decompression with large-volume paracentesis as a means of improving renal perfusion in patients with tense ascites, the clinician should be cautious about paracenteses >0.5 L, especially without the support of concomitant albumin infusion. Ascitic fluid may rapidly reaccumulate at the expense of intravascular volume, putting the patient at risk due to inadequate preload. Positive end-expiratory pressure (PEEP), as well as high intrathoracic pressure associated with mechanical ventilator support, may compromise cardiac output and renal perfusion. If possible, PEEP should be minimized and ECV expanded in high-risk patients.

There are animal data to suggest that hyperalimentation may increase the risk of ARF. However, the benefits of nutritional support seem to far outweigh this risk. Minimizing protein intake to between 0.6 and 0.8 g/kg/d during periods of very high risk may be prudent.

Supportive Therapy

Nonoliguric patients presenting with ARF have fewer complications, including a decreased dialysis requirement and improved survival.[19] Although conversion of an oliguric patient to nonoliguric has less certain benefit, it can often be accomplished by repleting volume (if deficient) and using high-dose loop diuretics (*eg*, furosemide, 200 mg IV or continuous infusions at 10 to 40 mg/h). Loop diuretics may have the theoretical advantage of decreasing tubular cell metabolic activity (thus lessening the oxygen requirement) but do not appear to alter the course of ARF. Although a renal vasodilator dose of dopamine (1.5 to 2.5 μg/kg/min) may stimulate urine volume, it does not improve GFR, shorten the duration of ARF, or decrease dialysis requirements.[20] In addition, dopamine may induce significant arrhythmia and possibly intestinal ischemia. If used, dopamine should be initiated early, given simultaneously with a loop diuretic, and promptly abandoned if an increase in urine volume does not occur within 24 h.

Hyperalimentation preserves lean muscle mass, decreases protein breakdown, improves wound healing, and may improve immune competence. It appears to improve renal tubular cell regeneration in animals with ATN and improve survival in critically ill patients, particularly those with multiple complications.[21] Enteral alimentation is preferred whenever possible. Regardless of the route, the hyperalimentation formula must be individualized and reevaluated daily in patients with ARF. Essential amino acid preparations offer no special advantage.

Potential drug toxicity must be avoided by adjusting antibiotic and other drug dosing in patients with renal failure.[22] This includes potential dietary sources of potassium (salt substitutes, oral tobacco products) and phosphorus (dairy products), as well as the magnesium and aluminum contained in antacids. Decreased renal excretion of normeperidine and NAPA (metabolites) may produce serious toxicity even though their parent drugs (meperidine and procainamide) are metabolized by the liver.[23,24] Finally, decreased protein binding (presumably displaced by uremic toxins) may accentuate the toxicity of morphine and phenytoin in any patient with renal failure.[25,26]

Uremic bleeding is best treated by RBC transfusion, raising the hemoglobin to 10 g/dL. Adjunctive therapies include IV estrogen (0.6 mg/kg/d for 5 days), cryoprecipitate infusion (10 U) and vasopressin (desmopressin acetate, 0.3 μg/kg every 12 h).[27]

The treatment of hyperkalemia is outlined in Table 5. When the serum potassium is <6 mEq/L, little therapy is required other than discontinuing the occult sources of dietary potassium. As the potassium rises above 6 mEq/L and/or peaked T waves appear, volume expansion (as tolerated),

Table 5. *Treatment of Acute Hyperkalemia**

Serum K+, mEq/L	ECG Changes	Treatment	Onset	Duration
6 mEq/L	Peaked T wave	Expand ECV; loop diuretics; sodium polystyrene sulfonate	Hours	Hours to days
7 mEq/L	Prolonged PR Widened QRS	Glucose/insulin (2 g/U) Albuterol (10 to 20 mg inhalation)	Minutes	Hours
8 mEq/L	Sine wave	Calcium (100 mg slow IV)	Minutes	<1 h

*Note: The correlation between the serum potassium and the ECG changes is variable. The ECG changes are likely a better indicator of therapeutic urgency.

Table 6. *Available Options for RRT*

Technique	Intermittent	Continuous
Peritoneal dialysis (PD)	Intermittent PD	Continuous cycler PD
Hemodialysis (HD)	IHD SLED	Continuous HD SLED
Ultrafiltration (UF)	Intermittent UF	SCUF
Hemofiltration (HF)	— —	Continuous arteriovenous HF CVVH
Hemodiafiltration (HDF)	— —	Continuous arteriovenous HDF CVVHDF

loop diuretics, and oral sodium polystyrene sulfonate powder are appropriate. (Sodium polystyrene sulfonate via rectum is reported to cause colonic necrosis.) Although somewhat slow to act, these treatments actually increase potassium excretion. When more urgent therapy is needed for hyperkalemia (>7 mEq/L), driving potassium intracellularly with glucose and insulin (25 to 50 g dextrose with 10 to 20 U of regular insulin) or the ß-agonist albuterol (5 to 20 mg [1.0 to 4.0 mL] inhaled) is indicated.[28] Albuterol usually works within 30 min, will lower the serum potassium by 0.6 to 1.0 mEq/L, and lasts for ≥2 h. Calcium therapy (10 mEq IV over 5 min) is reserved for hyperkalemia-induced heart block, the sine wave, or of course ventricular arrest. Its effect is immediate but short-lived (<30 min). Other maneuvers to remove potassium from the body (such as diuretics or sodium polystyrene sulfonate) must be initiated promptly as well. Dialysis (usually hemodialysis) can also be used to remove potassium.

Renal Replacement Therapy

Many patients with ARF will recover renal function within days and not require dialysis. However, if the duration of ARF is prolonged, or if hyperkalemia, ECV overload, refractory acidosis, or uremic symptoms (serositis, encephalopathy, bleeding) occur, some form of renal replacement therapy (RRT) may be necessary. The major goals of RRT in ARF are to maintain the patient's survival and support nonrenal organ function while awaiting recovery of renal function. Its two main objectives are (1) to control ECV by removing excess fluid (ultrafiltration), and (2) to control azotemia by removing excess solute. Depending on a patient's needs, these two objectives can be accomplished separately or simultaneously, intermittently or continuously, by peritoneal or hematogenous access. The available options for RRT are outlined in Table 6.

Peritoneal dialysis (PD) plays a relatively minor role as a RRT in the ICU (Fig 4). Nevertheless, it offers several advantages including simplicity, hemodynamic stability, and freedom from anticoagulation. Peritoneal access is achieved through a surgically or percutaneously placed catheter. Automated cyclers easily accomplish the exchange of dialysate. However, even with frequent dialysate exchanges and very hypertonic dialysate (4.25 g/dL dextrose), PD clearance of solute (urea clearance ≅18 mL/min)

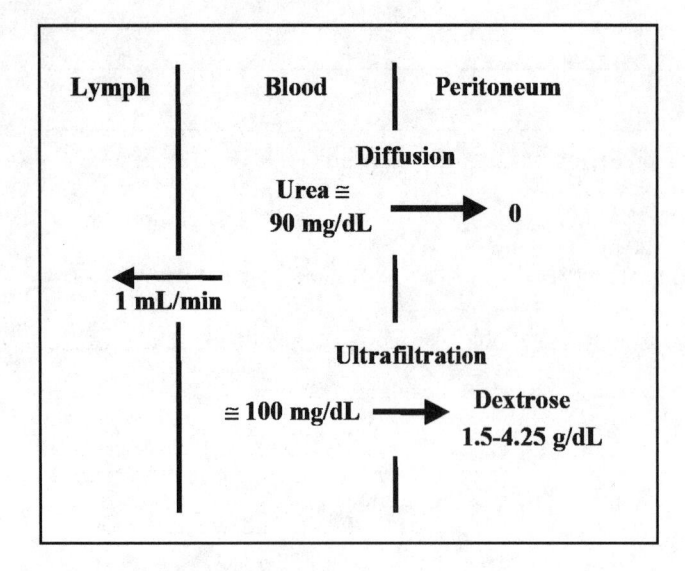

Figure 4. Peritoneal dialysis. Solute removal by diffusion down an electrochemical gradient from blood to dialysate. Hypertonic dialysate creates the force for ultrafiltration.

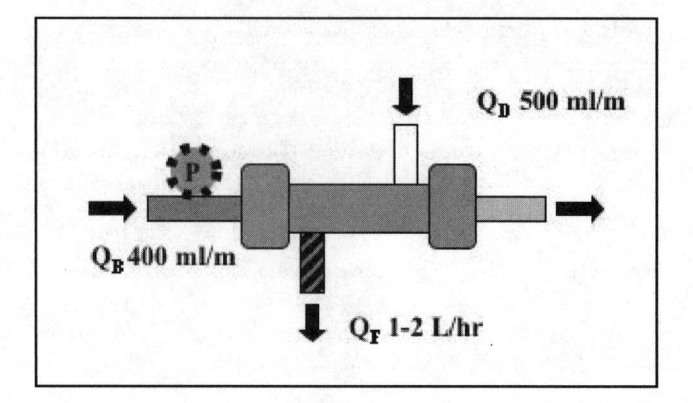

Figure 5. Intermittent hemodialysis (IHD). Blood flows (Q_B) at 350-500 mL/min through an hemodialyzer cartridge. Dialysate flows (Q_D) at 500-800 mL/min in the opposite dirrection (countercurrent). Solute removal is by diffusion down an electrochemical gradient. Ultrrafiltration results from a pressure gradient applied across a semipermeable membrane. Ultra-filtrate flow (Q_F) is limited to 1-2 L/hr because of hypotension. The major clinical application of IHD is rapid solute clearance.

and ultrafiltration (UF) rates (6 to 8 L/d) are limited. In addition, the intraperitoneal volume of dialysate can compromise respiration, and glucose loads and protein losses can be excessive. Therefore, PD appears better suited for the less catabolic, less uremic, and relatively normovolemic patient. We use it almost exclusively in patients who previously used PD and have a superimposed illness requiring ICU admission.

Intermittent hemodialysis (IHD) remains the most frequently utilized RRT in United States. Patient blood and dialysate, separated by a semipermeable membrane, run countercurrently through an artificial dialyzer in an extracorporeal circuit (Fig 5). A percutaneously placed, dual-lumen central venous catheter allows blood flows (Q_B) of 300 to 400 mL/min. Solute removal is accomplished by diffusion down an electrochemical gradient maintained by continuous dialysate flow of 500 to 800 mL/min. UF is driven by the transmembrane pressure (TMP). The membrane permeability (a product of pore size and surface area) limits the molecular size of solute clearance and the rate of UF at any given TMP. Typical membranes used for IHD restrict clearance to relatively small solutes (molecular weight <5,000 d) manifested by urea clearances of 200 to 250 mL/min. Volume removal is limited only by signs or symptoms of acute volume depletion as UF rates begin to exceed 1.5 L/h. The major clinical benefit of IHD is rapid solute clearance.

The hemodialysis membrane is not simply a passive structure but may, depending on its composition, induce significant biochemical effects. For example, cellulose-based dialysis membranes (cellulose acetate, cuprophane) can activate complement, induce coagulation factor XII, and induce functional defects in neutrophils.[29] This may increase susceptibility to infection, cause leukoagglutination, exacerbate renal injury, and delay recovery from ARF. Excellent clinical studies[30-32] demonstrate not only a lower rate of recovery from ARF but also a higher patient mortality when these so-called bioincompatible membranes are compared with "synthetic" membranes (*eg*, polysulfone, polyamide, polyacrylonitrile, polymethyl methacrylate) in the treatment of ARF. This mandates the use of synthetic, biocompatible membranes for all extracorporeal RRT in the ICU. In addition, the impact of dialysis dose on the survival of patients with ARF must be reexamined, because previous data suggesting no effect were generated at a time when only bioincompatible membranes were available.

While the issues of bioincompatibility relate to all forms of extracorporeal RRT, other problems are unique to IHD. Rapid solute removal can cause confusion, disorientation and other mental status changes termed *disequilibrium syndrome*. Hypoxemia (as much as a 10-mm Hg decrease in Pao_2) is expected. Air embolism and bleeding can occur with any central venous access catheter.

But the most frequent complication of IHD is hypotension. In a patient with ARF, in whom the kidney has lost the ability to autoregulate blood flow, even mild hypotension can induce oliguria, produce significant renal ischemia, and delay functional recovery. Other serious difficulties may arise if cerebral, myocardial, splanchnic, and peripheral perfusion are compromised.

Several factors contribute to hemodialysis-induced hypotension, including rapid ultrafiltration, rapid solute loss (decreasing intravascular osmolality, resulting in extracellular-to-intracellular fluid shift), changes in cardiac output and systemic vascular resistance, and the use of acetate as a dialysate buffer. These effects can be minimized by slowing Q_B, lengthening dialysis times, using intradialytic hypertonic crystalloids or colloids IV, temporarily suspending dialysate flow ("bypass"), lowering the dialysate temperature to 35°C, and buffering with HCO_3-based dialysate. Nevertheless, hypotension remains the major potential complication of IHD and is the major incentive for use of continuous renal replacement therapies (CRRTs).

Isolated UF (*ie*, without simultaneous dialysis [diffusion]) can provide substantial fluid losses without hypotension. The absence of dialysate flow limits solute removal to the minimum generated by convection alone. This protects intravascular volume while producing several liters of net UF daily. This technique has several clinical applications. It can be utilized emergently to treat acute pulmonary edema or as an adjunct to IHD, enhancing fluid removal either immediately adjacent to or isolated from a dialysis treatment. *Slow continuous ultrafiltration* (SCUF) (Fig 6) is particularly suited to a patient who has excessive IV fluid requirements with marginal urinary output, *eg*, a patient with severe cardiac or hepatic disease who needs parenteral nutrition. However, because of its inability to simultaneously control azotemia, SCUF has largely been replaced by continuous hemofiltration techniques.

Hemofiltration (HF) (Fig 7) overcomes the inability of SCUF to effectively remove solute. First, the permeability of the membrane filter is increased to the point where sieving coefficients approach 1 for most molecules up to a molecular weight of 25,000 d. Therefore, 1 L of ultrafiltrate equals 1 L of clearance for those molecules

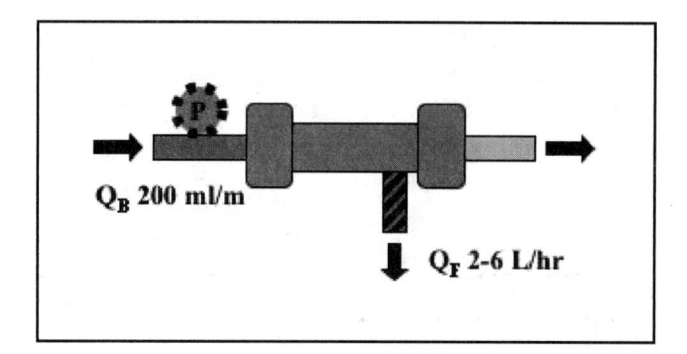

Figure 6. Slow continuous ultrafiltration (SCUF). Blood flow (Q_B) is generally slower than intermittent hemodialysis. No dialysate flows. Ultrafiltration volumes (Q_F) can approach 2-6 L/hr without hemodynamic instability. The primary clinical utility of SCUF is rapid ultrafiltration in a patient without need for solute removal.

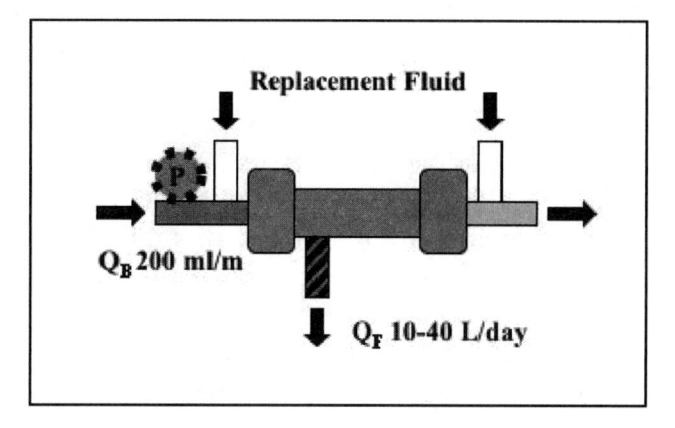

Figure 7. Continuous venovenous hemofiltration (CVVH). Highly permeable hemodialysis membranes allow high ultrafiltration rates (Q_F) necessitating replacement fluid. Solute removal is by convective transport. CVVH provides excellent solute and volume control without hemodynamic instability.

(*ie*, clearance rate equals UF rate). Second, the volume of UF (and therefore clearance) is increased several-fold (*eg*, 2 to 3 L/h, >40 L/d). Because the therapy is continuous, this quantity of UF enables solute clearance to approach and even surpass that of IHD on a daily or weekly basis. Of course, this massive rate of UF threatens hemodynamic stability. Therefore, replacement fluid is necessary as a substitute to ultrafiltrate. It is these two changes—increased membrane permeability and the need for replacement fluid—that distinguish HF from SCUF.

Replacement fluid is a simple crystalloid solution adjusted for the patient's individual needs. Generally, calcium, magnesium, and bicarbonate are added to 0.45 to 0.9% saline solution based on frequent laboratory evaluation (every 6 to 12 h).

Often, potassium and phosphorus also require replacement. The rate of administration depends on the patient's ECV and is adjusted to achieve the desired net hourly UF (net UF = actual UF – replacement volume). Replacement fluid can be administered either pre- or postfilter. Predilution improves UF rates and thus solute clearance, and lessens the need for anticoagulation. On the other hand, as UF volumes increase, logistics usually necessitate both pre- and postfilter infusion of replacement fluid. High volumes of room-temperature replacement fluid may induce hypothermia.

As solute clearance is equal to the UF rate, the efficacy of HF as a treatment of uremia is directly dependent on the daily UF volume. Increasing UF volume to 35 mL/kg/h will control azotemia in all but the most severely catabolic patients. If necessary, this convective clearance can be supplemented with a diffusive component by simply adding dialysate flow through the membrane. The dialysate utilized is either a lactate-based peritoneal dialysis solution or a basic crystalloid solution with bicarbonate added. Dialysate flow rates (usually 1 to 2 L/h) are much lower than with IHD. Adding this diffusion component transforms HF to hemodiafiltration (HDF) (Fig 8). However, at UF rates demonstrated to favorably influence survival (35 mL/kg/h), HDF is rarely, if ever, required.

Continuous arteriovenous hemofiltration or hemodiafiltration using the patient's own arteriovenous pressure gradient has largely been replaced by *continuous venovenous hemofiltration* (CVVH) or *continuous venovenous hemodiafiltration* (CVVHDF) requiring a blood pump. CVVH/CVVHDF avoids an arterial puncture and because it is pump-driven, Q_B is usually higher and more constant. This improves UF rates (and therefore clearance rates) and may modify the need for anticoagulation, although anticoagulation is required for these and all extracorporeal RRTs. Continuous heparin (infused prefilter) or regional citrate anticoagulation are both acceptable.[33]

The very porous membrane used for HF allows convective transport not only of small molecules such as urea, but also of larger molecules (so-called *middle molecules*) thought to contribute to the chronic uremic syndrome. Whether this has any impact on ARF or its survival is unknown. Perhaps the most intriguing feature of HF is its ability to remove even larger molecules (by filtration or adsorption), such as the proinflammatory cytokines tumor necrosis factor, interleukin-1 (IL-1), and IL-6. As mentioned, this offers the hope that HF may abrogate the systemic inflammatory response so often a feature of multiorgan failure and be useful as a primary therapy of sepsis, independently of its ability to treat renal failure. However, despite the removal of anti-inflammatory mediators such as IL-10, plasma levels of these cytokines usually remain constant, likely because of increased synthesis.[34] This might be overcome when short-term ultra-high-volume hemofiltration (35 L/4 h) is used as a "salvage" therapy for patients with refractory septic shock.[35] Nevertheless, to date there is no convincing evidence to support the use of HF as a treatment of sepsis alone.

Several adjustments to IHD can improve its inherent hemodynamic instability. These include slowing blood and dialysate flow rates to 200 and 100 mL/min, respectfully. Of course, both maneuvers will decrease the effectiveness of solute clearance, but this can be offset by longer dialysis times. Nocturnal hemodialysis employs these principles in patients with end-stage renal disease who, by dialyzing for 8 h per night, 6 to 7 nights per week, significantly improve not only solute clearance but also ECV and blood pressure control, mineral balance, and nutritional parameters while avoiding hypotensive episodes. This technique is gaining wider acceptance as a treatment for ARF as well.[36] Termed *sustained low-efficiency dialysis* (SLED) or *extended daily dialysis*, it is usually applied either continuously or for 8 to 12 h daily, thus avoiding immobilization and the inevitable

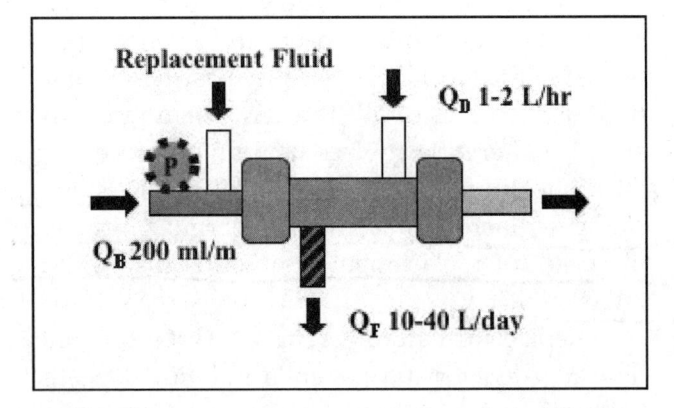

Figure 8. Continuous venovenous hemodiafiltration (CVVHDF). The addition of dialysate flow (Q_F) enhances the solute clearance of CVVH.

interruptions to continuous RRT (*eg*, surgery, procedures, radiology, etc). SLED is technically easier than CVVH/CVVHDF, as standard hemodialysis machines can be adapted to the lower flows and replacement fluid is unnecessary. Each contributes to generally lower cost. In addition, newer volumetric machines tightly control TMP, which permits the safe short-term use of highly permeable/high-flux dialysis membranes. This, coupled with a longer duration of dialysis, allows significant clearance of higher-molecular-weight solutes. Control of hypervolemia with hemodynamic stability is easily achieved with SLED.

CVVH/CVVHDF and SLED offer several theoretical advantages over IHD, including hemodynamic stability, more constant volume control and plasma solute concentrations, and higher weekly solute clearance. In addition, some clinicians suggest that IHD may actually prolong the course of ARF and adversely affect renal recovery and even patient survival. This could be related to episodes of hypotension, bioincompatibility of the dialysis membrane, or a relatively ineffective or inadequate dialysis. The topic of intensity or adequacy of dialysis has been at issue for some time. Although early studies[37,38] failed to demonstrate a significant survival benefit when patients with ARF underwent aggressive dialysis, these studies suffered from small sample size and several confounding variables including the use of bioincompatible membranes. More recently, three studies have directly correlated patient survival in ARF to the "dose" of RRT, regardless of the type of therapy. Schiffl and colleagues[39] demonstrated improved survival with IHD daily vs every other day. Ronco and colleagues[40] showed a survival benefit with CVVH UF rates at 35 or 45 mL/kg/h vs 25 mL/kg/h. Finally, Paganini and colleagues[41] directly correlated survival with the dose of RRT regardless of which RRT treatment was utilized. This latter study was particularly enlightening as it evaluated the influence of severity of illness on ARF requiring dialysis. At the extremes of illness (where patients either universally recovered or universally died despite therapy), dialysis dose appeared to have no effect. In the middle ranges of severity of illness, however, the dose of dialysis had a significant impact on survival. *These data suggest that when treating ARF with RRT, the dose delivered is more important than the modality selected.*

Direct comparison of CRRT vs IHD is difficult.[42] Uncontrolled trials and a recent meta-analysis suggest a slight survival advantage for CRRT.[43] However, most patients treated with IHD have historically received inadequate therapy. Slow and recirculating blood flow through central venous catheters, intradialyzer clotting due to inadequate anticoagulation, and early discontinuation or "bypass" of dialysis because of episodes of hypotension all likely contribute to this phenomenon. In addition, the weekly solute clearance of IHD can approach that of CRRT only if IHD is administered daily,[44] a practice not common in the United States until recently. On the other hand, CRRT has been applied to generally sicker patients, and this severity of illness appears to explain the excess in gross mortality attributed to CVVH in many studies.[45] A recent controlled trial directly comparing CRRT with IHD failed to demonstrate a survival advantage, although there was a slightly better renal recovery rate with CRRT.[46] Because the UF/clearance rates of IHD and CRRT in this study were relatively low, the fundamental question of which treatment is superior remains unanswered.

With no clear survival advantage established, the clinician is free to target a particular RRT to any given patient. When rapid solute control is necessary, *eg*, in a patient with severe hyperkalemia (rhabdomyolysis) or hyperuricemia (tumor lysis), IHD is most suitable. UF without dialysis (intermittently or SCUF) is best if volume overload without azotemia is the primary clinical problem. For hypotensive patients, we prefer either CVVH (particularly with sepsis and multisystem organ failure) or SLED. CVVH is also indicated when hepatic failure or head trauma complicate ARF. We primarily apply PD in the ICU only to those patients previously using PD who are not compromised by abdominal or respiratory problems. With extracorporeal techniques, filters with biocompatible or synthetic membranes should always be used.

Regardless of the particular RRT selected, the clinician must ensure an adequate dose of dialysis. Currently, no measure of dialysis adequacy allows comparison of different RRTs applied to patients with ARF.[47] Nevertheless, the data cited above suggest that survival in dialysis-requiring ARF is directly related to dialysis dose, *ie*, more is better. We therefore suggest the following "dosing guideline": IHD, 5 to 7 days weekly; CVVH or CVVHDF, ≥35 mL/kg/h UF; SLED, 8 to 12 h daily. This guideline should ensure the objectives of adequate solute and volume control in the vast majority of patients requiring RRT in the ICU.

Prognosis and Recovery

In most clinical series, mortality from ARF continues to average 50%. Mortality in nonoliguric patients may be as low as 25%; with oliguric ARF, it approaches 70%. The major determinants of outcome include preexisting renal function, precipitating event, the severity of comorbid conditions, and the number of complications. ARF associated with ventilatory failure, sepsis, trauma, abdominal catastrophe, and burns carries a mortality rate of 70 to 90%, but the mortality rate is 25 to 30% for patients with ARF caused by aminoglycosides, radiographic contrast, or other drug reactions.[48,49]

Mortality from ARF approaches 100% if three or more major organ systems have failed simultaneously. Mortality is highest in the very young and very old. The dose of dialysis (solute removal) appears to directly improve survival, while the severity of azotemia and the choice of dialysis modality do not. Again, the use of biocompatible dialysis membranes improves survival in those patients requiring dialysis.

Infection is the most common cause of death and is usually due to overwhelming sepsis from resistant Gram-negative bacteria or yeast. Other common causes of death are cardiovascular compromise (*eg*, strokes and myocardial infarction), respiratory failure (often with nosocomial pneumonia), and GI bleeding.

If the patient with ARF survives, recovery is usually prompt and sufficient to achieve dialysis independence (although as many as 50% of patients have decrements in GFR–or defects in urinary acidification and concentrating ability). Oliguria (if present) averages 10 to 14 days. Urinary volume recovers gradually during the next 3 to 7 days. Fluid therapy is needed to support this obligatory diuretic phase. Although the BUN and creatinine levels continue to rise during this phase, dialysis can usually be discontinued. Most survivors regain renal function within 30 days; rarely, a patient requires 60 to 90 days to recover. In one large series, 95% of survivors regained renal function, almost all within 30 days.[50] Those patients who have delayed or no recovery are usually older, have preexisting renal insufficiency, or suffer severe ischemic insults to the kidney.

References

1. Doty JM, Saggi BH, Sugarman HJ, et al. Effect of increased renal venous pressure on renal function. J Trauma 1999; 47:1000-1003
2. Espinel CH, Gregory AW. Differential diagnosis of acute renal failure. Clin Nephrol 1980; 13:73-77
3. Brosins FL, Lau K. Low fractional excretion of sodium in acute renal failure: role timing of the test and ischemia. Am J Nephrol 1986; 6:450-457
4. Diamond JR, Yoburn DC. Nonoliguric acute renal failure associated with a low fractional excretion of sodium. Ann Intern Med 1982; 96:597-600
5. Kaplan AA, Kohn OF. Fractional excretion of urea as a guide to renal dysfunction. Am J Nephrol 1992; 12:49-54
6. Liano F, Junco E, Pascual J, et al. Epidemiology of acute renal failure: a prospective, multicenter, community-based study. Kidney Int 1996; 53:811-818
7. Reid GM, Muther RS. Nitroprusside-induced acute azotemia. Am J Nephrol 1987; 7:313-315
8. Gines A, Escorsell A, Gines P, et al. Incidence, predictive factors, and treatment of the hepatorenal syndrome with ascites. Gastroenterology 1993; 105:229-236
9. Epstein M. Hepatorenal syndrome: emerging perspectives of pathophysiology and therapy. J Am Soc Nephrol 1994; 4:1735-1753
10. Uriz J, Gines P, Cardenas A, et al. Terlipressin plus albumin infusion: an effective and safe therapy of hepatorenal syndrome. J Hepatol 2000; 33:43-48
11. Angeli P, Volpin R, Gerunda G, et al. Reversal of type 1 hepatorenal syndrome with the administration of midodrine and octreotide. Hepatology 1999; 29:1690-1697
12. Merten GJ, Burgess WP, Gray LV, et al. Prevention of contrast-induced nephropathy with sodium bicarbonate: a randomized controlled trial. JAMA 2004; 291:2328-2334
13. Tepel M, van der Giet M, Schwarzfeld C, et al. Prevention of radiographic-contrast-agent-induced reductions in renal function by acetylcysteine. N Engl J Med 2000; 343:180-184

14. Hadjis T, Grieff M, Locknat D, et al. Calcium metabolism in acute renal failure due to rhabdomyolysis. Clin Nephrol 1993; 39:22-27
15. Brezis M, Rosen SN. Hypoxemia of the renal medulla—its implications for disease. N Engl J Med 1995; 332:647-655
16. Schrier RW, Wang W. Acute renal failure and sepsis. N Engl J Med 2004; 351:159-169
17. Bonventre JV. Mechanisms of ischemic acute renal failure. Kidney Int 1993; 43:1160-1178
18. Toback FG. Regeneration after acute tubular necrosis. Kidney Int 1992; 41:226-246
19. Anderson RJ, Linas SL, Berns AS, et al. Nonoliguric acute renal failure. N Engl J Med 1977; 296:1134-1138
20. Bellomo R, Chapman M, Finfer S, et al. Low-dose dopamine in patients with early renal dysfunction: a placebo-controlled randomised trial. Australian and New Zealand Intensive Care Society (ANZICS) Clinical Trials Group. Lancet 2000; 356:2139-2143
21. Fiaccadori E, Lombardi M, Leonardi S, et al. Prevalence and clinical outcome associated with preexisting malnutrition in acute renal failure: a prospective cohort study. J Am Soc Nephrol 1999; 10:581-593
22. Aronoff GR, Berns JS, Brier ME, et al. Drug prescribing in renal failure: dosing guidelines for adults. 4th ed. Philadelphia, PA: American College of Physicians, 1999
23. Szeto HH, Inturrisi CE, Saal S, et al. Accumulation of normeperidine, an active metabolite of meperidine, in patients with renal failure or cancer. Ann Intern Med 1977; 86:738-741
24. Bauer LA, Black D, Gensler A, et al. Influence of age, renal function and heart failure on procainamide clearance and N-acetylprocainamide serum concentrations. Int J Clin Pharmacol Ther Toxicol 1989; 27:213-216
25. Aronoff GR, Berns JS, Brier ME, et al. Drug prescribing in renal failure: dosing guidelines for adults. 4th ed. Philadelphia, PA: American College of Physicians, 1999; 19
26. Borga O, Hoppel C, Odar-Cederlof I, et al. Plasma levels and renal excretion of phenytoin and its metabolites in patients with renal failure. Clin Pharmacol Ther 1979; 26:306-314
27. Soundararajan R, Golper TA. Medical management of the dialysis patient undergoing surgery. In: Rose BD, ed. UpToDate [CD-ROM]. Wellesley, MA: UpToDate, 2001
28. Montoliu J, Lens XM, Revert L. Potassium-lowering effect of albuterol for hyperkalemia in renal failure. Arch Intern Med 1987; 147:713-717
29. Cheung AK. Biocompatibility of hemodialysis membranes. J Am Soc Nephrol 1990; 1:150-161
30. Schiffl H, Lang SM, Konig A, et al. Biocompatible membranes in acute renal failure: a case-controlled study. Lancet 1994; 344:570-572
31. Hakim RM, Wingard RL, Parker RA. Effect of the dialysis membrane in the treatment of patients with acute renal failure. N Engl J Med 1994; 331:1338-1342
32. Himmelfarb J, Tolkoff Rubin N, Chandran P, et al. A multicenter comparison of dialysis membranes in the treatment of acute renal failure requiring dialysis. J Am Soc Nephrol 1998; 9:257-266
33. Monchi M, Berghmans D, Ledoux D, et al. Citrate vs heparin for anticoagulation in continuous venovenous hemofiltration: a prospective randomized study. Intensive Care Med 2004; 30:260-265
34. De Vriese AS, Colardyn FA, Philippe JJ, et al. Cytokine removal during continuous hemofiltration in septic patients. J Am Soc Nephrol 1999; 10:846-853
35. Honore PM, Jamez J, Wauthier M, et al. Prospective evaluation of short-term, high-volume isovolemic hemofiltration on the hemodynamic course and outcome in patients with intractable circulatory failure resulting from septic shock. Crit Care Med 2000; 28:3581-3587
36. Marshall MR, Golper TA, Shaver MJ, et al. Sustained low-efficiency dialysis for critically ill patients requiring renal replacement therapy. Kidney Int 2001; 60:777-785
37. Conger JD. A controlled evaluation of prophylactic dialysis in post-traumatic acute renal failure. J Trauma 1975; 15:1056-1063
38. Gillum DM, Dixon BS, Yanover MJ, et al. The role of intensive dialysis in acute renal failure. Clin Nephrol 1986; 25:249-255
39. Schiffl H, Lang SM, Fischer R. Daily hemodialysis and the outcome of acute renal failure. N Engl J Med 2002; 346:305-310
40. Ronco R, Bellomo R, Homel P, et al. Effects of different doses in continuous veno-venous haemofiltration on outcomes of acute renal failure: a prospective randomized trial. Lancet 2000; 355:26-30
41. Paganini EP, Tapolyai M, Goormastic M, et al. Establishing a dialysis therapy patient outcome

link in intensive care unit acute dialysis for patients with acute renal failure. Am J Kidney Dis 1996; 28(suppl 3):S81-S89

42. Karsou SA, Jaber BL, Pereira BJ. Impact of intermittent hemodialysis variables on clinical outcomes in acute renal failure. Am J Kidney Dis 2000; 35:980-991

43. Kellum JA, Leblanc M, Angus DC, et al. Continuous versus intermittent renal replacement therapy: is there a difference? (abstract) Crit Care Med 1999; 27:A63

44. Clark WR, Mueller BA, Kraus MA, et al. Extracorporeal therapy requirements for patients with acute renal failure. J Am Soc Nephrol 1997; 8:804-812

45. Swartz RD, Messana JM, Orzol S, et al. Comparing continuous hemofiltration with hemodialysis in patients with severe acute renal failure. Am J Kidney Dis 1999; 34:424-432

46. Mehta RL, McDonald B, Gabbai FB, et al. A randomized clinical trial of continuous versus intermittent dialysis for acute renal failure. Kidney Int 2001; 60:1154-1163

47. Evanson JA, Himmelfarb J, Wingard R, et al. Prescribed versus delivered dialysis in acute renal failure patients. Am J Kidney Dis 1998; 32:731-738

48. Spurney RF, Fulkerson WJ, Schwab SJ. Acute renal failure in critically ill patients: prognosis for recovery of kidney function after prolonged dialysis support. Crit Care Med 1991; 19:8-11

49. McCarthy JT. Prognosis of patients with acute renal failure in the intensive care unit: a tale of two eras. Mayo Clin Proc 1996; 7:117-126

50. Morgera S, Kraft AK, Siebert G, et al. Long-term outcomes in acute renal failure patients treated with continuous renal replacement therapies. Am J Kidney Dis 2002; 40:275-279

Notes

Notes

Poisonings and Overdoses

Janice Zimmerman, MD, FCCP

Objectives:

- To describe physical examination and laboratory findings suggestive of intoxications
- To outline measures for the resuscitation and stabilization of the overdose patient
- To discuss use of interventions to decrease absorption of poisons and enhance elimination
- To review indicated interventions and antidotes for poisons and substances of abuse likely to be encountered in the ICU

Key words: antidotes; overdose; poisoning; substance abuse; toxicology

---

Intentional and accidental poisonings and substance abuse can result in the need for critical care support. In many cases, only supportive care is necessary until the effects of the toxin diminish. However, some poisonings require specific antidotes or interventions to decrease morbidity and mortality. General management principles of poisonings and substance abuse that are pertinent to intensive care management are presented, as well as interventions for specific overdoses that the intensivist is likely to encounter. Little evidence-based information is available and current recommendations are based on animal data, volunteer studies, case reports, pharmacologic data, and/or consensus opinion.

Clinical Presentation

Patients with possible overdose may be asymptomatic or present with life-threatening toxicities. The absence of symptoms on initial examination does not preclude potential deterioration and development of more severe symptoms. Life-threatening toxicities that often require intensive management include coma, seizures, respiratory depression, hypoxemia, arrhythmias, hypotension, hypertension, and metabolic acidosis.

Diagnosis

The diagnosis of the exact substance involved in an overdose or poisoning should not take precedence over resuscitation and stabilization of the patient (see "Management"). However, the initial evaluation of the patient may identify characteristic signs and symptoms that will enable the physician to make a specific diagnosis quickly and assist in directing optimal therapy.

History

Accurate information regarding the substance ingested, the quantity taken, and the time of ingestion should be collected, if possible. Establishing the time of ingestion is important to assess the significance of presenting symptoms. Drugs that may be accessible to the patient should be determined.

Physical Examination

Vital signs and the neurologic examination are particularly helpful in the initial evaluation of a patient. Tables 1 and 2 list drugs associated with changes in vital signs and neurologic alterations. Blood pressure may not be helpful in determining the toxin because of other systemic influences. Tachypnea is also fairly nonspecific and may be a compensatory response to metabolic acidosis or hypoxemia. Although the initial neurologic examination may be pertinent, it is also important to follow changes in neurologic function over time. Hypoactive bowel sounds may be associated with narcotic or anticholinergic agents, and hyperactive bowel sounds may result from poisoning with organophosphates.

Toxidromes

Findings on physical examination may enable the physician to characterize the poisoning into a classic "toxidrome." This classification may allow the physician to direct diagnostic evaluation and define appropriate therapy (Table 3).

Table 1. Clues to Diagnosis in Poisoning: Vital Signs

Vital Sign	Increased	Decreased
Blood pressure	Amphetamines/cocaine Anticholinergics Ephedrine Sympathomimetics	Antihypertensives Cyanide Cyclic antidepressants Ethanol Narcotics Organophosphates/carbamates Sedative/hypnotics
Heart rate	Amphetamines/cocaine Anticholinergics Carbon monoxide Cyanide Cyclic antidepressants Ethanol Sympathomimetics Theophylline	Barbiturates β-Blockers Calcium channel blockers Cholinergics Digitalis glycosides Sedative/hypnotics Organophosphates/carbamates γ-Hydroxybutyrate
Respiratory rate	Amphetamines Anticholinergics Carbon monoxide Hydrocarbons Organophosphates/carbamates Salicylates Theophylline	Alcohols Barbiturates γ-Hydroxybutyrate Narcotics Sedative/hypnotics
Temperature	Amphetamines/cocaine Anticholinergics β-Blockers Cyclic antidepressants Salicylates Sympathomimetics Theophylline	Barbiturates Carbon monoxide Ethanol Hypoglycemic agents Narcotics Sedative/hypnotics

Laboratory Examination

Effective use of laboratory data supplements the history and physical examination. An arterial blood gas measurement will detect hypoxemia, hypercarbia, and significant acid-base disorders. In combination with electrolytes, a significant anion-gap acidosis may be diagnosed. The detection of an osmolal gap (>10) through comparison of the measured osmolality with calculated osmolality—(2 × sodium + glucose/18) + (BUN/2.8)—may indicate the presence of methanol, ethanol, ethylene glycol, acetone, or isopropyl alcohol. An ECG should be obtained in unstable patients and when cardiotoxic drug ingestion is suspected.

Qualitative toxicology screens are performed on urine samples. These tests report only the presence or absence of a substance or class of drugs and are limited by the testing available at an institution. Qualitative toxicology screens are helpful in evaluating coma of unknown cause, distinguishing between toxicosis and psychosis, and (rarely) choosing a specific antidote. Qualitative test results seldom change the initial management of poisoned patients. Quantitative analyses provide serum levels and may direct specific therapies in selected cases. Quantitative levels that are particularly helpful in the patient with unknown poisoning are acetaminophen and salicylate levels. Other quantitative levels that may be useful include carbamazepine, carboxyhemoglobin, ethanol, methanol, ethylene glycol, theophylline, phenytoin, lithium, barbiturates, digoxin, and cyclic-antidepressant levels. Cyclic antidepressant levels confirm antidepressant ingestion, but the levels correlate poorly with toxicity.

Table 2. *Clues to Diagnosis in Poisoning: Neurologic Findings*

Vital Sign	Increased	Decreased
Pupils	*Pinpoint (Miotic)* Barbiturates (late) Cholinergics Narcotics (except meperidine) Organophosphates Phenothiazine Phencyclidine	*Dilated (Mydriatic)* Alcohol Anticholinergics Antihistamines Barbiturates Ethanol Meperidine Phenytoin Sympathomimetics
Nystagmus	Alcohols Carbamazepine Carbon monoxide	Phencyclidine Phenytoin Sedative/hypnotics
Seizures	Amphetamines Anticholinergics Carbon monoxide Cocaine Cyanide Cyclic antidepressants γ-Hydroxybutyrate Isoniazid	Lithium Organophosphates Phencyclidine Phenothiazines Salicylates Strychnine Theophylline

Table 3. *Toxidromes*

Poisoning Syndrome	Symptoms
Cholinergic (SLUDGE)	Salivation, lacrimation, urination, defecation, GI upset, emesis. Also, bradycardia, fasciculations, confusion, miosis
Anticholinergic	Dry skin, hyperthermia, mydriasis, tachycardia, delirium, thirst, urinary retention
Sympathomimetic	Hypertension, tachycardia, seizures, CNS excitation, mydriasis, diaphoresis
Narcotic	Miosis, respiratory depression, depressed level of consciousness, hypotension hyporeflexia
Sedative/hypnotic	Depressed level of consciousness, respiratory depression, hypotension, hyporeflexia

Management

Resuscitation and Stabilization

The initial priorities are airway, breathing, and circulation. Intubation may be necessary to support oxygenation and ventilation or to protect the airway. Hypotension from toxins is more commonly due to venous pooling, rather than myocardial depression, and should be initially treated with isotonic fluids, rather than vasopressor agents. Oxygen should be routinely administered to the poisoning victim, pending assessment of oxygenation by arterial blood gas or pulse oximetry.

In the patient with a depressed level of consciousness, the following additional interventions should be considered:

- 50% glucose (25 to 50 g)
- Thiamine (100 mg IV)
- Naloxone (0.4 to 2 mg IV), especially with classic findings of miosis and respiratory depression
- Flumazenil is not routinely recommended. Consider administration in patients who have a clinical course compatible with a sedative overdose. Flumazenil is contraindicated in known cyclic-antidepressant overdoses and in chronic benzodiazepine users because of the risk of seizures.

Nonspecific Therapy

After stabilization, nonspecific interventions may be considered to decrease absorption of toxin from the GI tract or to enhance elimination. GI decontamination can be attempted with gastric emptying procedures (induced emesis, gastric lavage), adsorption of drugs (activated charcoal), and decreasing transit time in the GI tract (cathartics, whole bowel irrigation).

Induced Emesis: Induced emesis with ipecac is not recommended in adults or children. Ipecac is effective in inducing vomiting but is not necessarily effective in recovering toxins. Contraindications to the use of ipecac include hydrocarbon or corrosive ingestion, absent gag reflex, depressed mental status, a risk for CNS depression or seizures, and pregnancy. Potential complications include aspiration pneumonitis, Mallory-Weiss tear, and protracted emesis, that delays the use of activated charcoal.

Gastric Lavage: Gastric lavage is performed in the adult with a 36F to 40F Ewald tube inserted orally. Lavage is performed with aliquots of 100 to 200 mL of normal saline solution or water. Some studies indicated that the greatest benefit of lavage in obtunded patients occurs within 1 h of ingestion, but more recent studies have failed to confirm any benefit. Current recommendations suggest that gastric lavage should not be used routinely, and should be considered only in life-threatening cases of ingestion when lavage can be instituted within 1 h of ingestion. The airway must be protected in patients with depressed level of consciousness. Lavage is contraindicated in acid or alkali ingestions because of possible esophageal perforation and in the presence of a severe bleeding diathesis. Complications of lavage include aspiration pneumonitis, esophageal perforation, and cardiovascular instability.

Activated Charcoal: Activated charcoal is probably the best intervention in poisonings and should be administered in most cases of orally ingested toxins. The greatest benefit is within the first hour after ingestion. The appropriate dose of charcoal (1 g/kg) may be administered by an orogastric or nasogastric tube if patient cooperation is limited. Substances not adsorbed by activated charcoal include iron, lithium, cyanide, strong acids or bases, alcohols, and hydrocarbons. The only contraindication to the use of charcoal is known or suspected GI perforation.

Current recommendations for decreasing GI absorption of toxins emphasize the use of activated charcoal despite lack of proven benefit. In patients who are critically ill on hospital presentation or who have a potentially life-threatening ingestion, gastric lavage plus activated charcoal can be considered, although the benefit of lavage has not been established.

Cathartics: Cathartics have been routinely administered with charcoal, based on the assumption that they decrease GI transit time, help limit drug absorption, and serve as an adjunct to charcoal therapy. However, there is no evidence of efficacy. Sorbitol is the most commonly used cathartic. Care must be taken with the very young and with elderly patients because electrolyte abnormalities can ensue due to diarrhea.

Whole Bowel Irrigation: Whole bowel irrigation involves large volumes of polyethylene glycol electrolyte solution given over time (1 to 2 L/h) to mechanically cleanse the bowel. This method has been recommended for ingested substances that are not adsorbed by activated charcoal (*ie*, iron and lithium), ingestions of sustained-release or enteric-coated products, and ingestions of illicit drug packets. This method may not be practical for many patients; further study is required to determine any benefit in toxic ingestions. Contraindications to this intervention include ileus, GI obstruction or perforation, hemodynamic instability, and intractable vomiting; CNS or respiratory depression and inability to cooperate are relative contraindications.

Enhanced Elimination: Measures to increase elimination of toxic substances attempt to utilize the normal detoxification mechanisms performed by the liver and kidney. Multiple doses of charcoal for drugs with an enterohepatic circulation may have the greatest potential utility. This technique may be helpful in poisonings with barbiturates, carbamazepine, quinine, dapsone, and theophylline. Although multiple doses of charcoal have been used in poisonings with cyclic antidepressants, digoxin and phenytoin, proof of effectiveness is lacking. The dosing regimen has not been standardized, but currently not <12.5 g/h or an equivalent amount at other intervals is recommended. Smaller doses administered more frequently may decrease the occurrence of vomiting. Repeat doses of charcoal should not contain a cathartic. Adequate gastric emptying must be assured before administration of a subsequent dose.

Forced diuresis to accelerate renal excretion of drugs has little clinical effect and may predispose to volume overload. Alkaline diuresis is effective in promoting the elimination of barbiturates and salicylates. Two ampules of sodium bicarbonate can be added to 1 L of dextrose 5% in water solution, and the rate of administration should be determined by the patient's ability to handle the fluid load and the maintenance of urine pH > 7. Acidification of urine has been proposed for ingestions involving phencyclidine, strychnine, amphetamines, and quinine. However, the metabolic consequences of acidification weigh against any clinical usefulness of this measure. Dialysis may be considered for life-threatening ingestions involving water-soluble substances of low molecular weight. Drug overdoses in which dialysis may be beneficial include alcohols, amphetamines, phenobarbital, lithium, salicylates, theophylline, and thiocyanate. Hemoperfusion is useful with the same compounds that are dialyzable and involves the passing of blood through a filtering device that contains charcoal or a synthetic resin as an absorbent. Charcoal hemoperfusion may be helpful in elimination of carbamazepine, phenobarbital, phenytoin, and theophylline. Hemodialysis and hemoperfusion are efficient methods of removing poisons but are costly, require trained personnel, and may be associated with complications. Use of continuous arteriovenous or venovenous hemoperfusion in poisoning has been reported on a limited basis.

Specific Therapy

Although management of many toxic ingestions involves only the nonspecific therapy outlined above, some toxins have specific interventions or antidotes. Table 4 lists toxins and their respective antidotes. Specific poisonings are discussed in detail below. Attention should be directed to managing those poisonings that most frequently result in death: analgesics, sedatives and hypnotics, antidepressants, stimulants and street drugs, cardiovascular drugs, and alcohols.

Specific Drug Poisonings

Acetaminophen

Knowledge of appropriate management of acetaminophen ingestions is important to prevent significant toxicity and mortality. Acetaminophen levels should be obtained in all multiple drug overdoses ≥4 h after ingestion. The Rumack-Matthew nomogram determines the need for N-acetylcysteine (NAC) therapy (140 mg/kg oral loading dose; 70 mg/kg orally every 4 h for 72 h) if the level plots above the "possible hepatic toxicity" line. An intravenous formulation of NAC (Cumberland Pharmaceuticals Inc.) is now available in the United States. It is administered as a loading dose of 150 mg/kg IV over 15 min and maintenance dose of 50 mg/kg over 4 h followed by 100 mg/kg over 16 h. In a safety study, 17% developed an anaphylactoid reaction. NAC serves as a substitute for glutathione, which normally metabolizes toxic metabolites of acetaminophen. Activated charcoal adsorbs acetaminophen and many co-ingestants. Charcoal interferes only slightly with the effectiveness of NAC, and the dose of NAC does not require adjustment. NAC is most effective in the first 8 h but is recommended up to 24 h after a significant ingestion. It is also reasonable to administer NAC > 24 h after ingestion if toxic levels of acetaminophen are present. Late administration of NAC may be potentially beneficial in fulminant hepatic failure due to

Table 4. *Antidotes and Interventions for Specific Toxins*

Toxin	Antidote or Intervention
Acetaminophen	N-acetylcysteine
Arsenic/mercury/gold/lead	BAL (dimercaprol)
Benzodiazepines	Flumazenil
β-Blocker	Glucagon, calcium (?), pacing
Calcium channel blocker	Calcium, glucagon, pacing
Carbon monoxide	100% oxygen, hyperbaric oxygen
Coumarin derivatives	Vitamin K_1
Cyanide	Nitrites, thiosulfate, hydroxocobalamin
Cyclic antidepressants	Blood alkalinization
Digoxin	Digoxin-specific Fab fragments
Ethylene glycol	Ethanol, fomepizole
Heparin	Protamine
Oral hypoglycemic agents/insulin	Glucose 50%, somatostatin
Iron	Deferoxamine
Isoniazid	Pyridoxine
Lithium	Hemodialysis
Methanol	Ethanol
Narcotics	Naloxone
Nitrites	Methylene blue
Organophosphates/carbamates	Atropine, pralidoxime
Salicylates	Urinary alkalinization, hemodialysis
Theophylline	Multiple-dose charcoal, hemoperfusion

Reprinted with permission from Critical Care Refresher Course, 2003. DesPlaines, IL: Society of Critical Care Medicine, 2003.

acetaminophen toxicity. The nomogram is useful only for single acute ingestions, and there are no firm guidelines for administration of NAC in chronic ingestions or multiple ingestions over time. A course of NAC should be strongly considered if hepatic enzymes are elevated at presentation. Antiemetics are frequently needed to improve tolerance of oral NAC. The local Poison Control Center should be contacted for other NAC regimens, such as shorter courses of therapy.

Recommendations for management of extended-release forms of acetaminophen include determination of acetaminophen levels 4 and 8 h after ingestion and initiation of NAC if either level is potentially toxic.

Alcohols

Ethylene glycol and methanol ingestions can result in significant morbidity and mortality. Clinical manifestations, metabolic derangements, and management are similar for both alcohols.

Cardiopulmonary and neurologic symptoms may include pulmonary edema, hypotension, ataxia, seizures, and coma. Abdominal pain, nausea, and vomiting are frequent. Visual disturbances (blurred vision, photophobia, blindness, optic disc hyperemia) suggest methanol toxicity, and the finding of urinary calcium oxalate crystals may indicate ethylene glycol ingestion. Significant symptoms may be delayed up to 24 h after methanol ingestion. Both ingestions are classically characterized by an anion gap metabolic acidosis and an osmolal gap. An anion gap metabolic acidosis may not be present initially if sufficient time has not elapsed for metabolism to toxic acids or high levels of ethanol prevent metabolism of other alcohols. An osmolar gap may not be present in late presentations if the alcohol has already been metabolized to acid. Many institutions are unable to provide blood levels of methanol or ethylene glycol in a timely manner, and treatment is initiated based on the clinical history and acid-base status.

Treatment of ethylene glycol and methanol ingestion includes the following:

- Maintenance of a secure airway
- Gastric lavage may be considered within 1 h of ingestion.
- Activated charcoal if other substances have potentially been ingested (does not adsorb alcohols)
- 50% glucose if indicated
- Thiamine, folate, multivitamin supplement
- Folinic acid (leucovorin) 50 mg can be administered every 4 to 6 hours for 24 hours in methanol ingestions to provide the cofactor for formic acid elimination.
- Hydration to maintain urine output.
- Ethanol orally or IV to maintain blood level at 100 to 150 mg/dL—ethanol is preferentially metabolized by alcohol dehydrogenase. A loading dose is followed by a maintenance infusion.
- Fomepizole (4-methylpyrazole), an inhibitor of alcohol dehydrogenase that does not cause CNS depression, may substitute for ethanol.
- Hemodialysis for visual impairment, renal failure, pulmonary edema, significant or refractory acidosis, level of >25 mg/dL
- Bicarbonate for acidosis is advocated by some clinicians.

Isopropyl alcohol is more potent than ethanol and results in similar manifestations at lower doses. Isopropyl alcohol ingestions are characterized by an osmolar gap and ketonemia/ketonuria but no metabolic acidosis. Treatment is supportive and may require intubation and mechanical ventilation for respiratory depression. Hemodialysis is reserved for evidence of hypoperfusion and failure to respond to supportive therapy.

Amphetamines/Methamphetamines

Amphetamines, methamphetamines, and related agents cause release of catecholamines, which results in a sympathomimetic toxidrome characterized by tachycardia, hyperthermia, agitation, hypertension, and mydriasis. Hallucinations (visual and tactile) and acute psychosis are frequently observed. Acute adverse consequences include myocardial ischemia and arrhythmias, seizures, intracranial hemorrhage, stroke, rhabdomyolysis, renal failure, necrotizing vasculitis, and death.

An amphetaminelike drug, 3-4-methylenedioxymethamphetamine, is a designer drug associated with "rave" parties. It is commonly known as ecstasy, XTC, E, and MDMA, and acts as a stimulant and hallucinogen. It increases release of serotonin and inhibits serotonin reuptake in the brain. Bruxism and jaw clenching are clues to use of ecstasy. Complications are usually a result of drug effects and nonstop physical activity. Hyponatremia and liver injury progressing to fulminant failure have also been reported.

Management of amphetamine intoxication is primarily supportive. Gastric lavage has little role, since absorption after oral ingestion is usually complete at the time of presentation. The patient should be carefully assessed for complications, including measuring of core temperature, obtaining an ECG, and evaluating laboratory data for evidence of renal dysfunction and rhabdomyolysis. IV hydration for possible rhabdomyolysis is warranted in individuals with known exertional activities pending creatine phosphokinase results. Benzodiazepines, often in high doses, are useful for control of agitation.

Benzodiazepines

Benzodiazepine overdoses rarely result in death unless other sedating drugs (*eg*, alcohol, narcotics) are also ingested. A benzodiazepine receptor antagonist, flumazenil, is available as a diagnostic tool and adjunctive treatment. Flumazenil should not be considered a substitute for intubation in patients with significant respiratory depression. Its use is contraindicated in suspected cyclic-antidepressant overdoses and in patients physically dependent on benzodiazepines because of the risk of seizures. The initial dose of flumazenil is 0.2 mg over an interval of 30 s, followed by doses of 0.3 mg and 0.5 mg every minute up to a cumulative dose of 3 mg. Resedation is likely due to the short half-life of flumazenil (0.7 to 1.3 h) compared with benzodiazepines. Flunitrazepam is a potent benzodiazepine banned in the United States that is associated with rape. It may not be detected by most urine drug screens.

β-Blockers

β-Adrenergic blockers produce toxicity primarily through bradycardia and hypotension although depressed level of consciousness may occur with lipid soluble agents (propranolol, timolol, metoprolol and acebutolol). Hypotension often results from negative inotropic effects rather than bradycardia. Glucagon is considered the initial drug of choice because it produces chronotropic and inotropic effects and does not act via β-receptors. An initial dose of 2 to 5 mg of glucagon is given IV and an infusion of 2 to 10 mg/h can be initiated, adjusted for desired clinical effects, and then tapered over 12 h as indicated. The goal of treatment is improvement in blood pressure and perfusion rather than an increase in heart rate. Transcutaneous pacing and transvenous pacing may be considered in cases refractory to glucagon. Additional drugs that have had variable efficacy in β-blocker overdoses include atropine, epinephrine, isoproterenol, and dopamine. Phosphodiesterase inhibitors such as milrinone, intra-aortic balloon pump, or cardiopulmonary bypass may be considered if there is no response to these interventions. In some cases, calcium and insulin euglycemia have been reported to be beneficial.

Calcium Channel Blockers

Calcium-channel-blocker overdose should be considered in the hypotensive, bradycardic patient, particularly if there is a history of use of antihypertensive agents. In the presence of hemodynamic instability, 10 mL of 10% calcium chloride should be administered IV. Calcium is effective in reversing negative inotropic effects and conduction abnormalities in ~50% of overdoses. Higher doses of calcium and continuous infusions may be required for beneficial effects. As in β-blocker overdose, glucagon may have beneficial effects. Transcutaneous and transvenous pacing are additional options in refractory cases. Successful treatment has also been reported with amrinone and insulin euglycemia (insulin 0.1 to 10 U/kg/h and glucose 10 to 75 g/h).

Carbon Monoxide

Carbon monoxide is a colorless, odorless gas that has 240 times greater affinity for hemoglobin as oxygen. Carboxyhemoglobin reduces oxygen-carrying capacity and also shifts the oxyhemoglobin dissociation curve to the left. Carbon monoxide also exerts direct cellular toxic effects. The clinical manifestations of carbon monoxide poisoning are nonspecific. The most common findings are headache, dizziness, and nausea; more severe exposure can result in chest pain, disorientation, seizures, coma, dyspnea, weakness, arrhythmias, and hypotension. Although the diagnosis of carbon monoxide poisoning is confirmed by an increased venous or arterial carboxyhemoglobin level, decisions for aggressive therapy with 100% oxygen should be based primarily on a clinical history suggestive of exposure. High-flow oxygen or intubation with administration of 100% oxygen should be initiated as soon as possible while confirmatory tests are obtained. An ECG, chest radiograph, and arterial blood gas measurement should be obtained to assess severity of toxicity. The finding of metabolic acidosis implies significant exposure with inadequate oxygen availability at the tissue level. The use of hyperbaric oxygen in the setting of carbon monoxide poisoning is debated but may be considered for any patient with a depressed level of consciousness, loss of consciousness, neurologic findings other than headache, cardiac ischemia or arrhythmia, carboxyhemoglobin level >25 to 40%, or persistent symptoms after normobaric oxygen treatment for 4 to 6 h. A recent clinical trial suggests that hyperbaric oxygen decreases the incidence of postexposure cognitive deficits.

Cocaine

Significant morbidity and mortality are associated with cocaine use by all routes, including nasal insufflation, IV administration, smoking, and oral ingestion. Toxicities include intracranial hemorrhage (subarachnoid and intraparenchymal), cerebrovascular accidents, seizures, noncardiogenic pulmonary edema, arrhythmias, hypertension, myocardial ischemia, barotrauma, bronchospasm, bowel ischemia, hyperthermia, and rhabdomyolysis. These potential morbidities should be considered in any critically ill cocaine abuser, and treatment should be initiated as indicated. Chest pain thought to be ischemic usually responds to nitroglycerin and/or benzodiazepines. Aspirin should be administered. Phentolamine is considered a second-line agent for chest pain. Thrombolysis for myocardial infarction should be considered only when other interventions have failed and immediate angiography and angioplasty are not available. In severe hypertension, labetolol may be the drug of choice because it has both α- and β-adrenergic blocking properties. In most cases, IV fluid hydration should be instituted until rhabdomyolysis can be excluded. Rhabdomyolysis is enhanced by high environmental temperatures and increased physical activity. The agitation and combativeness frequently associated with cocaine use can usually be controlled with benzodiazepines. If frank psychosis is present, neuroleptics such as haloperidol are indicated, although there is a potential concern of lowering the seizure threshold.

Cyanide

Cyanide exposure is rare, but may occur in occupational settings involving metal extraction, electroplating, chemical synthesis, and firefighting. Cyanide inhibits cytochrome oxidase, which halts oxidative phosphorylation. Metabolic acidosis and decreased oxygen consumption result. Symptoms include nausea and vomiting, agitation, and tachycardia. Serious poisonings can result in seizures, coma, apnea, hypotension, and arrhythmias. Additional complications include rhabdomyolysis, hepatic necrosis, and ARDS. Diagnosis may be difficult in the absence of an exposure history. A cyanide antidote kit (Taylor Pharmaceuticals; San Clemente, CA) is used for management:

- Amyl nitrite pearls are an immediate source of nitrite to induce methemoglobinemia. Methemoglobin has a higher affinity for cyanide than cytochrome oxidase.
- 10% sodium nitrite IV to induce methemoglobinemia
- 25% sodium thiosulfate IV enhances conversion of cyanide to thiocyanate, which is excreted by the kidneys.

Hydroxocobalamin has also been used for cyanide poisoning and relies on the formation of nontoxic cyanocobalamin (vitamin B_{12}). Mixed evidence exists for use of hyperbaric oxygen in cyanide poisoning.

Cyclic Antidepressants

Antidepressant overdoses account for the third largest number of deaths from poisoning in the United States. Toxicities include arrhythmias, seizures, depressed level of consciousness, and hypotension. Life-threatening events occur within the first 6 h of hospitalization; most often, they occur within 2 h of presentation. Serum levels may confirm ingestion but do not correlate with toxicity. Altered mental status is the best predictor of a significant ingestion and risk of complications. Cyclic antidepressants slow sodium influx into myocardial cells, resulting in intraventricular conduction delays, wide complex arrhythmias, and negative inotropy. The ECG may be normal in significant ingestions or demonstrate a QRS > 0.10 s or amplitude of the terminal R wave in aVR ≥ 3 mm.

Management should include the following measures:

- Maintain a secure airway.
- Stabilize vital signs.
- ECG monitoring
- Consider gastric lavage.
- Activated charcoal administration
- Alkalinization of blood and sodium loading with sodium bicarbonate to pH of 7.45 to 7.55 for prolonged QRS or wide complex arrhythmias. If effective, maintain an infusion for 4 to 6 hours and then taper.
- MgSO$_4$ for *torsades de pointes*.
- Benzodiazepines for seizures.
- Norepinephrine or phenylephrine for refractory hypotension rather than dopamine.

Sodium bicarbonate uncouples the cyclic antidepressant from the myocardial sodium channels and alkalinization with bicarbonate may be superior to hyperventilation. In an animal study, hypertonic saline solution was most effective in treatment of a wide QRS complex. Hypertonic saline has also been reported to be effective in refractory cases. Bicarbonate may also be beneficial for hypotension associated with myocardial depression that is unresponsive to other interventions. Physostigmine is not indicated in cyclic antidepressant overdose.

γ-Hydroxybutyrate

γ-Hydroxybutyrate (GHB) is a naturally occurring metabolite of γ-aminobutyric acid, which was banned in 1991 due to reported toxicities. Clinical effects of GHB ingestion may include hypothermia, loss of consciousness, coma, respiratory depression including arrest, seizurelike activity, bradycardia, hypotension, and death. Concomitant use of alcohol results in synergistic CNS and respiratory effects. More recently, γ-butyrolactone (GBL), 1,4-butanediol (BD), and gamma hydroxyvalerate, which are precursors of GHB, have been abused with resultant manifestations similar to GHB. The benefit of activated charcoal is unknown because of the rapid absorption of these substances. Although patients usually recover spontaneously in 2 to 96 h, supportive therapy with airway protection and mechanical ventilation may be necessary. Use of physostigmine to reverse CNS effects is not recommended. A GHB withdrawal syndrome of agitation and delirium has been reported in high-dose, frequent abusers.

Isoniazid

Isoniazid toxicity produces seizures (often intractable), an anion-gap metabolic acidosis, coma, and hepatic toxicity. The treatment of choice is intensive supportive care and the use of pyridoxine (vitamin B$_6$) 5 g IV or a dose equivalent to the amount of isoniazid ingested). Hemoperfusion or hemodialysis may be considered, particularly in patients with renal insufficiency.

Lithium

Although arrhythmias are reported, neurologic abnormalities are the major manifestation of acute and chronic lithium toxicity. CNS manifestations include lethargy, dysarthria, delirium, seizures, and coma. Symptoms of GI distress, polyuria, and polydipsia may be present. A decreased anion gap is suggestive of a severely elevated lithium level. Patients who chronically ingest lithium are more prone to toxic effects. A serum lithium level should be assessed at presentation and 2 h later to assess for increasing concentration. Serum lithium levels of >2.5 to 4 mmol/L may be considered life-threatening, depending on the clinical findings. Whole bowel irrigation may be considered in serious toxicity because lithium is not adsorbed by charcoal. Volume resuscitation should be aimed at restoring adequate urine output, but forced diuresis is not effective in enhancing lithium excretion. Diuretics can worsen toxicity and should be avoided. Hemodialysis is indicated in life-threatening toxicity, which may include renal dysfunction, severe neurologic dysfunction, volume overload or levels of ≥4 mmol/L in acute ingestion or ≥2.5 mmol/L in chronic ingestions. Owing to redistribution between intracellular and extracellular compartments, a rebound increase in lithium level can occur 6 to 8 h after dialysis. Improvement in neurologic status lags behind the decrease in serum lithium level. Continuous arteriovenous and venovenous hemodiafiltration have also been used to remove lithium and may be associated with less rebound. Sodium polystyrene sulfonate has been suggested to decrease lithium absorption, but evidence of clinical benefit is lacking and complications of hypokalemia, hypernatremia, and fluid overload may result.

Narcotics

Naloxone should be used to reverse the morbidity of respiratory depression and depressed level of consciousness associated with narcotic overdose. An initial dose of 2 mg should be administered IV unless the patient is known to be addicted, in which case lower initial doses should be used to prevent sudden withdrawal symptoms. Doses >2 mg may be required to reverse the effects of propoxyphene, codeine, pentazocine, methadone, oxycodone, hydrocodone, and fentanyl. Naloxone can be administered at doses up to 10 mg and occasionally up to 20 mg. Naloxone can also be administered by the intramuscular, sublingual, and endotracheal routes if IV access is not established. Continuous infusion may be necessary because all narcotics have a longer half-life than naloxone. The initial hourly infusion dose should be one half to two thirds of the amount (in milligrams) that was needed to initially reverse the respiratory depression. Noncardiogenic pulmonary edema may also occur with narcotics and can be managed with supportive care that may require intubation and mechanical ventilation.

Organophosphates/Carbamates/Nerve Gas

Organophosphate and carbamate poisoning producing a cholinergic syndrome is uncommon in the United States but prevalent in developing countries. Some nerve gases (sarin) that may be used in terrorist attacks produce similar toxicity. Cholinergic poisoning exerts potential deleterious effects on three systems: (1) the muscarinic (parasympathetic) system, inducing bronchorrhea, bradycardia, and salivation, lacrimation, urination, defecation, GI upset, and emesis (the "SLUDGE" syndrome; Table 3); (2) the nicotinic autonomic system, resulting in muscle weakness; and (3) the CNS, including confusion, slurred speech, and central respiratory depression. Pulmonary toxicity from bronchorrhea, bronchospasm, and respiratory depression is the primary concern. Both IV atropine and pralidoxime (30 mg/kg bolus followed by >8 mg/kg/h infusion recommended by the World Health Organization) are indicated. Atropine does not reverse nicotinic manifestations; therefore, patients with significant respiratory muscle weakness require the use of pralidoxime. Large amounts of atropine may be required, and the initial dose is usually 2 to 4 mg, repeated every 2 to 5 min as needed. A continuous infusion of atropine can be used. The end point of atropinization is clearing of secretions from the tracheobronchial tree. An intermediate syndrome of respiratory paralysis, bulbar weakness, proximal limb weakness, and decreased reflexes may develop 24 to 96 h after resolution of the cholinergic crisis.

Salicylates

Salicylates are found in many over-the-counter preparations. Patients with chronic rather than acute ingestions of salicylates are more likely to require intensive care. Symptoms of salicylate poisoning include tinnitus, nausea and vomiting, and depressed level of consciousness. In addition, fever, an anion-gap metabolic acidosis, coagulopathy, prolonged prothrombin time, transient hepatotoxicity, and noncardiogenic pulmonary edema may be present. The clinical presentation of salicylate toxicity may be mistaken for sepsis. A salicylate level should be measured initially and may need to be repeated to assess for continued absorption (especially with enteric-coated products). The Done nomogram used to estimate the severity of an acute salicylate overdose may not reliably correlate with observed toxicity. Acidemia predisposes to more severe toxicity because more drug crosses the blood-brain barrier. Gastric lavage may be considered for significant ingestions, and activated charcoal should be administered. Alkalinization of the urine (pH ≥ 7.5) is indicated to enhance salicylate excretion if serum levels are >35 mg/dL. Supplemental potassium is often needed. Hemodialysis may be indicated with levels of >100 mg/dL, refractory seizures, persistent alteration in mental status, or refractory acidosis.

Selective Serotonin Reuptake Inhibitors

Poisoning with selective serotonin reuptake inhibitors (SSRIs) is usually less severe than poisoning with cyclic antidepressants. Acute overdoses may result in nausea, vomiting, dizziness, and less commonly, CNS depression and arrhythmias. There are reports of cardiac toxicity responding to administration of sodium bicarbonate. Therapeutic doses, overdoses of SSRIs alone, or SSRI overdoses in combination with other agents can cause serotonin syndrome, which may be life-threatening. This syndrome may be precipitated by SSRIs, monoamine oxidase inhibitors, serotonin precursors (L-tryptophan), lithium, meperidine, and nonselective serotonin reuptake inhibitors (*eg*, imipramine, meperidine, trazodone). Clinical manifestations include altered mental status (agitation, coma), autonomic dysfunction (blood pressure fluctuation, hyperthermia, tachycardia, diaphoresis, diarrhea), and neuromuscular abnormalities (tremor, rigidity, myoclonus, seizures). Management of an overdose should include activated charcoal, but the benefit of gastric lavage has not been determined. Intensive supportive care may be necessary, including cooling, sedatives, anticonvulsants, and mechanical ventilation. The role of other agents, such as serotonin antagonists (propranolol, cyproheptadine, methysergide), bromocriptine, or dantrolene in the treatment of serotonin syndrome is not well established. Most cases of serotonin syndrome resolve in 24 to 72 h.

Theophylline

Theophylline toxicity is characterized by nausea, vomiting, and agitation. More serious complications include arrhythmias and seizures. Toxicity is more likely to occur following chronic theophylline use compared with an acute overdose in an individual not taking theophylline. Activated charcoal should be administered to decrease GI absorption. An initial theophylline level should be obtained, as well as a subsequent level 1 h later. Unfortunately, sustained-release preparations of theophylline may form conglomerates in the stomach and allow for continued absorption, despite aggressive interventions. Hypokalemia is commonly present in theophylline overdose and should be treated aggressively to prevent any contribution to the initiation of arrhythmias. Seizures are often poorly responsive to phenytoin but may respond to benzodiazepines. Any patient with a life-threatening complication and/or a level of >60 mg/L with chronic ingestion or a level of >80 to 90 mg/L with an acute ingestion should be considered for hemoperfusion or hemodialysis. Multiple doses of charcoal are indicated to enhance elimination of theophylline in patients with less severe manifestations.

Valproic Acid

Acute valproic acid (VPA) intoxication is an increasing problem due to greater utilization. CNS depression is the most common manifestation in acute overdose. Higher drug levels are associated with an increased incidence of coma and respiratory depression requiring intubation. Cerebral edema has been reported 48 to 72 h after ingestion and may be related to hyperammonemia that can occur in the absence of hepatotoxicity. Massive VPA ingestions can result in refractory hypotension. Pancreatitis has been associated with both chronic ingestion and acute overdose. Metabolic abnormalities include hypernatremia, anion gap metabolic acidosis, hypocalcemia, and acute renal failure. Serial VPA levels should be obtained due to delayed peak serum levels in overdose. An ammonia level should also be obtained in patients with altered level of consciousness. Activated charcoal is administered if the patient presents early after ingestion. Whole bowel irrigation has been proposed but further studies are needed to determine any indication for use in VPA ingestions. Although a potential enterohepatic recirculation of drug suggests that multiple dose activated charcoal may be beneficial, routine use is not currently recommended. Hemoperfusion, combined hemodialysis-hemoperfusion, or high flux hemodialysis may be considered in patients with persistent hemodynamic instability or metabolic acidosis. No antidote exists for VPA toxicity. L-carnitine has been proposed for supplementation in patients with VPA toxicity and hyperammonemia.

Herbal Medicine/Dietary Supplements

Herbal medicines are the most common form of alternative therapy in the United States, and can be marketed without testing for safety or efficacy. Poisoning may result from product misuse, from contamination of the product, or through interaction with other medications. Cardiac toxicity may result from aconitine and cardiac glycosides. Aconitine or related compounds are common ingredients in Asian herbal medications. Symptoms include paresthesias, hypersalivation, dizziness, nausea, vomiting, diarrhea, and muscle weakness. Sinus bradycardia and ventricular arrhythmias can occur. No antidote is available, but atropine may be considered for bradycardia or hypersalivation. Cardiac glycosides or digoxinlike factors can be found in many herbal preparations, particularly teas and laxatives. Toxicity is similar to digoxin toxicity, with visual disturbances, nausea, vomiting, and arrhythmias. A digoxin level should be obtained but may not correlate with clinical findings because numerous cardiac glycosides will not cross-react in the digoxin immunoassay. With significant toxicity, digoxin-specific antibodies should be administered. CNS stimulation is characteristic of preparations containing ephedrine and pseudoephedrine, which are often found in products marketed as "herbal ecstasy." A typical sympathomimetic syndrome can result with tachycardia, hypertension, mydriasis, and agitation. Seizures, stroke, myocardial infarction, arrhythmias, liver failure, and death have also been reported. Supportive care is indicated similar to management of other sympathomimetic syndromes. Ginkgo biloba has been reported to result in spontaneous bleeding including subdural hematomas, which may be due to antiplatelet activating factor effects. Treatment for bleeding includes supportive care and blood products as needed. Garlic may also result in bleeding as a result of inhibition of platelet aggregation, and ginseng has been associated with hypoglycemia. Kava-containing dietary supplements are possibly associated with hepatic failure requiring transplantation. Contaminants found in some products, such as mercury, arsenic, lead, antihistamines, etc, may cause toxicities.

Suggested Readings

American Academy of Clinical Toxicology; European Association of Poisons Centres and Clinical Toxicologists. Position statement: gastric lavage. J Toxicol Clin Toxicol 1997; 35:711–719

American Academy of Clinical Toxicology; European Association of Poisons Centres and Clinical Toxicologists. Position statement: single-dose activated charcoal. J Toxicol Clin Toxicol 1997; 35:721–724

American Academy of Clinical Toxicology; European Association of Poisons Centres and Clinical Toxicologists. Position statement: whole bowel irrigation. J Toxicol Clin Toxicol 1997; 35:753–762

American Academy of Clinical Toxicology; European Association of Poison Centres and Clinical Toxicologists. Position Statement and practice guidelines on the use of multi-dose activated charcoal in the treatment of acute poisoning. J Toxicol Clin Toxicol 1999; 37:731–751

Ang-Lee MK, Moss J, Yuan C-S. Herbal medicines and perioperative care. JAMA 2001; 286:208–216

Barceloux DG, Bond GR, Krenzelok EP, et al. American Academy of Clinical Toxicology practice guidelines on the treatment of methanol poisoning. J Toxicol Clin Toxicol 2002; 40:415–446

Barceloux DG, Krenzelok EP, Olson R, et al. American Academy of Clinical Toxicology practice guidelines on the treatment of ethylene glycol poisoning. J Toxicol Clin Toxicol 1999; 37:537–560

Bardin PG, van Eden SF, Moolman JA, et al. Organophosphate and carbamate poisoning. Arch Intern Med 1994; 154:1433–1441

Brent J, McMartin K, Phillips S, et al. Fomepizole for the treatment of ethylene glycol poisoning. N Engl J Med 1999; 340:832–838

Brent J, McMartin K, Phillips S, et al. Fomepizole for the treatment of methanol poisoning. N Engl J Med 2001; 344:424–429

Brok J, Buckley N, Gluud C. Interventions for paracetamol (acetaminophen) overdose. Cochrane Database Syst Rev 2002; (3):CD003328

Bryan TM, Skop BT, Mareth ER. Pathophysiology and management of the serotonin syndrome. Ann Pharmacother 1996; 30:527–533

De Smet PAGM. Herbal remedies. N Engl J Med 2002; 347:2046–2056

Glauser J. Tricyclic antidepressant poisoning. Cleve Clin J Med 2000; 67:704–719

Hall AH, Rumack BH. The treatment of acute acetaminophen poisoning. J Intensive Care Med 1986; 1:29–32

Isbister GK, Bowe SJ, Dawson A, et al. Relative toxicity of selective serotonin reuptake inhibitors (SSRIs) in overdose. J Toxicol Clin Toxicol 2004; 42:277–285

Kalant H. The pharmacology and toxicology of "ecstasy" (MDMA) and related drugs. CMAJ 2001; 165:917–928

Lange RA, Hillis LD. Cardiovascular complications of cocaine use. N Engl J Med 2001; 345:351–358

Leiken JB, Thomas RG, Walter FG, et al. A review of nerve agent exposure for the critical care physician. Crit Care Med 2002; 30:2346–2354

Li J, Stokes SA, Woeckner A. A tale of novel intoxication: a review of the effects of gamma-hydroxybutyric acid with recommendations for management. Ann Emerg Med 1998; 31:729–736

Martin TG. Serotonin syndrome. Ann Emerg Med 1996; 28:520–526

McKinney PE, Rasmussen R. Reversal of severe tricyclic antidepressant-induced cardiotoxicity with intravenous hypertonic saline solution. Ann Emerg Med 2003; 42:20–24

Mokhesi B, Leiken JB, Murray P, et al. Adult toxicology in critical care: Part I. General approach to the intoxicated patient. Chest 2003; 123:577–592

Mokhesi B, Leiken JB, Murray P, et al. Adult toxicology in critical care: Part II. Specific poisonings. Chest 2003; 123:897–922

Pond SM, Lewis-Driver DJ, Williams GM, et al. Gastric emptying in acute overdose: a prospective randomized controlled trial. Med J Aust 1995; 163:345–349

Saper RB, Kales SN, Paquin J, et al. Heavy metal content of ayurvedic herbal medicine products. JAMA 2004; 292:2868–2873

Sztajnkrycer MD. Valproic acid toxicity: overview and management. J Toxicol Clin Toxicol 2002; 40:789–801

Trujillo MH, Guerrero J, Fragachan C, et al. Pharmacologic antidotes in critical care medicine: a practical guide for drug administration. Crit Care Med 1998; 26:377–391

Weaver LK, Hopkins RD, Chan KJ, et al. Hyperbaric oxygen for acute carbon monoxide poisoning. N Engl J Med 2002; 347:1057–1067

Yuan TH, Kerns WP, Tomaszewski CA, et al. Insulin-glucose as adjunctive therapy for severe calcium channel antagonist poisoning. J Toxicol Clin Toxicol 1999; 37:463–474

Zed PJ, Krenzelok EP. Treatment of acetaminophen overdose. Am J Health Syst Pharm 1999; 56:1081–1093

Zimmerman JL. Poisonings and overdoses in the ICU: general and specific management issues. Crit Care Med 2003; 31:2794–2801

Zimmerman JL, Rudis M. Poisonings. In: Parrillo JE, Dellinger RP, eds. Critical care medicine. St. Louis, MO: Mosby, 2001; 1501–1524

Notes

Electrolyte Disorders: Derangements of Serum Sodium, Calcium, Magnesium, and Potassium

Richard S. Muther, MD

Objectives:

- To review the basic physiology affecting sodium, water, calcium, magnesium, and potassium balance
- To recognize the common critical care syndromes and causes of deranged serum cations
- To become facile with the acute treatment of disordered cation balance

Key words: hypercalcemia; hyperkalemia; hypermagnesemia; hypernatremia; hyperosmolality; hypocalcemia; hypokalemia; hypomagnesemia; hyponatremia; hypo-osmolality

Sodium

Water balance is measured by changes in osmolality. Osmolality is the number of osmotically active particles (osmoles) per liter of solution. (Osmolarity is expressed per kilogram). Hypo-osmolality indicates an excess of water relative to osmoles; hyperosmolality indicates water deficiency. The serum osmolality [in milliosmols per liter (mOsm/L)] can be calculated by the following formula:

$$\text{Serum osmolality} = 2(Na^+ + K^+) + (glucose/18) + (urea/2.8)$$

where mOsm is milliosmol, Na is sodium, and K is potassium; glucose and urea are given in mg/dL. The molecular weight of glucose is 180; urea, 28. Conversion from mg/dL to mOsm/L yields 18 and 2.8.

One can see that serum osmolality is primarily due to the serum concentration of sodium and potassium (and their accompanying anions), glucose and urea. Of these, the serum sodium is most powerful, accounting for nearly 95% of serum osmolality. Therefore, *in most clinical circumstances, the serum sodium can be used as a surrogate for osmolality*. The serum sodium concentration has no direct relationship to the total body sodium, but rather, is an indicator of water balance relative to sodium.

Tonicity refers to the osmotic force (ability to move water across a semipermeable membrane) exerted by osmotically active particles. Hypotonic solutions will lose water to, and hypertonic solutions will gain water from an isotonic solution. Not all osmoles are equivalent in tonicity. Urea, for example, readily crosses cell membranes and exerts no tonic force. Glucose will induce water movement from most cells. The major extracellular osmole, sodium, is responsible for the variation in serum tonicity in most cases and, as such, is largely responsible for the volume of extracellular fluid (ECV). Therefore, *an excess of body sodium causes water movement into the extracellular space and obligates an increase in ECV, though not an increase in sodium concentration.*

Hyponatremia is not always equivalent to hypo-osmolality (Fig 1). By stimulating water movement into the ECV, hyperglycemia physiologically lowers serum sodium by 1.6 mEq/100 mg/dL glucose, causing hyponatremia with hyperosmolality. The same is true for hypertonic mannitol. Other molecules increasing serum osmolality, such as ethanol, isopropyl alcohol, ethylene glycol, and methanol, do not cause hyponatremia because of their small size and high membrane permeability (ie, they do not create an osmotic force or tonicity). They will, however, cause an osmolar gap

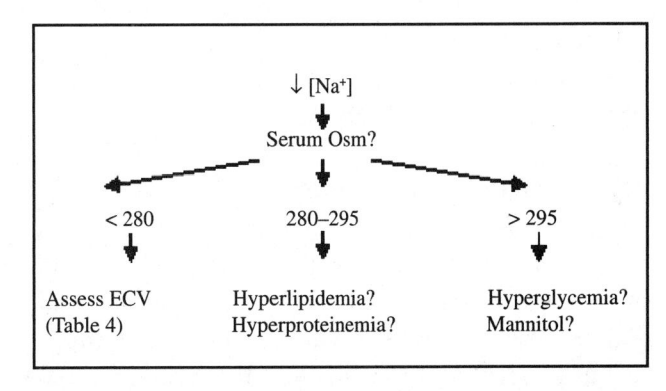

Figure 1. "Pseudohyponatremia" applies when hyponatremia does not reflect hypo-osmolality.

Table 1. *Differential Diagnosis of an Elevated Osmolar Gap**

With Anion-Gap Acidosis	Without Acidosis
Ethylene glycol	Isopropyl alcohol
Methanol	Diethyl ether
Formaldehyde	Mannitol
GFR < 10 mL/min	Severe hyperproteinemia
Paraldehyde	Severe hyperlipidemia

*The osmolar gap = measured − calculated osmolality. Calculated serum osmolality = 2(Na^+ + K^+) + glucose (mg/dL)/18 + BUN(mg/dL)/2.8.

Table 2. *Characteristics of Sodium and Water Balance**

	Sodium	Water
Distribution	Extracellular volume	Total body water
Assessment	Physical examination	Serum osmolality
	Urinary Na, FENa	Serum sodium
		UOsm, COsm
Regulation	GFR	Thirst
	Aldosterone	ADH
	"Third factors"	Renal handling of water

*UOsm, urinary osmolality. COsm, osmolar clearance.

defined as a >20-mOsm/L difference between the calculated and measured serum osmolality (Table 1). Hyperproteinemia (usually >10 g/dL) and hyperlipidemia cause an increase in the solid phase of the blood volume, causing "hyponatremia" as the sodium present is indexed to an artificially increased volume. The serum osmolality does not change. This pseudohyponatremia usually accounts for small changes in serum sodium (*eg*, 1 mEq sodium/460 mg/dL lipid).

In most clinical situations (pseudohyponatremia excepted), the serum sodium is directly related to the serum osmolality such that hyponatremia indicates an excess and hypernatremia a deficiency of water relative to total body sodium. The characteristics of body sodium and water balance are outlined in Table 2.

Regulation of Sodium Balance

As the major extracellular cation and osmole, sodim largely determines ECV. Changes in total body sodium are reflected as changes in the ECV and are best assessed clinically by physical findings. Therefore, rales, jugular venous distention, edema, and an S3 gallop indicate excess ECV and body sodium. Tachycardia, hypotension, flat neck veins in the supine position, dry mucous membranes, and skin tenting indicate ECV and body sodium depletion. In neither case will the serum sodium concentration necessarily change. Thus, *neither the total body sodium nor ECV is directly related to the serum sodium concentration.*

Ordinarily, renal sodium loss balances dietary sodium intake. The renal excretion of sodium is dependent on the glomerular filtration rate (GFR), aldosterone, and a variety of "third factors" that affect renal tubular reabsorption of filtered sodium. These include natriuretic peptides (atrial natriuretic peptide, brain natriuretic peptide), the renin angiotensin system, norepinephrine, prostaglandins, and intraglomerular and peritubular Starling forces. The GFR in turn is dependent on renal blood flow, the transglomerular capillary hydrostatic and oncotic pressures and the permeability of the glomerular capillary wall. The afferent and efferent glomerular arteriolar sphincters largely determine intraglomerular Starling forces (transglomerular capillary hydrostatic pressure and transglomerular capillary oncotic pressure). Aldosterone enhances distal tubular sodium reabsorption coupled to hydrogen ion (H^+) and potassium secretion. Normally, approximately 99% of filtered sodium is reabsorbed. The 1% excreted sodium is best measured by the fractional excretion of sodium (FENa).

Regulation of Water Balance

Thirst, antidiuretic hormone (ADH), and the kidneys control water balance. Hypothalamic receptors for hyperosmolality and hypovolemia stimulate thirst and ADH secretion. While hyperosmolality is the more common stimulus, hypovolemia is more potent. For example, a hypovolemic patient will continue to secrete ADH despite hypoosmolality and hyponatremia. ADH exerts its primary effect by enhancing renal water reabsorption across the collecting tubule, thus concentrating the urine (Fig 2). This passive reabsorption of water is dependent on the presence of a more highly concentrated renal medullary interstitium caused by active sodium and chloride reabsorption from the ascending limb of Henle. Sodium (but not water) reabsorption from the late ascending limb and early distal tubule dilutes the filtrate and

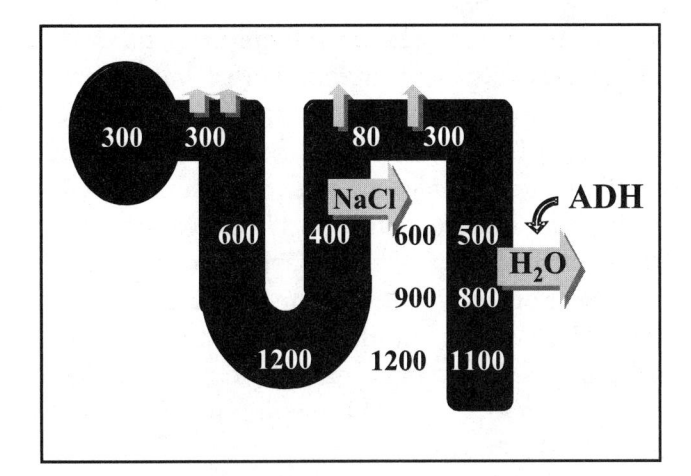

Figure 2. The renal handling of water. Water reabsorption (urinary concentration) requires the presence of ADH and a concentrated medullary interstitium provided by active Na$^+$ and Cl$^-$ reabsorption in the ascending limb of Henle. Water excretion (urinary dilution) occurs in the absence of ADH. GFR and proximal tubular reabsorption affect urinary concentration and dilution by controlling the delivery of glomerular filtrate to the loop and distal nephron. (Numbers reflect osmolality.)

Table 3. *Signs and Symptoms of ECV Depletion Roughly Correlate to a Percentage of TBW**

ECV Depletion	Mild	Moderate	Severe
TBW depletion	5%	10%	15%
Symptoms	"Dry"	Lethargy	Stupor
Heart rate	80	100	120
BP	Normal	Orthostatic	Shock
Jugular vein	Normal	<5 cm H$_2$O	Flat
Skin	Normal		Tenting

*The severity of symptoms and the urgency of replacement are affected by the acuity of the underlying disease.

generates free water. Free water excretion occurs in the absence of ADH. Both the GFR and proximal tubular reabsorption rate affect free water excretion (urine dilution) and reabsorption (urine concentration) as these factors control the quantity of glomerular filtrate delivered to the downstream nephron segments.

Clinical Disorders of Sodium Balance (Disorders of the ECV)

ECV Depletion: Hemorrhage, GI sodium loss, or renal sodium loss can deplete the ECV. Usually the sodium loss is isotonic. For example, the sodium concentration in diarrhea is approximately 120 mEq/L. In emesis, depending on the pH, it varies from 60 to 120 mEq/L. Coupled with insensible losses, therefore, the serum sodium changes little in most cases where GI sodium loss depletes the ECV. In fact, the predominant electrolyte disturbance is hypokalemia, which is associated with metabolic acidosis in cases of diarrhea, metabolic alkalosis with vomiting, or a balanced acid-base status where diarrhea and vomiting coexist.

Diuretics are the most common cause of renal salt wasting. Again, these are isosmotic losses, usually not associated with changes in the serum sodium concentration. Certainly, severe hyponatremias are reported with diuretics, but these are idiosyncratic (in the case of thiazide diuretics) or associated with an underlying disorder of sodium retention such as heart failure. Hypoaldosteronism will cause renal sodium loss and isotonic ECV depletion. If coupled to glucocorticoid deficiency, mild hyponatremia can occur. Various renal tubular defects can also cause "salt-losing" nephropathy. This is not uncommon, but it is usually relatively mild with several types of chronic interstitial nephritis. Very rare causes of renal sodium loss include Bartter's syndrome and renal tubular acidosis (RTA). Again, the volume lost in these cases is approximately isosmolar so that serum sodium concentration is either unchanged or mildly decreased. The major clinical feature is ECV depletion, determined by physical examination.

Basic fluid therapy for ECV depletion is isotonic crystalloid. When blood and/or colloid are needed, they are converted to "crystalloid equivalents" at a ratio of 3:1. The volume of replacement can be estimated by a percentage of total body water. (The effect of sodium is on total body water [TBW], although its distribution is extracellular.) Mild, moderate, or severe volume losses approximate 5, 10 or 15% of TBW depending on the rapidity with which they occurred (Table 3). The rate of replacement depends on the degree of hemodynamic instability.

ECV Expansion: The classic causes of ECV excess are the "edematous disorders": congestive heart failure (CHF), cirrhosis (with ascites), and nephrosis (nephrotic syndrome). Renal failure (decreased GFR) and hyperaldosteronism are other causes of sodium retention. Physical findings of ECV excess such as rales, jugular venous distension, ascites, and edema are usually present. When mild, the serum sodium is usually normal in these syndromes. When hyponatremia does occur, it is a marker of disease severity.

Several mechanisms are responsible for the renal sodium retention seen in these edematous disorders. The GFR is often low as a result of poor cardiac output or decreased oncotic pressure. Aldosterone excess and its effect to increase distal tubular sodium reabsorption is a secondary result. Increased levels of circulating or regionally generated angiotensin II cause preferential constriction of the efferent glomerular sphincter, lowering the hydrostatic pressure while raising the oncotic pressure in the peritubular capillary, thus enhancing proximal renal tubular sodium retention. These factors override the increased production and effects of natriuretic peptides such that the urinary sodium and FENa are extremely and inappropriately low.

The basic fluid therapy for patients with ECV excess is salt and water restriction.

Clinical Disorders of Water Balance

Hyponatremia: As a surrogate for serum osmolality, the serum sodium reflects changes in water balance relative to total body sodium. Therefore, after excluding pseudohyponatremia, one can best approach hyponatremia based on the patient's ECV (Table 4).

Hyponatremia occurs with ECV depletion whenever free water intake accompanies GI or renal sodium loss. The most common example is a GI illness with continued oral or IV water (without salt) replacement. Another example is diuretic-associated hyponatremia. Although it is usually mild, severe hyponatremia can occur, particularly with thiazide-type diuretics. Thiazides limit free water excretion by inhibiting distal tubular sodium reabsorption. ECV depletion appropriately stimulates ADH secretion and water reabsorption, contributing to the hyponatremia. Loop diuretics, on the other hand, gradually diminish medullary interstitial solute and osmolarity, thereby limiting the osmolar gradient for water reabsorption so that hyponatremia is less commonly a side effect of these agents. Elderly women and patients taking nonsteroidal anti-inflammatory drugs (NSAIDs) are particularly prone to thiazide-induced hyponatremia. Polydipsia and hypokalemia contribute to the pathogenesis. Treatment is to discontinue thiazides, restrict water, and replace potassium.

Isotonic saline solution is indicated for those patients with moderate to severe volume depletion. Care must be taken to avoid too rapid a correction of hyponatremia. Because ADH secretion is abrogated as saline solution is replaced, a physiologic water diuresis will correct the hyponatremia promptly. Hypertonic saline solution is rarely necessary.

Hyponatremia with a normal ECV occurs whenever the addition of free water to the ECV exceeds the renal capacity to excrete water. In normal patients, 10 to 15 L of water intake is required

Table 4. *Differential Diagnosis of Hyponatremia and Hypo-osmolality**

	Hypovolemia (↓ ECV)		Euvolemia (Normal ECV)		Hypervolemia (↑ ECV)
Diagnosis	Vomiting, diarrhea, fistula	Diuretics, hypo-aldosteronism, RTA,	Polydipsia, malnutrition	SIADH, hypothyroid, hypocortisol	CHF, cirrhosis/ascites, nephrotic syndrome, renal failure
UOsm, mOsm/L	>300	300	<100	>100	>300[†]
UNa, mEq/L	<20	>20	>30	>30	<10[†]
Other findings	Hypokalemia: vomiting, diarrhea, diuretics, RTAsteronism Hyperkalemia: hypoaldosteronism Metabolic alkalosis: Vomiting, diuretics Metabolic acidosis: diarrhea, hypoaldo-steronism		Hypokalemia: SIADH, polydipsia Hyperkalemia: hypocortisol Hypouricemia		
Fluid Therapy	Isotonic saline solution		Restrict H₂O		Restrict H₂O and saline solution

*UOsm = urine osmolality; UNa = urine sodium.
[†]Excludes renal failure.

to cause significant hyponatremia. Extreme polydipsia (psychogenic polydipsia) is rare, but hyponatremia can occur with significantly less water intake if ADH secretion is stimulated or its renal tubular effect is enhanced by certain drugs (Table 5). Chronic malnutrition or "low osmolar syndrome" is a much less dramatic cause of hyponatremia. These disorders will have appropriately dilute urine (specific gravity, <1.010; urinary osmolality, <200).

The syndrome of inappropriate antidiuretic hormone (SIADH) also causes hyponatremia in euvolemic patients. In fact, edema is an exclusion criterion for SIADH, as are hypothyroidism and cortisol deficiency. Features include hypo-osmolality with relatively high urinary osmolality (less than maximally dilute urine or >100 mOsm/L) and hyponatremia with relatively high urinary sodium (>30 mEq/L). Excluding the edematous disorders (heart, liver, and kidney disease) is also a prerequisite for the diagnosis of SIADH.

The basic fluid therapy for polydipsia or SIADH is sodium and water restriction. Drugs that inhibit ADH effect are useful therapeutic adjuncts. These include demeclocycline, phenytoin, lithium, and loop diuretics (by limiting medullary interstitial osmoles).

Hyponatremia marks the severity of the edematous disorders, particularly CHF. The decrease in "effective" intravascular volume stimulates thirst, increases ADH secretion, limits GFR, and enhances proximal renal tubular reabsorption of sodium and water, thus limiting delivery of glomerular filtrate to the diluting ascending limb. The result is increased intake and limited excretion of free water. Hyponatremia is also commonly seen in patients with cirrhosis (particularly those with ascites) and nephrotic syndrome. The urinary sodium is low (<20 mEq/L) and the urinary osmolarity is high (>300 mOsm/L), mimicking ECV depletion, although with very different physical findings. Basic fluid therapy for these disorders is salt and water restriction with diuretics.

Hypernatremia: Because thirst provides excellent protection against hyperosmolality, hypernatremia is unusual unless access to water is impaired. Therefore, hypernatremic patients are usually elderly, have a decreased mental status, or are in some way incapacitated. The fact that hypernatremia mandates hypertonicity ensures cellular dehydration, particularly of the brain. Therefore, hypernatremic patients are usually quite ill. Because hypernatremia is synonymous with hyperosmolality, a water deficit relative to sodium is always present. Therefore, an approach to the hypernatremic patient based on his or her salt balance (ECV) is appropriate (Table 6, Fig 3).

Hypernatremia in patients with decreased ECV occurs with osmotic cathartics and diuretics. The osmotic effect ensures that water will be lost in excess of sodium and potassium (because of the presence of another osmole). This occurs with lactulose or sorbitol in the intestinal tract or in the urine with hyperglycemia, mannitol, low-molecular-weight proteins (from hyperalimentation), and urea (postobstructive diuresis). The osmotic effect also causes variable salt depletion. Fluid therapy for these patients, therefore, requires water (to correct the free water deficit) and isotonic saline solution (to correct the decreased ECV).

Table 5. *Differential Diagnosis of SIADH*

Drugs
    Amitriptyline
    Bromocriptine
    Carbamazepine
    Chlorpropamide
    Cisplatin
    Cyclophosphamide
    Haloperidol
    MAO inhibitors
    Methylenedioxymethamphetamine
    NSAIDs
    Serotonin reuptake inhibitors (fluoxetine, etc)
    Thioridazine
    Thiothixene
    Vincristine/vinblastine
Malignancy
    Small cell lung
    Other lung
    Pancreas
    Several others
CNS Diseases
    Cerebrovascular accident
    Infection
    Trauma
Pulmonary
    Pneumonia
    Atelectasis
    Asthma
    Pneumothorax
Major Surgery
    Transphenoidal

Table 6. *Differential Diagnosis of Hypernatremia**

	Hypovolemia (↓ ECV)		Euvolemia (Normal ECV)		Hypervolemia (↑ ECV)
Diagnosis	GI loss: vomiting, diarrhea, fistula	Renal loss: hyperglycemia, mannitol, high-protein feedings, postobstructive diuresis	Sweating, hypodipsia	Central DI, nephrogenic DI	Hypertonic NaHCO$_3$, hypertonic saline solution, sea water ingestion
UOsm, mOsm/L	>800	300–800	>800	<300†	>800
UNa, mEq/L	<20	>30	<20	<20	>30
Other Findings	Hypokalemia: vomiting, diarrhea, diuresis Metabolic alkalosis: vomiting			UOsm after AVP: central DI, 400–800†, nephrogenic DI, no change	
Fluid Therapy	Combined water and saline solution		Water	Water	

*UOsm = urine osmolality; UNa = urine sodium; AVP = aqueous vasopressin, 5 U subcutaneously.
†Urine osmolality varies with partial vs complete DI.

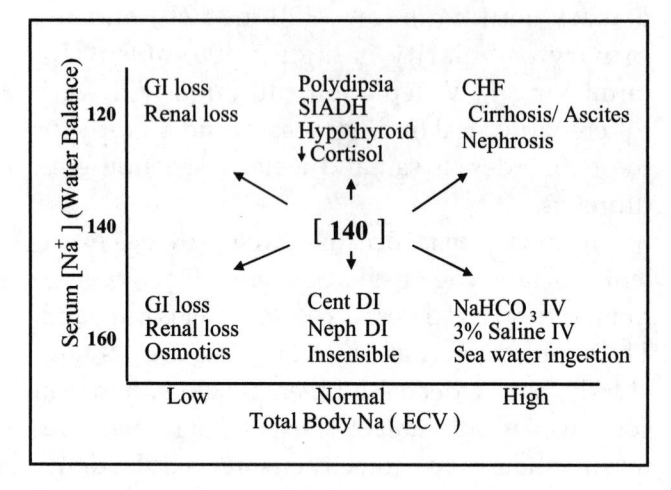

Figure 3. Differential diagnosis of hypo- and hypernatremia based on water balance relative to total body sodium (ECV). Cent = central; Neph = nephrogenic.

Table 7. *Differential Diagnosis of Central and Nephrogenic DI*

Central DI	Nephrogenic DI
Trauma	Drugs
Neurosurgery	Lithium
Transphenoidal	Demeclocycline
Pituitary infarction	Amphotericin
Sheehan's	Cisplatin
Cerebrovascular accident	Glyburide
Shock	Hypercalcemia
Neoplasm	Hypokalemia
Meningitis/encephalitis	Tubulointerstitial nephritis
Drugs	Obstructive uropathy
Phenytoin	Diuretic-phase acute tubular necrosis
Ethanol	
Familial	

Euvolemia with hypernatremia indicates isolated loss of free water. This can occur with massive insensible losses such as severe sweating or hyperventilation or, rarely, with primary hypodipsia. The most common cause of euvolemic hypernatremia, however, is diabetes insipidus (DI). These patients have an inappropriately low ADH level (central DI) or a blunted ADH effect (nephrogenic DI). The urinary osmolality is inappropriately low (<300 mOsm/L), despite hypernatremia. Patients with central DI will respond to parenteral administration of ADH by increasing urinary osmolality and decreasing urinary volume. Both central and nephrogenic DI can occur in either partial or complete forms and, therefore, a broad range of urinary osmolalities can be seen following water deprivation or ADH. The differential diagnosis of both central and nephrogenic DI is listed in Table 7.

The rarest clinical salt and water problem is hypernatremia with increased ECV. This occurs with massive administration of hypertonic bicarbonate or hypertonic saline solution, or rarely in those with salt-water ingestion. The urinary osmolality is high and the patients are appropriately excreting increased urinary sodium. Treatment is obviously to restrict the salt and administer free water and diuretics as needed.

Figure 3 plots the common derangement of body salt (disorders of the ECV) and water (disorders of serum osmolality). Most of the clinical syndromes seen in critically ill patients are actually combinations of separate salt (ECV) and water

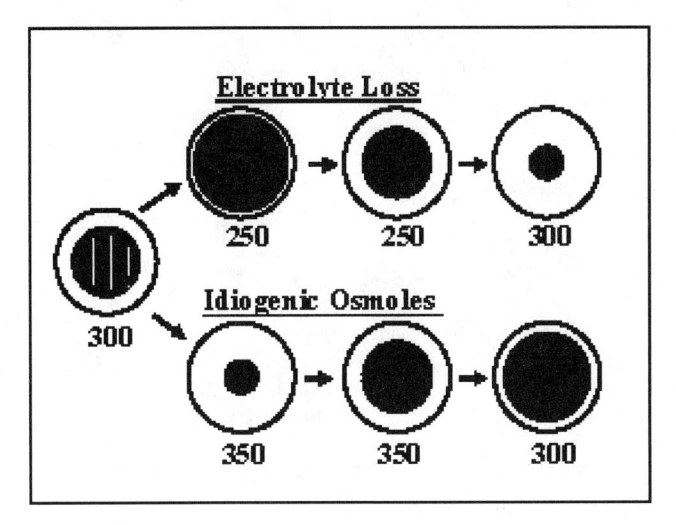

Figure 4. Acute change in serum osmolality effects intracerebral swelling or shrinkage. Within days, a new steady state is reached by brain electrolyte loss (in response to hypo-osmolality) or the generation of osmoles (in response to hyperosmolality). Too-rapid correction of serum osmolality will similarly effect a change in cerebral volume.

problems. When this occurs, it is helpful to approach each patient as if he has two separate problems. First, define the nature and treatment of the ECV problem. Next, identify the water (osmolality) problem and its treatment. Finally, sum and administer the therapies. This approach will simplify even the most severe derangement of fluid and electrolytes.

Treatment Issues

The serum osmolality is the major determinant of brain water and therefore brain volume (Fig 4). Abrupt hypo-osmolality causes brain edema; abrupt hyperosmolality causes brain shrinkage. The more rapidly this occurs, the more likely symptoms will occur and the more urgent is the need for therapy. Over time, adaptation to changes in osmolality occurs. With chronic hypo-osmolality, the brain loses electrolytes (osmolytes), thus lowering intracellular osmolality to that of plasma. With hyperosmolality, the brain will generate osmoles (idiogenic osmoles), thus raising intracerebral osmolality. Both adaptations tend to return brain osmolality toward plasma osmolality and brain volume towards normal as a new steady state is reached. Any subsequent change in plasma osmolality (ie, those induced by therapy) will cause brain swelling or shrinkage once again. Potential complications of this include altered mental status, seizures, coma, or the most serious complication, central pontine myelinolysis. Therefore, slow correction is the rule for severe degrees of either hypo- or hypernatremia.

For asymptomatic patients with hyponatremia, simple water restriction and observation are adequate. If the patient is hyponatremic and ECV depleted, isotonic saline solution can be given. Again, because ADH secretion is volume sensitive, too-rapid correction can occur as saline solution is administered; thus, frequent monitoring of the serum Na is required.

For patients who are severely symptomatic with hyponatremia, hypertonic (3%) saline solution is indicated to increase the serum Na by not more than 0.5 to 1 mEq/L/h and not more than 12 mEq/L in a 24-h period. One can calculate the sodium deficit in these patients as follows:

$$\text{Na deficit} = (\text{desired Na} - \text{current Na}) \times \text{TBW}$$

TBW is approximately 60% of body weight in men and 50% of body weight in women and in the elderly. Using this formula, a 70-kg man with a serum Na of 103 mEq/L would need 504 mEq of Na to raise his serum Na to 115 mEq/L (12 mEq/L × 42 L). This is approximately 3.3 L of isotonic saline solution (154 mEq/L) or approximately 1 L of 3% saline solution (513 mEq/L). Again, close observation for too-rapid correction or signs of fluid overload is mandatory in these patients.

For hypernatremia, the water deficit can be calculated as follows:

$$\text{Water deficit} = [(\text{current Na} \div \text{target Na}) - 1] \times (0.6 \times \text{body weight in kg})$$

For example, a 60-kg man with a serum Na of 175 mEq/L needs 9 L of free water to correct his serum Na to 140 mEq/L [(175 ÷ 140) = 1 × 36 L = 9L]. As with hyponatremia, correction should not exceed 0.5 to 1 mEq/L/h and not more than 12 mEq/L in a 24-h period in severely hypernatremic patients.

An excellent approach to fluid therapy for either hypo- or hypernatremia is to determine the effect of 1 L of a given fluid on serum [Na$^+$] as outlined by the following formula:

$$\text{Change } [Na^+] = \{(\text{infusate } Na^+ + K^+) - \text{serum } [Na^+]\}/(\text{TBW} + 1)$$

Table 8. *Sodium Content and Percent Distribution Into the ECV of 1 L of Crystalloid Solutions*

Infusate	Na+ (mEq)	% in ECV
Dextrose 5% in water	0	40
0.2% normal saline solution	34	55
0.45% normal saline solution	77	73
Lactated Ringer's solution	130	97
0.9% normal saline solution	154	100

In our above example, 1 L of dextrose 5% in water would decrease the patient's serum [Na+] by 4.7 mEq/L [(0 − 175) ÷ 37 = 4.7]. By this formula, it would require 7.5 L to decrease his serum Na+ from 175 mEq/L to 140 mEq/L. This formula easily adjusts for any potassium administered. Use of this formula requires knowledge of the Na+ content of commonly prescribed IV fluids. These are outlined in Table 8, along with their percent distribution into the ECV.

Calcium

Calcium balance is depicted in Figure 5. Approximately 400 mg (30 to 35% of an average daily intake of 1,200 mg) is absorbed from the intestinal tract. Daily excretion of this amount occurs in the urine and stool (150 to 200 mg/d in each). Vitamin D is the major factor controlling absorption. The fat-soluble vitamin D_3 is absorbed from the diet, 25-hydroxylated in the liver (to calcefediol), and 1-hydroxylated by the kidney to 1,25 dihydroxy vitamin D (calcitriol), the active form of the vitamin. Parathyroid hormone (PTH) and hypophosphatemia primarily stimulate the formation of calcitriol. Malabsorption, liver disease, and renal disease may cause vitamin D deficiency.

PTH preserves serum calcium by stimulating osteoclast resorption of bone, increasing renal tubular reabsorption of filtered calcium, and stimulating the production of calcitriol, which enhances intestinal absorption of calcium. PTH secretion is stimulated by ionized hypocalcemia and suppressed by hypercalcemia and hypomagnesemia. It is primarily the combined action of PTH and vitamin D on bone that controls serum calcium.

In the blood, approximately 40 to 50% of calcium is in the ionized or physiologically active form. In critically ill patients, total serum calcium is a poor predictor of ionized calcium. Albumin binding, alkalosis, and the presence of chelators such as citrate, phosphate, or lactate can significantly influence the ionized fraction with relatively little alteration of total calcium (Table 9). In fact, *pseudohypercalcemia* refers to the elevation of serum total calcium due to hyperalbuminemia. Similarly, low levels of serum albumin will lower serum total calcium. In neither case will the active or ionized calcium change. This direct relationship of total calcium to albumin can be quantitated: Δ albumin 1 g/dL = Δ total calcium 0.8 g/dL. Direct measurement of ionized calcium by ion-specific electrodes may be necessary in certain cases.

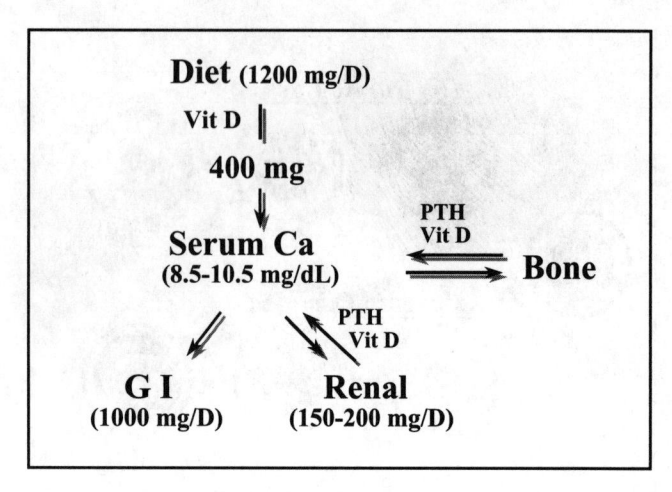

Figure 5. Calcium balance.

Hypercalcemia

Hypercalcemia (Table 10) can occur with excessive GI absorption (milk alkali syndrome, excess vitamin D) or with increased renal reabsorption of filtered calcium (hyperparathyroidism, thiazides). However, clinically significant hypercalcemia most often occurs with accelerated bone resorption. In hyperparathyroidism, direct osteoclast activation by PTH causes hypercalcemia. PTH or PTH-related peptides (PTHrP) can also be produced by several malignancies (lung, ovary, kidney, bladder). Osteoclast-activating factor, produced by myeloma cells, also causes hypercalcemia. Hypercalcemia caused by direct lytic involvement of bone is seen with several cancers (breast, prostate). Immobilization can cause hypercalcemia by increasing bone resorption, particularly in young patients or those with Paget's disease. Hypercalcemia is common in the recovery phase of rhabdomyolysis-induced acute renal failure. Severe hypercalcemia [>14 mg/dL (3.5 mmol/L)] usually

Table 9. *Common Clinical Conditions That Dissociate Total (TCa) and Ionized (ICa) Calcium**

Condition	TCa	ICa	Explanation	Degree
Hypoalbuminemia	↓	N	Decreased protein binding	Δ Alb 1.0 mg/dL = Δ TCa 0.8 mg/dL
Hyperalbuminemia	↑	N	Increased protein binding	Δ Alb 1.0 mg/dL = Δ TCa 0.8 mg/dL
Multiple myeloma	↑	N	Ca binding to globulin	
Respiratory alkalosis	N	↓	Increased albumin binding	Δ pH 0.1 = Δ ICa 0.16 mg/dL
Hyperparathyroidism	N	↑	Decreased albumin binding	
Hyperphosphatemia	N	↓	Chelation	
Hypercitratemia	N	↓	Chelation	

*N = normal; Alb = albumin.

Table 10. *Common Causes of Hypercalcemia*

Increased GI absorption
    Vitamin D intoxication
    Ectopic vitamin D
        Lymphoma
        Sarcoidosis
        Histoplasmosis
        Tuberculosis
Increased bone resorption
    Primary hyperparathyroidism
    Ectopic PTH, PTHrP
    Osteolytic metastases
    Multiple myeloma (osteoclast-activating factor)
    Immobilization
    Posthypocalcemic (*eg*, rhabdomyolysis)
Increased renal reabsorption
    Hyperparathyroidism
    Thiazide diuretics

requires a combination of factors, including excessive osteoclast-stimulated bone resorption, increased renal tubular calcium reabsorption (due to PTH, PTHrP, or volume depletion), and immobilization. This combination is most often seen in patients with malignancy in the ICU setting.

The clinical manifestations of hypercalcemia include anorexia, constipation, and abdominal pain progressing to weakness, lethargy, obtundation, and even coma as the serum calcium increases to 16 mg/dL. Polyuria due to nephrogenic DI may produce volume depletion, which in turn stimulates renal tubular calcium reabsorption and aggravates hypercalcemia. Renal insufficiency is common with acute and/or severe hypercalcemia. A shortened QT interval, bradycardia, and heart block may occur, particularly in patients taking digitalis.

Treatment of mild hypercalcemia (<12 mg/dL) may require only simple hydration, restriction of dietary calcium, and treatment of the underlying disease. As serum calcium increases above 12 mg/dL or the patient becomes symptomatic, specific anticalcemic therapy may be required (Table 11). IV saline solution (3 to 4 L/d) and furosemide (80 to 160 mg/d) can produce a modest decrement in serum calcium by enhancing renal calcium excretion. When using saline solution and furosemide, one should achieve a minimum urinary output of 100 mL/h. Corticosteroids (hydrocortisone 200 to 300 mg/d IV or prednisone 40 to 80 mg/d, po) are effective when hypercalcemia is caused by excess vitamin D (vitamin D intoxication, sarcoidosis, lymphoma) or multiple myeloma.

More aggressive treatment is required for serum calcium >14 mg/dL. Although relatively weak, calcitonin (4 to 8 U/kg q6-12h) can work within hours to lower serum calcium. Calcitonin is also a potent analgesic and therefore particularly suited for patients with bone pain. Usually, treatment with mithramycin (25 μg/kg IV) or the bisphosphonates (etidronate, 7.5 mg/kg IV; pamidronate, 30 to 90 mg IV; zolendronic acid, 4 to 8 mg IV) will also be necessary. Mithramycin will begin to lower serum calcium within hours, with its nadir effect at 48 to 72 h. The effect typically persists for several days, but repeat dosing is often necessary. The effect of bisphosphonate therapy is usually slower but more prolonged, with a nadir in serum calcium at 7 days and a duration of several weeks. Zolendronic acid (4 to 8 mg IV) is likely superior to pamidronate. A constant infusion of gallium nitrate (200 mg/m^2/d for 5 days) will normalize serum calcium in 70 to 80% of hypercalcemic patients. The onset, however, is relatively slow and the nadir is usually at 8 to 10 days. Use of gallium is limited by its nephrotoxicity. The use of oral (too weak) and IV (too dangerous) phosphate is no longer recommended for treatment of hypercalcemia.

Table 11. *Treatment of Hypercalcemia**

Therapy	Dose	Onset	Duration	Efficacy	Toxicity
NS	3–6 L/D	Hours	Hours	1–2 mg/dL	Excess ECV
Furosemide	80–160 mg/d	Hours	Hours	1–2 mg/dL	ECV depletion
Hydrocortisone	200 mg/d	Hours	Days	Mild‡	↑BP, ↓K, ↑glucose
Calcitonin	4–8 U/kg	Hours	Hours	1–2 mg/dL	Nausea, thrombopenia
Mithramycin	25 µg/kg	12 h	Days	1–5 mg/dL	Marrow, liver, kidney
Pamidronate	30–90 mg/wk	Days	1–4 wk	1–5 mg/dL	Fever
Zolendrate§	4–8 mg	Days	Weeks	1–5 mg/dL	
Gallium	200 mg/m²	Days	Days to weeks	1–5 mg/dL	Fever

* NS = normal saline solution; K, potassium.
† Expected decrease in serum calcium.
‡ Effective for hypercalcemia of vitamin D excess or ectopic vitamin D syndromes.
§ Preferred bisphosphonate.

Hemodialysis or peritoneal dialysis with a zero-calcium dialysate is rarely necessary but can be used to treat severe hypercalcemia.

Hypocalcemia

Hypocalcemia (Table 12) can be seen with vitamin D deficiency, PTH deficiency or resistance, or binding by various intravascular or tissue chelators. Malabsorption of calcium and vitamin D is most commonly from small-bowel resection or inflammation (*eg*, Crohn's disease). Liver disease (decreased synthesis of calcefediol) or renal disease (decreased synthesis of calcitriol) may also cause vitamin D deficiency. Hypoparathyroidism most often occurs postthyroidectomy, but rarely is due to a familial multiglandular condition. Suppression of PTH release is usually due to hypomagnesemia (see below) but may accompany severe hypermagnesmia, sepsis, burns, pancreatitis, or rhabdomyolysis. Hypomagnesemia also causes PTH resistance. Rapid or massive blood or plasma transfusion may cause calcium chelation by citrate, an effect also seen when citrate is used as an alternative anticoagulant for hemodialysis. The most common calcium chelator, however is phosphorus, and this hypocalcemic syndrome may occur in patients with major tissue damage (burns, rhabdomyolysis), tumor lysis syndrome, or acute and chronic renal failure.

The clinical signs of hypocalcemia include perioral paresthesia, muscular spasms, tetany, and even seizures. Chvostek's and Trousseau's signs do not usually develop unless the serum calcium falls below 6 mg/dL. Several studies suggest that ionized hypocalcemia and elevated PTH are associated with an increased mortality. Prolongation of the QT interval is common. Bradycardia and hypotension are indications for emergent therapy.

Because treatment of hypocalcemia with calcium alone is only transiently effective, one must identify and correct the underlying cause. Mild or asymptomatic hypocalcemia requires only an

Table 12. *Common Causes of Hypocalcemia*

Decreased GI absorption
    Vitamin D deficiency
        Malabsorption
        Hepatic failure
        Renal failure
    Malabsorption syndromes
Decreased bone resorption
    Hypoparathyroidism
        Postthyroidectomy
        Familial
        Hypomagnesemia
        Sepsis
        Burns
        Pancreatitis
        Rhabdomyolysis
    PTH resistance
        Hypomagnesemia
        Pseudohypoparathyroidism
    Osteoblastic metastases
Intravascular or tissue chelation
    Citrate
        Transfusion
        Anticoagulation
    Albumin
    Fat embolus
    Hyperphosphatemia
        Burns
        Rhabdomyolysis
        Tumor lysis
        Renal failure

increase in dietary calcium. IV calcium (100 to 200 mg IV over 10 min followed by 100 mg/h constant infusion) should be reserved for symptomatic patients or those with serum calcium <6 mg/dL. Calcium gluconate (90 mg elemental calcium per 10 mL ampule) is preferred to limit vein irritation and extravasation. Calcium infusion should be avoided in patients with severe hyperphosphatemia. Serum calcium should initially be monitored every 4 h. Once the serum calcium is >7 mg/dL, it usually can be maintained with oral calcium supplements (0.5 to 1.0 g tid). The addition of vitamin D3 (25,000 to 50,000 units three times weekly), calcefediol (25-[OH]D3) (50 to 300 μg/d) or calcitriol (1,25 (OH)2 D3) (0.25 to 1 μg/d) will be necessary in those patients with vitamin D deficiency. Thiazide diuretics, by inducing intravascular volume contraction, increase proximal tubular calcium reabsorption and can serve as a therapeutic adjunct. Finally, the hypocalcemia of magnesium depletion cannot be corrected until magnesium losses are replaced.

Magnesium

One third of the approximately 360 mg (30 mEq) daily dietary magnesium is absorbed (Fig 6). Renal excretion accounts for most of the daily magnesium loss, but some GI secretion occurs as well. Like calcium, magnesium is primarily an intracellular cation stored in bone (55%) and skeletal muscle (30%). Less than 1% of total body magnesium is in the extracellular fluid (ECF). Unlike calcium, however, no hormones control magnesium balance, and the serum magnesium is not readily exchangeable with tissue stores. Therefore, loss of magnesium can lead rather quickly to hypomagnesemia, and there is little protection against hypermagnesemia when renal excretion is impaired.

Hypermagnesemia

Hypermagnesemia occurs primarily in patients with renal insufficiency or in those receiving excess magnesium by IV (treatment of preeclampsia), rectal (magnesium-containing enemas), or oral (antacids, laxatives) routes. The latter occurs more commonly when absorption is enhanced by GI inflammation (ulcer, gastritis, colitis). Excess

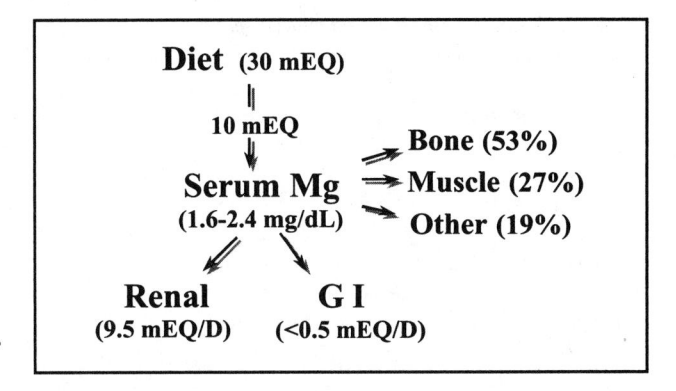

Figure 6. Magnesium balance.

Table 13. *Clinical Manifestations of Hypo/hypermagnesemia Related to the Serum Level*

Serum Level (mg/dL)	Manifestations
>12	Muscle paralysis, complete heart block, cardiac arrest
>7	Somnolence, respiratory depression, hypocalcemia, bradycardia, hypotension
>4	Lethargy, hyporeflexia
1.6–4	Usually asymptomatic
<2	"Normomagnesemic magnesium depletion"
<1.6	Weakness, anorexia, hypokalemia, hypocalcemia
<1.2	Tetany, positive Chvostek's and Trousseau's signs, wide QRS, peaked T
<0.8	Convulsions, prolonged PR, ventricular arrhythmia

dietary magnesium will not cause hypermagnesemia unless renal function is impaired.

The signs and symptoms of hypermagnesemia are related to the plasma level (Table 13). Lethargy and hyporeflexia can occur at levels >4 mg/dL. Respiratory depression, bradycardia, and hypotension are usually seen at >7 mg/dL. A serum magnesium >12mg/dL can cause muscle paralysis, complete heart block, and cardiac arrest. In these cases, IV calcium (100 to 200 mg of elemental calcium over 5 to 10 min) can be life-saving. Dialysis can also be used when renal function is impaired. Milder symptoms and magnesium levels <8 mg/dL require only volume expansion and discontinuing exogenous magnesium.

Hypomagnesemia

Hypomagnesemia occurs in 12% of hospitalized patients but in 40 to 60% of ICU patients. It

Table 14. *Common Causes of Hypomagnesemia*

GI losses
    Malabsorption
    Diarrhea
    Gastric suction
    Prolonged dietary restriction
Renal losses
    Excessive IV fluids
    Postobstructive diuresis
    Recovery-phase acute tubular necrosis
    Drugs
        Diuretics
        Aminoglycosides
        Alcohol
        Amphotericin
        Cyclosporine
        Platinum
    Ketoacidosis
    Bartter's syndrome
    Renal tubular acidosis
Increased cellular uptake
    Refeeding
    Recovery from hypothermia
    Insulin
    Rapid tumor growth
    Rhabdomyolysis
    Pancreatitis

predicts excess mortality in acutely ill and postoperative adult patients and in neonates with ventilatory failure. Treatment of hypomagnesemia improves survival in some studies of endotoxic shock (rats), patients with acute myocardial infarction (MI), and postoperative patients with left ventricular dysfunction.

GI and renal losses account for most cases of magnesium depletion (Table 14). Extreme diarrhea or malabsorption can readily deplete serum magnesium; prolonged vomiting or gastric secretion induces hypomagnesemia more gradually. Because of obligate daily losses of magnesium in the stool and urine, a 1- to 2-week period of not eating or not receiving magnesium in IV fluids will cause hypomagnesemia in most patients.

Renal magnesium wasting occurs with excessive diuresis (IV fluids, postobstructive, diuretic phase of acute renal failure), diuretic drugs (loop and thiazide diuretics) and with several drugs (Table 14). Renal magnesium loss can easily be distinguished from GI losses by demonstrating an elevated fractional excretion of magnesium (FEMg > 1.5%) in a hypomagnesemic patient. The calculation must account for the plasma (P) protein binding of magnesium as follows:

$$FEMg = (UMg \times PCr \times 100)/[(0.7 \times PMg) \times UCr]$$

where UMg is urinary magnesium, PCr is plasma creatinine, PMg is plasma magnesium, and UCr is urinary creatinine.

Hypomagnesemia can result with increased cellular uptake from several causes, including refeeding, insulin therapy, or tissue injury (rhabdomyolysis). Acute pancreatitis can cause hypomagnesemia by saponification.

The clinical manifestations of magnesium depletion are roughly correlated with the plasma level (Table 13). Weakness, anorexia, and neuromuscular irritability can progress to respiratory depression and convulsions in severe cases. The cardiac toxicity is highly dependent on concurrent myocardial perfusion such that severe arrhythmias may occur with seemingly mild hypomagnesemia in the setting of acute MI. Hypokalemia (due to renal potassium wasting) and hypocalcemia (due to altered PTH resistance and release) occurs in as many as 40% of magnesium-deficient patients (trication deficiency). Neither the hypokalemia nor hypocalcemia of magnesium deficiency can be corrected without magnesium repletion. In fact, hypokalemia and hypocalcemia in the ICU patient often corrects with magnesium administration, even in normomagnesemic patients (normomagnesemic magnesium depletion).

Treatment of hypomagnesemia includes correcting the underlying GI or renal cause. Serious complications such as ventricular ectopy, hypokalemia, or hypocalcemic tetany require IV magnesium sulfate (1 g [8 mEq] IV stat followed by 6 g over 24 h). Because serum levels normalize before tissue stores are repleted, renal losses of magnesium usually continue, necessitating daily magnesium replacement (6 to 8 g magnesium sulfate) for 3 to 5 days. Milder cases of hypomagnesemia can be treated by slow-release tablets (Table 15). Amiloride will increase magnesium absorption in the cortical collecting tubule and is an excellent adjunct to magnesium therapy.

The use of magnesium to prevent arrhythmias and improve survival in patients with acute MI remains controversial and is not routinely recommended. However, in high-risk patients, 16 mEq (8 mmol/L, 192 mg) of magnesium IV over 5 to 15 min prior to reperfusion (thrombolysis or angioplasty) with 128 mEq (64 mM, 1,536 mg)

Table 15. *Treatment of Hypomagnesemia*

Serum Mg (mg/dL)	Clinical Situation	Treatment	Elemental Mg mg	mM	mEq
≥1.6	Chronic depletion	Magnesium oxide 400 mg bid	241	10	20
≥1.6	Prolonged IV fluids	MgSO$_4$ 4 g/d IV	400	16	32
1.2–1.6	Minimal signs/symptoms	MgSO$_4$ 8 g/d IV	800	32	64
<1.2	Hyperreflexia, myoclonus	MgSO$_4$ 6 g IV q6-8h	600	25	50
<1.2	Ventricular arrhythmias	MgSO$_4$ 2 g IV over 15 min	200	8	16

over the ensuing 24 h appears to decrease the incidence of arrhythmia and left ventricular dysfunction and improve mortality. It is contraindicated in patients with a greater than first-degree heart block or bradycardia, as magnesium can delay atrioventricular conduction.

Potassium

Although 2% of total body potassium is in the ECF, serum potassium is in dynamic equilibrium with intracellular stores. Movement into and out of cells is controlled by the adrenergic nervous system, insulin, and alterations in pH. Daily dietary intake (100 mEq) is matched by daily renal (90 mEq) and GI (10 mEq) excretion. Like calcium and magnesium, alterations in serum potassium are best explained by changes in intake, cellular shift, and renal excretion (Fig 7).

Hyperkalemia

The causes of hyperkalemia are outlined in Table 16. Because the kidney is able to substantially increase potassium excretion (up to 300 mEq daily), excess dietary potassium rarely causes hyperkalemia. However, in patients with even mild renal impairment, excessive potassium intake may be an important cause of hyperkalemia. Besides oral potassium supplements, occult sources of potassium include potassium penicillin, salt substitutes, stored blood, and oral (chewed) tobacco products.

Hyperkalemia is often due to release of cellular potassium. Nonselective β-blockers (*eg*, propranolol) may elevate serum potassium by this mechanism. Aldosterone deficiency increases serum potassium by causing an intra- to extracellular potassium shift and by decreasing renal excretion. Insulin deficiency and hypertonicity (*eg*, hyperglycemia) independently cause cellular-to-serum

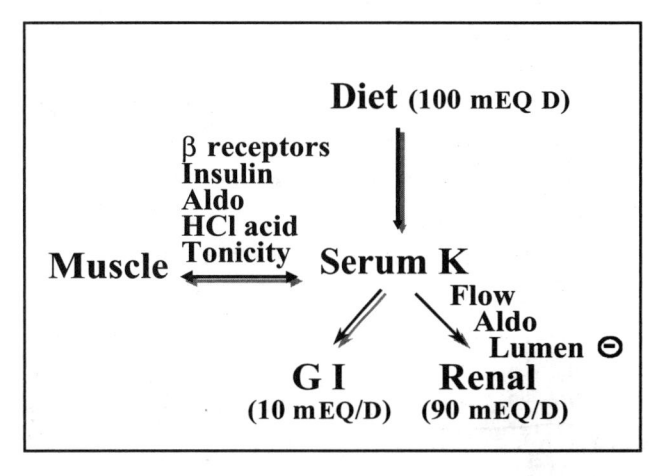

Figure 7. Potassium balance. Aldo = aldosterone.

shift of potassium, which explains the hyperkalemia (and the prompt resolution with therapy) so often seen in diabetic ketoacidosis. Hyperchloremic acidosis (but not organic acidoses—*eg*, ketoacidosis, lactic acidosis) is also associated with hyperkalemia due to cellular shifts. In these cases, the serum potassium increases by an average of 0.5 mEq/L for each 0.1 decrement in pH. Finally, cell lysis can present a potentially huge potassium burden to the ECF. Thus, life-threatening hyperkalemia can be seen with rhabdomyolysis, tumor lysis syndrome, massive hemolysis, and occasionally with succinylcholine, particularly with simultaneous renal insufficiency.

The most common causes of hyperkalemia are related to decreased renal excretion. Because the renal tubules not only reabsorb nearly all potassium filtered at the glomerulus, but also secrete most of the 90 mEq of potassium excreted daily, hyperkalemia rarely develops from renal failure (low GFR) *per se*. Rather, "renal" hyperkalemia is usually due to some defect in tubular potassium secretion. Tubular secretion of potassium requires aldosterone, good-functioning distal and collecting tubular cells, and an adequate delivery of filtered sodium and water to these nephron segments.

Thus, any cause of hypoaldosteronism (hyporeninemia, isolated aldosterone deficiency, angiotensin-converting enzyme inhibitors [ACEIs] or angiotensin-receptor blockers, heparin) predisposes to hyperkalemia. Hyperkalemia frequently accompanies tubulointerstitial renal diseases (particularly chronic pyelonephritis, analgesic nephropathy, sickle-cell disease, transplant rejection, and obstructive uropathy) despite relative preservation of renal function (GFR > 20 mL/min). The failure to simultaneously secrete hydrogen ion allows hyperchloremic (nonanion-gap) acidosis frequently to accompany hyperkalemia (type IV RTA). Finally, several drugs cause hyperkalemia by inhibiting tubular potassium secretion. In addition to potassium-sparing diuretics (spironolactone, triamterene, and amiloride), cyclosporine, tacrolimus, high-dose trimethoprim, pentamidine, NSAIDs, and ACEIs all share this potential complication.

Pseudohyperkalemia is the release of potassium when blood clots in a test tube. Patients with severe leukocytosis (>100,000) or thrombocytosis (>400,000) are particularly prone to this phenomenon. This diagnosis is confirmed by a simultaneously drawn serum (red-top) and plasma (green-top) potassium level.

The toxicity of hyperkalemia is neuromuscular and cardiac. Paresthesias and weakness may progress to flaccid paralysis. ECG changes include peaked T waves in the precordial leads followed by decreased R-wave amplitude, widened PR interval, widened QRS complex, and finally loss of the P wave and the development of the sine wave. Heart block or ventricular standstill may occur at any point. The correlation between the serum potassium and the ECG is quite variable.

The treatment of hyperkalemia is outlined in Table 17. When the serum potassium is <6 mEq/L, little therapy is required other than discontinuing the occult sources of dietary potassium listed in Table 16. As the potassium rises to >6 mEq/L and/or peaked T waves appear, volume expansion (as tolerated), loop diuretics, and oral sodium polystyrene sulfonate powder (Kayexalate; Sanofi Winthrop Pharmaceuticals; New York, NY) are appropriate. (Kayexalate via rectum is reported to cause colonic necrosis.) Although somewhat slow to act, these treatments actually increase potassium excretion. When more urgent therapy is needed for hyperkalemia (>7 mEq/L), driving potassium intracellularly with glucose and insulin (25 to 50 g dextrose with 10 to 20 U of regular insulin) or the β-agonist albuterol (5 to 20 mg [1.0 to 4.0 mL] inhaled) is indicated. Albuterol usually works within 30 min, will lower the serum potassium by 0.6 to 1.0 mEq/L, and lasts for 2 h or more. Calcium therapy (10 mEq IV over 5 min) is reserved for hyperkalemia-induced heart block, the sine wave, or of course ventricular arrest. Its effect is immediate but short-lived (<60 min). Other maneuvers to remove potassium from the body (such as diuretics or Kayexalate) must be promptly initiated as well. Dialysis (usually hemodialysis) can also be employed to remove potassium.

Table 16. *Common Causes of Hyperkalemia*

Excess intake (usually only with renal insufficiency)
    Potassium supplements
    Salt substitutes
    Potassium penicillin
    Stored blood
    Oral tobacco products
Intra- to extracellular shift
    $β_2$-blockers
    Aldosterone deficiency
    Insulin deficiency
    Hypertonicity
    Succinylcholine
    Hyperchloremic acidosis
    Cell lysis
        Tumor lysis syndrome
        Hemolysis
        Rhabdomyolysis
Decreased renal excretion
    Decreased GFR (<5 mL/min)
    Decreased tubular secretion
        Hypoaldosteronism
            Primary
            Hyporeninemic
            Heparin
            ACEIs/angiotensin-receptor blockers
        Tubulo-interstitial nephritis
            Analgesic nephropathy
            Pyelonephritis
            Sickle-cell nephropathy
            Renal transplant nephropathy
            Obstructive nephropathy
        Drugs
            Amiloride
            Spironolactone
            Triamterene
            Cyclosporine
            Tacrolimus
            Trimethoprim
            Pentamidine
            NSAIDs

Table 17. *Treatment of Hyperkalemia*

Serum K (mEq/L)	ECG Δ	Treatment	Onset	Duration	Mechanism
<6	None	Avoid NSAIDs Restrict dietary K			
>6	Peaked T Prolonged PR	ECV expansion Loop diuretic IV Kayexalate po	Hours 1–2 h 2–4 h	Hours Hours	Renal excretion GI excretion
>7	Widened QRS	Glucose/insulin IV Albuterol (inhaled) NaHCO$_3$ IV*	Minutes Minutes Minutes	Hours Hours Hours	Redistribution Redistribution Redistribution
>8	Sine wave	Calcium	1–3 min	<1 h	Cardiac

*Most useful with simultaneous hyperchloremic acidosis.

Hypokalemia

The causes of hypokalemia are listed in Table 18. Significant GI loss of potassium is usually colonic (diarrhea, cathartic abuse) and accompanied by a hyperchloremic acidosis. Although gastric juice contains very little potassium (10 mEq/L), vomiting or gastric suction often causes hypokalemia due to concurrent volume contraction, secondary hyperaldosteronism, and renal potassium wasting. This also explains the renal hydrogen ion secretion and the seemingly "paradoxic aciduria" of contraction alkalosis. Renal artery stenosis (secondary hyperaldosteronism) causes hypokalemia due to urinary potassium loss. Renal wastage is also seen when nonreabsorbable anions (*eg*, carbenicillin) are filtered into the urine, increasing distal potassium secretion. Any process increasing tubular flow (diuretics, diuretic phase of acute renal failure, postobstructive diuresis) will enhance tubular potassium secretion. Renal tubular acidosis (type I and II) and Bartter's syndrome are rare causes of renal hypokalemia. Hypomagnesemia is a more common cause of hypokalemia due to renal potassium loss.

Hypokalemia caused by extra- to intracellular shift usually accompanies refeeding or treatment of hyperglycemia with insulin. Hypokalemia may cause a wide range of clinical manifestations. Muscle weakness (including respiratory muscles), myalgias, cramps, and even rhabdomyolysis can occur. Gastroparesis, ileus, and constipation are common features. Hypokalemia may also cause nephrogenic DI, renal phosphate wasting, and acidification defects due to decreased ammonia production. The most serious hypokalemia toxicity, however, is cardiac. Isolated premature ventricular contractions, ventricular tachycardia, delayed conduction, enhancement of digitalis toxicity, and various ECG changes (U waves, flat T waves, ST-segment depression, and atrioventricular block) may all occur.

Potassium replacement can be done via the enteral or IV route. Potassium with chloride or other anions (citrate, bicarbonate, phosphate) is effective orally or via a gastric tube and can be given with impunity as long as renal function is normal. With

Table 18. *Common Causes of Hypokalemia*

GI losses
    Diarrhea
    Cathartics
    Enteric fistula
    Villous adenoma
Extra- to intracellular shift
    Insulin therapy
    Refeeding
    β-Agonists
    Periodic paralysis
Renal losses
    Hyperaldosteronism
        Adrenal adenoma
        Cushing's syndrome
        Vomiting/gastric suction
        Renal artery stenosis
        Exogenous steroids
        Licorice
    Nonabsorbable anions
        Carbenicillin
        Ticarcillin
        Piperacillin
        Ketones
    Increased urine flow
        Diuretics
        Renal tubular acidosis
        Bartter's syndrome
Magnesium depletion

more severe degrees of hypokalemia or in patients symptomatic from hypokalemia, rapid correction may be accomplished intravenously. When potassium is >2mEq/L and there are no ECG changes, 10 mEq/h is sufficient; 40 mEq/h can be given with cardiac monitoring if the serum potassium is <2 mEq/L. Peripheral infusions should be concentrated to ≤60 mEq/L and administered through as large a vein as possible. Central infusions are best administered into the superior vena cava.

One must remember the necessity of treating coexistent magnesium depletion in hypokalemic patients.

Annotated Bibliography

Sodium

Adrogue HJ, Madias NE. Hypernatremia. N Engl J Med 2000; 342:1493–1499

Adrogue HJ, Madias NE. Hyponatremia. N Engl J Med 2000; 342:1581–1589

Faber MD, Kupin WL, Heilig CW, et al. Common fluid electrolyte and acid-base problems in the intensive care unit: selected issues. Semin Nephrol 1994; 14:8–22

A particularly good review.

Oster JR, Singer I. Hyponatremia, hypoosmolality and hypotonicity: tables and fables. Arch Intern Med 1999; 159:333–336

Rose BD. Hypoosmolal states. In: Clinical physiology of acid-base and electrolyte disorders. 4th ed. New York, NY: McGraw-Hill, 1994; 651–694

Zaloga, GP, Kirby RR, Bernards WC, et al. Fluids and electrolytes. In: Civetta JM, Taylor RW, Kirby RR, eds. Critical care. 3rd ed. Philadelphia, PA: JB Lippincott, 1997; 413–441

An excellent review with the critical care practitioner in mind.

Calcium

Akmal M, Bishop JE, Telfer N, et al. Hypocalcemia and hypercalcemia in patients with rhabdomyolysis with and without acute renal failure. J Clin Endocrinol Metab 1986; 63:137–142

Belezikian JP. Management of acute hypercalcemia. J Clin Endocrinol Metab 1993; 77:1445–1449

Outlines aggressive therapy of hypercalcemia based on pathophysiology.

Binstock ML, Mundy GR. Effect of calcitonin and glucocorticoids in combination on the hypercalcemia of malignancy. Ann Intern Med 1980; 93:269–272

Major P, Lortholary A, Hon J, et al. Zolendronic acid is superior to pamidronate in the treatment of the hypercalcemia of malignancy: a pooled analysis of two randomized controlled clinical trials. J Clin Oncol 2001; 19:558–567

Perlia CP, Gubisch NJ, Walter J, et al. Mithramycin treatment of hypercalcemia. Cancer 1970; 25:389–394

Rosol TJ, Capen CC. Mechanisms of cancer-induced hypercalcemia. Lab Invest 1992; 67:680–702

Excellent discussion of hormonal causes of hypercalcemia in cancer patients.

Suki WN, Yium JJ, Von Minden M, et al. Acute treatment of hypercalcemia with furosemide. N Engl J Med 1970; 283:836–840

Demonstrates the importance of isotonic hydration with furosemide as adjunctive therapy for hypercalcemia.

Magnesium

Alfrey AC. Normal and abnormal magnesium metabolism. In: Schrier RW, ed. Renal and electrolyte disorders. 4th ed. Boston, MA: Little Brown, 1992; 371–404

Broner CW, Stidham GL, Westenkirchner DF, et al. Hypermagnesemia and hypocalcemia as predictors of high mortality in critically ill pediatric patients. Crit Care Med 1990; 18:921–928

Emphasizes the importance of electrolyte disorders in critically ill patients.

Rubeiz GJ, Thill-Baharozian M, Hardie D, et al. Association of hypomagnesemia and mortality in acutely ill medical patients. Crit Care Med 1983; 21:203–209

Salem M, Munoz R, Chernow B. Hypomagnesemia in critical illness: a common and clinically important problem. Crit Care Clin 1991; 7:225–252

Woods KL, Fletcher S. Long-term outcome after intravenous magnesium sulfate in inspected acute myocardial infarction: the second Leister intravenous magnesium intervention trial (LIMIT-2). Lancet 1994; 343:816–819

Treatment of acute MI with magnesium may improve survival.

Potassium

Blumberg A, Wiedmann P, Shaw S, et al. Effect of various therapeutic approaches on plasma potassium and major regulating factors in terminal renal failure. Am J Med 1988; 85:507–512

The combination of insulin and glucose is more effective than bicarbonate in treating "renal" hyperkalemia.

DeFronzo RA. Hyperkalemia and hyporeninemic hypoaldosteronism. Kidney Int 1980; 17:118–134

A complete and excellent review.

Fulop M. Serum potassium in lactic acidosis and ketoacidosis. N Engl J Med 1979; 300:1087–1089

Clarifies the mechanism and therapy of hyperkalemia in patients with metabolic acidosis.

Gabow PA, Peterson LN. Disorders of potassium metabolism. In: Schrier RW, ed. Renal and electrolyte disorders. 4th ed. Boston, MA: Little Brown, 1992; 231–285

An excellent outline of renal hyperkalemia.

Hamill RJ, Robinson LM, Wexler HR, et al. Efficacy and safety of potassium infusion therapy in hypokalemic critically ill patients. Crit Care Med 1991; 19:694–699

Kruse JA, Carlson RW. Rapid correction of hypokalemia using concentrated intravenous potassium chloride infusions. Arch Intern Med 1990; 150:613–617

The safety and efficacy of high-dose IV potassium.

Montoliu J, Lens XM, Revert L. Potassium-lowering effect of albuterol for hyperkalemia in renal failure. Arch Intern Med 1987; 147:713–717

Albuterol is safe and effective for short-term therapy for hyperkalemia.

Notes

Hemodynamic Monitoring

Jesse B. Hall, MD, FCCP

Hemodynamic monitoring may be defined as the collection and interpretation of various parameters that inform determination of: (1) the etiology of a state of hypoperfusion and/or (2) the response of the cardiopulmonary unit to interventions such as fluid therapy, vasoactive drugs, or adjustments in positive pressure ventilation. For many patients, adequate monitoring is achieved by routine vital signs along with collection of data such as input/output, physical examination, and urine electrolytes. In other patients, invasive measurements are made, including use of arterial catheters, central venous catheters (CVC), and right heart catheters (RHC). These catheters provide for continuous transduction of pressure in either the arterial or venous circuit and sampling of blood for determination of oxygen saturation. Simultaneous determination of arterial and mixed venous blood gases also permits determination of oxygen content, oxygen delivery, oxygen consumption, arteriovenous oxygen content difference, and calculation of cardiac output by Fick determination.

The use of invasive methods of assessing hemodynamics—arterial and right heart catheters—grew during the evolution of critical care medicine despite a lack of prospective trials demonstrating efficacy and improved patient outcome. Indeed, one retrospective study suggested that use of the RHC is associated with an independent negative effect on survival. This study has been criticized largely on the basis of design—it was retrospective, and thus even reasonably sophisticated methods of case matching may have failed to control for the inevitable differences in patient status and hence prognosis that might contribute to decisions to perform invasive monitoring. However, prospective trials have been undertaken and one recent large multicenter study evaluating the use of RHC for high-risk surgical patients failed to demonstrate either a benefit or detriment to its use. It is important to note that in order for trials of invasive monitoring to demonstrate benefit, investigators must identify a patient population at risk for or exhibiting a hemodynamic state amenable to interventions that will improve outcome—monitoring alone is unlikely to confer benefit. Moreover, for many conditions—sepsis, the acute respiratory distress syndrome (ARDS)—the proper fluid and vasoactive drug interventions remain to be defined. For these conditions, trials have been designed and implemented that test not only the monitoring modality but the proper intervention as well (eg, randomizing patients with ARDS to either a RHC or CVC and then further to either a "fluid liberal" or "fluid conservative" management strategy).

Differential Diagnosis of Hypoperfused States and Bedside Assessment

A useful and readily applicable bedside algorithm at the time of resuscitation of patients with circulatory inadequacy is—is this low- or high-output hypotension? If the former, is the heart full or not? And when fluid resuscitation has occurred, is the response definitive or has low-output shock now taken on the characteristics of high-flow shock (eg, septic shock with initial hypovolemia, now fluid-resuscitated)? Often this simple algorithm succeeds in fully resuscitating the patient. If not, further information gathering from invasive monitoring and/or echocardiography is appropriate (Table 1).

Alternatives to Pulmonary Artery Catheterization

Given uncertainties concerning the benefits of invasive monitoring with the RHC, recent literature has emphasized alternative approaches. In the most significant recent trial evaluating resuscitation of patients with early severe sepsis and septic shock, RHC was not used but rather patients were randomized to routine care vs early goal-directed therapy (EGDT) guided by arterial blood pressure, right atrial pressure, right atrial oxygen saturation (as a surrogate of mixed venous blood saturation) and urine volume. Outcomes were improved with EGDT despite no use of RHC, suggesting the use of the cardiac output to determine the adequacy of the circulation in patients with sepsis may be less useful than the concentration of effluent blood returning from the systemic circulation.

There has also been considerable study of the use of the arterial pressure waveform alone as an indicator for the adequacy of intravascular volume and response to fluid challenge. Numerous studies have shown that responders and nonresponders to fluid challenge are not well defined by the baseline right atrial pressure or pulmonary artery occlusion pressure (Fig 1). This relates to many factors to be discussed below.

However, patients with spontaneous respirations will typically exhibit drops in right atrial pressure during inspiration related to swings in intrathoracic pressure that has been shown to correlate with relative hypovolemia and "preload reserve," making this observation useful in determining the need for further fluid resuscitation. In addition, patients undergoing

Table 1. *Rapid Formulation of an Early Working Diagnosis of the Etiology of Shock*

Defining Features of Shock		
Blood pressure	⇓	
Heart rate	⇑	
Respiratory rate	⇑	
Mentation	⇓	
Urine output	⇓	
Arterial pH	⇓	
	High Output Hypotension *Septic Shock*	*Low Cardiac Output* *Cardiogenic and Hypovolemic*
Is Cardiac Output Reduced?	No	Yes
Pulse pressure	⇑	⇓
Diastolic pressure	⇑	⇓
Extremities digits	Warm	Cool
Nailbed return	Rapid	Slow
Heart sounds	Crisp	Muffled
Temperature	⇑ or ⇓	⇔
White cell count	⇑ or ⇓	⇔
Site of infection	++	−
	Reduced Pump Function *Cardiogenic Shock*	*Reduced Venous Return* *Hypovolemic Shock*
Is the Heart Too Full?	Yes	No
Symptoms clinical context	Angina ECG	Hemorrhage dehydration
Jugular venous pressure	⇑	⇓
S_3, S_4, gallop rhythm	+++	−
Respiratory crepitations	+++	−
Chest radiograph	Large heart ⇑ upper lobe flow Pulmonary edema	Normal
What Does Not Fit?		

Overlapping etiologies (septic cardiogenic, septic hypovolemic, cardiogenic hypovolemic)
Short list of other etiologies

High output *hypotension*	*High right atrial* *pressure hypotension*	*Nonresponsive* *hypovolemia*
Liver failure	Pulmonary hypertension	Adrenal insufficiency
Severe Pancreatitis	(most often pulmonary embolus)	Anaphylaxis
Trauma with significant SIRS	Right ventricular infarction Cardiac tamponade	Spinal shock
Thyroid storm		
Arteriovenous fistula		
Paget's disease		

Get more information	Echocardiography, right heart catheterization

mechanical ventilation often have respiratory excursion of arterial blood pressure as demonstrated below (Fig 2).

The result of these cyclical changes in tidal volume is to cause a cyclical change in stroke volume that is detectable on the arterial pressure waveform and signals the existence of hypovolemia (Fig 3).

Empiric investigation has shown that when a greater than 13% increase in the pulse pressure change between maximal (Ppmax) and minimal (Ppmin) pulse pressure exists, patients are highly likely to respond to fluid challenge:

$$\Delta PP (\%) = 100 \times ((Ppmax - Ppmin) / (Ppmax + Ppmin/2))$$

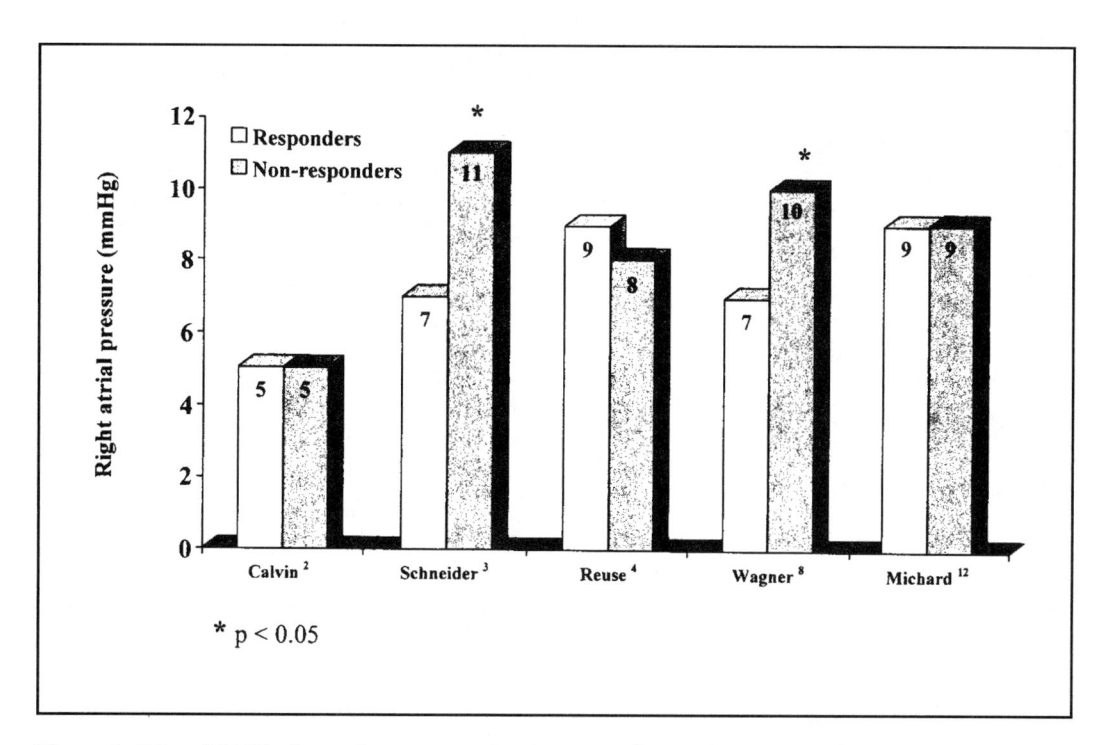

Figure 1. Mean MAP before volume expansion in responders and nonresponders.

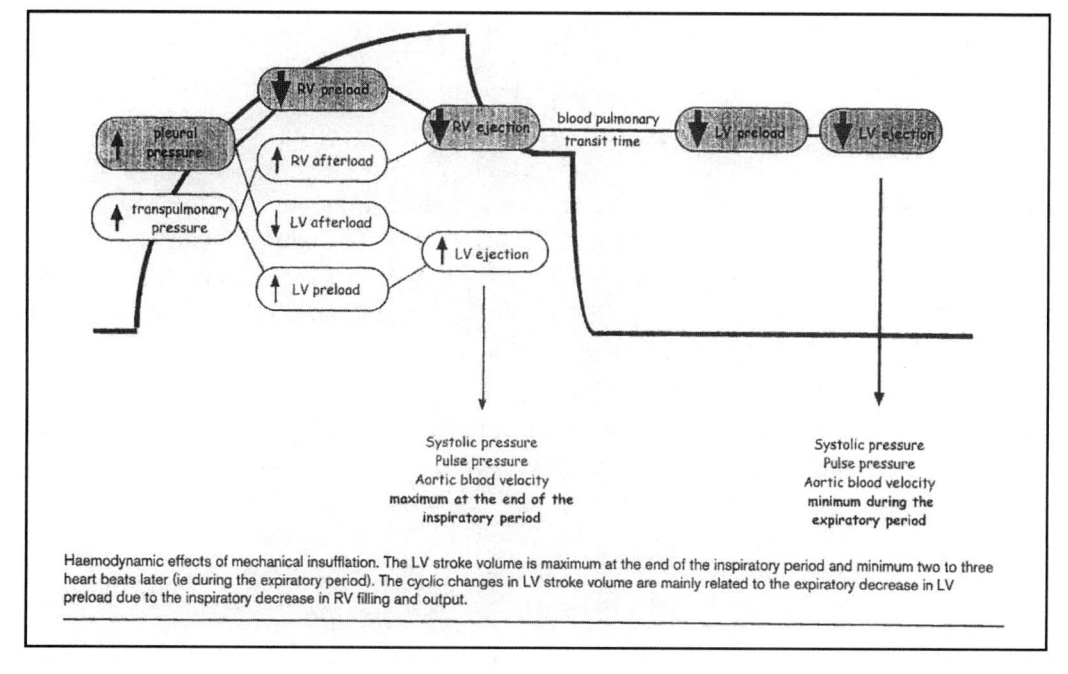

Figure 2. Haemodynamic effects of mechanical insufflation. The LV stroke volume is maximum at the end of the inspiratory period and minimum two to three heart beats later (ie during the expiratory period). The cyclic changes in LV stroke volume are mainly related to the expiratory decrease in LV preload due to the inspiratory decrease in RV filling and output.

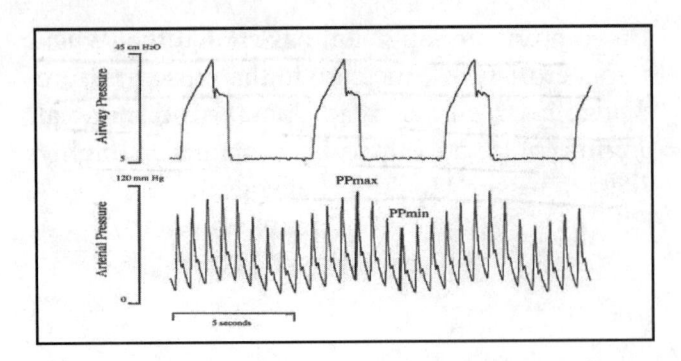

Figure 3.

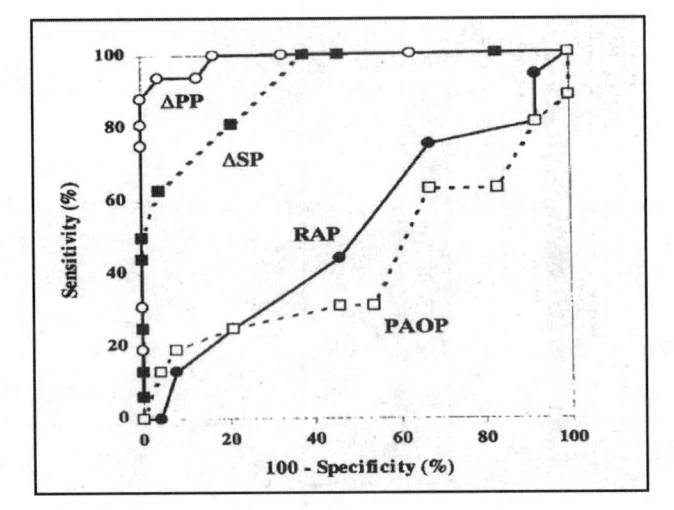

Figure 4.

The receiver operator curve for the pulse pressure variation using this threshold and other measures or cardiac preload in patients with sepsis and hypoperfusion are shown in Figure 4.

While not validated on large groups of patients, this approach is attractive and could eventually prove to be more useful than measurements of right atrial or pulmonary capillary wedge pressure.

Pulmonary Artery Catheterization

Indications and Complications

Rather than offer a list of many conditions that may require PA catheterization, the reader is guided to the statement above recommending formulation of questions concerning the etiology of hypoperfusion or the response to therapy, and answer these questions if possible with clinical data, including volume or drug challenges. When this approach is inadequate, PA catheterization is to be considered. Complications of the procedure are given in Table 2.

Table 2. *Complications of Pulmonary Artery (PA) Catheterization*

I. Complications related to central vein cannulation
II. Complications related to insertion and use of the PA catheter
    A. Tachyarrhythmias
    B. Right bundle branch block
    C. Complete heart block (pre-existing left bundle branch block)
    D. Cardiac perforation
    E. Thrombosis and embolism
    F. Pulmonary infarction due to persistent wedging
    G. Catheter-related sepsis
    H. Pulmonary artery rupture
    I. Knotting of the catheter
    J. Endocarditis, bland and infective
    K. Pulmonic valve insufficiency
    L. Balloon fragmentation and embolization

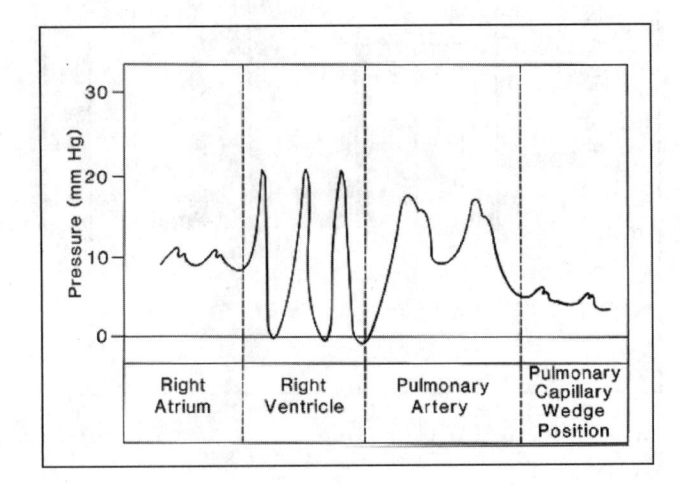

Figure 5.

Interpretation of Pressure Waveforms

Under most conditions, the waveforms obtained as the PA catheter (PAC) is advanced through the right atrium, right ventricle, and into the pulmonary artery to a wedged position are readily identified as characteristic of each segment of the circulation as it is traversed, as demonstrated in Figure 5. While waveform recognition is extremely helpful in positioning the catheter, and often makes the use of fluoroscopic techniques unnecessary, it is essential for the measurement and interpretation of waveforms displayed during PA catheterization to be correlated to the ECG tracing so that specific components of the waveform can be identified and various pitfalls in measurement of intravascular pressure can be avoided.

The Normal Pressure Waveform: In sinus rhythm, the atrial pressure waveform is characterized by two major positive deflections (A and V waves) and two negative deflections (X and Y descents) (Fig 6). A third positive wave, the C wave, is sometimes seen. The A wave results from atrial systolic contraction and is followed by the X descent as the atria relax following contraction. The C wave results from closure of the atrioventricular valves and interrupts the X descent. After the X descent, the V (ventricular) wave is generated by passive filling of the atria during ventricular systole. Lastly, the Y descent reflects the reduction in atrial pressure as the atrioventricular valves open. In correlating these waveforms to the ECG, the first positive pressure wave to follow the P wave is the A wave. The right atrial A wave is usually seen at the beginning of the QRS complex, provided that atrioventricular conduction is normal. The peak of the right atrial V wave normally occurs simultaneously with the T wave of the ECG, provided that the Q-T interval is normal.

The pulmonary artery waveform has a systolic pressure wave and a diastolic trough. A dicrotic notch due to closure of the pulmonic valve may be seen on the terminal portion of the systolic pressure wave. Like the right atrial V wave, the PA systolic wave typically coincides with the electrical T wave. The PA diastolic pressure (Ppad) is recorded as the pressure just before the beginning of the systolic pressure wave.

The Ppw tracing contains the same sequence of waves and descents as the right atrial tracing. However, when the atrial waveform is referenced to the ECG, the mechanical events arising in the left atrium (Ppw) will be seen later than those of the right atrium, because the left atrial pressure waves must travel back through the pulmonary vasculature and a longer length of catheter (Fig 7). Therefore, in the Ppw tracing the A wave usually appears after the QRS complex and the V wave is seen after the T wave. As such, the systolic pressure wave in the PA tracing *precedes* the V wave of the Ppw tracing. An appreciation of the latter relationship is critical when tracings are being analyzed to ensure that balloon inflation has resulted in a transition from an arterial (PA) to atrial (Ppw) waveform, and to detect the presence of a "giant" V wave in the Ppw tracing.

Common Problems Producing Erroneous Pressure Waveforms: Of the many problems causing artifact or erroneous tracings, the most commonly encountered are overdamping, catheter whip, overwedging, incomplete wedging, and Zone I catheter conditions.

Overdamping results from air bubbles within the catheter system or kinking, clotting, and fibrin deposition along the catheter course; many times these problems can be resolved by catheter flushing.

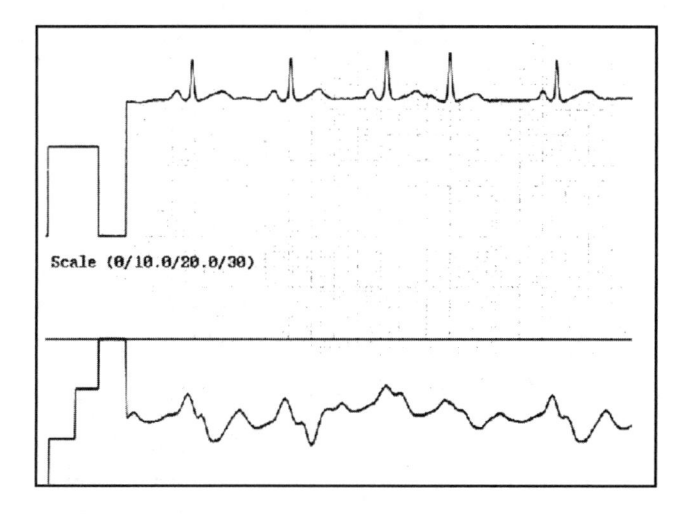

Figure 6.

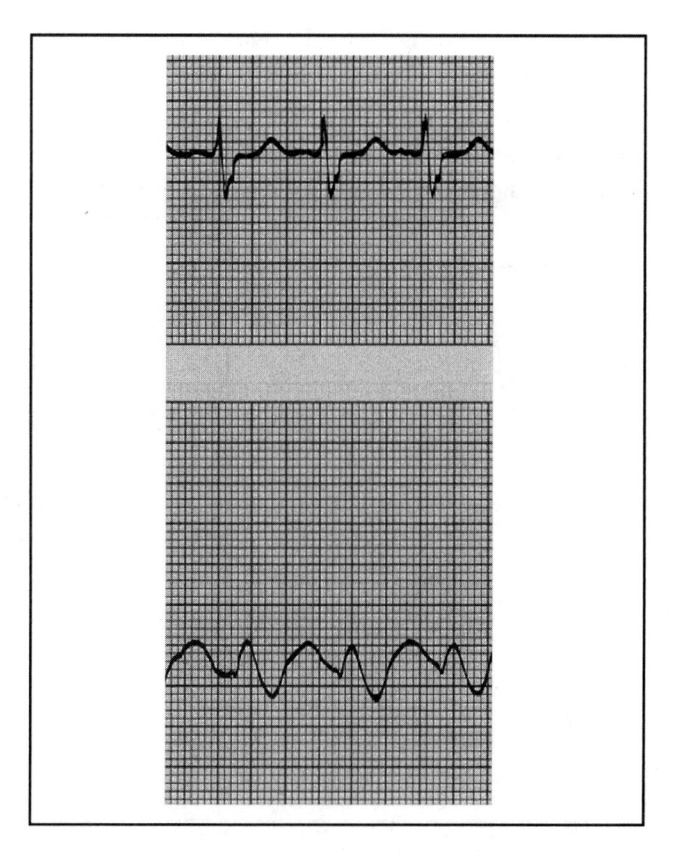

Figure 7.

The main effect of overdamping on the pressure waveform is to artifactually lower the systolic pressure and raise the diastolic pressure with consequent effects on interpretation (Fig 8).

Catheter whip arises from cardiac contractions causing shock transients transmitted to the catheter. The results on the right ventricular or pulmonary arterial waveforms are an exaggerated diastolic pressure in some cycles, highlighting the need to avoid readings obtained by electronic systems.

Overwedging (Fig 9) is signaled by a rise in recorded pressure with balloon inflation as the balloon herniates over the catheter tip or the tip is pushed into the vessel wall with continued fluid ingress elevating the measured pressure. Overwedging requires repositioning of the catheter.

Incomplete wedging (Fig 10) and Zone I positioning of the catheter can be subtle but are important to identify since erroneous and often overestimation of Ppw occur.

Zone I conditions of the lung refer to those segments of the lung in which alveolar pressure exceeds pulmonary vascular pressure and hence there is no flow (Fig 11).

This phenomenon is uncommon when the catheter is floated into position since this typically results in Zone II or III positioning. It would be more likely to result from forceful positioning of the catheter, hypovolemia emerging after placement, or with large increases in PEEP. This condition should be considered when changes in Ppw

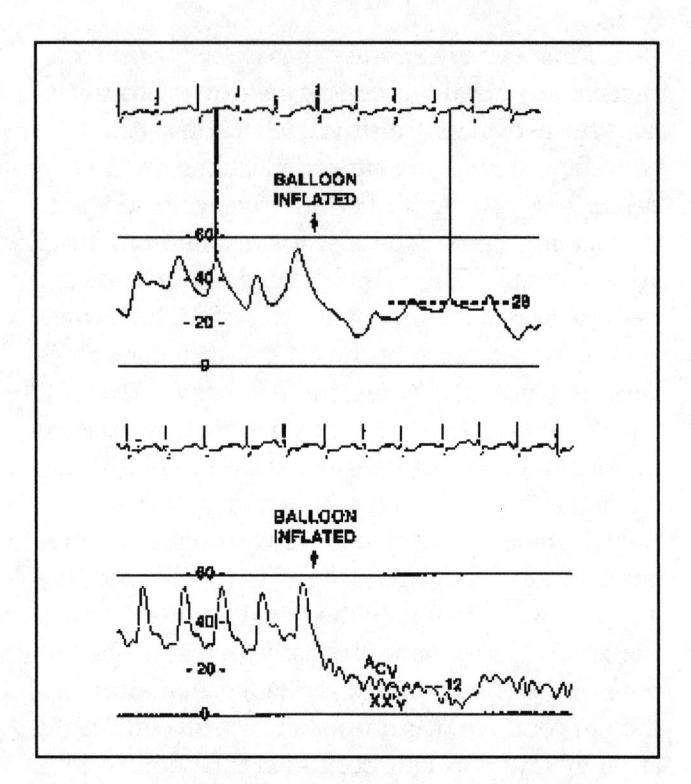

Figure 10. Incomplete wedge pressure (Ppw). Top: With balloon inflation, there is a decrease in pressure to a value that approximates pulmonary artery diastolic pressure (Ppad). The clinical setting (ARDS) is usually associated with a large Ppad-Ppw gradient. Review of the tracings indicates that there is a single positive wave coinciding with the electrocardiographic T wave after balloon inflation, a pattern inconsistent with a left atrial waveform. Bottom: Waveforms after the catheter had been retracted, the balloon inflated, and the catheter floated to a full wedge position. Now, there is a large Ppad-Ppw gradient and the tracing after balloon inflation is consistent with a left atrial waveform. The incomplete wedge tracing yielded an incorrect measurement of the wedge pressure as 28 mm Hg, substantially higher (in a very clinically relevant sense) than the true wedge pressure of approximately 12 mm Hg.

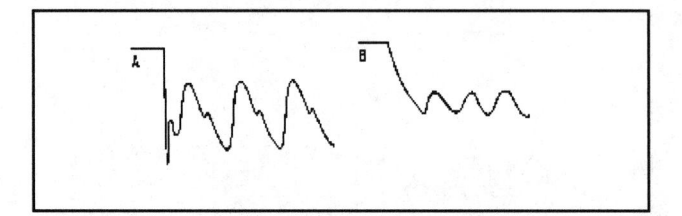

Figure 8. Rapid flush test: A) appropriately damped system; B) over damped system.

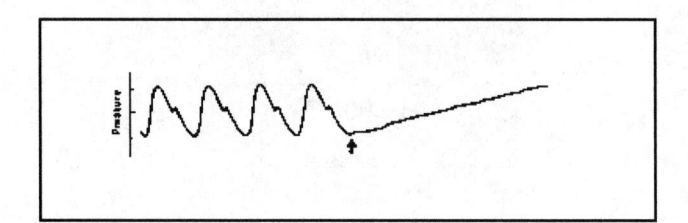

Figure 9.

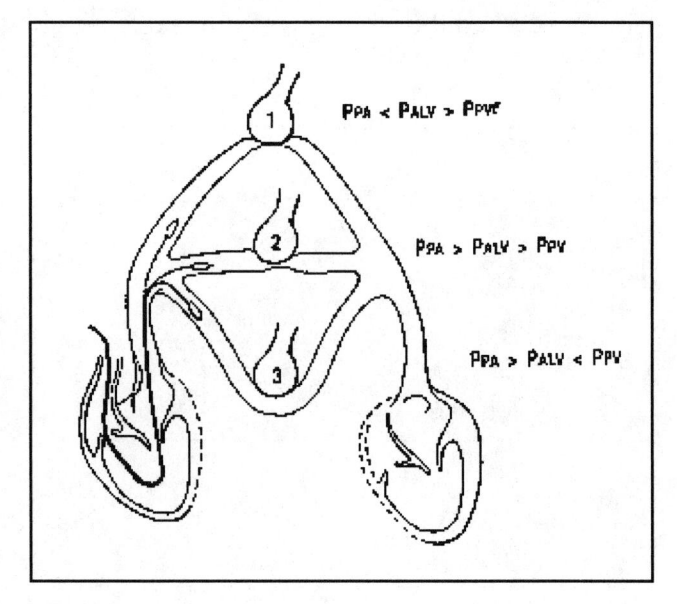

Figure 11. Lung zones.

track PEEP changes exactly or when the excursion in pulmonary artery systolic pressures with respiration exceed those Ppw significantly (Fig 12).

The Correlation of Pressure to Ventricular Preload and Volume: The use of Ppw as a measure of left ventricular end-diastolic pressure and hence preload depends on the Ppw closely reflecting pulmonary venous, left atrial, and left ventricular pressures, that is, with minimal pressure gradient across the system. One potential confounder to interpretation of intravascular pressures is the fluctuation in intrathoracic pressure related to the respiratory cycle. The effect of varying intrathoracic pressure on the wedge (Ppw) pressure is seen in Figure 13. The top line is a Ppw tracing and the bottom in the intrapleural (Ppl) pressure. In this example the patient is receiving assisted ventilation. Arrows indicate end expiratory pressures. Negative deflections in Ppl and Ppw pressures result from inspiratory muscle activity, and subsequent positive deflections represent lung inflation by the ventilator. At end expiration, the respiratory system has returned to its relaxed state and Ppl is back to baseline (−2 cm H$_2$O). Transmural wedge pressure remains approximately constant throughout the ventilating cycle. Since Ppl is not usually measured clinically, it is necessary that Ppw be recorded at a point where Ppl can be reliably estimated (*ie*, end-exhalation, assuming no expiratory muscle activity).

The correlation of pressure to volume is further complicated by a variety of conditions that cause the ventricle to be effectively stiff (diastolic dysfunction or pericardial disease) or conditions that cause juxta-cardiac pressure to rise related to positive pressure ventilation (PEEP, intrinsic PEEP [PEEPi], active expiratory effort) (Fig 14).

The effects of PEEP in conditions such as ARDS are often blunted, since the stiff lungs of these patients do not distend greatly with high ventilator pressures and hence minimal increases in juxta-cardiac pressure are encountered. However, in cases in which PEEPi exists in chronic obstructive pulmonary disease (COPD)/asthma patients undergoing mechanical ventilation, or in agitated/obstructed patients with very active expiratory muscle effort, cardiovascular effects may be large. This effect is shown in Figure 15, where the increase in blood pressure and cardiac output despite a fall in wedge pressure and esophageal pressure is shown during a brief interruption in positive pressure ventilation in a patient with COPD.

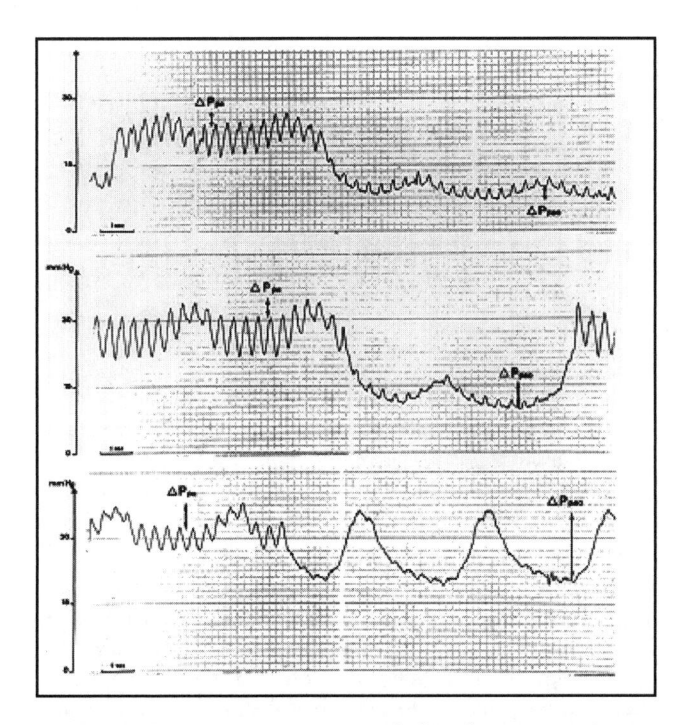

Figure 12. Pressure tracings recorded in the same patient at different levels of end-expiratory pressure-zero (ZEEP) on the top panel, 15 cm H$_2$O in the center panel, and 20 cm H$_2$O in the bottom panel.

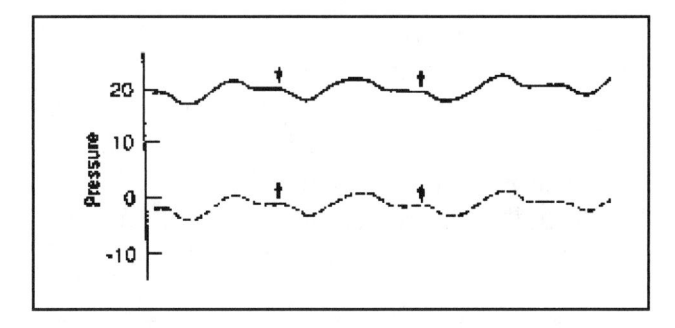

Figure 13.

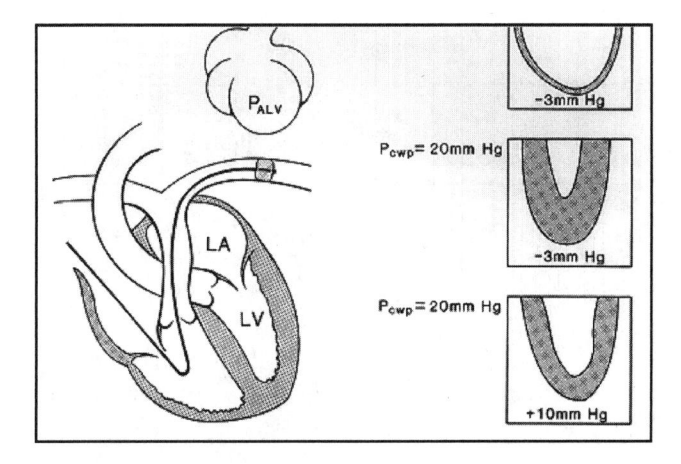

Figure 14.

This constellation of problems is best avoided by:

- Awareness of their existence
- Reading pressure tracings at end expiration
- Considering measures (sedation, ventilator adjustment, paralysis) that diminish or eliminate PEEPi
- Considering a ventilator disconnect in patients with severe airflow obstruction and PEEPi to demonstrate limitation to venous return
- Using a fluid challenge when effective "diastolic" dysfunction may be present, to determine "preload reserve"

In determining the response to a fluid challenge, it is necessary to note that a minimum of 500 mL of crystalloid is required and even then small effects on cardiac output and arterial blood pressure are typically seen. One study has suggested that the use of a drop in the right atrial pressure with respiration is a useful indicator of preload reserve.

Specific Disorders: Tricuspid regurgitation is encountered in conditions with direct valvular injury (*eg*, endocarditis) and generally in right heart failure. It is characterized by a prominent and broad V wave and a steep Y descent; the latter is often most useful for making this diagnosis (Fig 16). It is useful to note tricuspid regurgitation not only for its implications for underlying disorders but also because it will confound thermal dilution cardiac output determination.

Mitral regurgitation is characterized by a giant V wave that may confound distinction between the PA and Pwp tracings (Fig 17). Significant mitral regurgitation may be present without a giant V wave (ascribed to enlarged and compliant left atrium which does not exhibit a large pressure excursion with the additional volume) and a number of conditions can cause a giant

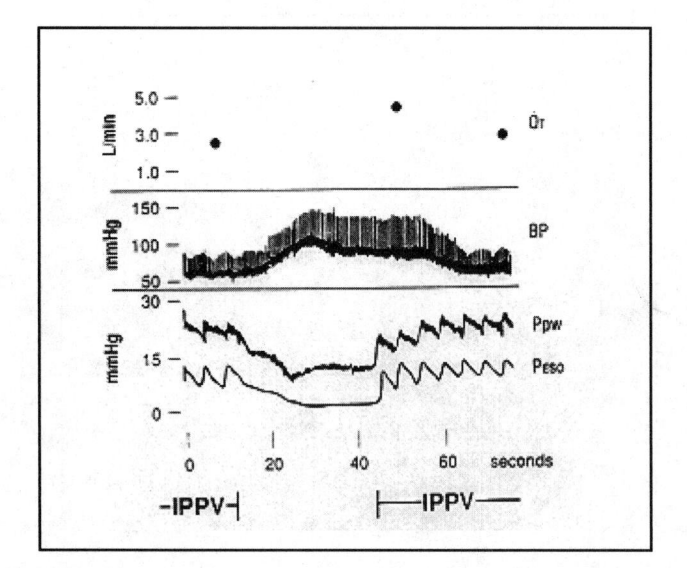

Figure 15.

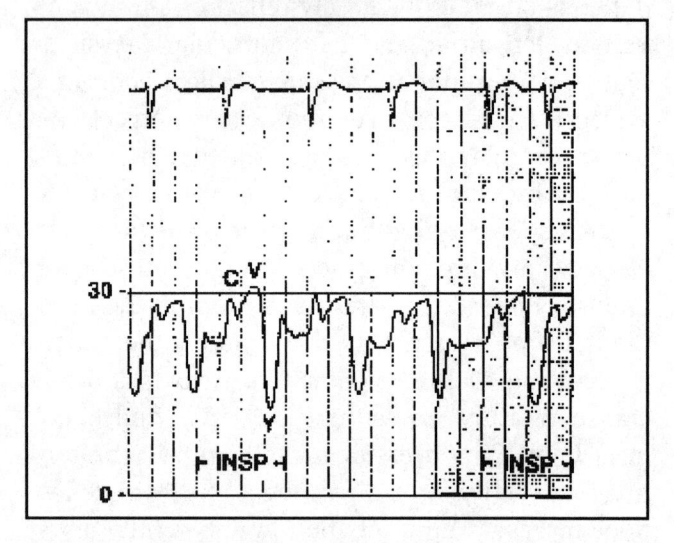

Figure 16. Giant V wave in right atrial waveform indicates tricuspid regurgitation.

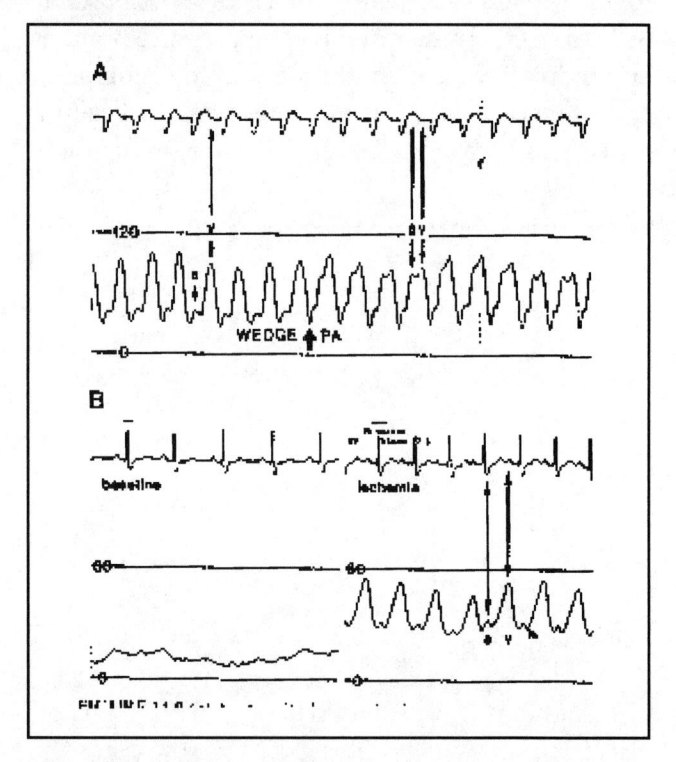

Figure 17. A) Acute mitral regurgitation with giant V wave in pulmonary wedge tracing. The pulmonary artery (PA) tracing has a characteristic bifid appearance due to both a PA systolic wave and the V wave. Note that the V wave occurs later in the cardiac cycle than the PA systolic wave, which is synchronous with the T wave of the electrocardiogram. B) Intermittent giant V wave due to ischemia of the papillary muscle. Wedge tracings are from same patient at baseline and during ischemia. Scale in mm Hg.

V wave in the absence of mitral regurgitation (hypervolemia, VSD).

Right ventricular infarction is characterized by an elevated right ventricular end-diastolic pressure at initial passage of the catheter with narrow pulse pressures when there is hemodynamic compromise. This same pattern can also be present in conditions causing acute right heart failure secondary to increases in pulmonary vascular resistance (eg, pulmonary embolus) but in these latter conditions there will be a large PAD-Ppw gradient reflecting the increase in pulmonary vascular resistance.

Interpretation of Flows and Parameters of Oxygen Delivery

In most clinical settings, cardiac output is determined by thermal dilution. In addition to a number of technical conditions making the measurement unreliable, tricuspid regurgitation may be present and cause underestimation (usually) or overestimation (rarely) of cardiac output. Under this circumstance, determination of cardiac output by Fick may be useful.

Determination of whether a measured flow is adequate is usually best judged by peripheral parameters of perfusion (eg, urine volume, presence of lactic acidosis) or by the mixed venous oxygen saturation (Svo_2). Low Svo_2 (< 60 %) strongly suggests inadequate oxygen delivery and anemia, hypoxemia, or inadequate cardiac output should be sought and corrected. Interpretation of a high Svo_2 in high-output states is difficult. Accordingly, the greatest utility of modified catheters which permit continuous monitoring of Svo_2 is in circumstances in which there is risk for it to be low and therapy can be directed at early recognition of this phenomenon (eg, postoperative cardiac surgery patients).

Echocardiography

Many of the problems of relating measured pressures to ventricular preload can be addressed by cardiac imaging by echo. In addition, this diagnostic tool is useful for identifying a host of structural abnormalities. It should be considered as an adjunct to pulmonary artery catheterization. As technology permits more continuous monitoring by transesophageal route, its use in the ICU is likely to expand.

Useful Applications of Echocardiography in the ICU

- Identification of ischemia
- Correlation of pressure to volume and identification of diastolic dysfunction
- Characterization of valve lesions, VSD, ASD
- Identification of pericardial disease
- Identification of right-left heart interactions in acute right heart failure

Selected Reading

Connors AF, Speroff T, Dawson NV, et al. The effectiveness of right heartcatheterization in the initial care of critically ill patients. JAMA 1996; 276:889-897

Fuchs RM, Heuser RR, Yin FC, et al. Limitations of pulmonary wedge V wavesin diagnosing mitral regurgitation. Am J Cardiol 1982; 49:849-854

Leatherman JW, Marini JJ. Clinical use of the pulmonary artery catheter. In:Hall JB, Schmidt GA, eds. Principles of critical care. 2nd ed. New York, NY: McGraw Hill, 1998; 155-177

Magder S, Georgiadis G, Cheone T. Respiratory variations in right atrial pressure predict the response to fluid challenge. J Crit Care 1992; 7:76-85

Michard F, Boussat S, Chemla D, et al. Relation between respiratory changes in arterial pulse pressure and fluid responsiveness in septic patients with acute circulatory failure. Am J Respir Crit Care Med 2000; 162:134-138

Michard F, Teboul JL. Predicting fluid responsiveness in ICU patients. Chest 2002; 121:2000-2008

Michard F, Teboul JL. Using heart-lung interactions to assess fluid responsiveness during mechanical ventilation. Crit Care 2000; 4:282-289

Perret C, Tagan D, Feihl F, et al. The pulmonary artery catheter in clinical care. Oxford, England: Blackwell Science, 1996; 347

Russell JA, Phang TP. The oxygen delivery/consumption controversy: approaches to management of the critically ill. Am J Respir Crit Care Med 1994; 149: 533-537

Shah KB, Rao TLK, Laughlin S, et al. A review of pulmonary artery catheterizations in 6,245 patients. Anesthesiology 1984; 61:271

Teboul JL, Besbes M, Andrivet P, et al. A bedside index assessing the reliability of pulmonary artery occlusion pressure measurements during mechanical ventilation with positive end-expiratory pressure. J Crit Care Med 1992; 7:22-29

Notes

Hypothermia, Hyperthermia, and Rhabdomyolysis

Janice L. Zimmerman, MD, FCCP

Objectives:

- To understand the physiologic responses associated with hypothermia
- To outline supportive measures and rewarming techniques for management of hypothermia
- To describe predisposing factors for heat stroke, the clinical manifestations, and cooling methods
- To discuss the clinical presentations and management of malignant hyperthermia and neuroleptic malignant syndrome
- To describe etiologies, clinical presentation, and treatment of rhabdomyolysis

Key words: heat stroke; hyperthermia; hypothermia; malignant hyperthermia; neuroleptic malignant syndrome; rhabdomyolysis

Temperature Regulation

The balance between heat production and heat loss normally maintains the core body temperature at 36.6 ± 0.38°C (97.9 ± 0.7°F). Heat is produced from the dissolution of high-energy bonds during metabolism. At rest, the trunk viscera supply 56% of heat; during exercise, muscle activity may account for 90% of generated heat. Heat production may increase two- to fourfold with shivering and more than sixfold with exercise. Most heat loss (50 to 70%) normally occurs through radiation. Conduction of heat through direct contact with cooler objects or loss of heat due to convection accounts for a smaller percentage of heat loss. Evaporation of sweat from the skin is the major mechanism of heat loss in a warm environment.

The anterior hypothalamus is responsible for the perception of temperature and initiation of physiologic responses. Information is received from temperature-sensitive receptors in the skin, viscera, and great vessels, as well as receptors located in the hypothalamus. When a temperature increase is sensed, hypothalamic modulation results in increased sweating (a cholinergically mediated response), cutaneous vasodilation, and decreased muscle tone. Conversely, a decrease in temperature results in decreased sweating, cutaneous vasoconstriction, and increased muscle tone and shivering. These homeostatic mechanisms deteriorate with age.

Hypothermia

Definition and Etiologies

Hypothermia is defined as the unintentional lowering of core body temperature (tympanic, esophageal, or rectal) to <35°C (<95°F). Multiple factors may lead to increased heat loss, decreased heat production, or impaired thermoregulation (Table 1). Hypothermia may be characterized as primary (accidental), due to exposure to cold temperatures, or secondary, resulting from a disease process, such as myxedema or sepsis. Exposure is often found in hypothermic patients, along with underlying chronic disease processes or impairment from ethanol, drugs, or mental illness. Immersion hypothermia is often distinguished from nonimmersion hypothermia, because it occurs more rapidly and is more often accompanied by asphyxia. Hypothermia is frequently noted in trauma patients and is associated with increased mortality rates.

To facilitate management and anticipate physiologic changes, hypothermia can be classified by the degree of temperature reduction. Mild hypothermia refers to core temperatures of 32 to 35°C (90 to 95°F); moderate hypothermia, 28 to 32°C (82 to 90°F); and severe hypothermia, <28°C (<82°F).

Pathophysiology

General Metabolic Changes: Hypothermia produces multisystemic involvement that varies with core temperature (Table 2). The initial response to cold is cutaneous vasoconstriction, which results in shunting of blood from colder extremities to the body core. Vasodilation secondary to ethanol can prevent this normal compensatory response. Vasoconstriction fails at temperatures <24°C (<75°F), and the rate of heat loss increases due to relative vasodilation. Heat production is increased two- to fivefold by the onset of shivering with core temperatures of 30 to 35°C (86 to 95°F). Shivering continues until glycogen stores are depleted, which usually occurs when the body temperature reaches 30°C (86°F).

Cardiovascular System: An initial tachycardia is followed by progressive bradycardia. The pulse rate decreases by 50% when core temperature reaches 28°C (82°F). Bradycardia is secondary to alterations in conductivity and automaticity that are generally refractory to standard treatment (*eg*, atropine). Cardiac function and blood pressure also decline proportionately as the core temperature decreases. Systemic vascular resistance predictably increases.

Hypothermia produces a variety of myocardial conduction abnormalities. Atrial fibrillation is common and usually converts to sinus rhythm spontaneously during rewarming. At temperatures of <29°C (<84°F), ventricular fibrillation (VF) can occur spontaneously or be induced by movement or invasive procedures (*eg*, central line, nasogastric tube). Asystole occurs at temperatures <20°C (<68°F). VF and other arrhythmias are extremely refractory to defibrillation and drug treatment until the core temperature increases to ~30°C (~86°F).

Although many ECG abnormalities have been described, the most characteristic of hypothermia is the J wave (also called the Osborne wave) at the junction of the QRS complex and ST segment (Fig 1). The J wave can occur in patients with core temperatures of <32°C (<90°F), and it is almost always present at temperatures of <25°C (<77°F). It has been observed that the size of the J wave may be inversely correlated with temperature. The presence of this wave is not pathognomonic for hypothermia, nor does it have prognostic value. It is important to distinguish J waves from ST segment elevation indicating myocardial infarction. Prolongation of the P–R, QRS, and Q–T intervals may be noted.

Other Organ Systems: As temperature decreases, tidal volume and respiratory rate will decrease. The cough reflex may be blunted, and cold-induced bronchorrhea may contribute to atelectasis. Hypoxemia may develop early depending on the circumstances (*eg*, water immersion, aspiration). Although renal blood flow and glomerular filtration rate decrease in hypothermia, there is an initial cold-induced diuresis due to the relative central hypervolemia resulting from peripheral vasoconstriction. Additional contributory factors include the inhibition of antidiuretic hormone release and renal tubular concentrating defects. Ethanol exacerbates the diuresis. With warming, volume depletion may become evident.

With mild hypothermia, victims may exhibit confusion, lethargy, or combativeness. Below a core temperature of 32°C (90°F), the patient is usually unconscious with diminished brainstem

Table 1. *Factors Predisposing to Hypothermia*

Increased heat loss
    Environmental exposure
    Skin disorders
        Burns
        Dermatitis
        Psoriasis
    Vasodilation
        Alcohol
        Drugs (phenothiazines)
    Iatrogenic
        Heat stroke treatment
        Environmental cold (operating suite)
Decreased heat production
    Endocrine disorders
        Hypopituitarism
        Hypothyroidism
        Hypoadrenalism
    Insufficient fuel
        Hypoglycemia
        Anorexia nervosa
        Malnutrition
        Extreme exertion
    Neuromuscular inefficiency
        Extremes of age
        Inactivity
        Impaired shivering
Impaired thermoregulation
    Peripheral dysfunction
        Neuropathies
        Spinal cord transection
        Diabetes
    Central dysfunction
        CNS hemorrhage/trauma
        Cerebrovascular accident
        Drugs
            Sedatives
            Alcohols
            Cyclic antidepressants
            Narcotics
        Neoplasm
        Parkinson's disease
        Anorexia nervosa
Miscellaneous states
    Sepsis
    Pancreatitis
    Carcinomatosis
    Uremia
    Sarcoidosis

Table 2. *Manifestations of Hypothermia**

Core Temp (°C)	Musculoskeletal	Neurologic	Other
Mild Hypothermia			
36	Shivering begins	Slurred speech	
34	Maximal shivering	Increased confusion	
33	Decreased shivering	Stupor	Decreasing BP; respiratory alkalosis, cold diuresis
Moderate Hypothermia			
32	Shivering nearly absent; onset of muscle rigidity	Pupils dilated	Arrhythmias; J waves on ECG
30		DTRs absent	Severe hypoventilation
28	Extreme muscle rigidity	No voluntary movement	Shock; inaudible heart sounds
Severe Hypothermia			
26			
24	Patient appears dead		Severe risk of VF; minimal cardiac activity
22			
20		Isoelectric EEG	Asystole
18		Isoelectric EEG	Asystole

*DTR = deep tendon reflex. To convert Celsius to Fahrenheit temperature, multiply by 9/5, then add 32.

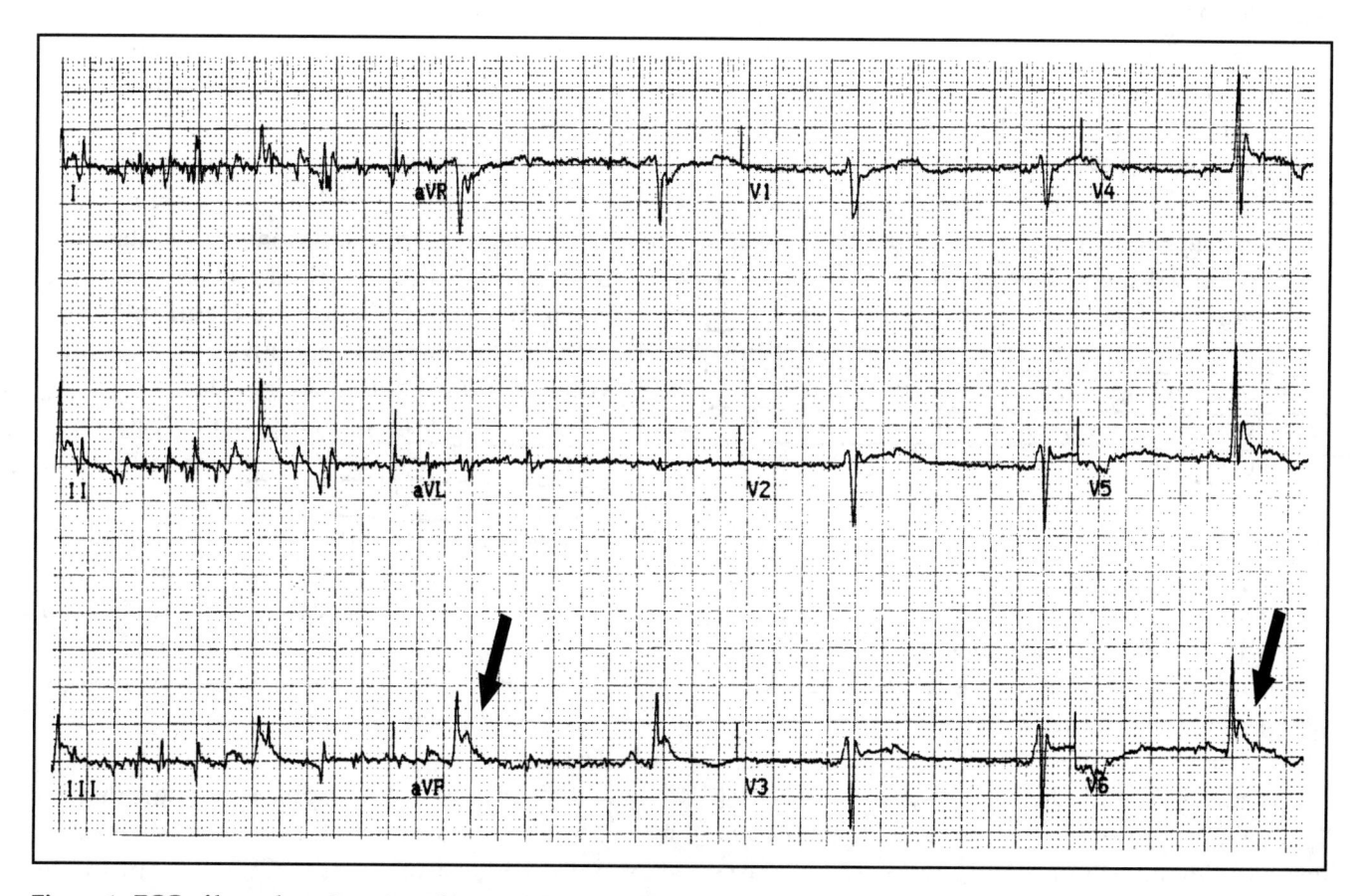

Figure 1. ECG of hypothermic patient showing J wave (arrow).

function. Pupils dilate below a core temperature of 30°C (86°F). Intestinal motility decreases at <34°C (<93°F), resulting in the common finding of ileus. Hepatic dysfunction affects the generation of glucose as well as drug metabolism.

Laboratory Findings: The physiologic changes described are reflected by clinical laboratory tests. An increased hematocrit is usually found, with normal or low platelet and WBC counts. The increase in hematocrit is due to hemoconcentration and splenic contraction. However, restoration of intravascular volume and warming often result in a mild anemia. Platelet and WBC counts may drop as temperatures decrease due to sequestration. Platelet dysfunction occurs with hypothermia and may compromise hemostasis. Although disseminated intravascular coagulation (DIC) may develop, initial coagulation studies (prothrombin time, partial thromboplastin time) are often normal as these laboratory measurements are performed on warmed blood. Electrolytes are variable and no consistent changes are predictable. Increased values of BUN and creatinine result from hypovolemia. Hyperglycemia is common as a result of catecholamine-induced glycogenolysis, decreased insulin release, and inhibition of insulin transport. Hypoglycemia may be evident in malnourished and alcoholic patients. Hyperamylasemia is common and may be related to a preexisting pancreatitis or pancreatitis induced by hypothermia. The acid-base status is difficult to predict in hypothermia, but factors, such as respiratory acidosis, lactate generation from shivering, decreased acid excretion, and decreased tissue perfusion, contribute to acidemia. There is general agreement that arterial blood gas values do not need to be corrected for temperature. However, the Pao_2 should be corrected to evaluate oxygen delivery and the alveolar-arterial gradient.

Diagnosis

The clinical manifestations of hypothermia vary with the etiology, acuteness of onset, severity, and duration. It is imperative to recognize early signs of mild hypothermia, especially in the elderly. These patients may present with confusion, lethargy, impaired judgment, and the unusual manifestation of "paradoxical undressing." More severe hypothermia results in manifestations that are easily recognizable: muscle rigidity, decreased reflexes, decreased respiratory rate, bradycardia, hypotension, and even the appearance of death. The clinical suspicion of hypothermia should be confirmed with an accurate core temperature measurement. Any low temperature (35°C or 95°F) should be checked with a thermometer capable of registering lower temperatures. A rectal probe is most practical even though it may lag behind core changes. The probe should be inserted to an adequate depth (approximately 15 cm), avoiding cold fecal material. An esophageal probe is an alternative, but readings may be falsely elevated in the intubated patient who receives heated oxygen. Thermistors in bladder catheters provide readings similar to intravascular devices. Reliability of tympanic temperature devices has not been established in hypothermia.

Management

Hospital Management: The severity of hypothermia, clinical findings, and comorbid conditions of the patient determine the aggressiveness of resuscitation techniques. The following measures should be instituted as indicated.

1. *Airway management.* Intubation is often necessary for airway protection and/or delivery of supplemental oxygen. The orotracheal route is preferred because of the risk of traumatic bleeding with the nasal route. However, muscle rigidity may preclude orotracheal intubation. Blind nasotracheal intubation in a patient with spontaneous respirations may be facilitated by topical vasoconstrictors and a smaller endotracheal tube. Endotracheal tube cuff pressures should be monitored after rewarming, because volume and pressure will increase.
2. *Supplemental oxygen.* Pulse oximetry cannot be relied on to guide therapy in conditions of hypothermia and hypoperfusion.
3. *Cardiopulmonary resuscitation.* Cardiopulmonary resuscitation should be initiated if the patient is pulseless (assess for 30 to 45 s) or has a nonperfusing rhythm, such as asystole or ventricular fibrillation. Chest wall compression is often difficult.
4. *ECG monitoring.*
   - *In bradycardia:* Avoid pharmacologic manipulation and pacing.
   - *In VF:* Initial defibrillation should be attempted, even if the temperature is <30 to

32°C (<86 to 90°F). If unsuccessful, institute rewarming. Avoid IV drugs until the temperature increases to ~30°C (~86°F) and then use the lowest effective dose. Dosing intervals should be increased in hypothermic patients. Epinephrine and vasopressin have improved coronary artery perfusion pressure in hypothermic animals. The efficacy of amiodarone has not been established in hypothermia, but it is a reasonable initial antiarrhythmic drug. Magnesium sulfate has also been used successfully. Lidocaine has limited efficacy and procainamide may increase the incidence of VF.
- *In asystole:* Follow advanced cardiac life support guidelines, and administer pharmacologic agents when the temperature approaches 30°C (86°F).
5. *Core temperature monitoring.*
6. *Rewarming (see below).*
7. *IV fluids.* All patients require fluids for hypovolemia. Warm normal saline solution containing glucose is a reasonable choice. Increased fluid requirements are often necessary during rewarming to prevent or treat hypotension that may occur with vasodilation. Lactated Ringer's solution should be avoided because of impaired hepatic metabolism of lactate.
8. *Vasopressor drugs.* Hemodynamic instability should first be managed with volume replacement. Vasopressor drugs have a minimal effect on constricted vessels and increase the risk of dysrhythmias.
9. *Nasogastric or orogastric tube.* Insert to relieve gastric distention.
10. *Urinary catheter.*
11. *Venous access.* Peripheral venous catheters are preferred. Central venous lines (subclavian, internal jugular) are not routinely recommended, because they may precipitate dysrhythmias.
12. *Laboratory studies.* Studies should include complete blood count, prothrombin time, partial thromboplastin time, electrolytes, creatine kinase level, and arterial blood gases. Thyroid function evaluation, toxicology screen, and blood cultures are obtained as warranted.
13. *Search for associated conditions* requiring urgent intervention, such as hypoglycemia, sepsis, adrenal insufficiency, and hypothyroidism.

Rewarming Methods: Choices and controversies—Although warming is the primary treatment for hypothermia, controversy exists as to the optimal method, duration, and rate of rewarming. Rapid rewarming has not been proven to improve survival. No controlled studies comparing rewarming methods exist and rigid treatment protocols cannot be recommended. Three types of rewarming techniques exist: passive external rewarming (PER), active external rewarming (AER), and active core rewarming (ACR).

PER is the least invasive and the slowest method. It involves placing the patient in a warm environment, providing an insulating cover, and allowing the body to regain heat. This technique should be applied as the sole method only in patients with mild hypothermia and as an adjunct in moderate and severe hypothermia. The patient must be able to generate heat for PER to be effective. Rewarming rates with PER in mild hypothermia range from 0.5 to 2.0°C/h (1 to 3.6°F/h).

AER involves the external application of heat, such as warming blankets, heating pads, radiant heat lamps, or immersion in warm water. Currently, forced-air warming devices are the most effective and practical means of applying AER, particularly in the perioperative period. A potential disadvantage of this method is the theoretical concern of "after-drop." When a heat source is applied, peripheral vasodilation occurs and colder peripheral blood is transported to the relatively warmer core, thereby reducing the core temperature. After-drop has been hypothesized to increase the incidence of VF. In response to this concern, it has been suggested that heat be applied only to the thorax, leaving the extremities vasoconstricted. The advantages of AER are its ease of institution, ready availability, low cost, and noninvasiveness. Earlier studies showing high mortality when AER was utilized are not supported by more recent experience. AER is often combined with ACR techniques in patients with moderate or severe hypothermia.

ACR is the most rapid and most invasive method and involves the application of heat to the body core. ACR is indicated in patients with a core temperature of <28°C (<82°F) or with an arrested cardiac rhythm. Techniques for ACR include heated humidified oxygen, heated IV fluids, thoracic lavage, peritoneal lavage, gastric/rectal lavage, hemodialysis, continuous arteriovenous/venovenous rewarming, and cardiopulmonary bypass.

One of the simplest methods to institute is warm, humidified, inhaled oxygen (42 to 45°C, or 107.6 to 113°F), which prevents further respiratory heat loss and may result in a modest heat gain. A rewarming rate of 1 to 2.5°C/h (2 to 4.5°F/h) can be expected. This technique should be used routinely on most victims of moderate to severe hypothermia. Heated IV fluids (40 to 42°C. or 104 to 107.6°F) are also easy to institute. Although gastric, bladder, or rectal lavage with warm fluids are simple procedures, there is little information regarding efficacy of these methods. Gastric lavage may predispose to aspiration, and it cannot be performed during chest compressions. They should be used only as an adjunct until more effective rewarming methods can be initiated.

For patients with severe hypothermia, more invasive ACR is preferred: peritoneal lavage, thoracic lavage, hemodialysis, continuous arteriovenous/venovenous rewarming, and cardiopulmonary bypass. These procedures require specialized equipment and intensive care. However, they are very efficient at rewarming and, in the case of cardiopulmonary bypass, may provide for hemodynamic stabilization of the patient. Peritoneal lavage can be instituted through a peritoneal dialysis catheter, using dialysate heated to 40 to 45°C (104 to 113°F). Closed thoracic lavage involves placement of anterior and posterior chest tubes, infusion of heated saline (40 to 42°C, or 104 to 107.6°F) through the anterior tube, and gravity drainage from the posterior tube. Hemodialysis, utilizing a two-way-flow catheter, may be best suited for hemodynamically stable patients. Continuous arteriovenous/venovenous rewarming utilizes a modified fluid warmer with 40°C (104°F) water infused through the inner chamber. Cardiopulmonary bypass (femoral-femoral or atrial-aortic) is the most invasive and labor-intensive technique for rewarming. It has the advantage of providing complete hemodynamic support and rapid rewarming rates (1 to 2°C every 3 to 5 min).

The choice of rewarming methods may combine techniques, such as truncal AER with ACR, using heated oxygen and IV fluids. Availability of resources may be a decisive factor in choosing the method of rewarming. In all cases, complications of rewarming, such as DIC, pulmonary edema, compartment syndromes, rhabdomyolysis, and acute tubular necrosis, must be anticipated.

Future Therapies

Intravenous fluids heated to 65°C (149°F) have been utilized in animal studies and demonstrated rewarming rates of 2.9–3.7°C/h with minimal intimal injuries. Diathermy (ultrasound or low frequency microwave radiation) involves the conversion of energy waves into heat. It can deliver large amounts of heat to deep tissues. Further investigation is needed to determine optimum clinical use.

Outcome From Hypothermia

There are currently no strong predictors of death or permanent neurologic dysfunction in severe hypothermia. Therefore, there are no definitive indicators to suggest which patients can or cannot be resuscitated successfully. Core temperature before rewarming and time to rewarming do not predict outcome. Severe hyperkalemia (>10 mEq/L) may be a marker of death. In general, resuscitative efforts should continue until the core temperature is 32°C (90°F). However, the decision to terminate resuscitation must be individualized based on the circumstances.

Hyperthermia

Heat Stroke

Definition: Heat stroke is a life-threatening medical emergency that occurs when homeostatic thermoregulatory mechanisms fail. This failure usually results in elevation of body temperature to >41°C (>105.8°F), producing multisystem tissue damage and organ dysfunction. Two syndromes of heat stroke occur: classic heat stroke (nonexertional) and exertional heat stroke. Classic heat stroke typically affects infants and elderly individuals with underlying chronic illness. The occurrence of classic heat stroke is usually predictable when heat waves occur. The syndrome develops over several days and results in significant dehydration and anhidrosis. Exertional heat stroke typically occurs in young individuals, such as athletes and military recruits exercising in hot weather. These individuals usually have no chronic illness, and this syndrome occurs sporadically and often unpredictably. Dehydration is less severe, and ~50% of individuals will have profuse sweating.

Predisposing Factors: Heat stroke results from increased heat production and/or decreased heat loss (Table 3). Environmental factors of high heat and humidity contribute to heat production, as well as limit heat loss. Sympathomimetic drugs, such as cocaine and amphetamines, increase muscle activity and may also disrupt hypothalamic regulatory mechanisms. Numerous drugs interfere with the ability to dissipate heat. Drugs with anticholinergic effects, such as cyclic antidepressants, antihistamines, and antipsychotics, inhibit sweating and disrupt hypothalamic function. Ethanol may contribute to heat stroke by several mechanisms: vasodilation resulting in heat gain, impaired perception of the environment, and diuresis. β-adrenergic blockers may impair cardiovascular compensation and decrease cutaneous blood flow. Factors that increase the risk of death, as identified in the July 1995 heat wave in Chicago, include being confined to bed because of medical problems and living alone.

Diagnosis: The diagnosis of heat stroke requires a history of exposure to a heat load (either internal or external), severe CNS dysfunction, and elevated temperature (usually >40°C, or >104°F). The absolute temperature may not be critical, because cooling measures are often instituted before the patient is admitted to a health-care facility. Sweating may or may not be present.

Clinical Manifestations: Profound CNS dysfunction is a defining characteristic of heat stroke. Dysfunction may range from bizarre behavior, delirium, and confusion to decerebrate rigidity, cerebellar dysfunction, seizures, and coma. These changes are potentially reversible, although permanent deficits can occur. Lumbar puncture results may show increased protein, xanthochromia, and lymphocytic pleocytosis.

Tachycardia, an almost universal cardiovascular finding in heat stroke, occurs in response to peripheral vasodilation and the need for increased cardiac output. The peripheral vascular resistance is usually low unless severe hypovolemia is present. Compensatory vasoconstriction occurs in the splanchnic and renal vascular beds. If the patient is unable to increase cardiac output, hypotension develops. A variety of ECG changes have been described in heat stroke, including conduction defects, increased Q-T interval, and nonspecific ST-T changes.

Tachypnea may result in a significant respiratory alkalosis. However, victims of exertional heat stroke usually have lactic acidosis. Hypoglycemia may be present in exertional heat stroke victims owing to increased glucose utilization and impaired hepatic gluconeogenesis. Hypoglycemia may be present in exertional heat stroke victims as a result of increased glucose utilization and impaired hepatic gluconeogenesis. Rhabdomyolysis and renal failure occur more commonly with exertional heat stroke and may be caused by myoglobinuria, thermal parenchymal damage, or decreased renal blood flow due to hypotension. Hematologic effects include hypocoagulability, which may progress to DIC. Hepatic injury results in cholestasis and elevation of transaminase levels.

An inflammatory response may cause or contribute to the clinical manifestations of heat stroke. Increased concentrations of endotoxin, tumor necrosis factor, soluble tumor necrosis factor receptor, and interleukin-1 have been demonstrated in heat stroke victims. Interleukin-6 and nitric oxide metabolite concentrations correlate with the severity of illness. Endothelial cell activation/injury is suggested by findings of increased concentrations of circulating intercellular adhesion molecule-1, endothelin, and von Willebrand-factor antigen.

Table 3. *Predisposing Factors for Heat Stroke*

Increased Heat Production
    Exercise
    Fever
    Thyrotoxicosis
    Hypothalmic dysfunction
    Drugs (sympathomimetics)
    Environmental heat stress
Decreased Heat Loss
    Environmental heat stress
    Cardiac disease
    Peripheral vascular disease
    Dehydration
    Obesity
    Skin disease
    Anticholinergic drugs
    Ethanol
    β-blockers

Electrolyte concentrations are variable in heat stroke. Hyperkalemia can result from rhabdomyolysis, but hypokalemia occurs more commonly. Hypocalcemia can occur, particularly with rhabdomyolysis, but usually does not require therapy.

Differential Diagnosis: The history and physical findings usually indicate the diagnosis of heat stroke. In the absence of adequate history, other processes to be considered include CNS infection, hypothalamic lesions, thyroid storm, and other hyperthermic syndromes, such as neuroleptic malignant syndrome.

Treatment: Along with resuscitative measures, immediate cooling should be instituted for any patient with a temperature of >41°C (>105.8°F). Two methods of cooling have been used: conductive cooling and evaporative cooling. Because definitive human studies are lacking, the optimal cooling method remains controversial.

Direct cooling by enhancing conduction of heat from the body is accomplished by immersing the patient in cold water. Skin massage to prevent cutaneous vasoconstriction in the limbs has been recommended. Shivering can result in an undesirable increase in heat production. This method requires considerable staff time and makes it difficult to treat seizures and perform other resuscitative measures. Variants of this method include ice-water soaks and application of ice packs to the axillae, groin, and neck.

Evaporative cooling is a widely used practical cooling method. The patient is placed nude on a stretcher and sprayed with warm (not cold) water. Air flow is created with use of fans to enhance evaporative cooling. This method allows personnel to institute other resuscitative measures while cooling occurs. Other cooling methods, such as peritoneal lavage, iced gastric lavage, or cardiopulmonary bypass, have not been effectively tested in humans. Antipyretics are not indicated and dantrolene is ineffective.

In addition to cooling, most patients will require intubation for airway protection. Supplemental oxygen should be instituted for all patients. The type and quantity of IV fluids should be individualized based on assessment of electrolytes and volume status. Overaggressive hydration may result in cardiac decompensation during cooling, especially in the elderly. Hypotension usually responds to cooling as peripheral vasodilation decreases. Vasopressor agents that result in vasoconstriction can decrease heat exchange and are not recommended for initial management of hypotension. A thermistor probe should be used for monitoring of core temperature during cooling efforts. Cooling should be stopped at 38.0 to 38.8°C (100.4 to 102°F) to prevent hypothermic overshoot.

Outcome: With appropriate management, the survival rate from heat stroke approaches 90%. However, morbidity is related to the duration of hyperthermia and to underlying conditions. Advanced age, hypotension, coagulopathy, hyperkalemia, acute renal failure, and prolonged coma are associated with a poor prognosis. Elevated lactate levels are associated with a poor prognosis in classic heat stroke but not exertional heat stroke. In retrospective studies, rapid cooling (<1 h) was associated with a decreased mortality.

Malignant Hyperthermia

Definition: Malignant hyperthermia (MH) is a drug- or stress-induced hypermetabolic syndrome characterized by hyperthermia, muscle contractures, and cardiovascular instability. It results from a genetic defect of calcium transport in skeletal muscle. The primary defects are postulated to be impaired reuptake of calcium into the sarcoplasmic reticulum, increased release of calcium from the sarcoplasmic reticulum, and a defect in the calcium-mediated coupling contraction mechanism. Sustained muscle contraction results in increased oxygen consumption and heat production. It is genetically transmitted as an autosomal-dominant trait and occurs in 1 in 50 to 1 in 150,000 adults who receive anesthesia.

Triggers: Halothane and succinylcholine have been involved in the majority of reported cases of MH. Additional potentiating drugs include muscle relaxants, inhalational anesthetic agents, and drugs, such as ethanol, caffeine, sympathomimetics, parasympathomimetics, cardiac glycosides, and quinidine analogs. Less commonly, MH can be precipitated by infection, physical or emotional stress, anoxia, or high ambient temperature.

Clinical Manifestations: Manifestations of MH usually occur within 30 min of anesthesia in 90% of cases. However, onset of the syndrome may occur postoperatively. Muscle rigidity begins in the muscles of the extremities or the chest. In patients receiving succinylcholine, the stiffness most commonly begins in the jaw. The development of masseter spasm after administration of a paralyzing agent should be considered an early sign of possible MH. Tachycardia is another early, although nonspecific, sign. Monitoring of arterial blood gases or end-tidal CO_2 may detect an early increase in CO_2. Hypertension and mottling of the skin also occur. The increase in temperature usually occurs later, but it is followed rapidly by acidosis, ventricular arrhythmias, and hypotension. Laboratory abnormalities include increased sodium, calcium, magnesium, potassium, phosphate, creatine kinase, and lactate dehydrogenase levels. Lactate levels are increased and arterial blood gases indicate hypoxemia and an increase in $Paco_2$.

Treatment: Once the diagnosis of MH is entertained, the inciting drug should be discontinued immediately. The most effective and safest therapy is dantrolene, which prevents release of calcium into the cell by the sarcoplasmic reticulum. Uncoupling of the excitation contraction mechanism in skeletal muscle decreases thermogenesis. Dantrolene should be administered by rapid IV push, beginning at a dose of 2.5 mg/kg and repeated every 5 min until the symptoms subside or the maximum dose of 10 mg/kg has been reached. Decreasing muscle rigidity should be evident within minutes. Subsequent doses of 1 mg/kg every 4 to 6 h should be continued for 36 to 48 h. If dantrolene is ineffective or slowly effective, evaporative cooling methods can also be utilized. Calcium channel blockers are of no benefit in MH and should not be used to treat arrhythmias.

The Malignant Hyperthermia Association of the United States provides a hotline for assistance in managing MH (800) MH-HYPER, (800) 644-9737, or (315) 464-7079 if outside the United States. The organization also maintains a Web site with useful information online: www.mhaus.org.

Neuroleptic Malignant Syndrome

Definition: Neuroleptic malignant syndrome (NMS) is an idiosyncratic reaction, usually to neuroleptic drugs, characterized by hyperthermia, muscle rigidity, alterations in mental status, autonomic dysfunction, and rhabdomyolysis. It may occur in up to 1% of all patients taking neuroleptic agents; it affects the young more than the old, and affected individuals are more likely to be male than female. The pathogenesis is unknown, but it is thought to be related to CNS dopamine antagonism and altered hypothalamic temperature set point.

Triggers: Although the majority of cases have been associated with haloperidol, the following agents have been associated with NMS: butyrophenones (*eg*, haloperidol); phenothiazines (*eg*, chlorpromazine, fluphenazine); thioxanthenes (*eg*, thiothixene); dopamine-depleting agents (*eg*, tetrabenazine); dibenzoxazepines (*eg*, loxapine); and withdrawal of levodopa/carbidopa or amantadine. Rechallenge with an inciting drug may not result in recurrence of NMS kinase. Various diagnostic criteria have been proposed (Table 4), but NMS remains a clinical diagnosis based on exposure to neuroleptic agents or other dopamine antagonists in association with characteristic manifestations.

Clinical Manifestations: NMS usually occurs 1 to 3 days after initiating a neuroleptic agent or changing the dose, and the syndrome may last for a period of 1 to 3 weeks. Hyperthermia is universally present, and the average maximal temperature is 39.9°C (103.8°F). However, NMS has been reported to occur without temperature elevation. Autonomic dysfunction includes tachycardia, diaphoresis, blood pressure instability, and arrhythmias. Autonomic dysfunction may precede changes in muscle tone. A general increase in muscle tone or tremors occurs in >90% of patients. Early manifestations of changes

Table 4. *Diagnostic Criteria for NMS**

Major Criteria
    Fever
    Muscle rigidity
    ↑ Creatinine kinase
Minor Criteria
    Tachycardia
    Abnormal blood pressure
    Tachypnea
    Altered consciousness
    Diaphoresis
    Leukocytes

*Diagnosis of NMS is suggested by the presence of all three major criteria or by the presence of two major and four minor criteria.

in muscle tone include dysphagia, dysarthria, or dystonia. Altered mental status occurs in 75% and can range from agitation to coma. Rhabdomyolysis occurs frequently with elevations of creatine kinase and may lead to serious electrolyte abnormalities. WBC counts are often increased (10,000-40,000/mm^3) and may demonstrate a left shift. DIC has also been reported. Volume depletion or renal injury from rhabdomyolysis can result in elevated BUN and creatinine levels.

Various diagnostic criteria have been proposed (Table 4), but NMS remains a clinical diagnosis based on exposure to neuroleptic agents or other dopamine antagonists in association with characteristic manifestations.

Treatment: Dantrolene is the most effective agent for reducing muscle rigidity and decreasing temperature. It is given in the same doses as described for MH. In addition, dopamine agonists have been reported to have beneficial effects in NMS. These drugs include bromocriptine (2.5 to 10 mg tid), amantadine (100 mg bid), and levodopa/carbidopa. Supportive therapies must also be instituted as indicated. Complications may include respiratory failure, cardiovascular collapse, renal failure, arrhythmias, or thromboembolism. The Neuroleptic Malignant Syndrome Information Service (www.nmsis.org) maintains a hotline for medical professionals (888) 667-8367 if assistance is needed.

Rhabdomyolysis

Definition

Rhabdomyolysis is a clinical and laboratory syndrome resulting from skeletal muscle injury with release of cell contents into the plasma. Rhabdomyolysis occurs when demands for oxygen and metabolic substrate exceed availability. This syndrome may result from primary muscle injury or secondary injury due to infection, vascular occlusion, electrolyte disorders, or toxins. Table 5 provides an overview of causes of rhabdomyolysis.

Manifestations

Clinical manifestations of rhabdomyolysis consist of myalgias, muscle swelling and tenderness, discoloration of the urine, and features of the underlying disease. However, overt symptoms or physical findings may not be present. Laboratory evaluation reflects muscle cell lysis with elevation of muscle enzyme levels (creatine kinase, lactate dehydrogenase, aldolase, and aspartate aminotransferase), hyperkalemia, hyperphosphatemia, and hypocalcemia. Coagulation abnormalities consistent with DIC may occur. Renal failure may result secondary to release of myoglobin and other toxic muscle components. A urine dipstick positive for blood and an absence of RBCs on microscopic examination suggest the presence of myoglobinuria.

Treatment

The treatment of rhabdomyolysis is aimed at treating the underlying disease and preventing complications. Maintenance of intravascular volume and renal perfusion is the most important aspect of preventing renal failure. Volume resuscitation should target a urine output of 2 to 3 mL/kg/h. Although increased urine output is beneficial, other interventions to prevent renal failure are more controversial. Alkalinization of the urine may be helpful, but clinical relevance has not been established. The greatest benefit of administering sodium bicarbonate may be restoration of

Table 5. *Causes of Rhabdomyolysis*

Traumatic	Infections	Toxins/Drugs	Metabolic Disorders
Crush syndrome	Coxsackievirus	Alcohol	Enzyme deficiencies
Muscle compression	Gas gangrene	Amphetamines	Hyperosmolar states
Hyperthermic syndromes	Hepatitis	Carbon monoxide	Hypokalemia
Burns	Influenza B virus	Cocaine	Hypomagnesemia
Electrical injury	Legionella	Phencyclidine	Hypophosphatemia
Exertion	Salmonella	Snake/spider venom	Inflammatory muscle disease
Seizures	Shigella	Statins	Thyroid disease
Vascular occlusion	Tetanus	Steroids	Vasculitis

intravascular volume rather than a change in pH. Treatment with bicarbonate should be individualized, based on the patient's ability to tolerate the sodium and fluid load. Loop diuretics and osmotic diuretics have been advocated to be protective of the kidneys, but convincing clinical data are lacking. Loop diuretics theoretically can worsen renal tubular acidosis, which is thought to potentiate myoglobin-induced nephropathy. Diuresis should not be attempted without adequate volume replacement.

Electrolyte abnormalities should be anticipated and treated expeditiously. The most life-threatening abnormality is hyperkalemia. Hypocalcemia does not usually require treatment and empiric administration of calcium may exacerbate muscle injury.

The patient must be closely observed for the development of a compartment syndrome. Monitoring of intracompartmental pressures may be required. Fasciotomy is often recommended for intracompartmental pressures of >30 to 35 mm Hg.

Suggested Readings

Hypothermia

Braun R, Krishel S. Environmental emergencies. Emerg Med Clin North Am 1997;15: 451–476

Danzl DF, Pozos RS. Accidental hypothermia. N Engl J Med 1994; 331:1756–1760

Delaney KA, Howland MA, Vassallo S, et al. Assessment of acid-base disturbances in hypothermia and their physiologic consequences. Ann Emerg Med 1989; 18:72–82

Gentilello LM. Advances in the management of hypothermia. Surg Clin North Am 1995; 75:243–256

Gentilello LM, Cobean RA, Offner PJ, et al. Continuous arteriovenous rewarming: rapid reversal of hypothermia in critically ill patients. J Trauma 1992; 32:316–327

Giesbrecht GG, Bristow GK. Recent advances in hypothermia research. Ann N Y Acad Sci 1997; 813: 663–675

Hanania NA, Zimmerman JL. Accidental hypothermia. Crit Care Clin 1999; 15:35–49

Kornberger E, Schwarz B, Linder KH, et al. Forced air surface rewarming in patients with severe accidental hypothermia. Resuscitation 1999; 41:105–111

Krismer AC, Lindner KH, Kornberger R, et al. Cardiopulmonary resuscitation during severe hypothermia in pigs: does epinephrine or vasopressin increase coronary perfusion pressure? Anesth Analg 2000; 90: 69–73

Schaller MD, Fischer AP, Perret CH. Hyperkalemia, a prognostic factor during acute severe hypothermia. JAMA 1990; 264:1842–1845

Thornton D, Farmer JC. Hypothermia and hyperthermia. In: Parrillo JE, Dellinger RP, eds. Critical care medicine.

2nd ed. St. Louis, MO: Mosby, 2000; 1525–1538 Vassal T, Benoit-Gonin B, Carrat F, et al. Severe accidental hypothermia treated in an ICU: prognosis and outcome. Chest 2001; 120:1998–2003

Walpoth BH, Walpoth-Aslan BN, Mattle HP, et al. Outcome of survivors of accidental deep hypothermia and circulatory arrest treated with extracorporeal blood warming. N Engl J Med 1997; 337:1500–1505

Hyperthermia

Balzan MV. The neuroleptic malignant syndrome: a logical approach to the patient with temperature and rigidity. Postgrad Med J 1998; 74:72–76

Bouchama A, De Vol EB. Acid-base alterations in heatstroke. Intensive Care Med 2001; 27:680–685

Bouchama A, Knochel JP. Heat stroke. N Engl J Med 2002; 346:1978–1988

Carbone JR. The neuroleptic malignant and serotonin syndromes. Emerg Med Clin North Am 2000; 18: 317–325

Caroff SN, Mann SC. Neuroleptic malignant syndrome. Med Clin North Am 1993; 77:185–202

Caroff SN, Rosenburg H, Mann SC. et al. Neuroleptic malignant syndrome in the perioperative setting. Am J Anesthesiol 2001; 28:387–393

Chan TC, Evans SD, Clark RF. Drug-induced hyperthermia. Crit Care Clin 1997; 13:785–808

Denborough M. Malignant hyperthermia. Lancet 1998; 352:1131–1136

Gaffin SL, Gardner JW, Flinn SD, Cooling methods for heatstroke victims. Ann Intern Med 2000; 132:678

Hubbard RW, Gaffin SL, Squire DL. Heat-related illness. In: Auerbach PS, ed. Wilderness medicine: management of wilderness and environmental emergencies. 4th ed. St Louis, MO: Mosby, 2001; 195

Pelonero AL, Levenson JL, Pandurangi AR. Neuroleptic malignant syndrome: a review. Psychiatric Services 1998; 49:1163–1172

Tomarken JL. Malignant hyperthermia. Ann Emerg Med 1987; 16:1253–1265

Viejo LF, Morales V, Puñal P, et al. Risk factors in neuroleptic malignant syndrome: a case-control study. Acta Psychiatr Scand 2003; 107:45–49

Weiner JS, Khogali M. A physiological body-cooling unit for treatment of heat stroke. Lancet 1980; 1:507–509

Yarbrough B, Vicario S. Heat illness. In: Marx JA, Hockberger RS, Walls RM, eds. Emergency medicine: concepts and clinical practice. 5th ed. St Louis, MO: Mosby, 2002; 1997–2009

Rhabdomyolysis

Allison RC, Bedsole L. The other medical causes of rhabdomyolysis. Am J Med Sci 2003; 326:79–88

Reilly KM, Salluzzo R. Rhabdomyolysis and its complications. Res Staff Phys 1990; 36:45–52

Holt SG, Moore KP. Pathogenesis and treatment of renal dysfunction in rhabdomyolysis. Intensive Care Med 2001; 27:803–811

Thompson PD, Clarkson P, Karas RH. Statin-associated myopathy. JAMA 2003; 289:1681–1690

Notes

Notes

Pulmonary Hypertension and Critical Illness

Brian K. Gehlbach, MD

Objectives:

- Discuss the pathophysiology of right ventricular dysfunction in the setting of acute and chronic pulmonary hypertension.
- Describe the causes of acute pulmonary hypertension.
- Discuss the use of fluids and vasoactive drugs in the management of acute right ventricular failure.
- Discuss ventilatory management of the patient with acute right ventricular failure.

Key words: ARDS; pulmonary arterial hypertension; pulmonary hypertension

---

This article reviews important principles in the management of patients with acute and chronic pulmonary hypertension. The specific treatment of diseases that cause pulmonary hypertension—for example, pulmonary embolism—is beyond the scope of this review. Similarly, surgical therapies such as atrial septostomy, right ventricular assist devices, and transplantation are not considered.

Pulmonary Hypertension and the Right Ventricle

Animal models suggest that under normal resting conditions, the right ventricle performs only a minor role in maintaining cardiac output. Right ventricular work is significantly less than that of the left ventricle because of the much lower resistance of the pulmonary vascular circuit relative to the systemic circulation. Pulmonary vascular resistance falls even further in response to an increase in cardiac output as the increase in pulmonary blood flow recruits new vessels and dilates existing ones. As a result, pulmonary artery pressure changes very little in response to a fourfold increase in cardiac output, as when a healthy individual performs strenuous exercise.

In contrast to the left ventricle, the thin-walled, crescent-shaped right ventricle has a low tolerance for acute increases in afterload, such as occurs in a large pulmonary embolism. As a result, the right ventricle is typically unable to sustain acute increases in mean pulmonary artery pressure to ≥40 mm Hg. When pulmonary vascular resistance rises acutely, there is a decrease in right ventricular ejection and an increase in end-diastolic pressure and volume. Further increases in end-diastolic volume result in a shift of the interventricular septum into the left ventricle, impairing its function and filling. The net result of these effects is a reduction in cardiac output and coronary perfusion pressure, impairing oxygen delivery to the right ventricular myocardium at the same time that its demand for oxygen has significantly increased. The resulting ischemia further impairs systolic performance, causing a further reduction in right ventricular ejection and progressive dilatation and failure, initiating a downward spiral that, uninterrupted, leads to death.

Understanding this phenomenon of ventricular interdependence is crucial to avoiding misguided attempts to improve cardiac performance through the liberal administration of fluids, which serves only to increase right ventricular end-diastolic volume and worsen its function. In contrast to acute increases in right ventricular afterload, more gradual increases are better tolerated by the right ventricle and result in hypertrophy.

Acute Pulmonary Hypertension

While massive pulmonary embolism is a well-recognized cause of acute pulmonary hypertension and right ventricular failure, there are many other causes (Table 1). Air embolism has a variety of causes but chiefly occurs in hospitalized patients following the insertion or manipulation of central venous catheters or as a complication of various neurosurgical, orthopedic, or cardiac surgeries. Fat embolism most commonly follows trauma to the pelvis or long bones (accidental or surgical) but may be seen in other settings as well, including in patients with sickle-cell disease and

Table 1. Causes of Acute Pulmonary Hypertension

Pulmonary thromboembolism
Other embolism
    Air
    Fat
    Tumor
Acute lung injury/ARDS
Sepsis
Surgical resection of pulmonary vascular bed
Drugs
After cardiac surgery*
Hypoxemia
Hypercapnea
Acute-on-chronic pulmonary hypertension

*Etiology unclear; many cases likely related to effects of cardiopulmonary bypass.

Table 2. World Health Organization Classification of Pulmonary Hypertension

1. Pulmonary arterial hypertension
   A. Idiopathic
   B. Familial
   C. Associated with collagen vascular disease, congenital systemic-to-pulmonary shunts, portal hypertension, HIV, drugs and toxins, various other etiologies
2. Pulmonary hypertension with left-heart disease
3. Pulmonary hypertension associated with lung disease and/or hypoxemia
4. Pulmonary hypertension due to chronic thrombotic and/or embolic disease
5. Miscellaneous (sarcoidosis, histiocytosis X, lymphangiomyomatosis, compression of pulmonary vessels)

acute chest syndrome. Neurologic dysfunction and a petechial rash may accompany the development of acute hypoxemic respiratory failure and acute pulmonary hypertension but are not invariably present.

Acute pulmonary hypertension frequently complicates the acute respiratory distress syndrome (ARDS) but its precise prevalence is unknown. The etiology is likely multifactorial and includes hypoxic vasoconstriction; microthrombosis; inflammatory mediator release; and in patients treated with high levels of positive end-expiratory pressure (PEEP), compression of extra-alveolar vessels due to alveolar overdistension.

While evidence exists that sepsis may lead to acute pulmonary hypertension even in the absence of acute lung injury, this is rarely of great clinical consequence unless the patient also has acute lung injury or preexisting pulmonary vascular disease. In such cases, patients with sepsis may be particularly vulnerable to right ventricular failure due to cytokine-induced ventricular dysfunction, decreased coronary artery perfusion from systemic hypotension, and increased myocardial work as the right ventricle attempts to increase its cardiac output.

Acute-on-Chronic Pulmonary Hypertension

The intensivist is frequently involved in the care of patients with preexisting pulmonary hypertension. While some patients may present to the ICU with a known diagnosis of pulmonary hypertension, in others this condition is recognized when the right ventricle fails to meet the demands of the acute illness. The possibility that the patient's pulmonary hypertension may have a chronic basis is suggested by the presence of right ventricular hypertrophy on echocardiography or by mean pulmonary artery pressures that are >40 mm Hg.

The causes of pulmonary hypertension are numerous and grouped into five broad categories based on common etiologic and clinical features (Table 2). Most patients with suspected chronic pulmonary hypertension should undergo right-heart catheterization. This procedure not only confirms the diagnosis and quantifies its severity but also provides important additional information relating to the etiology, severity, and vasoreactivity of the disease. While the diagnosis of pulmonary arterial hypertension has historically conferred a dismal prognosis, the therapies available for the treatment of this condition have expanded considerably over the past decade. While the treatment of patients with pulmonary arterial hypertension is best undertaken in collaboration with physicians with considerable expertise in this area, the intensivist should be familiar with the medications used to treat such patients (Table 3). Calcium-channel blockers are appropriate therapy only for the small subset of patients who respond positively to acute vasoreactivity testing at right-heart catheterization, and they are not appropriate for critically ill patients with right-heart failure.

Table 3. US Food and Drug Administration-Approved Medications for Pulmonary Arterial Hypertension

Drug	Route of Administration	Functional Class	Major Adverse Effects	Other Considerations
Epoprostenol (prostanoid)	IV	III–IV	Flushing, headache, nausea, diarrhea, jaw pain, arthralgias	Longest experience with use; medication needs to be kept cold; short half-life with risk of cardiovascular collapse with infusion interruption
Iloprost (prostanoid)	Inhaled	III–IV	Flushing, headache, nausea, jaw pain, cough, hypotension	No need for indwelling catheter; requires 6 to 9 inhalations/day; ↑ risk of syncope
Treprostinil (prostanoid)	Subcutaneous	II–IV	Infusion site pain, headache, diarrhea, nausea, flushing, jaw pain	Infusion site pain is limiting; no need for IV catheter
Bosentan (endothelin receptor antagonist)	Oral	III–IV	Hepatocellular injury, edema, flushing, headache, decreased hemoglobin	Monitor liver function tests monthly and CBC every 3 mo; avoid in pregnancy, liver disease
Sildenafil (phosphodiesterase-5 inhibitor)	Oral	I–IV	Headache, flushing, dyspepsia	Avoid nitrates

Treatment of Acute Right Ventricular Failure

Fluid Therapy

While the right heart is sensitive to decreased preload in the setting of right ventricular ischemia and infarction, overly vigorous fluid resuscitation in the setting of acute right ventricular failure may be harmful. Many patients with acute right ventricular failure already exhibit evidence of increased right-sided pressures at presentation. In such patients, further fluid administration causes an increase in the right ventricular end-diastolic volume and a shift of the interventricular septum into the left ventricle, impairing its filling and function. Right ventricular performance may worsen as ischemia is provoked by increased wall tension and decreased coronary artery perfusion from systemic hypotension. While a trial of volume is usually reasonable in the resuscitation of patients in shock, in the case of a suspected right-heart syndrome the trial should employ small, discrete boluses (*eg*, 250 mL at a time) and a decision made whether to continue the therapy based on whether any improvement in cardiac output, urine output, or central venous saturation occurs.

Vasoactive Drug Therapy

Catecholamines: Dobutamine and norepinephrine are the drugs of choice in acute right-heart failure due to massive pulmonary embolism and likely in other causes of right-heart failure requiring the administration of catecholamines. Dobutamine increases the cardiac output by improving right ventricular contractility and reducing pulmonary vascular resistance. Animal data and limited studies in humans indicate that norepinephrine improves right ventricular performance by increasing mean arterial pressure and thereby improving coronary artery perfusion of the ischemic right ventricle. While left ventricular afterload is also increased, this effect is not important so long as left ventricular function is not significantly impaired. Dobutamine is typically administered at doses of between 5 and 10 µg/kg/min and norepinephrine at doses of between 2 and 20 µg/min.

Vasopressin: Few data are available regarding the use of vasopressin in acute right ventricular failure. In one study, vasopressin caused pulmonary vascular constriction and decreased right ventricular contractility. At the present time, vasopressin should be considered inferior to dobutamine and norepinephrine in the patient requiring circulatory support for right-heart failure.

Phosphodiesterase Inhibitors: Amrinone and milrinone act as both inotropes and vasodilators and, in small studies, have shown promise in the treatment of acute right-heart syndromes. Both agents have long half-lives, are difficult to titrate, and can provoke hypotension. As a result, their use in acute right-heart failure has been limited. The selective type 5 phosphodiesterase inhibitor sildenafil, used in the management of patients with pulmonary arterial hypertension, has shown promise in attenuating acute pulmonary embolism-induced pulmonary hypertension. Data on its use in ARDS are quite limited.

Inhaled Nitric Oxide: Inhaled nitric oxide causes selective pulmonary capillary and arteriolar dilation wherever alveoli are effectively ventilated. This has the effect of both decreasing pulmonary vascular resistance and improving matching of ventilation and perfusion, thereby decreasing blood flow to shunted areas and improving oxygenation. Inhaled nitric oxide is therefore a theoretically attractive therapy for acute right-heart failure, particularly in the setting of ARDS. Unfortunately, while numerous studies have demonstrated short-term beneficial effects of inhaled nitric oxide on oxygenation and pulmonary hemodynamics, no survival benefit has ever been demonstrated. Considerable caution in its administration is warranted, as abrupt discontinuation may precipitate cardiovascular collapse. This may occur during disconnection from the ventilator (inadvertent or intentional), or if the supply source is exhausted. Inhaled nitric oxide is effective at reducing pulmonary artery pressures following cardiac surgery.

Prostaglandins: For unstable class IV patients with pulmonary arterial hypertension, IV epoprostenol is indicated, although initiating therapy in the acutely hypotensive patient can be problematic and may require the administration of inotropic agents. Similar to inhaled nitric oxide, inhaled prostacyclin analogues have been shown in small studies to improve oxygenation in patients with ARDS without improving clinical outcomes.

Endothelin Receptor Antagonists: To date, almost no data exist regarding the use of endothelin receptor antagonists such as bosentan in the critically ill patient with acute right-heart failure.

Ventilator Management

Intubation and mechanical ventilation, while potentially lifesaving, have the potential to precipitate cardiovascular collapse in the patient with acute right-heart failure. The reasons for this are multiple and include not only reduced venous return and increased right ventricular afterload due to positive pressure ventilation, but also reduced preload caused by the sympatholytic effects of sedatives and narcotics used to facilitate intubation and mechanical ventilation. The use of sedatives and narcotics should therefore be minimized at the time of intubation whenever possible.

Hypercapnea, a common and typically well-tolerated consequence of lung protective ventilatory strategies, causes a rise in pulmonary artery pressure and should be avoided if possible in patients with right-heart–limited circulations. Hypoxemia causes pulmonary arterial vasoconstriction and should similarly be avoided.

Tidal volumes should be limited in patients with acute right-heart syndromes. One reason for this proscription is to avoid reductions in venous return caused by high intrathoracic pressure, although the effects of mechanical ventilation on right ventricular preload are difficult to predict in the patient with acute right-heart failure. Large tidal volumes also increase right ventricular afterload, probably through the compression of extra-alveolar vessels.

The effects of PEEP in right-heart failure are complex and highly variable. PEEP may reduce right ventricular afterload when its application is associated with substantial lung recruitment. However, if the PEEP administered causes overdistension of normal lung and compression of extra-alveolar vessels, right ventricular afterload may increase. In general, high levels of PEEP are harmful. Given the inherent difficulty in assessing the effects of PEEP on the circulatory status of patients with right-heart failure, an approach that generally tries to limit PEEP to the least level that allows adequate oxygenation on a nontoxic fraction of inspired oxygen is appropriate. Table 4 suggests an approach to the mechanical

Table 4. *Ventilator Management in Acute Right-Heart Failure*

Avoid hypoxemia
Avoid hypercapnea
Seek the lowest tidal volume that allows adequate elimination of carbon dioxide
Seek the least PEEP that allows adequate oxygenation on a nontoxic fraction of inspired oxygen; avoid intrinsic PEEP

---

ventilatory management of patients with acute right-heart failure.

Annotated Bibliography

Gomberg-Maitland M, Preston IR. Prostacyclin therapy for pulmonary arterial hypertension: new directions. Semin Respir Crit Care Med 2005; 26:394–401
Recent review of this important class of medications used to treat pulmonary arterial hypertension.

Jardin F, Genevray B, Brun-Ney D, et al. Dobutamine: a hemodynamic evaluation in pulmonary embolism shock. Crit Care Med 1985; 13:1009–1012

Jardin F, Vieillard-Baron A. Monitoring of right-sided heart function. Curr Opin Crit Care 2005; 11:271–279
Useful review of monitoring of right-sided heart function focusing on the use of echocardiography.

Lee SH, Channick RN. Endothelin antagonism in pulmonary arterial hypertension. Semin Respir Crit Care Med 2005; 26:402–408
Recent review of this important new class of medications used to treat pulmonary arterial hypertension.

Lee SH, Rubin LJ. Current treatment strategies for pulmonary arterial hypertension. J Intern Med 2005; 258:199–215
An excellent review of the state-of-the-art treatment of pulmonary arterial hypertension.

Leather HA, Segers P, Berends N, et al. Effects of vasopressin on right ventricular function in an experimental model of acute pulmonary hypertension. Crit Care Med 2002; 30:2548–2552
Suggests that vasopressin may be detrimental in the treatment of right ventricular failure.

Mebazaa A, Karpati P, Renaud E, et al. Acute right ventricular failure: from pathophysiology to new treatments. Intensive Care Med 2004; 30:185–196
Recent review of acute right ventricular failure, from pathophysiology to diagnosis to treatment.

McIntyre KM, Sasahara AA. The hemodynamic response to pulmonary embolism in patients without prior cardiopulmonaory disease. Am J Cardiol 1971; 28:288–294

Molloy WD, Lee KY, Girling L, et al. Treatment of shock in a canine model of pulmonary embolism. Am Rev Respir Dis 1984; 130:870–874

Squara P, Dhainaut JF, Artigas A, et al. Hemodynamic profile in severe ARDS: results of the European Collaborative ARDS Study. Intensive Care Med 1998; 24:1018–1028
Large prospective study that evaluated pulmonary hemodynamic variables in 424 of 586 patients with ARDS.

Taylor RW, Zimmerman JL, Dellinger RP, et al. Low-dose inhaled nitric oxide in patients with acute lung injury: a randomized controlled trial. JAMA 2004; 291:1603–1609
One of several studies showing short-term physiologic improvement but no improvement in clinical outcomes with the use of inhaled nitric oxide.

Notes

Acute Respiratory Distress Syndrome

Jesse B. Hall, MD, FCCP

The acute respiratory distress syndrome (ARDS) and the related acute lung injury (ALI) syndromes are forms of Type I or acute hypoxemic respiratory failure (AHRF). This form of lung dysfunction rises from diseases causing collapse and/or filling of alveoli with the result that a substantial fraction of mixed venous blood traverses nonventilated airspaces, effecting a right-to-left intrapulmonary shunt (Fig 1, panel b). In addition to the adverse consequences upon gas exchange, interstitial and alveolar fluid accumulation result in an increase in lung stiffness, imposing a mechanical load with a resulting increase in the work of breathing (Fig 1, panel a). Uncorrected, the gas exchange and lung mechanical abnormalities may eventuate in tissue hypoxia, respiratory arrest, and death (Fig 2). When this form of respiratory failure arises from acute lung injury with diffuse alveolar damage and flooding, it is termed ARDS.

Classification and Definition

To a first approximation, the disorders causing AHRF may be divided into diffuse lesions, such as pulmonary edema, and focal lung lesions, such as lobar pneumonia (Table 1). Since the distribution of airspace involvement may have implications for the response to interventions, such as positive end-expiratory pressure (PEEP), this nosology is of both therapeutic and didactic value.

Low-pressure pulmonary edema, termed *ARDS* as a clinical entity, results from injury to the lung microcirculation sustained from direct lung insults (*eg*, aspiration, inhalation, or infectious agents) or indirectly by systemic processes (*eg*, sepsis, traumatic shock with large volume blood product resuscitation). The former is termed "pulmonary" ARDS and the latter "extrapulmonary" ARDS. Some studies have suggested different lung mechanical properties between these entities and a different response to ventilator maneuvers directed at alveolar recruitment.

In addition to the distinction between pulmonary and extrapulmonary forms of ARDS/ALI, it is also useful to distinguish between the early phases of acute lung injury and events occurring subsequently (Fig 3).

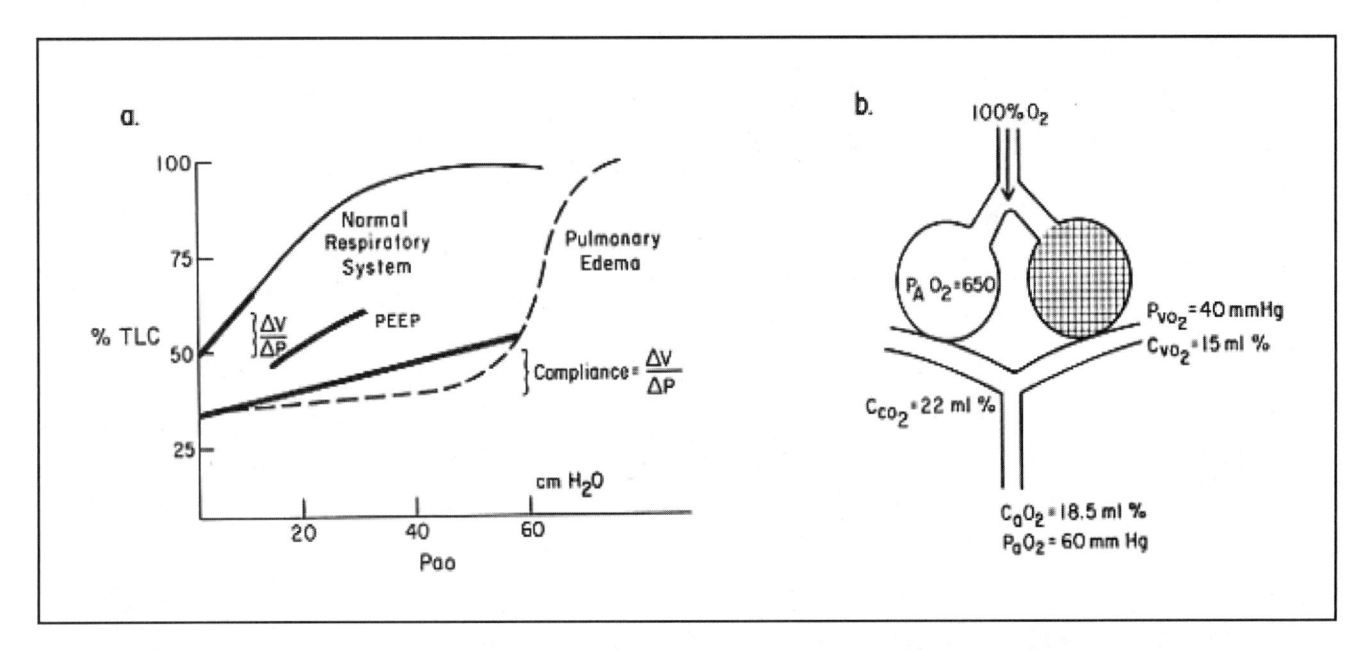

Figure 1.

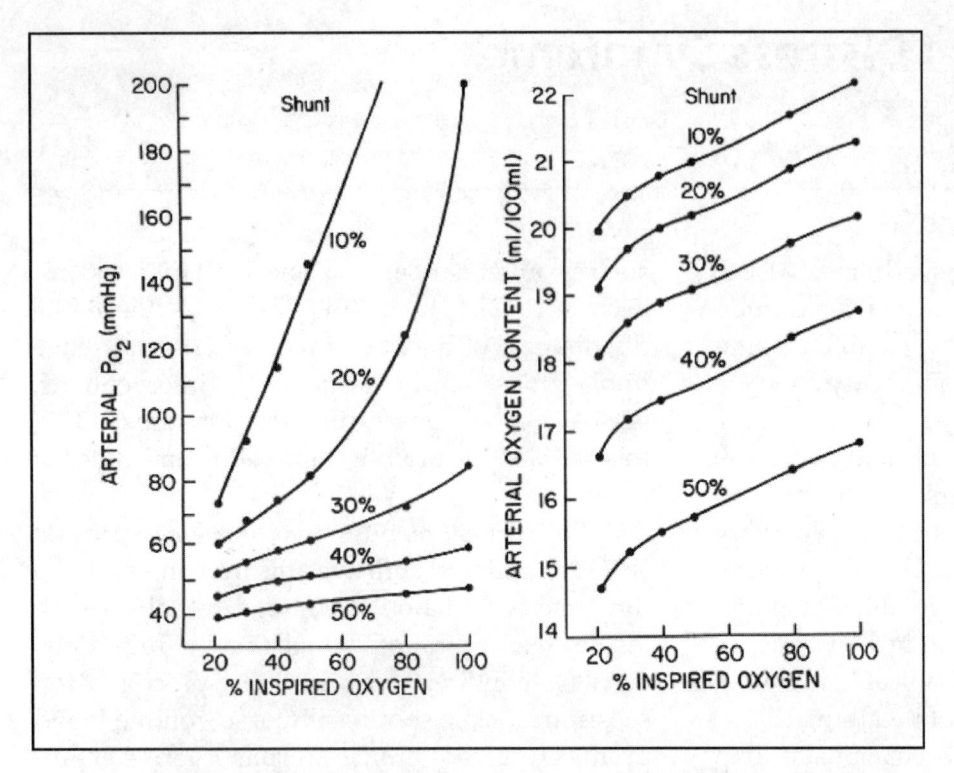

Figure 2. Left panel: The impact of shunt fraction on oxygenation—note that when shunt is 30% and above, the response to oxygen as judged by arterial P_{O_2} is minimal. Right panel: Even though the arterial P_{O_2} changes with oxygen are minimized by large shunt fraction, the increase in arterial oxygen content are large given the steep slope of the hemoglobin-oxygen dissociation curve in this range.

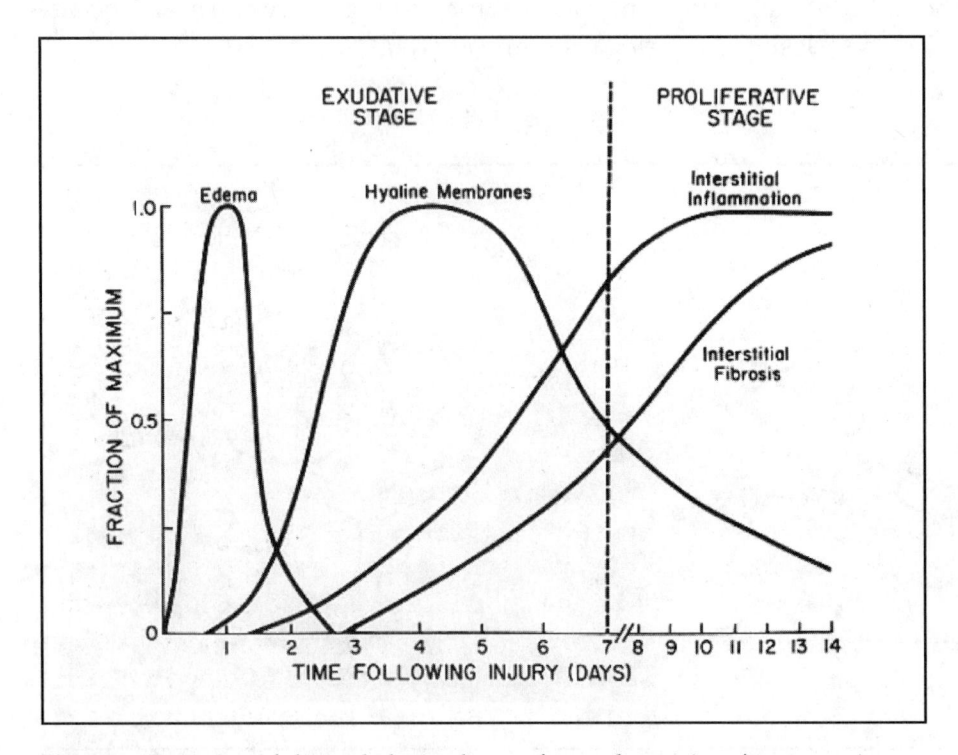

Figure 3. Depiction of the pathologic phases of acute lung injury/acute respiratory distress syndrome.

Table 1. *Causes of Acute Hypoxic Respiratory Failure*

Homogenous Lung Lesions (producing pulmonary edema)
    Cardiogenic or Hydrostatic Edema
        Left ventricular (LV) failure
        Acute LV ischemia
        Accelerated or malignant hypertension
        Mitral regurgitation
        Mitral stenosis
        Ball-valve thrombus
        Volume overload, particularly with co-existing renal and cardiac disease
    Permeability or Low-Pressure Edema (ARDS)
        Most Common
            Sepsis and sepsis syndrome
            Acid aspiration
            Multiple transfusions for hypovolemic shock
        Less Common
            Near drowning
            Pancreatitis
            Air or fat emboli
            Cardiopulmonary bypass
            Pneumonia
            Drug reaction or overdose
            Leukoagglutination
            Inhalation injury
            Infusion of biologics (*eg*, interleukin 2)
            Ischemia-reperfusion (*eg*, post-thrombectomy, post-transplant)
    Edema of Unclear or "Mixed" Etiology
        Re-expansion
        Neurogenic
        Post-ictal
        Tocolysis-associated
    Diffuse Alveolar Hemorrhage
        Microscopic angiitis
        Collagen vascular diseases
        Goodpasture's syndrome
        Severe coagulopathy and bone marrow transplant
        Retinoic-acid syndrome
Focal Lung Lesions
    Lobar Pneumonia
    Lung Contusion
    Lobar Atelectasis (acutely)

By light microscopy, early ARDS/ALI is characterized by flooding of the lung with proteinaceous fluid and minimal evidence of cellular injury. By electron microscopy, changes of endothelial cell swelling, widening of intercellular junctions, increased numbers of pinocytotic vesicles, and disruption and denudation of the basement membrane are prominent. This early phase of diffuse alveolar damage (DAD) has been termed **exudative** and is a period of time during which pulmonary edema and its effects are most pronounced, and intrapulmonary shunt is a primary problem dictating ventilatory strategies.

Over the ensuing days, hyaline membrane formation in the alveolar spaces is prominent, and inflammatory cells become more numerous. The latter phase of DAD is dominated by disordered healing. This can occur as early as 7 to 10 days after initial injury and often exhibits extensive pulmonary fibrosis, not dissimilar microscopically to patients with longstanding pulmonary fibrosis. This has been termed the **proliferative** phase of DAD. Pulmonary edema may not be as prominent in this latter phase of lung injury, and the clinician managing the patient is challenged by the large dead space fraction and high minute ventilation requirements. These patients may also exhibit progressive pulmonary hypertension—even if the pulmonary circulation was normal at baseline, slightly improved intrapulmonary shunt which is less responsive to PEEP, further reduction in lung compliance, and a tendency toward creation of Zone I conditions of the lung if the patient develops hypovolemia.

Patients with ARDS/ALI have a large number of underlying medical and surgical etiologies and there has been broad recognition of a need for specific definitions of these entities. The widely applied definitions offered by a joint American-European Consensus Conference published in 1994 are given in Table 2.

Scoring systems have also been used to grade patients with ALI/ARDS. Despite the large derangements in lung physiology in these patients, initial measurements of gas exchange and lung mechanics have not been very useful to predict mortality in these patients. One recent report, however, indicated that the dead space fraction measured during the first day of mechanical ventilation was a powerful determinant of survival—the odds ratio for mortality associated with each increase of dead-space fraction of .05 was 1.45 (95% CI 1.15-1.83, $p = .002$) (Fig 4).

Treatment

This discussion will focus upon ventilator and circulatory strategies for patients with ARDS/ALI, but it cannot be overemphasized that, simultaneously, a search for and treatment of the underlying cause of the lung failure must be conducted. Absent an identification and treatment of the underlying process(es) causing lung

Table 2. *The 1994 American-European Consensus Conference Definitions of Acute Lung Injury and the Acute Respiratory Distress Syndrome**

	Timing	Oxygenation	CXR	Ppw
ALI Criteria	Acute onset	Pao$_2$/Fio$_2$ <300 mm hg (regardless of PEEP level)	Bilateral infiltrates	<18 mm Hg or no clinical evidence right atrial hypertension
ARDS Criteria	Acute onset	Pao$_2$/Fio$_2$ <200 mm hg (regardless of PEEP level)	Bilateral infiltrates	<18 mm Hg or no clinical evidence right atrial hypertension

*CXR = chest radiograph; Ppw = pulmonary capillary wedge pressure; Fio$_2$ = fraction inspired oxygen; PEEP = positive end-expiratory pressure.

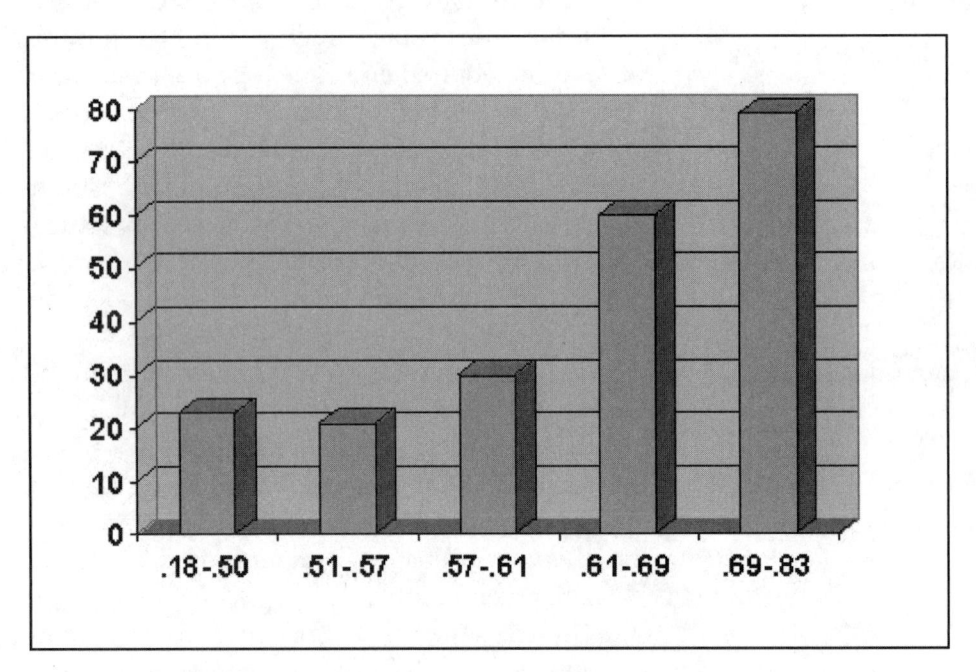

Figure 4. The observed mortality according to the quintile of dead-space fraction in 179 patients with ARDS (from Nuckton et al; N Engl J Med, 2002; 346:1281).

injury, supportive therapy alone will likely ultimately result in mounting complications and irreversible organ failures.

Ventilatory Management of ARDS

Lung Mechanics, Ventilator-Induced Lung Injury, and Ventilator-Associated Lung Injury

Over the past decade or more, a body of knowledge has accrued from both bench and clinical investigations, which has motivated intensivists to reconsider how they ventilate patients with ARDS. Much of this work was based upon early observations that mechanical ventilation, using large tidal volumes and high inflation pressures, could cause lung injury in animals with normal lungs or worsen a baseline lung injury. This phenomenon was termed *ventilator-induced lung injury* (VILI). VILI is indistinguishable morphologically, physiologically, and radiologically from DAD caused by other etiologies of acute lung injury. VILI is unique because one can identify that mechanical ventilation is the cause of lung injury, and hence the term *ventilator-induced* lung injury. Ventilator-associated lung injury (VALI) is defined as lung injury that resembles ARDS and that occurs in patients on mechanical ventilation. VALI is invariably associated with pre-existing lung pathology, such as ARDS. However, while the experimental data is overwhelming in demonstrating the existence of VILI, one cannot be sure in any particular case whether and to what extent VALI is caused by a particular ventilator strategy, rather VALI is only *associated* with mechanical ventilation.

Studies in animal models of VILI have demonstrated that lung injury during mechanical ventilatory support appears related to the distending volume to which the lung is subjected, rather than the distending pressure as measured at the mouth. For instance, in animal experiments in which the chest is banded and mechanical ventilation is conducted with high airway pressures but low tidal volumes resulting from the restricted chest wall, lung injury is not present. Such observations have caused the term "volutrauma" to be coined for this form of microstructural injury, a refinement of the standard term "barotraumas" applied to the grosser forms of extra-alveolar air collections that are sought on routine radiographs obtained on patients undergoing mechanical ventilation.

In addition to the detrimental effects of overdistension, numerous investigations have suggested a protective or ameliorating effect of PEEP on VILI. This protective effect has been postulated to result from the action of PEEP to avoid alveolar collapse and reopening. In the aggregate, these studies offer a view of VILI that is portrayed in Figure 5—that during the respiratory cycle, alveolar opening and collapse occur if end-expiratory pressure is zero or only modestly positive, and depending on end inspiratory lung volume, alveolar overdistension may occur.

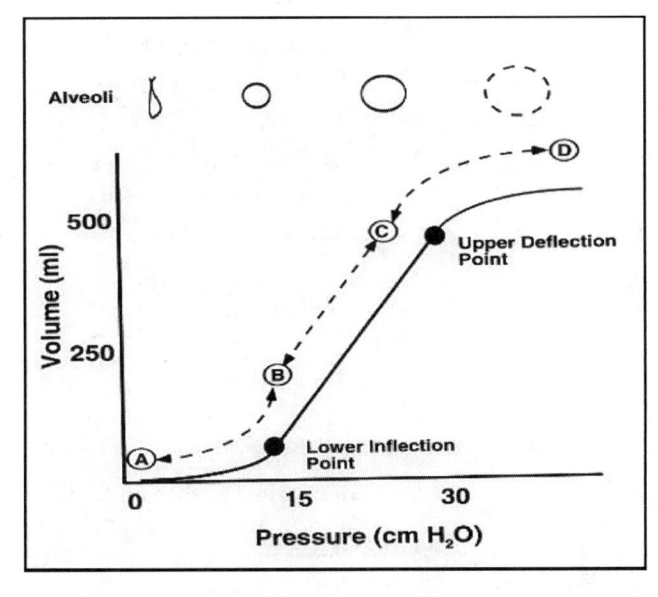

Figure 5. An idealized and simplified depiction of the pressure volume curve of the injured lung during inflation, with the state of alveolar collapse and inflation.

In both animal models of lung injury and patients with ARDS, the respiratory system inflation pressure volume (PV) curve exhibits a sigmoidal shape, with a lower inflection point (LIP) and an upper inflection point (UIP). Marked hysteresis is often noted when the inflation and deflation limbs are compared. The presence of the LIP is consistent with the edematous lung behaving as a two-compartment structure, with a population of alveoli exhibiting near normal compliance and another recruitable only at higher transpulmonary pressure. As transpulmonary pressure is raised to the LIP, effecting alveolar recruitment, lung compliance improves as reflected by the increase in the slope of the PV curve. Volume tends to increase in a nearly linear fashion as pressure is increased, until the UIP is reached, with a flattening of the curve taken to represent alveolar over-distension with the attendant risks of alveolar injury.

Clinical Studies of Ventilator Strategies for ARDS

These descriptions of VILI in animals and physiologic observations in patients resulted in strategies that have been tested at the bedside and demonstrated improved patient outcome. In the field of critical care medicine, this is one of the most substantive examples of bench-to-bedside transfer of knowledge that now provides an evidence-based approach to patient care.

Hickling reported a favorable impact on survival of tidal volume (VT) reduction and permissive hypercapnea in the management of patients with ARDS, comparing outcome to historical controls. These studies were limited by the lack of a randomized prospective controlled design, particularly in light of findings that the survival of patients with ARDS in the same timeframe is likely improving apart from the details of mechanical ventilatory support.

The first prospective randomized trial testing a strategy of limiting VT and utilizing PEEP to avoid alveolar recruitment-derecruitment (so-called "open lung" ventilation) was conducted by Amato and colleagues, who randomized patients with ARDS to two treatments: (1) assist-control ventilation with tidal volumes of 12 mL/kg, PEEP sufficient to maintain an adequate Sao_2 on $Fio_2 < 0.6$, and respiratory rates sufficient to maintain arterial carbon dioxide levels of 25 to 38 mm Hg, no efforts were made to control peak inspiratory or plateau airway pressures ("conventional" approach); or (2) pressure-controlled inverse ratio ventilation, pressure-support ventilation, or volume-assured pressure-support ventilation with tidal volumes less than 6 mL/kg, recruitment maneuver, peak pressures less than 40 cm H_2O, and PEEP titrated to maintain lung inflation above the lower inflection point ("open-lung" approach). Patients managed with the "open-lung" approach demonstrated a more rapid recovery of pulmonary compliance, decreased requirement for high F_{IO_2}, a lower rate of barotrauma, a higher rate of liberation from the ventilator, decreased death associated with respiratory failure, and a decreased mortality at 28 days (although not at hospital discharge).

While these results were striking, a number of concerns regarding this study deserve consideration. The number of patients included in the study was small (only 53). Furthermore, there were multiple treatment differences between the two groups, including PEEP strategy, V_T, P_{CO_2}, minute ventilation, lung recruitment maneuvers, and mode of ventilation. Importantly, mortality was extremely high in the conventional ventilation group (71%), and the early differences in mortality seen between the groups did not seem consistent with the two ventilator strategies differing by the accrual of progressive lung injury. Finally, patients with severe metabolic acidosis, a common feature of patients with overwhelming sepsis and ARDS, were excluded from study. Even if one accepts the results of this study, perhaps the benefit was simply due to V_T reduction, not to the PEEP strategy. Even if this PEEP strategy prevented VILI, the PEEP value selected from the LIP on inflation of edematous lungs from zero end expiratory pressure is considerably larger than the PEEP value required to maintain alveolar recruitment during tidal ventilation on PEEP. In addition, several other investigations evaluating the effect of V_T manipulation on outcome did not show a similar salutary effect of low V_T ventilation.

The controversy over proper tidal volumes for ventilation of patients with ARDS has been largely resolved by the performance of a trial conducted by the NIH-funded ARDSnet, a network of 10 centers in 24 hospitals comprising 75 intensive care units that enrolled 861 patients. Patients were randomized to a strategy of either 12 mL/kg V_T or 6 mL/kg V_T, based on ideal body weight. If plateau airway pressure (Pplat), used as a surrogate of end inspiratory lung "stretch," exceeded 30 cm H_2O pressure in the low V_T group, tidal volume was further reduced as necessary to reduce Pplat to this target value. The experimental protocol could be summarized, as shown in Table 3.

The trial stopped sooner than the anticipated endpoint, because the findings were striking. The strategy achieved a significant difference in tidal volumes as intended—the mean tidal volumes on days 1 to 3 were 6.2 and 11.8 mL/kg in the low and high groups, respectively ($p < .001$), associated with Pplat of 25 and 33 cm H_2O, respectively ($p < .001$). PEEP levels were minimally higher in the low V_T group from days 1 to 3 (averaging less than 1 cm H_2O and lower on day 7). The low V_T group had a modest increase in $Paco_2$ relative to the traditional group and a very modest decrease in pH; the potential for greater degrees of respiratory acidosis between the groups was minimized by the higher respiratory rates used in the low V_T group. The primary endpoint of the study, 28-day mortality, was significantly improved with low V_T ventilation, falling from 39.8% in the traditional group to 31.0% with low V_T ventilation ($p = .007$). In

Table 3. *ARDSnet Low Tidal Volume Protocol*

Variable	Protocol
Ventilator mode	Volume assist-control
Tidal volume	≤6 mL/kg predicted body weight*
Plateau airway pressure	≤30 cm H_2O
Vent rate/pH goal	6-35/min, adjusted to achieve arterial pH > 7.30 if possible
Inspiratory flow	Adjust for I:E of 1.1:1.3
Oxygenation	55 ≤ Pao_2 ≤ 80 mm Hg or 88 ≤ Sao_2 ≤ 95%
F_{IO_2}/PEEP combinations	.3/5, .4/5, .4/8, .5/8, .5/10, .6/10, .7/10, .7/12, .7/14, .8/14, .9/14, .9/16, .9/18, 1.0/18, 1.0/22, 1.0/24
Weaning	Attempt by PS when F_{IO_2}/PEEP <.4/8

*Predicted body weight for men = 50 + (2.3 × (height in inches − 60)) or 50 + (.91 × (height in cm − 152.4))
Predicted body weight for women = 45 + (2.3 × (height in inches − 60)) or 45 + (.91 × (height in cm − 152.4))

addition, the number of ventilator-free days in the first 28 days was greater in the low V_T group.

This trial is a benchmark and confirms earlier basic and clinical studies suggesting that low V_T ventilation can be protective for patients with ARDS and will improve outcome. Perhaps the best evidenced-based recommendation for routine management of patients with ARDS undergoing mechanical ventilation is to implement the ARDSnet protocol. While questions surround other elements of ventilatory strategy—the "best PEEP" level, the trade-off between F_{IO_2} and PEEP, the use of recruitment maneuvers, patient positioning—the current evidence strongly supports the use of the ARDSnet strategy pending additional information to guide these other components of ventilatory support.

Despite these very convincing data from a well-conducted trial and the peer-review of the report of this study, some have called the results into question. A recent metaanalysis by Eichacker and colleagues has suggested that the ARDSnet V_T trial may have "missed" the ideal V_T for these patients by not testing V_T in the range between 6 and 12 mL/kg, and that, while survival was better for patients with lower V_T, these results point more to the detrimental effects of very high tidal volumes and not to the superiority of lower tidal volumes. While this argument is interesting in a theoretical sense, there are really no data to support this contention, and most experts would agree that the ARDSnet trial indeed tested the general range of V_T used in managing these patients and that the results support the low V_T approach.

Practical Points for Managing the Patient With ALI/ARDS

Upon presentation, the patient should receive oxygen provided by a high-flow or rebreather mask, although these devices rarely achieve a tracheal F_{IO_2} much above 0.6 in dyspneic, tachypneic patients. The administration of supplemental oxygen is a diagnostic, as well as therapeutic, maneuver. Patients whose oxygenation improves dramatically with supplemental oxygen generally have a small shunt and a larger component of ventilation-perfusion mismatch (or hypoventilation). Even when the Pao_2 improves only slightly, indicating a large shunt, oxygen delivery may rise importantly, due to the steep nature of the hemoglobin saturation relationship at low Pao_2 (Fig 2). The role of noninvasive positive-pressure ventilation (NIPPV) has not been established in ARDS. Although we have used NIPPV successfully in this setting, we believe it is generally not a good choice and patients must be carefully selected. Since the course of ARDS is usually longer than patients will tolerate NIPPV, and since ARDS is so often associated with hemodynamic instability, coma, and multiorgan system failure (including ileus), we believe all but exceptional patients should be endotracheally intubated.

Intubation should be performed early and electively when it is clear that mechanical ventilation will be required, rather than waiting for frank respiratory failure. If hypoperfusion is present, as in the patient with hypotension, cardiovascular instability, or the hyperdynamic circulation of sepsis, oxygen delivery may be compromised not only by hypoxemia but by an inadequate cardiac output, as well. In this circumstance, sedation and muscle relaxation should be considered as a means to diminish the oxygen requirement of the skeletal muscles. Patients with extreme hypoxemia despite ventilator management as described below may also benefit from sedation or paralysis.

The initial ventilator settings should pursue the protocol given in Table 3. While the use of low V_T is strongly supported by current evidence, the proper PEEP level is less clear. Some intensivists recommend a "least PEEP" approach, using PEEP only as necessary to achieve adequate oxygenation and avoid toxic levels of F_{IO_2} (although these thresholds are not well established). Others would recommend higher PEEP levels with a goal of achieving maximal lung recruitment and avoiding mechanical events, such as collapse-reinflation that could lead to VALI. Some even advocate use of the PV curve of the lung measured during the respiratory cycle as a guide to this PEEP titration. A trial completed recently by ARDSnet, comparing the PEEP strategy as implemented in the low vs high tidal volume trial against a higher PEEP level, did not show a difference in survival; although, even though this study was prospective and randomized, a difference in age and severity of illness existed between the two cohorts, somewhat confounding interpretation.

Regardless of specific strategy, reducing PEEP, even for short periods of time, is often associated with alveolar derecruitment and, hence, rapid arterial hemoglobin desaturation. Thus, once endotracheal tube suctioning has been accomplished for diagnostic purposes, nursing and respiratory therapy staff should be instructed to keep airway disconnections to a minimum, or to use an in-line suctioning system that maintains sterility and positive pressure, usually via the suctioning catheter residing in a sterile sheath and entering the endotracheal tube via a tight-sealing diaphragm. These suctioning systems are generally effective for lesser levels of PEEP (<15 cm H_2O) but often leak if higher levels are attempted.

Innovative Therapies for ARDS

While the general strategy described above will provide adequate ventilatory support for the majority of patients with ALI/ARDS, a fraction of patients will have severe hypoxemia or other adverse consequences of these approaches, and innovative or salvage therapies have been reported in the literature. In general, these approaches are not supported by large prospective trials (or trials have been conducted without benefit seen), but they may have some role in individual patient management.

Prone Position: Multiple studies have shown that a substantial fraction of patients with ARDS exhibit improved oxygenation with prone positioning. Some studies suggest this maneuver enhances lower lobe recruitment and, thus, would have the potential to not only improve gas exchange but, perhaps, reduce VALI and ultimate patient outcome. A recent large prospective trial evaluated proning in patients with ALI/ARDS and did not see a benefit. In subset analysis, there did appear to be a trend to improved outcome in patients with more severe physiologic derangement. In addition, this study has been criticized for the relatively short periods of proning that were employed. Further studies of this strategy are ongoing.

High Frequency Ventilation: If excessive lung excursion is associated with injury to the lung, then it seems reasonable that ventilation with very small tidal volumes at high frequencies would be associated with the least possible VILI and would be associated with improved outcome. High-frequency jet ventilation (HFV) typically employs tidal volumes of 1 to 5 mL (or higher) and respiratory rates of 60 to 300 breaths/min. Gas exchange is poorly understood under these conditions but is thought to occur as much through augmented axial diffusion as through bulk flow. Unfortunately, multiple trials of high-frequency ventilation in adults have failed to demonstrate any benefit compared to mechanical ventilation. It is interesting to note that HFV has never been associated with either improved oxygenation, reduced barotrauma, or decreased days of mechanical ventilation. These are all outcomes that would be reasonably expected as a logical extension of the physiology and concerns driving open lung ventilation. That they have not been observed suggests that all previous investigations of HFV were conducted using the wrong guidelines for ventilation (*ie*, striving to maintain normocarbia) or that some other effect, not yet understood, precludes benefit from this technique. Future studies of HFV should compare this technique to ventilation using the low VT ventilation, as described in the ARDSnet trial, and will have to demonstrate benefit, compared to these strategies, to gain acceptance.

Extracorporeal Gas Exchange: The use of extracorporeal gas exchange (ECMO) to adequately oxygenate and ventilate the blood while allowing the lung to rest remains an attractive strategy for the management of patients with acute lung injury but has not been supported by clinical outcome studies. There is little apparent future for this technique in adult patients with ARDS. ECMO is best regarded at this time as heroic salvage therapy for patients with isolated respiratory failure in whom all other supportive measures have failed.

Inhaled Nitric Oxide: Nitric oxide (NO) is a potent endogenous vasodilator that, when given by inhalation, selectively vasodilates the pulmonary circulation. Inhaled NO (iNO) has several potentially salutary effects in ARDS: it selectively vasodilates pulmonary vessels that subserve *ventilated* alveoli, diverting blood flow to these alveoli (and away from areas of shunt). The first effect, the lowering of the pulmonary vascular resistance, accompanied by a lowering of the pulmonary artery pressure, appears maximal at very low concentrations (approximately 0.1 ppm) in patients with ARDS. The beneficial effects on oxygenation take place at somewhat higher inspired concentrations of NO (1-10 ppm). The rapid inactivation of iNO via hemoglobin binding prevents unwanted systemic hemodynamic side effects, but also mandates the continuous delivery of gas to the ventilator circuit. In the numerous studies evaluating the acute response to iNO, there has been a consistent finding of approximately 50% to 70% of patients improving oxygenation. However, two recent prospective trials have failed to demonstrate improved long-term outcome from iNO administration in ARDS ventilation, and thus this remains a salvage therapy at best.

Circulatory Management of ARDS

Debate has surrounded the proper circulatory management of patients with ARDS for decades. On the one hand, animal and some clinical studies suggest that edemagenesis can be reduced by reducing pulmonary microvascular pressures in acute lung injury, in a fashion similar to the management of cardiogenic pulmonary edema. Of course, since these microvascular pressures are normal in these patients despite their lung flooding, the possibility of reducing cardiac preload exists, thus engendering inadequate organ perfusion in a patient population known to be at risk of multiple organ failure and in whom outcome appears dictated in large part by the accrual of organ failures.

In addition, the proper monitoring tools for assessing the adequacy of the circulation in these patients and whether monitoring should include invasive hemodynamic measurement is equally controversial. It seems reasonable to state that mere monitoring with invasive measurements, that is not coupled to a strategy to achieve pre-defined goals, is not warranted.

It is difficult to make firm recommendations in the current state of knowledge. The ARDSnet is currently conducting a trial that enrolls and randomizes patients to management with either a central venous catheter or right heart catheter, and then each group is additionally randomized to receive a fluid liberal or fluid conservative strategy. It is hoped that information from this study will help guide the circulatory management of these patients and will determine how that strategy can be best conducted.

Management of Proliferative Phase ARDS

A subset of patients with ARDS will progress over the first week of mechanical ventilation to disordered healing and severe lung fibrosis. This is usually characterized by increasing airway pressures or a falling V_T on pressure-control ventilation, a further fall in lung compliance, less response to PEEP, a "honey-comb" appearance on the chest radiograph, progressive pulmonary hypertension, and rising minute ventilation requirements (>20 L/min). Barotrauma is a prominent feature and multiple organ failures often accrue. A number of observations regarding their supportive therapy should be made. Increased vascular permeability at this point in the course may be minimal, and strategies to reduce preload and edema are fraught with complications. Patients are prone to increases in Zone I lung conditions, and attempts to reduce the pulmonary capillary wedge pressure (Ppw) may result in increased dead space and hypoperfusion. Thus, seeking the lowest Ppw providing adequate cardiac output is no longer appropriate; instead, liberalization of fluid intake to provide a circulating volume in excess of that just adequate is a better strategy in this later phase of ARDS.

Interventions to directly influence the course of lung fibrosis are not well established, but high-dose corticosteroid therapy has its advocates. One recent prospective trial has shown an improved survival with the use of corticosteroids in late ARDS, but routine use in late ARDS remains controversial. The utility of corticosteroids was studied by ARDSnet in a randomized trial, and data from this study presented in abstract form. Survival differences were not seen related to corticosteroid therapy.

If corticosteroids are used in this setting, aggressive measures to monitor for ventilator-associated pneumonia are warranted. This complication of mechanical ventilation has a high incidence and high mortality in patients with ARDS. In view of the abnormal chest radiograph and gas exchange, multiple causes of fever and leukocytosis and high incidence of colonization of the airway, diagnosis is difficult and may be aided by various techniques to obtain protected specimens.

Long-term Sequelae of ARDS

There is a variability to recovery of lung function following acute lung injury. Patients may recover with minimal or no abnormality by routine lung function testing shortly after acute lung insult, or they may remain substantially impaired for a year or longer, if not permanently. In most studies, approximately a fourth of patients show no impairment at 1 year, a fourth moderate impairment, roughly half only mild impairment, and a very small fraction severe impairment. Exertional dyspnea is the most commonly reported respiratory symptom, although cough and wheezing are common as well. A reduced single-breath carbon monoxide-diffusing capacity is the most common pulmonary function abnormality. Spirometry and lung volumes tend to reveal mixed restrictive-obstructive abnormalities. Determining the prognosis after ARDS may be aided by obtaining complete lung functions at the time of discharge. Those patients with substantial abnormalities should be referred for appropriate follow-up. Herridge and colleagues also recently reported that lung dysfunction may be of only minor significance in terms of regaining general function, and that weight loss, neuromuscular weakness, and neuropsychiatric dysfunction related to critical illness or supportive management may be much more significant than respiratory dysfunction *per se*.

Selected Reading

Amato MB, Barbas CS, Medeiros DM, et al. Effect of a protective-ventilation strategy on mortality in the acute respiratory distress syndrome. N Engl J Med 1998; 338:347-354

Anzueto A, Baughman RP, Guntupalli KK, et al. Aerosolized surfactant in adults with sepsis induced acute respiratory distress syndrome. N Engl J Med 1996; 334:1417-1421

Bernard GR, Artigas A, Brigham KL, et al. The American-European Consensus Conference on ARDS: definitions, mechanisms, relevant outcomes, and clinical trial coordination. Am J Respir Crit Care Med 1994; 149:818-824

Brower RG, Lanken PN, MacIntyre N, et al. Higher versus lower positive end-expiratory pressures in patients with the acute respiratory distress syndrome. N Engl J Med 2004; 351:327-336

Brower RG, Rubenfeld GD. Lung-protective ventilation strategies in acute lung injury. Crit Care Med 2003; 31(suppl):S312-S316

Brower RG, Ware LB, Berthiaume Y, et al. Treatment of ARDS. Chest 2001; 120:1347-1367

Chastre J, Trouillet JL, Vuagnat A, et al. Nosocomial pneumonia in patients with acute respiratory distress syndrome. Am J Respir Crit Care Med 1998; 157:1165-1172

Dreyfuss D, Saumon G. Ventilator-induced lung injury: lessons from experimental studies. Am J Respir Crit Care Med 1998; 157:294-323

Eichacker PQ, Gerstenberger EP, Banks SM, et al. Meta-analysis of acute lung injury and acute respiratory distress syndrome trials testing low tidal volumes. Am J Respir Crit Care Med 2002; 166:1510-1514

Gattinoni L, Pelosi P, Suter PM, et al. Acute respiratory distress syndrome due to pulmonary and extra-pulmonary disease: different syndromes? Am J Respir Crit Care Med 1998; 158:3-11

Herridge MS, Cheung AM, Tansey CM, et al. One-year outcomes in survivors of the acute respiratory distress syndrome. N Engl J Med 2003; 348:683-693

Hickling KG. The pressure-volume curve is greatly modified by recruitment: a mathematical model of ARDS lungs. Am J Respir Crit Care Med 1998; 158:194-202

Meduri GU, Headley AS, Golden E, et al. Effect of prolonged methylprednisolone therapy in unresolving acute respiratory distress syndrome: a randomized controlled trial. JAMA 1998; 280:159-165

Nuckton TJ, Alonso JA, Kallet RH, et al. Pulmonary dead space fraction as a risk factor for death in the acute respiratory distress syndrome. N Engl J Med 2002; 346:1281-1286

O'Connor M, Hall JB, Schmidt GA, et al. Acute hypoxemic respiratory failure. In: Hall JB, Schmidt GA, Wood LDH, eds. Principles of critical care. New York, NY: McGraw-Hill Publishers, 1998; 537-559

Rubenfeld GD. Epidemiology of acute lung injury. Crit Care Med 2003; 31(suppl):S276-S284

Slutsky AR, Tremblay LN. Multiple system organ failure: is mechanical ventilation a contributing factor? Am J Respir Crit Care Med 1998; 157:1721-1725

Steinbrook R. How best to ventilate? Trial design and patient safety in studies of the acute respiratory distress syndrome. N Engl J Med 2003; 348:1393-1401

Stewart TE. Controversies around lung protective mechanical ventilation. Am J Respir Crit Care Med 2002; 166:1421-1422

The Acute Respiratory Distress Syndrome Network. Ventilation with lower tidal volumes as compared with traditional tidal volumes for acute lung injury and ARDS. N Engl J Med 2000; 342:1301-1308

Ware LB, Matthay MA. The acute respiratory distress syndrome. N Engl J Med 2000; 342:1334-1347

Notes

Notes

Weaning From Mechanical Ventilation

James K. Stoller, MD, MS, FCCP

Objectives:

- To review the frequency of weaning failure
- To discuss the logic of weaning, ie, questions to ask when approaching the ventilated patient
- To assess available predictors of weaning success and failure
- To describe the techniques of weaning and the evidence supporting their use
- To understand special considerations in weaning, *eg*, auto-positive end-expiratory pressure, imposed work of breathing, cardiac ischemia, the importance of psychological factors, routine interruption of sedation and of a systematic approach to weaning

Key words: auto-positive end-expiratory pressure; mechanical ventilation; pressure support; T-piece; weaning; work of breathing

Introduction

Weaning from mechanical ventilation is the process of freeing the patient from dependence on mechanical ventilatory assistance. The use of the term "weaning" must be distinguished from the term "extubation," which is the removal of the endotracheal tube. As is obvious at the bedside, but sometimes vague in studies that describe the outcomes of ventilated patients, the criteria for weaning differ from those of extubation, as some patients may be able to support normal ventilation but still require an endotracheal tube to provide airway protection.

This chapter will first review the frequency with which weaning fails, and will then discuss the weaning process, beginning with the logic of weaning. A discussion of weaning predictors follows, with emphasis on predictors of weaning success and of weaning failure. Available weaning predictors are assessed critically with specific attention to their diagnostic performance. Techniques of weaning are reviewed, followed by an analysis of available studies regarding the preferred approach to weaning patients from mechanical ventilation. Finally, special considerations in weaning, such as work of breathing measurements, the role of auto-positive end-expiratory pressure (PEEP), psychological factors, and management of sedation are addressed.

In the context that evidence-based guidelines for weaning and discontinuing ventilatory support were issued in late 2001 by a collective task force of the American College of Chest Physicians, the American Association for Respiratory Care, and the American College of Critical Care Medicine.[1] These guidelines are presented (Table 1) and cited where appropriate.

Logic of Weaning: Questions To Ask

The process of weaning proceeds by addressing two sequential questions: (a) Is the patient a candidate to begin weaning? (b) If the patient is deemed a candidate to wean, is weaning likely to succeed? This logic is reflected in 1 and 2 of the available evidence-based guidelines on weaning (Table 1). In this context, to initiate weaning, the following conditions must be satisfied:

Recommendations

- Improvement in the underlying process causing respiratory failure
- Adequacy of mental status and muscular strength, including
  - Resolution of the effects of sedating and paralyzing medications
  - Wakefulness sufficient to allow cooperation in weaning and to allow subsequent extubation, as well as ability to clear and handle secretions
- Hemodynamic stability, generally considered to be resolution of sepsis or the need for pressor support
- Normality of acid-base and electrolyte status, with special attention given to assuring restoration of baseline acid-base balance (ie, allowing hypercapnia if chronically present and avoiding new metabolic alkalosis) and to assuring the normality of electrolytes that affect muscle function (*eg*, phosphate, calcium, and potassium)

Table 1. *Recommendations from the Task Force for Evidence-Based Guidelines for Weaning and Discontinuing Ventilatory*

Recommendation 1: In patients requiring mechanical ventilation for >24 hours, a search for all the causes that may be contributing to ventilatory dependence should be undertaken. This is particularly true in the patient who has failed attempts at withdrawing the mechanical ventilatory. Reversing, all possible ventilatory and non-ventilatory issues should be an integral part of the ventilatory discontinuation process.

Recommendation 2: Patients receiving mechanical ventilation for respiratory failure should undergo a formal assessment of discontinuation potential if the following criteria are satisfied:
1. Evidence for some reversal of the underlying cause for respiratory failure.
2. Adequate oxygenation (*eg*, Pao_2/Fio_2 ratio > 150 to 200; requiring positive end-expiratory pressure [PEEP] ≤ 5 to 8 cm H_2O; Fio_2 ≤ 0.4 to 0.5); and pH (*eg*, ≥ 7.25);
3. Hemodynamic stability, as defined by the absence of active myocardial ischemia and the absence of clinically significant hypotension (*ie*, a condition requiring no vasopressor therapy or therapy with only low-dose vasopressors such as dopamine or dobutamine, <5 µg/kg/min); and
4. The capability to initiate an inspiratory effort.

The decision to use these criteria must be individualized. Some patients not satisfied all of the above criteria (*eg*, patients with chronic hypoxemia values below the thresholds cited) may be ready for attempts at the discontinuation of mechanical ventilation.

Recommendation 3: Formal discontinuation assessments for patients receiving mechanical ventilation for respiratory failure should be performed during spontaneous breathing rather than while the patient is still receiving substantial ventilatory support. An initial brief period of spontaneous breathing can be used to assess the capability of continuing onto a formal spontaneous breathing trial (SBT). The criteria with which to assess patient tolerance during SBTs are the respiratory pattern, the adequacy of gas exchange, hemodynamic stability, and subjective comfort. The tolerance of SBTs lasting 30 to 120 minutes should prompt consideration for permanent ventilator discontinuation.

Recommendation 4: The removal of the artificial airway from a patient who has successfully been discontinued from the ventilatory support should be based on assessments of airway patency and the ability of the patient to protect the airway.

Recommendation 5: Patients receiving mechanical ventilation for respiratory failure who fail an SBT should have the cause for the failed BST determined. Once reversible causes for failure are corrected, and if the patient still meets the criteria listed in Table 3, subsequent SBTs should be performed every 24 hours.

Recommendation 6: Patients receiving mechanical ventilation for respiratory failure who fail an SBT should receive a stable, non-fatiguing, comfortable form of ventilatory support.

Recommendation 7: Anesthesia/sedation strategies and ventilator management aimed at early extubation should be used in post-surgical patients.

Recommendation 8: Weaning/discontinuation protocols that are designed for nonphysician healthcare professionals (HCPs) should be developed and implemented by ICUs. Protocols aimed at optimizing sedation also should be developed and implemented.

Recommendation 9: Tracheotomy should be considered after a initial period of stabilization on the ventilator when it becomes apparent that the patient will require prolonged ventilator assistance. Tracheotomy then should be performed when the patient appears likely to gain one or more of the benefits ascribed to the procedure. Patients who may derive particular benefit from early tracheotomy are the following:
1. Those requiring high levels of sedation to tolerate translaryngeal tubes;
2. Those with marginal respiratory mechanics (often manifested as tachypnea) in whom a tracheostomy tube having lower resistance might reduce the risk of muscle overload;
3. Those who may derive psychological benefit from the ability to eat orally, communicate by articulated speech, and experience enhanced mobility; and
4. Those in whom enhanced mobility may assist physical therapy efforts.

Recommendation 10: Unless there is evidence for clearly irreversible disease (*eg*, high spinal cord injury or advanced amyotrophic lateral sclerosis), a patient requiring prolonged mechanical ventilatory support for respiratory failure should not be considered permanently ventilator-dependent until 3 months of weaning attempts have failed.

Recommendation 11: Critical care practitioners should familiarize themselves with facilities in their communities, or units in hospitals they staff, that specialize in managing patients who require prolonged dependence on mechanical ventilation. Such familiarization should include reviewing published peer-reviewed data from those units, if available. When medically stable for transfer, patients who have failed ventilator discontinuation attempts in the ICU should be transferred to those facilities that have demonstrated success and safety in accomplishing ventilator discontinuation.

Recommendation 12: Weaning strategies in the prolonged mechanical ventilation patient should be slow-paced and should include gradually lengthening self-breathing trials.

- Nutritional repletion
- Adequacy of oxygenation, *eg*, Pao_2 exceeding 60 mm Hg (8.0 kPa) with Fio_2 of <0.5 and PEEP of <5 cm H_2O.

When the aforementioned conditions are satisfied, it is reasonable to proceed with weaning. Attention then turns to assessing the likelihood that the weaning effort will succeed. In this regard, many different predictors of weaning have been proposed.[2,3]

Predictors of Weaning

Weaning prediction is the process of estimating the likelihood that weaning and/or extubation efforts will succeed or fail in a specific patient at a specific time. As with decision-making in clinical medicine in general, weaning success or failure is a dichotomous outcome (*ie*, the patient either does or does not wean) and the process of predicting weaning outcome involves applying a weaning predictor to estimate the probability of weaning or extubation failure or success.[2]

Many different weaning predictors have been proposed (Table 2).[2,3] Available univariate (single variable) predictors include measures of lung mechanics and work of breathing (*eg*, forced vital capacity, maximal inspiratory pressure), measures of gas exchange adequacy (*eg*, ratios of Pao_2/Fio_2 and Pao_2/Pao_2), and measures of the adequacy of systemic perfusion (*ie*, gastric intramural pH).

Tables 3 through 5 review the statistical performance of several commonly used univariate weaning predictors (*ie*, the minute ventilation of <10 L/min [Table 3], the forced vital capacity [Table 4], and the maximal inspiratory force of <–30 cm H_2O [Table 5]) and show that the positive predictive values of univariate weaning predictors generally exceed their negative predictive values. Remembering that the positive predictive value estimates the likelihood that the patient will wean if the predictor indicates success and that the negative predictive value estimates the likelihood of weaning failure if the predictor indicates failure, it can be concluded that univariate predictors are more reliable indicators of weaning success than they are of weaning failure. That is, the failure to satisfy the univariate weaning predictor does not confidently predict failure to wean; as shown by Krieger et al,[4] slavish attention to deferring weaning when a univariate weaning predictor

Table 2. *Proposed Univariate Predictors of Weanability*

Lung Mechanics and Work
  VC > 10 mL/kg
  V_T > 300 mL
  Maximal inspiratory force <–30 cm H_2O
  $P_{0.1}$ < 6 cm H_2O
  Dynamic compliance >25 mL cm H_2O
  Respiratory rate <25 breaths/min
  Minute ventilation <10 L/min
  MVV > 2 times minute ventilation
  Respiratory frequency/V_T < 105 breaths/min/L
  Oxygen cost of breathing <15%
  V_D/V_T < 0.60

Gas Exchange and Perfusion
  $P(A-a)o_2$ < 350 mm hg (46.7 kPa) on Fio_2 of 1.0
  Pao_2/Fio_2 > 238
  Pao_2/Pao_2 > 0.47
  Gastric pH > 7.30 and/or ↓ by <0.09 during weaning

VC, vital capacity; V_T, tidal volume; $P_{0.1}$, airway occlusion pressure; V_D/V_T, deadspace volume to tidal volume; MVV, maximum ventilatory ventilation; $P(A-a)o_2$, alveolar-arterial oxygen tension difference.

Table 3. *Minute Ventilation <10 L/min as a Univariate Weaning Predictor*

Study (date)	N	Sensitivity (%)	Specificity (%)	Positive Value	Negative Value
Sahn & Lakshminarayan (1973)[a]	100	92	100	100	71
Tahvanainen et al (1983)	47	45	78	89	25
Krieger et al (1989)[b]	269	NS	NS	93	15
Yang & Tobin (1989)	41	24	69	55	37

NS, not stated.
[a] Minute ventilation <10 L/min; maximal inspiratory pressure (MIP) <–30 cm H_2O; and maximal voluntary ventilation (MVV) >2 times minute ventilation; [b] minute ventilation <10 L/min and MIP <–30 cm H_2O.
Reproduced with permission from Stoller JK: Establishing clinical unweanability. *Respir Care* 1991; 36:186–198.

Table 4. *Vital Capacity (Measured in mL/kg) as a Univariate Weaning Predictor*

					Prediction Performance	
Study (Date)	Criterion	N	Sensitivity (%)	Specificity (%)	Positive Value	Negative Value
Milbern et al (1978)[a]	>15	33	25	0	58	0
Tahvanainen et al (1983)	>10	47	97	13	83	50
Pardee et al (1984)	>17	133	90	60	88	NS

NS, not stated.
[a] Vital capacity > 15 mL/kg and maximal inspiratory pressure <−25 cm H_2O.
Reproduced with permission from Stoller JK: Establishing clinical unweanability. *Respir Care* 1991; 36:186–198.

Table 5. *Maximal Inspiratory Pressure ≤−30 cm H_2O as a Univariate Weaning Predictor*

Prediction Performance

Study (date)	N	Patient Type	Sensitivity (%)	Specificity (%)	Positive Predictive Value	Negative Predictive Value
Sahn & Lakshmin-arayan (1973)[a]	100	Mean MV duration 37 hrs	92	100	100	71
Milburn et al. (1978)[b]	33	Mean MV 3.1 hrs	25	0	58	0
Tahvanainen et al. (1973)	47	Mean MV 5 days	68	0	74	0
DeHaven et al. (1986)	48	Mean MV 55 hrs	49	100	100	12
Krieger et al. (1989)	269	Mean age >70 yrs, MV 71 hrs	NS	NS	92	21
Yang & Tobin (1989)	41	NS	76	25	61	40

MV, mechanical ventilation; NS, not stated. [a] Maximal inspiratory pressure <−30 cm H_2O, minute ventilation <10 L/min, and maximal voluntary ventilation ≥2 minute ventilation; [b] maximal inspiratory pressure <−30 cm H_2O and vital capacity ≥15 mL/kg.
Reproduced with permission from Stoller JK: Establishing clinical unweanability. *Respir Care* 1991; 36:186–198.

is not met could unduly delay weaning (*ie*, in up to 41% of patients using the maximal inspiratory force of <−30 cm H_2O as the criterion).

To improve the capability to predict weaning success and failure, a number of multivariate weaning predictors have been developed and evaluated.[2,3,5] As reviewed in Table 6,[2,6-16] these multivariate predictors vary in content from simple combinations of univariate predictors (*eg*, maximal minute ventilation > twice minute ventilation, maximal inspiratory force of <−30 cm H_2O, and minute ventilation of <10 L/min) to more complex scoring systems that assess dozens of clinical variables and provide an overall score that is used to predict weanability (*eg*, the Adverse Factor and Ventilator Score[7] and the Burns Weaning Assessment Program[13]). In general, these multivariate indices demonstrate higher positive and negative predictive values than the univariate predictors; they are, therefore, more useful and reliable predictors, although their general failure to achieve perfect predictive capability should cause the astute clinician to regard them with circumspection in completely assuring or excluding weanability.

As a specific example of a widely used multivariate weaning predictor, the rapid shallow breathing index (otherwise known as the frequency to tidal volume ratio [f/Vт]) calculates the patient's spontaneous breathing frequency divided by the patient's spontaneous tidal volume in liters, both determined with the patient who does not receive mechanical ventilatory assistance (*ie*, breathing through an endotracheal tube connected to a respirometer). As first proposed by Yang and Tobin,[10] an f/Vт value of <105 was found to best discriminate between patients who were successfully weaned (defined as maintaining spontaneous breathing for >24 hrs after extubation) and who were not successfully weaned. This threshold value was developed from a "hypothesis-generating" set of 36 patients and subsequently validated in a "hypothesis-testing" set of 64 patients, in whom an f/Vт of >105 had an overall negative predictive value (the chance that a patient would fail to wean if f/Vт exceeded 105) of 0.95 and a

Table 6. *Summary of Selected Multivariate Indices for Weaning Prediction*

Study (Date) (Ref)	N	Index	Patient Type	Positive Predictive	Negative Predictive
Hilberman et al. (1976) (6)	124	Nurse assessments	Open-heart surgery	82%	67%
Krieger et al. (1984) (4)	269	NIF <−30 cm H_2O, V_E >10 L/min	>70 yrs old, on MV mean 71 hrs	93%	15%
Morganroth et al. (1984) (7)	11	Adverse factor and vent score	COPD, on MV >30 days	73%	97%[a]
Higgins et al. (1988) (8)	29	Vent dependence score	Post-OHS on MV >48 hrs	NS	NS
Yang & Tobin (1989) (9)	41	CROP score	NS (abstract)	87%	72%
Yang & Tobin (1991) (10)	100	CROP >13, Freq/V_T <105	On MV 8.2 ± 1.1 days	711%	70%[b]
Jabour et al. (1991) (11)	38	Weaning index <4	MICU on MV <3 days	96%	95%
Ashutosh et al. (1991) (12)	24	Neural network discriminant function	On MV 12.7 days	100%[b]	100%[b]
Burns et al. (1991) (13)	37	BWAP	Stable on MV >1 wk, felt ready to wean	—	97%
Scheinhorn et al. (1995) (14)	565	$P(A-a)o_2$, BUN, gender	On MV >6 wks	71%	67%
Epstein (1995) (15)	184	Freq/V_T >100	MICU on MV, f/V_T measured within 8 hrs of wean onset	83%	40%
Gluck et al. (1995) (16)	55	Score (5 variables), points >3	On MV ≥3 wks	83%	100%

NIF, negative inspiratory force; MV, mechanical ventilator; V_E, minute ventilation; COPD, chronic pulmonary obstructive disease; OHS, open-heart surgery; NS, not stated; BWAP, Burns Weaning Assessment Program; BUN, blood urea nitrogen; MICU, medical intensive care unit; V_T, tidal volume.
[a] Hypothesis-generating study, not confirmed in a separate data set; [b] hypothesis-testing data set included.

positive predictive value of 0.78. In the subset of 20 patients who received mechanical ventilation for >8 days, the negative and positive predictive values were slightly lower (0.89 and 0.64, respectively), emphasizing the increased difficulty of establishing unweanability in long-term, mechanically ventilated patients. Subsequent studies[1,15] have largely confirmed the usefulness of the rapid shallow breathing index, while also emphasizing its shortcomings in predicting weaning outcome when nonrespiratory factors are at play (*eg*, congestive heart failure or upper airway obstruction as causes).

At the same time, Vallverdu et al[17] have emphasized that the diagnostic accuracy of different weaning parameters differs according to the underlying cause of respiratory failure. Specifically, in a series of 217 consecutive patients with respiratory failure of various etiologies, the rapid shallow breathing index demonstrated highest diagnostic accuracy in predicting weaning success in patients with chronic obstructive pulmonary disease (COPD) (0.76), but lower accuracy in patients with neurologic disease (0.65) or miscellaneous causes of acute respiratory failure (0.66). In contrast, values of maximal inspiratory pressure and maximal expiratory pressure best distinguished patients who were successfully intubated vs those patients who failed extubation when the cause of respiratory failure was neurologic disease. Overall, the recent evidence-based guidelines report[1] concludes that "judging by areas under the receiving operator curves for all variables, none of these variables demonstrate more than modest accuracy in predicting weaning outcome." The putative reason is that in available studies, clinicians making weaning decisions have already considered the results of weaning predictors when choosing patients for weaning.

Techniques of Weaning

A variety of techniques for weaning patients from mechanical ventilation has been described,[3,18–21] including T-piece trials of increasing duration that interrupt periods of completely supported breaths, intermittent mandatory ventilation (IMV) weaning in which the IMV rate is decreased progressively, pressure-support weaning in which the level of pressure support is decreased progressively, and combinations of the above (*eg*, pressure-support weaning with an IMV back-up rate). Strategies in use have changed as available ventilatory modes have evolved. For example, a survey of technical directors of respiratory care departments conducted by Venus et al[22] in 1987 indicated that IMV was the primary mode of weaning employed by 72% of the respondents. A survey of practices in 47 Spanish ICUs by Esteban et al.[19] showed that in 195 patients who were being weaned, T-piece trials of increasing duration were used most commonly (24%), followed by synchronized IMV weaning (18%), pressure-support weaning (15%), and combined pressure-support with an IMV back-up rate (9%). Other combinations applied concurrently or in succession were used in 33%. Finally, in a recent randomized trial[22] of daily observation of spontaneous (T-piece) breathing vs "routine" weaning practice, the most common routine weaning mode was pressure-support with IMV (43%), followed by IMV alone (31%), pressure-support alone (15%), continuous positive airway pressure (CPAP) (5%), and other (6%).

Recent attention has focused on comparing available techniques of weaning. Three important studies have provided important insights. Each of the weaning techniques is described below, followed by a summary of the evidence supporting specific techniques of weaning.

T-Piece Trials

Also known as Briggs trials, T-piece trials allow the patient to breathe spontaneously through the endotracheal tube (or tracheostomy) connected to a T-piece set-up. CPAP can be applied to the T-piece circuit, although PEEP levels >5 cm H_2O would be unlikely during weaning trials, because adequate oxygenation on acceptably low levels of PEEP is considered a criterion for beginning weaning.

Intermittent Mandatory Ventilation Weaning

IMV weaning was first proposed in 1973 as a new and preferred weaning strategy.[23] With IMV weaning, a volume and frequency of breaths are set, and the frequency is decreased gradually until the patient has assumed most of the minute ventilation.

Pressure Support Ventilation

Unlike IMV, which is a volume-cycled mode of mechanical ventilation, pressure support ventilation[24] delivers gas at a set pressure level for a duration determined by the patient's inspiratory flow demands (*ie*, flow-cycled). Pressure support weaning involves the gradual diminution of the pressure level, allowing the patient gradually to assume more of the work of breathing (WOB).

Studies Comparing Weaning Modes

Three controlled trials [18,21,25] have contributed important insights and comparisons of available weaning strategies. Brochard et al.[18] conducted a randomized, controlled trial in which 109 patients who failed initial weaning attempts were randomized to one of three weaning strategies: (a) T-piece trials, in which progressively increasing intervals of spontaneous breathing through a T-piece were undertaken until the patient tolerated up to three T-piece trials lasting 120 mins (n = 35 patients); (b) synchronized IMV weaning, in which the IMV rate was decreased by 2 to 4 breaths/min twice

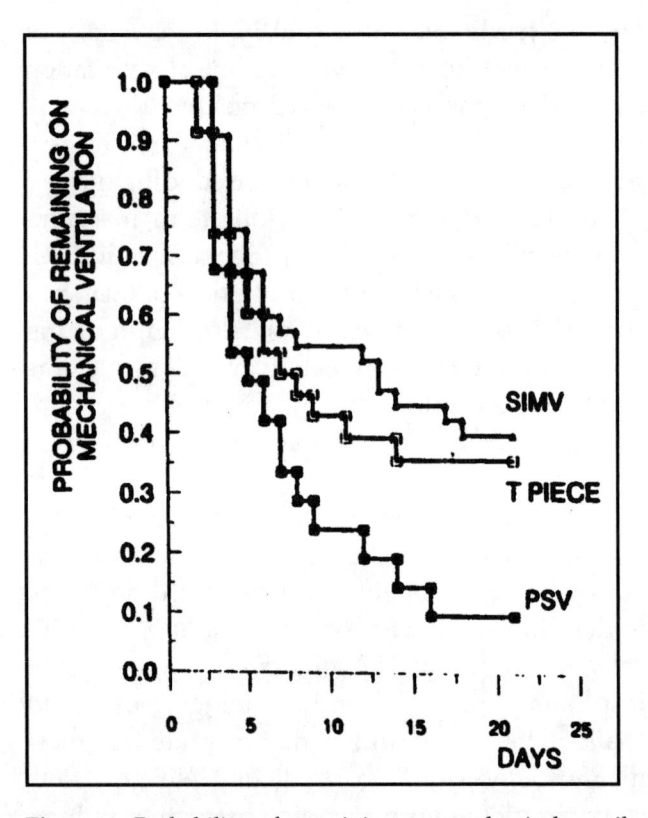

Figure 1. Probability of remaining on mechanical ventilation in patients with prolonged difficulties in tolerating spontaneous breathing. This probability was significantly lower for pressure-support ventilation (PSV) than for T-piece of synchronized intermittent ventilation (SIMV) (cumulative probability for 21 days, $p < 0.03$ with the log-rank test). Reproduced with permission from Brochard et al.[18]

daily, until the patient tolerated 24 hrs at an IMV rate of <4 (n = 43 patients); or (c) pressure-support weaning, in which the level of pressure was decreased by 2 or 4 cm H_2O twice daily until the patient could tolerate breathing at pressure-support of <8 cm H_2O for 24 hrs (n = 31 patients). The study concluded that pressure support was the preferred weaning mode (Figure 1) based on the following: (a) Fewer patients failed to wean with pressure-support than with the other modes (23% vs 43% [T-piece] and 42% [IMV], $p < 0.05$); (b) time-to-event analysis showed that the probability of requiring continued ventilatory support was lower with pressure support than with the other modes ($p = 0.03$); and (c) weaning duration was shorter with pressure support (mean 5.7 ± 3.7 days) than for the other modes pooled (mean 9.3 ± 8.2 days, $p < .05$).

In a second randomized trial of weaning modes, Esteban et al.[25] randomized 130 patients who had failed initial weaning attempts to one of four weaning modes: (a) IMV weaning, in which the rate was decreased by 2 to 4 breaths/min at least twice daily until the patient tolerated an IMV rate of <5 for 2 hrs (n = 29 patients); (b) pressure support weaning, in which the pressure was decreased by 2 to 4 cm H_2O at least twice daily until a pressure support level of 5 cm H_2O was tolerated for 2 hrs (n = 37 patients); (c) intermittent trials of spontaneous breathing, in which T-piece trials of increasing length were undertaken at least twice daily until the patient could tolerate 2 hrs of spontaneous breathing (n = 33 patients); and (d) once-daily T-piece trials, in which a single T-piece trial was undertaken daily until 2 hrs of spontaneous breathing were tolerated without distress (n = 31 patients). Unlike the study by Brochard et al,[18] this study concluded that a once-daily T-piece trial was the preferred strategy (Figure 2), based on the following findings: (a) The rate of successful weaning was higher with this technique than with IMV or pressure

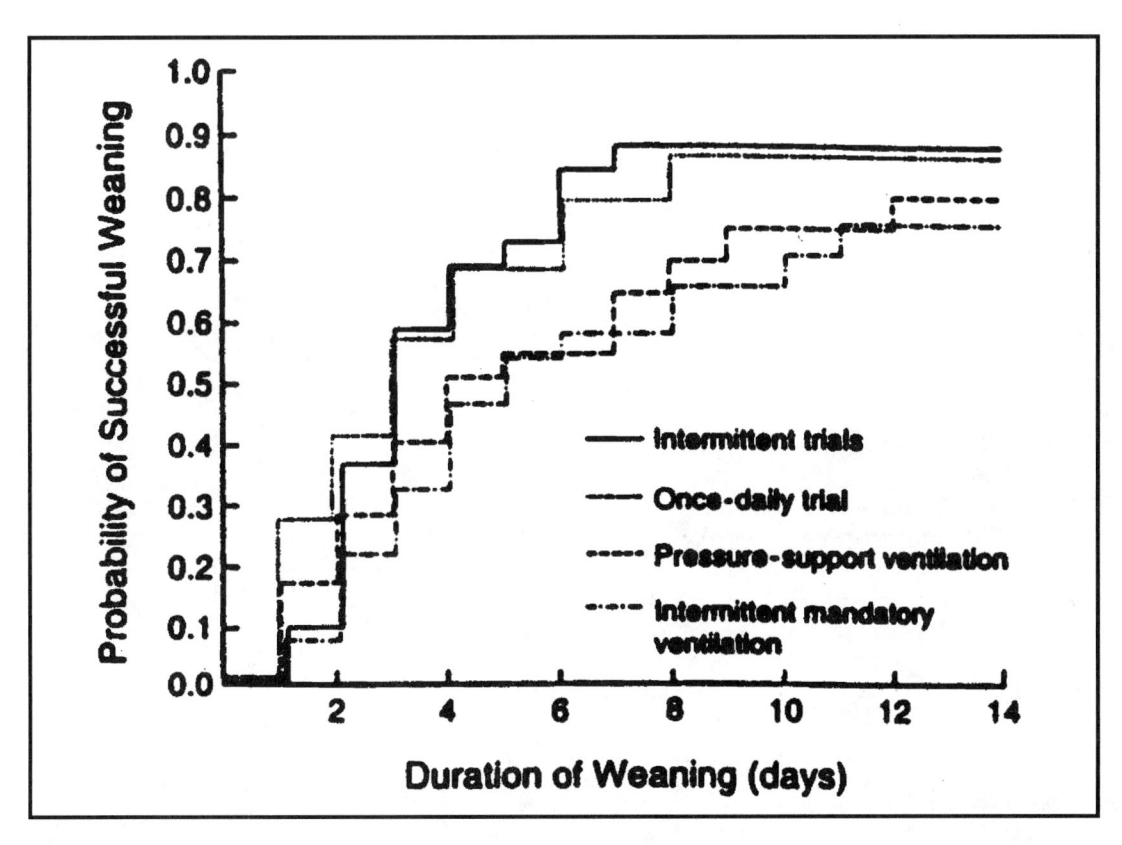

Figure 2. Kaplan-Meier curves of the probability of successful weaning with intermittent mandatory ventilation (IMV), pressure support ventilation (PSV), intermittent trials of spontaneous breathing (SB), and a once-daily trial of SB. After adjustment for baseline characteristics in a Cox proportional hazards model, the rate of successful weaning with a once-daily trial of SB was 2.83 times higher than that with IMV ($p < 0.006$) and 2.05 times higher than that with PSV ($p < 0.04$). Reproduced with permission from Esteban et al.[20]

support weaning; and (b) weaning was more rapid with once daily T-piece trials than with pressure support or IMV modes.

Finally, the most recent controlled trial of different weaning strategies by Ely et al[21] randomized patients to a once-daily respiratory assessment and trial of spontaneous breathing for up to 2 hrs with physician notification of a successful trial (n = 149 patients) versus usual care by the managing physicians (pulmonologist, cardiologist, or intensivist; n = 151 patients). As shown in Figure 3, this study shows that a strategy of conducting daily trials of spontaneous breathing is preferred because this approach was associated with shorter weaning time (median 1 vs 3 days, $p < 0.001$), shorter duration of mechanical ventilation (median 4.5 vs 6 days, $p < 0.003$), fewer total complications (20% vs 41%, $p < 0.001$), a lower rate of reintubation (4% vs 10%, $p = 0.04$), and lower ICU costs (median $15,740 vs $20,890, $p < 0.03$). Overall, these three studies show that contrary to early views and practices,[22] IMV weaning is the least likely to effect successful extubation and requires longer weaning than other available strategies, and that daily assessment of respiratory status and spontaneous breathing trials was associated with shorter weaning duration than usual practice. Attempts[26] to reconcile the discordant conclusions from the studies of Brochard et al and Esteban et al have attributed the differing results to differing definitions of weaning failure in the two studies (14 days on mechanical ventilation [Esteban et al] vs 21 days), and to different constraining conditions for attempting extubation with the compared weaning modes (ie, Brochard et al permitted extubation from 8 cm H_2O of pressure support vs 5 cm H_2O by Esteban et al and Brochard et al required IMV breathing on <4 breaths for 24 hrs before attempting extubation vs an IMV rate of <5 for 2 hrs by Esteban et al).

More recently, Esteban et al[27] examined whether a spontaneous breathing trial should last ≤2 hrs (ie, 30 mins) before extubation In a multicenter trial in which 526 patients were allocated randomly to 30- vs 120-min trials of spontaneous breathing, these investigators found no differences

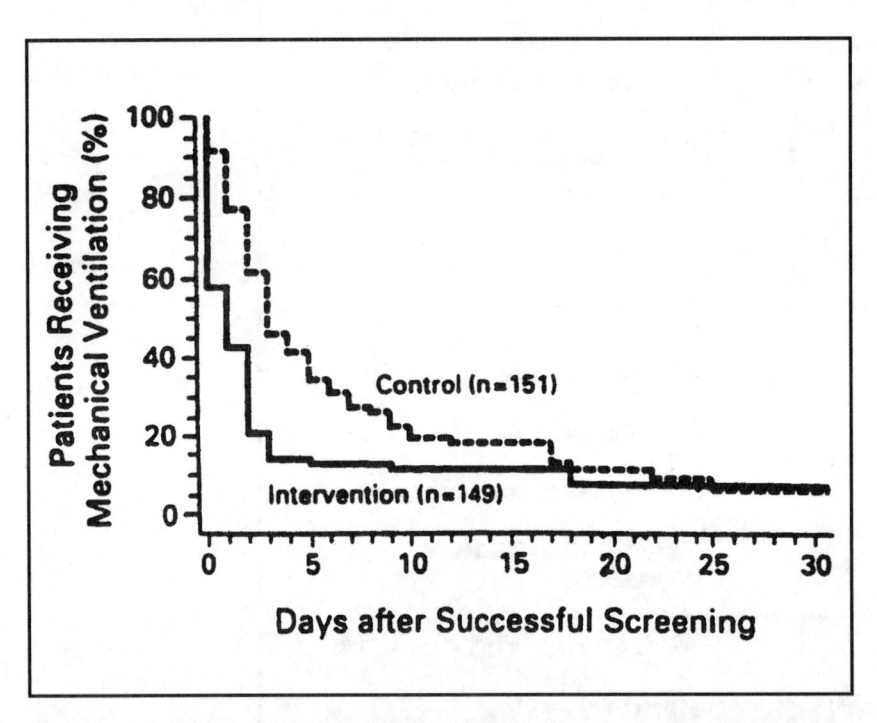

Figure 3. Kaplan-Meier analysis of the duration of mechanical ventilation after a successful screening test. After adjustment for the severity of illness at baseline (as measured by the APACHE II score), age, gender, race, location of the ICU, and duration of intubation before enrollment, a Cox proportional hazards analysis showed that mechanical ventilation was discontinued more rapidly in the intervention group than in the control group (relative risk of successful extubation, 2.13; 95% confidence interval, 1.55 to 2.92; $p < 0.001$). Reproduced with permission from Ely et al.[21]

between the two durations in rates of extubation failure or ICU or hospital mortality, but a longer length of hospital stay in the group undergoing a 2-hr trial. These findings, which have been confirmed by Perren et al,[28] endorse use of the shorter, 30-min period of spontaneous breathing before an extubation decision.

Finally, recent attention has turned to the value of noninvasive ventilation in accelerating extubation. Nava et al[29] conducted a randomized, controlled trial in which patients intubated because of acute ventilatory failure complicating COPD were randomized to a traditional pressure-support weaning approach versus a new strategy (in which patients were extubated after 48 hrs and managed thereafter with noninvasive ventilation). Patients managed with noninvasive ventilation experienced several advantages: (a) fewer days on mechanical ventilation; (b) fewer days in the ICU; (c) a higher weaning success rate on day 21; (d) a lower rate of nosocomial pneumonia; and (e) a higher survival rate at 60 days (92% vs 72%, $p = 0.0009$). These and other, more recent confirmatory results from Girault et al[30] suggest that early extubation with subsequent noninvasive ventilatory support may be a beneficial weaning strategy in patients with respiratory failure due to COPD.

Special Considerations in Weaning

To optimize the possibility of weaning, attention to several special considerations can be helpful in some clinical circumstances. These special considerations include: (a) the possibility of unsuspectedly high imposed WOB and the contribution of the endotracheal tube, (b) auto-PEEP as a source of increased inspiratory work in circumstances where dynamic hyperinflation accompanies airflow limitation, (c) occult cardiac ischemia as an impediment to weaning, (d) the importance of psychological readiness and motivation to wean, (e) the importance of routine daily cessation of sedative medications in patients receiving mechanical ventilation, and (f) the importance of implementing protocols by respiratory therapists and/or nurses to accelerate liberation from mechanical ventilation. Each of these special considerations is discussed below.

Work of Breathing and Role of the Endotracheal Tube

Measuring the inspiratory WOB by integrating the area under a pressure-volume curve has been advocated because elevated WOB predicts inspiratory muscle fatigue with subsequent weaning failure as an expected consequence. Various threshold values of WOB have been proposed (Table 7),[31-35] but few of these threshold values have been validated prospectively or compared head-to-head with other available weaning parameters. In a small, hypothesis-generating study of 17 patients, Fiastro et al[34] compared WOB with vital capacity, negative inspiratory force, tidal volume, and minute ventilation as weaning predictors and showed that as WOB values decreased <1.60 kg•m/min (16 joules/min), WOB better discriminated between patients with weaning success versus weaning failure than did the other more conventional measures. Until recently, the persisting uncertainty about a useful threshold value for WOB and the lack of methods for easy and widespread clinical measurement precluded adoption of WOB measurement for clinical practice outside of an investigative context. More recently, commercial devices that permit straightforward measurement of WOB have become available and have fostered enthusiasm

Table 7. *Proposed Work of Breathing (Transpulmonary) as a Weaning Predictor*

First Author (Date) (Ref)	No. of Patients	Threshold Value (kg • m/min)	Comment
Peters (1972) (31)	55	1.80	—
Proctor (1973) (32)	168	1.35	13.7% false-positive and false-negative rate with value
Henning (1977) (33)	28	1.70	—
Fiastro (1988) (34)	17	1.60	Better discriminator than vital capacity, tidal volume, minute ventilation, negative inspiratory force
Brochard (1989) (35)	8	0.8	—

for using WOB measurements in guiding weaning decisions. For example, Gluck et al[16] compared a weaning protocol using measurements of WOB and f/VT with a clinical approach using conventional weaning criteria (*eg*, minute ventilation, negative inspiratory force, tidal volume, and static compliance) in 23 ventilated patients. This study showed that the protocol incorporating WOB measurements would hasten weaning in at least 41% of instances and that the projected duration of weaning was shortened in these patients by 1.68 days.

Apart from appreciating the potential value of measuring WOB to enhance decision-making about weaning, clinicians should be attentive to sources of imposed WOB that can hamper weaning. That the endotracheal tube can contribute importantly to imposed WOB has been shown by Shapiro et al.[36] In a study of three normal volunteers breathing through endotracheal tubes of various caliber (6- to 10-mm inner diameter), these investigators showed that WOB rose precipitously as the caliber decreased and as minute ventilation rose. For subjects breathing through 6- and 7-mm inner diameter tubes at levels of minute ventilation routinely achieved clinically (15 to 25 L/min), the tension-time index approached values of 0.15 at which respiratory muscle fatigue is expected. Thus, use of larger caliber (*ie*, >7.5-mm inner diameter) endotracheal tubes and avoidance of nasotracheal intubation in patients experiencing weaning difficulty are advised. More recently, WOB measurements have been shown to be useful in helping to identify patients whose weaning difficulty is attributable to unsuspectedly high imposed WOB.[37] From a group of 116 surgical ICU patients on mechanical ventilation for >48 hrs, Kirton et al[37] identified 28 patients (24%) with oral endotracheal tubes of >8-mm inner diameter who developed marked tachypnea during a CPAP trial despite satisfying simple weaning criteria. WOB measurements in these 28 patients were performed and included a measurement of the work imposed by the endotracheal tube. Using a value of <0.8 joules/L as a WOB threshold, the investigators identified six patients with total WOB below this value, all of whom were successfully extubated. Of the remaining 22 patients whose total WOB measurements exceeded this threshold (mean WOB 1.6 ± 0.83 joules/L), 21 patients were found to have a major component of their total WOB imposed by the endotracheal tube, leaving their "physiologic" work of breathing below the threshold value. Extubation was successfully undertaken in all 21 (with subsequent reintubation for unrelated and unpredictable reasons in two patients), leading to the conclusion that high imposed WOB can unsuspectedly contribute to weaning failure and that WOB measurements directed at identifying the components of "imposed" and "physiologic" WOB can enhance decision-making in a subset of difficult-to-wean patients.

Auto-PEEP as a Source of Imposed Work of Breathing

Auto-PEEP is defined as PEEP that is present in the alveoli but not measured at the mouthpiece without special maneuvers,[38] *eg*, an end-expiratory hold. Synonyms for auto-PEEP include intrinsic PEEP, occult PEEP, endogenous PEEP, and unidentified PEEP. As shown by Brown and Pierson,[38] auto-PEEP occurs commonly among mechanically ventilated patients (39% of 62 patients assessed) and may produce high alveolar pressures at end-expiration (*ie*, up to 15 cm H_2O). Three varieties of auto-PEEP can be considered,[39] each of which may occur under distinct physiologic circumstances even though several types may coexist. The first type is auto-PEEP with dynamic hyperinflation and airflow limitation, which commonly accompanies COPD, both in spontaneously breathing and mechanically ventilated patients. Other types include auto-PEEP with dynamic hyperinflation but no airflow limitation (*eg*, during high minute ventilation or with a small endotracheal tube that hampers lung emptying) and auto-PEEP without dynamic hyperinflation (*eg*, due to expiratory muscle recruitment).

In considering weaning, the first type of auto-PEEP—auto-PEEP with dynamic hyperinflation and air flow limitation—is most significant because such auto-PEEP imposes an inspiratory threshold load that must be overcome by the inspiratory muscles before inspiration can begin.[38,40,41] Such auto-PEEP arises when lung emptying is impaired due to expiratory airflow resistance and expiratory flow limitation; end-expiratory lung volume then exceeds resting functional residual capacity; air is trapped at end-expiration and alveolar pressure exceeds downstream pressure (at the mouth) with resulting auto-PEEP. By imposing an inspiratory load, such auto-PEEP can be the source of imposed WOB. As shown by Petrof et al[40] and Smith and Marini,[41] application of external PEEP can decrease the inspiratory WOB by offsetting the inspiratory load imposed by the auto-PEEP. Levels of external PEEP, up to ~85% of the auto-PEEP, can lessen imposed WOB without increasing end-expiratory lung volume or lessening cardiac output. On this basis, clinicians should be attentive to the possibility of auto-PEEP in managing patients on mechanical ventilation. If found in a clinical circumstance favoring dynamic hyperinflation with airflow limitation (*ie*, in patients with COPD), careful application of external PEEP to levels not exceeding the level of auto-PEEP may be helpful to lessen imposed WOB and enhance weaning.

Other Special Considerations in Weaning

Besides giving attention to WOB imposed by the endotracheal tube and by auto-PEEP, clinicians should appreciate other potential impediments to weaning, including unsuspected cardiac ischemia,[42] the patient's anxiety and lack of psychologic readiness to wean,[43] and the lack of a systematic weaning routine in the ICU. Recent studies suggest that weaning can be accelerated by detection and treatment of cardiac ischemia, by providing biofeedback to lessen anxiety and to assure ventilatory targets, and by implementing a team to conduct regular weaning[44] and/or weaning protocols supervised by respiratory therapists and nurses,[45,46] at least in adults. Two recent studies[47,48] have examined the impact of implementing processes and protocols hospital-wide to enhance weaning outcomes. Specifically, Smyrnios et al showed that formation of a multidisciplinary weaning team to help supervise weaning throughout an academic medical center was associated with accelerated liberation from mechanical ventilation and shorter ICU and hospital length of stay.[47] More recently, Burns et al[48] instituted unit-specific outcomes managers to assure protocol adherence and showed that benefits after implementation included shorter duration of mechanical ventilation (mean 12 vs 14 days, $p < 0.0001$), shorter ICU length of stay (mean 16 vs 22 days, $p < 0.0008$), shorter hospital length of stay (mean 25 vs 30 days, $p < 0.0001$), and lower hospital mortality (31% vs 38%, $p = 0.02$).

In contrast to the results from several randomized trials in adults in which protocols implemented by respiratory therapists and/or nurses were associated with accelerated liberation from mechanical ventilation,[45,46] results from a recent trial in mechanically ventilated children (<18 years of age) failed to show that protocols shortened the duration of ventilator dependence.[49] While the precise reason for discordance with the results of the adult trials remains uncertain, it is possible that the already short duration of mechanical ventilation in control pediatric patients (median 2 days) makes it difficult to show significant acceleration of weaning.

Other interventions found to accelerate weaning were use of a collaborative, multidisciplinary weaning approach using a bedside weaning board and flow sheet[50] and respiratory therapists' using a handheld computer on which a weaning protocols is programmed.[51] The former intervention has been associated with a shortened ICU length of stay and a trend toward shortened time on mechanical ventilation in adults. Regarding the second,[51] compared with using a weaning protocol on paper, respiratory therapists' using a handheld computer with a weaning protocol was associated with a shorter time to beginning a weaning trial (mean 49.9 vs 72.5 hours, $p = 0.018$) and had a shorter ICU length of stay (mean 6.2 vs 7.7 days, $p = 0.018$). Finally, a recent randomized controlled trial has shown that daily interruption of sedative medications to reassess neurologic status and weaning readiness in adults is associated with a shortened duration of mechanical ventilation.[52]

Annotated References

1. The collective task force facilitated by the American College of Chest Physicians; the American Association for Respiratory Care, and the American College of Critical Care Medicine. Evidence-based guidelines for weaning and discontinuing ventilatory support. Chest 2001; 120(Suppl): 375S–484S
   This supplement presents a systematic review of available literature and recommendations.

2. Stoller JK. Establishing clinical unweanability. Respir Care 1991; 36:186–198
   This comprehensive review paper considers the diagnostic performance of various weaning predictors and considers whether predictors perform sufficiently well to assure weaning failure.
3. Lessard MR, Brochard LJ. Weaning from ventilatory support. Clin Chest Med 1996; 17:475–489
   This is an excellent recent review of weaning principles and techniques.
4. Krieger BP, Ershowsky PF, Becker DA, et al. Evaluation of conventional criteria for predicting successful weaning from mechanical ventilatory support in elderly patients. Crit Care Med 1989; 17:858–861
5. Tobin MJ, Yang K. Weaning from mechanical ventilation. Crit Care Clin 1990; 6:725–747
6. Hilberman M, Kamm B, Lamy M, et al. An analysis of potential physiological predictors of respiratory adequacy following cardiac surgery. J Thorac Cardiovasc Surg 1976; 71:711–720
7. Morganroth ML, Morganroth JL, Nett LM, et al. Criteria for weaning from prolonged mechanical ventilation. Arch Intern Med 1984; 144:1012–1016
8. Higgins TL, Kraenzler EJ, Blum JM. Evaluation of criteria for discontinuing mechanical ventilation following open heart surgery. Abstr. Chest 1988; 94(Suppl 1):40S
9. Yang KL, Tobin MJ. Decision analysis of parameters used to predict outcome of a trial of weaning from mechanical ventilation. Abstr. Am Rev Respir Dis 1989; 139:A98
10. Yang KL, Tobin MJ. A prospective study of indexes predicting the outcome of trials of weaning from mechanical ventilation. N Engl J Med 1991; 324:1445–1450
    This study reports the diagnostic performance of various indices of weaning in 100 patients who were clinically stable and deemed ready for a weaning trial. The frequency to tidal volume ratio (f/V_t) was found to be most discriminative, with values exceeding 105, indicating rapid shallow breathing and predicting weaning failure.
11. Jabour ER, Rabil DM, Truwit JD, et al. Evaluation of a new weaning index based on ventilatory endurance and the efficiency of gas exchange. Am Rev Respir Dis 1991; 144:531–537
12. Ashutosh K, Lee H, Mohan C, et al. Prediction criteria for successful weaning from respiratory support: Statistical and connectionist analyses. Crit Care Med 1992; 20:1295–1301
13. Burns SM, Fahey SA, Barton DM, et al. Weaning from mechanical ventilation: A method for assessment and planning. AACN Clin Issues Crit Care Nurs 1991; 2:372–389
14. Scheinhorn D, Hassenpflug, Artinian BM, et al. Predictors of weaning after six weeks of mechanical ventilation. Chest 1995; 107:500–505
15. Epstein SK. Etiology of extubation failure and the predictive value of the rapid shallow breathing index. Am J Respir Crit Care Med 1995; 152:545–549
16. Gluck EH, Barkoviak MJ, Balk RA, et al. Medical effectiveness of esophageal balloon pressure manometry in weaning patients from mechanical ventilation. Crit Care Med 1995; 23:504–509
17. Vallverdu I, Calaf N, Subirana M, et al. Clinical characteristics respiratory functional parameters, and outcomes of a two-hour T-piece trial in patients weaning from mechanical ventilation. Am J Respir Crit Care Med 1998; 158:1855–1862
18. Brochard L, Rauss A, Benito S, et al. Comparison of three methods of gradual withdrawal from ventilatory support during weaning from mechanical ventilation. Am J Respir Crit Care Med 1994; 150:896–903
19. Esteban A, Alia I, Ibanez J, et al. Modes of mechanical ventilation and weaning: A national survey of Spanish hospitals. Chest 1994; 106:1188–1193
    This study reports a survey of 47 Spanish intensive care units in which 195 patients were weaning. T-piece trials were the most common weaning mode used (24%), followed by synchronized intermittent mandatory ventilation(18%), and pressure-support (15%), with other combinations in the remainder.
20. Esteban A, Frutos F, Tobin MJ, et al. A comparison of four methods of weaning patients from mechanical ventilation. N Engl J Med 1995; 332:345–350
    This is one of the three recent, randomized, controlled trials of various strategies for weaning. The study concludes that once-daily trials of spontaneous breathing is preferred to intermittent mandatory ventilation and slightly better than pressure-support weaning.
21. Ely EW, Baker AM, Dunagan DP, et al. Effect on the duration of mechanical ventilation of identifying patients capable of breathing spontaneously. N Engl J Med 1996; 335:1864–1869
    This is a recently published, randomized, controlled trial of weaning strategies and shows that daily trials of spontaneous breathing with reporting of results to managing clinicians can accelerate weaning compared with standard practice.

22. Venus B, Smith RA, Mathru M. National survey of methods and criteria used for weaning from mechanical ventilation. Crit Care Med 1987; 15:530–533
23. Downs JB, Klein EF, Desautels D, et al. Intermittent mandatory ventilation: A new approach to weaning patients from mechanical ventilation. Chest 1973; 64:331–335

   This is one of the original descriptions of intermittent mandatory ventilation.
24. MacIntyre NR. Respiratory function during pressure support ventilation. Chest 1986; 89:677–682
25. Esteban A, Frutos F, Tobin MJ, et al. A comparison of four methods of weaning patients from mechanical ventilation. N Engl J Med 1995; 332:345–350

   This is one of the three recent randomized trials of weaning strategies. The investigators conclude that once-daily trials of spontaneous breathing is the preferred mode of weaning.
26. Tobin MJ. Problematic weaning. In: Critical Care Medicine: A Concise Review. Northbrook, IL, ACCP, 1995, pp 202–206
27. Esteban A, Alia I, Tobin MJ, et al. Effect of spontaneous breathing trial duration on outcome of attempts to discontinue mechanical ventilation. Am J Respir Crit Care Med 1999; 159:512–518
28. Perren A, Domenighetti G, Mauri S, et al. Protocol-directed weaning from mechanical ventilation: Clinical outcome in patients randomized for a 30-min or 120-min trial with pressure support ventilation. Intens Care Med 2002; 28: 1058-1063
29. Nava S, Ambrosino N, Clini E, et al. Non-invasive mechanical ventilation in the weaning of patients with respiratory failure due to chronic obstructive pulmonary disease. Ann Intern Med 1998; 128: 721–728
30. Girault C, Daudenthum I, Chevron V, et al. Non-invasive ventilation as a systematic extubation and weaning technique in acute-on-chronic respiratory failure: A prospective, randomized controlled study. Am J Respir Crit Care Med 1999; 160: 86-92
31. Peters RM, Hilberman M, Hogan JS, et al. Objective indications for respiratory therapy in post-trauma and postoperative patients. Am J Surg 1972; 124:262–269
32. Proctor HJ, Woolson R. Prediction of respiratory muscle fatigue by measurements of the work of breathing. Surg Gynecol Obstet 1973; 136:367–370
33. Henning RJ, Shubin H, Weil MH. The measurement of the work of breathing for the clinical assessment of ventilator dependence. Crit Care Med 1977; 5:264–268
34. Fiastro JF, Habib MP, Shon BY, et al. Comparison of standard weaning parameters and the mechanical work of breathing in mechanically ventilated patients. Chest 1988; 94:232–238
35. Brochard L, Harf A, Lorino H, et al. Inspiratory pressure support prevents diaphragmatic fatigue during weaning from mechanical ventilation. Am Rev Respir Dis 1989; 139:513–521
36. Shapiro M, Wilson RK, Cesar G, et al. Work of breathing through different sized endotracheal tubes. Crit Care Med 1986; 14:1028–1031
37. Kirton OC, DeHaven CB, Morgan JP, et al. Elevated imposed work of breathing masquerading as ventilator weaning intolerance. Chest 1995; 108:1021–1025
38. Ranieri VM, Grasso S, Fiore T, et al. Auto-positive end-expiratory pressure and dynamic hyperinflation. Clin Chest Med 1996; 17:379–394
39. Brown DG, Pierson DJ. Auto-PEEP is common in mechanically ventilated patients: A study of incidence, severity, and detection. Respir Care 1986; 31:1069–1074
40. Petrof BJ, Legaré M, Goldberg P, et al. Continuous positive airway pressure reduces work of breathing and dyspnea during weaning from mechanical ventilation in severe chronic obstructive pulmonary disease. Am Rev Respir Dis 1990; 141:281–289
41. Smith TC, Marini JJ. Impact of PEEP on lung mechanics and work of breathing in severe airflow obstruction. J Appl Physiol 1988; 65:1488–1499
42. Chatila W, Ani S, Guaglianone D, et al. Cardiac ischemia during weaning from mechanical ventilation. Chest 1996; 109:1577–1583
43. Holliday JE, Hyers TM. The reduction of weaning time from mechanical ventilation using tidal volume and relaxation biofeedback. Am Rev Respir Dis 1990; 141:1214–1220

   This paper describes a randomized, controlled trial showing that formal biofeedback (i.e., by providing feedback on tidal volume and on relaxation [with an electromyogram of the frontalis muscle]) was associated with a shortened duration of mechanical ventilation compared with usual visits and reassurance.
44. Cohen IL, Bari N, Strosberg MA, et al. Reduction of duration and cost of mechanical ventilation in an intensive care unit by use of a ventilatory management team. Crit Care Med 1991; 19:1278–1284
45. Kollef MH, Shapiro SD, Silver P, et al. A randomized controlled trial of protocol-directed versus

physician-directed weaning from mechanical ventilation. Crit Care Med 1997; 25:567–574

46. Marelich GP, Murin S, Battistella F, et al. Protocol weaning of mechanical ventilation in medical and surgical patients by respiratory care practitioners and nurses: Effect on weaning time and incidence of ventilator-associated pneumonia. Chest 2000; 118:459–467

47. Smyrnios NA, Connolly A, Wilson MM, et al. Effects of a multifaceted, multidisciplinary, hospital-wide quality improvement program on weaning from mechanical ventilation. Crit Care Med 2002; 30: 1224–1230

48. Burns SM, Earven S, Fisher C, et al. Implementation of an instiutional program to improve clinical and financial outcomes of mechanically ventilated patients: One-year outcomes and lessons learned. Crit Care Med 2003; 31: 2752–2763

49. Randolph AG, Wypij D, Venkataram ST, et al. Effect of mechanical ventilator weaning protocols on respiratory outcomes in infants and children: A randomized controlled trial. JAMA 2002; 288: 2561–2568

This paper describes a randomized controlled trial in which, unlike the findings in several available trials in adults, the use of weaning protocols in children did not accelerate liberation from mechanical ventilation.

50. Hennemann E, Dracup K, Ganz T, et al. Effect of a collaborative weaning plan on patient outcome in the critical care setting. Crit Care Med 2001; 29: 297–303

51. Iregui M, Ward S, Clinikscale D, et al. Use of a hand-held computer by respiratory care practitioners to improve the efficiency of weaning patients from mechanical ventilation. Crit Care Med 2002; 30: 2038–2043

50. Kress JP, Pohlman AS, O'Connor MF, et al. Daily interruption of sedative infusions in critically ill patients undergoing mechanical ventilation. N Engl J Med 2000; 342: 1471–1477

Notes

Notes

Trauma and Thermal Injury

David J. Dries, MSE, MD, FCCP

Objectives:

- To identify the multisystem manifestations of trauma
- To recognize common patterns of presentation for cardiopulmonary injury
- To recognize evolving management of secondary brain injury
- To identify patients at high risk for venous thromboembolism following injury
- To recognize burn injury of various degrees and associated treatment options
- To assess and manage inhalation injury
- To review the latest available data regarding the outcome of burn injury

Key words: blunt cardiac injury; duplex ultrasonography; hemothorax; inhalation injury; low-molecular-weight heparin; pneumothorax; secondary brain injury; venous thromboembolism

Trauma

Principal decision-making in the management of multiple organ injury rests with the trauma surgeon. The intensivist, however, is a critical component of the management team, particularly in the setting of blunt injury with multiple system dysfunction and less need for acute operative intervention. Certain types of injury have implications for all members of the trauma care team, both Emergency Department management and critical care support. All team members should, therefore, be able to identify and act immediately upon identification of injury and complications of initial treatment. The international process for injury identification and treatment is discussed in the *Advanced Trauma Life Support Course* published by the American College of Surgeons Committee on Trauma.

This chapter reviews recent developments and discusses common patterns of injury or complications of injury according to organ system.

Airway and Spine

The initial priority in the management of any injured patient is assessment and management of the airway. At the same time, care is taken to prevent movement of the cervical spine. All patients with blunt trauma are at risk for cervical spine injury. Patients with unknown cervical spine status and need of emergency airway control may be intubated safely by temporary removal of the immobilizing the cervical collar, while inline stabilization is maintained during intubation. After securing the airway, the collar is reapplied and the patient remains on log roll precautions until the complete spine status has been assessed. The choice of nasotracheal vs orotracheal intubation technique is based on provider preference and experience. Nasotracheal intubation, however, requires spontaneous respiration. In addition, no tubes should be passed through the nose of a patient who has midfacial trauma with a risk of cribriform plate fracture. When other means of airway control have failed, a surgical airway may be required.

Neurologic examination alone does not exclude a cervical spine injury. The integrity of the bony components of the cervical spine may be assessed in various ways. A variety of plain radiographs, CT scans, or MRI scans may be obtained. The following patients are excluded from examination: (1) those who cannot relate neurologic examination changes; (2) those who are unresponsive due to either primary injury or the effects of pain medication; and (3) those who receive muscle relaxants. Thus, recommendations were developed to determine the presence or absence of cervical spine instability.

The following recommendations were made for patients at risk for cervical spine injury:

- Patients who are alert, awake, and without mental status changes and neck pain and who have no distracting injuries or neurologic deficits may be considered to have a stable cervical spine and need no radiologic studies.
- All other patients should have at least a lateral view of the cervical spine, including the base of the occiput to the upper border of the first

thoracic vertebra; and anteroposterior view showing the spinous processes of the second cervical through the first thoracic vertebra; and an open mouth odontoid view indicating lateral masses of the first cervical vertebra and the entire odontoid process. Axial CT scans with sagittal reconstruction may be obtained for any questionable level of injury or any area which cannot be adequately visualized on plain radiographs.

- Flexion and extension views of the cervical spine may be appropriate in patients complaining of significant neck pain with normal plain radiograph results.
- Patients with neurologic deficits which may refer to a cervical spine injury require subspecialty consultation and MRI evaluation. MRI may also facilitate clearance of ligamentous injury.
- Patients with an altered level of consciousness secondary to traumatic brain injury or other causes may be considered to have a stable cervical spine if adequate three-view plain radiographs and thin-cut axial CT images through C1 and C2 are normal.
- Most recent work suggest that CT scans may facilitate evaluation of the cervical spine in any head-injured or intubated patient. More and more centers are adding CT scans of the cervical spine when scans of the head are obtained after injury.

Cervical spine injury following blunt trauma reportedly occurs at a frequency of 4 to 6%. In the literature of cervical spine injury, there is little supporting evidence that defines the criteria for determining who gets cervical spine radiographs and who does not. Long-term follow-up to identify all cases of cervical spine injury missed in the acute setting is frequently unavailable. The true incidence of cervical spine injury is thus not known. The three-view plain spine series (anteroposterior, lateral, and open mouth odontoid view), supplemented by thin-cut axial CT imaging with sagittal reconstruction through suspicious areas or in adequately visualized areas, provides a false-negative rate of <0.1%, if the studies are technically adequate and properly interpreted.

The lessons of cervical spine evaluation have also been applied to injuries to the thoracic and lumbar regions. While plain films in the majority of patients are adequate to screen in individuals with high-risk mechanisms, helical CT allows reconstruction of the thoracic and lumbar spine from various views. This information can be obtained in patients receiving chest and abdominal CT scanning protocols for other visceral injuries. A dedicated spine CT examination is no longer required. In our center, adjacent spine reconstructions are obtained in any patient receiving torso scans as a part of evaluation for injury. When the use of helical CT was compared to conventional radiographs of the thoracic and lumbar spine, improved sensitivity and specificity were obtained.

Tracheobronchial Injury

Tracheal or laryngeal disruption or fracture most commonly occurs at the junction of the larynx and the trachea. Signs and symptoms may include hoarseness, subcutaneous air, edema, or crepitus at the neck, but the patient may have minimal evidence of injury. The patient should be allowed to assume the position of comfort; this position may include sitting, if spinal injury is unlikely during the patient's initial assessment. Airway management by an experienced physician may include an awake tracheostomy. Cricothyroidotomy should be avoided.

Injury to the proximal trachea may be caused by blunt or penetrating trauma. Blunt injury to the cervical trachea occurs in <1% in all patients with blunt trauma to the trunk. Injury to the larynx is the most common blunt injury. A direct blow to the trachea may cause compression or fracture of the cartilaginous ring, hematoma formation, bleeding, or airway obstruction. Injury to the trachea may also occur from the shoulder restraint harness of a seat belt. Proximal tracheal injuries may be caused by gunshot wounds or stab wounds to the neck. Hemoptysis and airway obstruction are signs that indicate the need for urgent access to the airway. Patients with subcutaneous air or dissecting air within the cervical fascia should be suspected for tracheal and/or esophageal injury.

Patients presenting with massive subcutaneous or mediastinal emphysema are suspected to have a distal tracheal or bronchus injury. Hemoptysis, hemopneumothorax or a collapsed lung on plain chest radiograph confirms injury in the major intrathoracic airways. When chest tubes are placed and there is constant air loss, major airway disruption must be suspected. In this situation, bronchoscopy should be done as soon as possible to exclude a tracheal or large bronchial tear or proximal bronchial obstruction by a foreign body or secretions. Over 80% of traumatic tracheobronchial tears occur within 2.5 cm of the carina; lobar or segmental bronchi are seldom injured. Injury to the distal trachea is associated with severe compression trauma to the chest, particularly when the glottis is closed.

Airway control and ventilation may be difficult in these patients. A double lumen endotracheal tube may be required. Placement of these tubes requires skill and secretion management may be difficult. Surgical repair must be prioritized. If an airway can be established and maintained, other life-threatening problems, such as intraabdominal hemorrhage, may be addressed. Repair of distal tracheal or bronchial injuries typically requires a thoracotomy. Postoperative management of these patients has several components. Repeat bronchoscopy may be required for secretion control. Mechanical ventilation should be provided to minimize the pressure within the airways. Use of pressure control modes of ventilation may be optimal.

Intrabronchial bleeding, manifest as hemoptysis and air hunger, is poorly tolerated and may lead rapidly to death due to alveolar flooding. Bleeding is typically caused by injury to bronchial arteries or fistulas between pulmonary veins, pulmonary arterial branches, and the bronchus. These patients may rapidly become hypoxic before other evidence of respiratory failure is apparent. In general, these patients should be positioned to facilitate drainage of blood out of the trachea. The uninvolved lung must be free of blood, if possible. Nasotracheal suctioning or bronchoscopy may be necessary to keep the bronchial tree clear and the contralateral lung expanded. For severe bleeding, a double lumen endotracheal tube may be inserted to confine the bleeding and protect the uninvolved lung. Where severe bleeding continues, thoracotomy should be performed with clamping of the involved bronchus at the hilum.

Recognizing the paucity of literature on tracheobronchial injuries, Richardson reviewed a single institution experienced with a single lead surgeon in the management of tracheobronchial injuries. He divided injuries into those involving the larynx and trachea and those involving the mainstem bronchus. In all, 60 patients were treated from 1976 to 2001 for blunt and penetrating injuries. Six injuries involved the larynx and trachea while 27 tracheal wounds and 27 injuries to the mainstem bronchus were identified. Only one of six laryngotracheal wounds had a good result. One patient required tracheal resection and other required permanent tracheostomy. Of tracheal injuries, patients surviving tracheal resection and end-to-end anastomosis had good outcomes. Two granuloma complications were caused by use of permanent suture. One patient treated by a primary tracheal repair developed stenosis requiring resection. Of patients with injuries to the mainstem bronchus, 14 pneumonectomies were performed with eight survivors. Three of these patients developed stump leaks with empyema and three of these individuals had cor pulmonale on follow-up. Ten patients had repair of blunt mainstem bronchial injuries; in two cases, bronchial stenosis required pneumonectomy. Clearly, these patients frequently have suboptimal outcome. Where end-to-end tracheal repairs can be created and direct repair of mainstem bronchus injuries provided, improved outcome can be anticipated.

Rib and Pulmonary Parenchymal Injury

Rib fractures are frequently not detected on chest radiographs; the fracture may be documented by tenderness on physical examination. Pain control is essential for assuring adequate spontaneous ventilation. Where multiple adjacent rib segments are fractured, a flail chest may occur. The clinical manifestation of flail chest is paradoxical movement of the involved portion of the chest wall, ie, inward movement of the segments during inhalation. Frequently, flail chest is associated with contusion of the underlying lung, pain, and hypoxemia. Less common is pneumothorax associated with an open thoracic wound. Open pneumothorax is generally associated with soft tissue deficit requiring dressings or closure and chest tube placement to reexpand the involved lung. Another complication of rib injury is hemothorax. Massive hemothorax is suggested by physical examination and the chest radiograph.

Rapid loss of 1000 to 2000 mL of blood or ongoing blood loss of >200 mL/h through a chest tube is an indication for thoracotomy. In general, pneumothorax is associated with rib fractures and requires chest tube placement. Suction is applied routinely at approximately 20 cm H_2O. Any patient with a pneumothorax who requires a general anesthetic should have a chest tube in place. Perhaps the most feared complication of rib fracture is tension pneumothorax. Air is under pressure in the pleural space resulting hemodynamic embarrassment and pulmonary dysfunction. This emergency should not be diagnosed by a chest radiograph. This clinical diagnosis is based on absent breath sounds, respiratory distress, jugular venous distention, and cardiovascular compromise. The trachea may deviate away from the side, requiring tube thoracostomy. Needle catheter placement into the pleural space at the second intercostal level in the midclavicular line may be necessary for urgent decompression of the involved hemithorax.

A common result of rib and chest wall injury is pulmonary contusion. Patients with penetrating trauma may have areas of hemorrhage surrounding a missile tract. The patient sustaining pulmonary contusion from blunt trauma may have a more globular or diffuse pattern of injury. Pulmonary contusion is usually diagnosed on the basis of the history of blunt chest trauma and findings of localized opacification on chest radiographs. The extent of pulmonary contusion is usually underestimated on plain film radiographs. CT scans evaluate and quantify pulmonary contusions. A scan demonstrating a large contusion (>20%) increases the likelihood of prolonged ventilatory support for acute respiratory failure.

CT may also be useful in confirming the diagnosis of pulmonary contusion. One third of pulmonary contusions do not manifest on plain radiographs until 12 to 24 hours after injury. More frequently than previously noted, CT scans have also demonstrated traumatic pneumatocele and parenchymal lacerations to the lung. Hypoxia may be the first evidence of severe pulmonary contusion. If the contusion is large enough or is bilateral, a significant decrease in lung compliance may also occur with associated increase in shunt fraction. The overall mortality rate of patients with pulmonary contusion is 15 to 16%. When chest wall injury is associated with this problem, particularly flail chest, the mortality rate approaches 45%.

Treatment is directed primarily at maintaining ventilation and preventing pneumonia. Progressive respiratory therapy to promote deep breathing, coughing, and mobilization is critical. Pain relief is essential for chest wall injuries. To this end, epidural analgesia is superior to intrapleural medication administration or rib blocks. The patient should be euvolemic, not dehydrated. Mechanical ventilation may be required in the hypoxic patient. This therapy may also be necessary in the patient with shock, increased work of breathing, coma, or significant preexisting lung disease.

An intriguing clinical series from the University of Oregon Health and Science University describes use of absorbable prostheses for rib fracture fixation in ten patients. These individuals underwent rib fracture fixation with absorbable plates and screws. Indications included flail chest with failure to wean (five patients), acute pain with rib instability (four patients) and a significant chest wall defect. All patients with flail chest weaned successfully from mechanical ventilation. Patients with pain and instability reported subjective improvement or resolution of symptoms. The patient with a chest wall defect returned to full athletic activity within six months. Muscle sparing incisions were used and thoracoscopic assistance was employed in three cases. Two patients with screw fixation only developed loss of rib fracture reduction and one patient developed a wound infection. Given the frequency of rib fractures and the morbidity associated with this problem, absorbable plates are an option which warrants further evaluation for rib fracture repair in selected patients. This technique may be enhanced with further refinements in minimally invasive surgical methods.

ICU Resuscitation

Patients sustaining major trauma without brain injury surviving the first six hours after injury are at risk for multiple organ failure. A statistical model suggests that age, injury severity score and severity of shock are independent risk factors for this complication. The University of Texas Houston, Houston Medical School, has developed a shock resuscitation protocol applied to major torso trauma patients at known risk for multiple organ failure (Fig 1). This standardized process employs much of the contemporary thinking regarding protocol-driven resuscitation and comes from a group with an extensive database in this area.

Patients likely to require this resuscitation were those with injuries including two or more abdominal organs, two or more long bone fractures, a complex pelvic fracture, flail chest and/or major vascular injury. Blood loss is a marker of need for aggressive resuscitation. Where patients are anticipated to need six units of packed red blood cells or more during the first 12 hours after hospital admission and demonstrate an arterial base deficit ≥6 mEq/L during the first 12 hours after hospital admission, shock resuscitation is employed. Trauma victims 65 years of age or older are also at increased risk if they have any two of the previous criteria. Notably, patients with severe brain injury (Glasgow Coma Scale [GCS] score ≤8 or abnormal brain CT scan results) were not resuscitated by this protocol.

The resuscitation strategy employed is a goal-directed, rule-based process emphasizing hemoglobin and volume loading to attain and maintain oxygen delivery for the first 24 hours of hospital stay. A hierarchy of five therapies including red cell transfusion, lactated Ringers infusion, creation of Starling curves for oxygen transport determination, inotrope and vasopressor administration with data managed in a database.

Use of invasive hemodynamic monitoring and endpoints of resuscitation remain controversial. In the late 1980s, unrecognized flow-dependent oxygen consumption was a suspected cause of late organ failure and it was thought that oxygen delivery should be pushed until oxygen consumption reached a plateau. Shoemaker and coworkers, noting that survivors of severe injury increased oxygen delivery to supranormal levels compared with nonsurvivors, proposed that supranormal oxygen delivery be used as a resuscitation goal. In a series of publications, these workers provided data to support the concept that early optimization to supranormal oxygen delivery improved outcome. These publications prompted controversy, which has persisted for over 20 years and has led to a host of prospective trials offering conflicting results. More recently, Shoemaker seems to refute previous observations that early

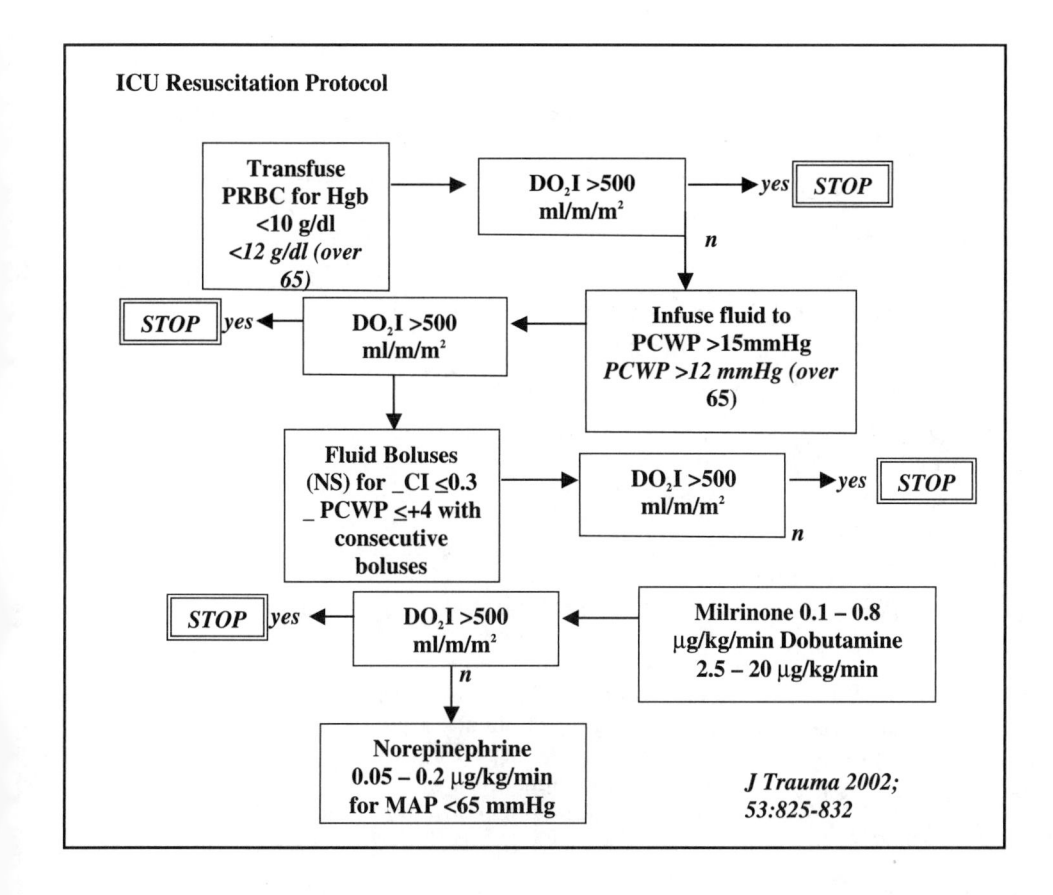

Figure 1.

optimization of hemodynamics to supernormal performance improves outcome in the setting of critical injury.

Moore and coworkers in Houston address this issue by comparing two cohorts of patients. The control patients were resuscitated to an oxygen delivery index of 600 mL/min/m^2 as compared to a more modest, but acceptable, resuscitation endpoint of 500 mL/min/m^2. Comparing a wide range of hemodynamic variables, these workers suggest that outcome with the more modest resuscitation goal was comparable in patients with critical injury and that patients could be resuscitated with a smaller resuscitation fluid volume for a lower target oxygen delivery index. Other observations from this group suggest that females have a comparable if not better response to resuscitation after trauma, and trauma during the later years of life is not inevitably associated with resuscitation futility. While acceptance of the invasive hemodynamic monitoring strategy and fluid resuscitation endpoints of Moore and coworkers is not uniform among the trauma community, this is some of the best recent data incorporating an ICU resuscitation strategy after injury. An interesting concern with such aggressive protocols is an increased recognition of abdominal compartment syndrome, both as a primary consequence of injury and as a secondary effect of resuscitation strategy. Clearly, we still need to strike a balance.

In an effort to optimize early blood resuscitation, a trauma exsanguination policy has been instituted in a number of institutions allowing expedient blood component product replacement during acute patient contact. Patients presenting *in extremis* typically receive noncross-matched blood in the resuscitation room while specific component replacement begins in the operating room and continues in the angiography suite or ICU. Ten units of Group O noncross-matched packed red blood cells, six units of platelets and four units of stored plasma are prepared in a typical protocol and dispensed as the initial response. Later, four units of fresh frozen plasma are thawed to replace the stored plasma and five more units of Group O blood can be immediately delivered at the request of the trauma surgeon. Continuation of the protocol dispenses additional components. This cycle may be repeated until discontinued by the trauma surgeon. In the opinion of its proponents, the institution of a massive transfusion policy for patients presenting in profound shock with blood product loss may be responsible for reduced transfusion requirements and may have avoided other complications of continued slow but steady losses by providing more rapid component therapy.

Damage Control

In use for over a decade, the concept of damage control has become an accepted, proven surgical method with wide applicability and success. Damage control is no longer confined the abdomen and its principles cross surgical disciplines including thoracic, urologic, orthopedic and vascular surgery. The concept is most often used in the massively injured exsanguinating patient with multiple competing surgical priorities (Tables 1–4). With growing experience and application, the technique continues to evolve. The group at the University of Pennsylvania Trauma Center first published on the contemporary experience with damage control in 1993. This experience included 24 abdominal injury patients. This group has noted an

Table 1. *Indications for Damage Control*

1. Inability to achieve hemostasis due to coagulopathy
2. Inaccessible major venous injury
3. Time-consuming procedure in a patient with suboptimal response to resuscitation
4. Management of extra-abdominal life-threatening injury
5. Reassessment of intraabdominal contents

Table 2. *Stages of Damage Control*

1. Abbreviated Resuscitative Surgery
   - Hemorrhage control
   - Control of fecal spillage
   - Packing
   - Temporary abdominal closure
   - Splinting, external fixation
2. Critical Care Unit Resuscitation
   - Rewarming
   - Control acidosis
   - Treat coagulopathy
   - End organ support
3. Definitive Reconstructive Surgery
   - Gastrointestinal continuity
   - Removal of packs
   - Abdominal closure
   - Definitive stabilization of fractures, other injuries

Table 3. *Complications of Damage Control*

Type	Rate
Wound Infection	5–100%
Abdominal Abscess	0–83%
Dehiscence	9–25%
Bile Leak	8–33%
Enterocutaneous Fistula	2–25%
Abdominal Compartment Syndrome	2–25%
Multisystem Organ Failure	20–33%
Mortality	12–67%

Table 4. *Damage Control Approach to Specific Organ Injury*

Organ	Treatment
Liver	Packing, embolization
Spleen	Splenectomy, *not splenorrhaphy*
Duodenum	Treat associated vascular injury drain succus
Pancreas	Treat associated vascular injury drain pancreatic bed
Urology	Rapid nephrectomy if hematoma expanding
	Pack stable hematoma
	Transurethral or suprapubic bladder catheter
	Ureteral stents (internal/external)
Pelvic Fracture	Pelvic compression (MAST pants, sheet)
	External fixator
	Embolization (5–10%)
Extremity Fracture	External fixator
	Temporary soft tissue coverage

improvement in survivability when abbreviated laparotomy and abdominal packing is combined with physiologic resuscitation and more extensive visceral repair at later operations.

The patient receiving damage control treatment is *in extremis* and undergoes a truncated laparotomy, followed by physiologic optimization in the ICU and eventual restoration of gastrointestinal, orthopedic or thoracic integrity at a subsequent operation. In general, the decision to proceed with a damage control approach comes from the operating surgeon prompted by the patient's presenting pathophysiology and response to resuscitation.

With the escalation of gun violence in the late 1980s and early 1990s, trauma centers accumulated significant experience in treating severely injured patients. They found that efforts to proceed with definitive repair at initial operation often led to patient demise despite control of anatomic bleeding. Many of the damage control techniques used today were developed during this period. Various descriptors have been used to describe the procedure: temporary abdominal closure, *"bailout surgery,"* abbreviated laparotomy, planned reoperation and staged laparotomy. *"Damage control"* is a term used by the United States Navy describing the capacity of a ship to absorb damage and maintain mission integrity. It has become the preferred descriptor of this modern, three-phase surgical approach to the catastrophically injured patient. Damage control is neither a bailout procedure nor an abandonment of proper surgical technique. It is a deliberate and calculated surgical approach requiring mature surgical judgment. The decision to use damage control is now often made on presentation on the basis of patient pathophysiology (coagulopathy, hypothermia and acidosis), subsequent response to fluid therapy, and magnitude of blood loss. Classic triggers for damage control are well described and may include pH < 7.30, transfusion of 10 or more units of packed red blood cells (estimated blood loss > 4 L) and temperature of 35°C or lower. Success with damage control requires its application prior to onset of profound acidosis when rapid control of hemorrhage, simultaneous resuscitation, and reversal of hypothermia can best limit coagulopathy.

Damage control philosophy has undergone maturation with involved personnel understanding the pathophysiology and supporting the steps necessary to reverse the cascade of events leading to resuscitation failure. It has become increasingly apparent that damage control does not simply describe the initial truncated operation but the entire process from the first moment of patient contact in the field until definitive repair has been successfully completed.

It has been impossible in the reports covering the evolution of damage control to quantify or describe maturation of surgical skill and technique. Perhaps the best indicator is the time in minutes from patient arrival to surgical control of bleeding. At present, no investigative group can provide these data. The fact that less blood is now given with comparable crystalloid volume may suggest earlier control of major bleeding. As experience with the damage control approach has evolved, surgeons are better prepared to recognize a compelling source of bleeding and move expeditiously to control it definitively or pack and proceed with angiographic embolization if appropriate.

Abdominal Closure

A variety of methods to accomplish temporary abdominal closure have evolved with damage control techniques. Most operators now do not close skin or fascia after the initial operation. A variety of temporary dressings including the "vacuum pack" technique are used for temporary abdominal closure in damage control patients. In our center, the nonadherent aspect of a small bowel bag is placed on the intestine with interposition of omentum between the dressing and intestine if at all possible. Our temporary abdominal dressing allows rapid and effective temporary abdominal coverage and increase in abdominal capacity. Controlled egress of fluid from the abdomen is permitted by drains, which are laid within the layers of the dressing, and the sterile barrier created in the operating room is maintained. Prior to use of temporary abdominal closure techniques, which increase the abdominal domain, intraabdominal hypertension was a common complication in patients receiving standard closure of the abdomen after massive fluid resuscitation (Table 5). During this earlier time period, abdominal compartment pressures were not routinely measured and abdominal compartment syndrome less well recognized as a cause of refractory shock.

Table 5. *Causes of Abdominal Hypertension**

Peritoneal tissue edema
    Diffuse peritonitis
    Severe abdominal trauma
Fluid overload secondary to hemorrhagic or septic shock
Retroperitoneal hematoma
Reperfusion injury after bowel ischemia
Inflammatory edema secondary to acute pancreatitis
Ileus and bowel obstruction
Intraabdominal masses
Abdominal packing for hemorrhage
Closure of the abdomen under tension
Intraabdominal fluid accumulations

*Modified from Wittman D. Compartment syndrome of the abdominal cavity. In: Irwin RS, Cerra FB, Rippe JM, eds. Intensive care medicine. Philadelphia, PA: Lippincott-Raven, 1999; 1890.

Contemporary approaches allow rapid detection of intraabdominal hypertension and abdominal compartment syndrome when clinical signs (distended abdomen, elevated peak inflation pressures, decreased urine output, elevated bladder pressures) are suggestive of its presence. The use of temporary abdominal closure does not eliminate the possibility of abdominal compartment syndrome but these techniques allow sufficient expansion of the abdominal domain that this problem is infrequent.

Abdominal Compartment Syndrome

Intraabdominal hypertension has a variety of physiologic effects. In experimental preparations, animals die from congestive heart failure as abdominal pressure passes a critical threshold. Increased intraabdominal pressure significantly decreases cardiac output and left and right ventricular stroke work and increases central venous pressure, pulmonary artery wedge pressure and systemic and pulmonary vascular resistance. Abdominal decompression reverses these changes. As both hemidiaphragms are displaced upward with increased intraabdominal pressure, decreased thoracic volume and compliance are seen. Decreased volume within the pleural cavities predisposes to atelectasis and deceases alveolar clearance. Pulmonary infections may also result. Ventilated patients with abdominal hypertension require increased airway pressure to deliver a fixed tidal volume. As the diaphragm protrudes into the pleural cavity, intrathoracic pressure increases with reduction of cardiac output and increased pulmonary vascular resistance. Ventilation and perfusion abnormalities result and blood gas measurements demonstrate hypoxemia, hypercarbia and acidosis. Elevation of intraabdominal pressure also causes renal dysfunction. Control of intraabdominal pressure leads to reversal of renal impairment. Intraabdominal pressure as low as 15 to 20 mm Hg may produce oliguria. Anuria is seen with higher intraabdominal pressures. Clearly, deterioration in cardiac output plays a role in diminished renal perfusion but even when cardiac output is maintained at normal or supranormal values by blood volume expansion, impairment of renal function persists in the setting of intraabdominal hypertension. Renal dysfunction is also caused by compression of the renal vein, which creates partial renal blood outflow obstruction. Compression of the abdominal aorta and renal arteries may contribute to increased renal vascular resistance. Direct pressure on the kidneys may also elevate cortical pressures.

Other organs affected by increased intraabdominal pressure include the liver where hepatic blood flow has been demonstrated to decrease with abdominal hypertension. It may be assumed that hepatic synthesis of acute phase proteins, immunoglobulins and other factors of host defense may be impaired by reduced hepatic flow. Other gastrointestinal functions may be compromised by increased intraabdominal pressure. Splanchnic hypoperfusion may begin with intraabdominal pressure as low as 15 mm Hg. Reduced perfusion of intraabdominal arteries, veins and lymphatics may create changes in mucosal pH, translocation, bowel motility and production of gastrointestinal hormones. Finally, intracranial hypertension is seen with chronic increase in intraabdominal pressure. Intracranial hypertension has been demonstrated to decrease when intraabdominal pressure is reduced in morbidly obese patients. Abdominal hypertension significantly increases intracranial pressures at intraabdominal pressures routinely used during laparoscopy.

A recent international conference has attempted to standardize definitions of intraabdominal hypertension and abdominal compartment syndrome. Intraabdominal pressure (IAP) should be expressed in "mm Hg" and measured at end expiration in the complete supine position after ensuring that abdominal muscle contractions are absent with a transducer zeroed at the level of the midaxillary line. The current reference standard for IAP measurement is the pressure measured via an indwelling urinary drainage catheter within the bladder. Using a bladder catheter, the aspiration port may be connected to a pressure transducer and intraabdominal pressure read from the bedside monitor. An alternative and less expensive technique is to read the height of the urine column in urinary catheter drainage tubing. (For either pressure measurement, 50 mL of sterile room temperature saline solution is instilled in the bladder, and a stabilization period of 30 to 60 s is allowed.) Abdominal perfusion pressure (APP) assesses not only severity of intraabdominal hypertension but also the adequacy of the patient's systemic perfusion. APP = mean arterial pressure (MAP) − IAP. Intraabdominal hypertension (IAH) is the pathologic evaluation of IAP. IAH is defined by sustained or repeated IAP ≥ 12 mm Hg or an APP ≤ 60 mm Hg. Grades of IAH have been proposed: Grade I: IAP between 12 and 15 mm Hg; Grade II: IAP between 16 and 20 mm Hg; Grade III: IAP between 21 and 25 mm Hg; and Grade IV: IAP > 25 mm Hg. IAH may be classified into two types. Acute intraabdominal hypertension develops within hours as a result of trauma, intraabdominal hemorrhage, or over days as a result of sepsis, capillary leak, or other critical illness. Chronic intraabdominal hypertension develops over months to years as a result of morbid obesity, intraabdominal tumor growth, chronic ascites, or pregnancy and is characterized by progressive abdominal wall adaptation to increase in IAP.

Abdominal compartment syndrome (ACS) is present when organ dysfunction occurs as a result of IAH. ACS is defined by sustained or repeated IAP > 20 mm Hg and/or APP < 60 mm Hg in association with new-onset single or multiple organ failure. ACS is not graded but rather considered as an all or none phenomenon. ACS may be further classified into three types. Primary ACS develops due to conditions associated with injury or disease in the abdominal/pelvic region requiring emergent surgical or angioradiographic intervention. Secondary ACS develops due to conditions outside the abdomen, such as sepsis, capillary leak, major burns, or other conditions requiring massive fluid resuscitation. Recurrent ACS develops following initial successful surgical or medical treatment of either primary or secondary ACS or following closure of a previous decompressive laparotomy.

Operative decompression is the method of choice in the patient with severe abdominal hypertension and evidence of intraabdominal organ dysfunction. After decompression, improvements in hemodynamics, pulmonary function, tissue perfusion and renal function have been demonstrated in a variety of clinical settings. To prevent hemodynamic decompensation during decompression, intravascular volume should be restored, oxygen delivery maximized and hypothermia and coagulation defects corrected. The abdomen should be opened under optimal conditions in the operating room including hemodynamic monitoring with adequate venous access and controlled ventilation. Adjunctive measures to combat expected reperfusion wash out from byproducts of anaerobic metabolism include prophylactic volume loading and use of vasoconstrictor agents to prevent sudden changes in blood pressure. After decompression, the abdomen and the fascial gap is left open using one of a variety of temporary abdominal closure methods.

Abdominal Organ Injury

The focus on management for intraabdominal organ injury remains nonoperative. The practitioner must be aware, however, of patients at greater risk for failure of that approach. Nonoperative management should be entertained only in hemodynamically stable patients. Identifying hemodynamically stable patients may be challenging in the setting of multiple injuries. A recent multicenter study of blunt splenic injury from the Eastern Association for the Surgery of Trauma (EAST) included over 1,400 patients (age <15 yr) from 26 centers. Nonoperative management was attempted in 61% of these patients with a resulting failure rate of 10.4%. Failure was associated with increasing age, Injury Severity Score (ISS), GCS, grade of splenic injury, and quantity of hemoperitoneum. Interestingly, other studies of nonoperative management of splenic injury suggest that many patients in high-risk categories can be managed nonoperatively, and that there is no increased mortality with failure of this approach.

Advances in nonoperative management have indicated differences between the spleen and liver. A high percentage of liver injuries appear to be manageable nonoperatively, and a somewhat lower proportion of liver injuries fail nonoperative management in comparison with blunt injury to the spleen. It has been speculated that liver injuries are more commonly associated with low-pressure venous injuries, and a greater proportion of spleen injuries are associated with arterial or arteriolar injury. Planned nonoperative management of the liver may be attempted in as many as 85% of patients with liver injuries; a failure rate of only 7% was found. In addition, significant improvement in outcome with nonoperative management was identified compared to operative management with respect to abdominal infection rates, transfusions, and length of hospital stay. Patients requiring operation due to hemodynamic instability may be successfully treated with packing. Evolution to nonoperative management in stable patients with high-grade injury results in lower mortality. In another major report from the University of Louisville, death secondary to blunt liver injury dropped from 8 to 2%; this improvement was attributed to improved methods of managing hepatic venous injuries. Proposed improvements in the management of hepatic venous injury include nonoperative management in stable patients and willingness to employ gauze packing in unstable individuals.

As nonoperative management of abdominal solid organ injury continues to advance, missed blunt bowel injury has received increased attention. The sensitivity of CT scanning in defining bowel injury has been assessed by a variety of investigators. Recent reports suggest that sensitivity with latest-generation CT scans is as high as 94% for bowel injury particularly if unexplained free fluid is considered a critical finding. A number of patients explored after CT scanning, however, have nontherapetic laparotomies for bowel hematomas or contusions.

Late-generation CT scanners, contrast-enhanced CT scans, and angiography support are changing the face of management for injury to the solid abdominal and retroperitoneal organs. As abdominal CT scans replace laparotomy as the definitive diagnostic procedure in injury, the contrast blush is a useful tool in identification of slow bleeding sites associated with lacerations to solid organs. In patients who are hemodynamically stable, these sites may then be embolized with a high degree of success in both the liver and the spleen. Aggressive application of CT scanning and angiographic intervention has increased the rate of salvage and decreased length of stay and resource consumption for patients with these solid organ injuries. It is important to note that patients with significant solid organ injury may present without significant free intraperitoneal blood. Therefore, up to 5% of these patients with significant trauma may not be appreciated with abdominal ultrasound, which is designed to examine the abdomen for the fluid stripe indicative of free intraperitoneal blood. Many investigators now recommend that abdominal ultrasound not be used as the sole diagnostic modality in stable patients at risk for blunt solid organ injury. Finally, it appears that the approach to blunt organ injury may vary with the type of hospital treating the patient. A recent multicenter study in Pennsylvania suggested that patients treated at Level II trauma centers had a higher rate of operative treatment and lower rate of failure for nonoperative management than Level I trauma centers. Mortality for patients managed nonoperatively was lower at Level I trauma centers. Level I trauma centers were also more likely to repair rather than remove the spleen.

Perforation of the gastrointestinal tract, whether due to blunt or penetrating injury, is being managed with direct repair rather than diverting ileostomy or colostomy in an increasing number of patients. Indications for consideration of primary repair of injury perforating the gastrointestinal tract include good response to resuscitation, lack of acidosis, limited blood loss, limited fecal spillage and a small number of associated injuries. Where additional life-threatening injuries which complicate evaluation or limit available time for primary bowel repair are present, immediate control of spillage from the gut is appropriate with diversion of the fecal stream at the primary operation or during staged repair in the patient receiving damage control management.

Traumatic Brain Injury

Traumatic brain injury accounts for 40% of all deaths from acute injuries. It is the single most important factor in determining the outcome of various forms of trauma. Two hundred thousand victims with such injuries require hospitalization each year and often are permanently disabled. Many more persons suffer mild traumatic brain injury resulting in a physician visit or temporary disability. Individuals at greatest risk for traumatic brain injury are typically young and at the beginning of potentially productive life. Thus, loss of potential income, cost of acute care, and continued expenses of rehabilitation and medical care are enormous. These realities mandate aggressive attention to the management of brain injury. Clinical factors associated with poorer outcome with head injury include:

- Midline shift on CT scan
- Systolic blood pressure <90 mm Hg
- Intracranial pressure (ICP) >15 mm Hg
- Age >55 years
- Glasgow Coma Scale score <8

Notably, head injury outcomes are determined by the number of secondary insults, not the injuries to other organ systems or body regions.

Given these realities, the most important concept in the recent treatment of brain-injured patients is the distinction between primary and secondary brain injury. Primary injury is that injury which occurs at the time of the traumatic incident and includes brain lacerations or other mechanical injuries to the brain at the moment of impact. After impact, the brain continues to be injured by various mechanisms including the mechanical injury from cerebral edema or intracranial hematomas, ischemia from hypotension, cerebral edema or cerebral vascular dysregulation, hypoxia from inadequate ventilation, and secondary damage from a wide array of inflammation mediators. While prevention is the only strategy to avert primary brain injury, secondary injury can be prevented or at least blunted. Thus, the management of traumatic brain injury now includes increasing emphasis on the prevention of secondary insults.

The most important feature of the initial neurologic examination, the Glasgow Coma Scale, is designed to identify rapidly the severity of patient injury. Patients with GCS scores of 13 to 15 are considered to have mild head injuries. These individuals have an excellent prognosis and may not require hospitalization. They have a 3% chance of deteriorating into coma and serial neurologic exams make this deterioration easy to detect. Individuals with GCS scores of 8 to 12 have moderate head injury. These patients do not have normal neurologic examinations, but the severity of their injuries usually is not appreciated until the full GCS score is obtained. This group of patients has a 20% chance of declining into coma (GCS score of ≤8). Patients with severe head injury have the worst prognosis and require the most immediate care. All of these individuals require head CT scanning; except for select subpopulations, all of them require intra-cranial pressure (ICP) monitoring. As a group, there is a >50% chance of an increased ICP; their depressed clinical examinations often preclude detection of changing neurologic status until their condition reaches catastrophic deterioration.

Evacuation of mass lesions has been the traditional focus of brain injury management throughout this century. The goal of removing space-occupying lesions is to prevent cerebral herniation. In previous studies among patients who talk and die, undetected hematomas were the principal cause of death. These are examples of patients who survive primary brain injury with the ability to talk and interact at some level but who later succumb to preventable secondary brain injury. Cerebral herniation, representing the compression of critical neurologic centers against the retaining structures of the skull, is the common final pathway in these patients. Once herniation (regardless of the type) has occurred, patient outcome is dramatically affected. Studies over the last 50 years have demonstrated that once herniation occurs and the patient slips into coma, the mortality rate reaches 33 to 41%, compared with mortality rates of 0 to 21% in patients who present with herniation before coma. Once herniation occurs and the patient progresses to coma, hematomas must be evaluated within hours to avoid a significant risk of mortality.

After evacuation of mass lesions, emphasis is given to monitoring and control of ICP. ICP monitoring was introduced over 40 years ago as a means to quantify the study of brain swelling and cerebral edema. While the study of ICP initially focused on prevention of herniation by preventing swelling, it was soon apparent that keeping ICP from rising was a desirable end. As ICP rises, cerebral perfusion decreases and the threat of brain ischemia increases. Data are now emerging, however, that even in patients with adequate cerebral perfusion pressure (CPP), high ICP is associated with poor outcome. In the past, a variety of guidelines have been proposed for the optimal ICP level for treatment. Most current data place 25 mm Hg as the highest acceptable level for ICP at which treatment must begin. Modern methods of ICP monitoring include the ventriculostomy and intraparenchymal fiberoptic or strain-gauge devices. Subarachnoid bolts and epidural monitoring are used rarely or in select patient populations. Ventriculostomy carries an increased risk of infection and a slightly increased risk of bleeding. It is, however, the gold standard for ICP measurement.

Experimental work beginning in the mid-1980s demonstrated that ischemia is a significant threat to the head-injured patient. Ischemia had long been recognized as a factor in the outcome of head injury, but recent work has changed the paradigm through which head injury was viewed. Up to this time, the treatment priority has been control of cerebral edema and prevention of cerebral herniation. Any technique reducing ICP was thought to be good for the head-injured patient. By giving equal attention to ischemia, the current approach to the head-injured patient has evolved.

Ischemia is common following head injury. Autopsy findings have indicated that 60% of head-injured patients had ischemia. Cerebral blood flow on the first day after injury is less than half that of healthy individuals and may approach the ischemic threshold. In normal gray matter, cerebral blood flow is 50 mL/100 g/min of tissue, and in white matter, cerebral blood flow is 18 mL/100 g/min of tissue. Typical blood flow to gray matter within the first 8 hrs after head injury is 30 mL/100 g/min of tissue, and in individuals with more severe injuries, cerebral blood flow as low as <20 mL/100 g/min of tissue has been noted.

Improved recent understanding of cerebral blood flow coincides with multiple studies demonstrating disastrous consequences of hypotension in the setting of head injury. An increased death rate in head-injured patients with hypotension was documented in the National Traumatic Coma Data Bank where the two most important factors related to outcome from head injuries were time spent with ICP of >20 mm Hg and time spent with systolic pressure of <90 mm Hg. These data suggest that patients with only a single episode of systolic blood pressure of <90 mm Hg have a significantly worse outcome than those individuals who never experience this degree of hypotension.

Recent head injury management, therefore, places maintenance of adequate CPP as a goal equivalent to prevention of high ICP. The autoregulatory mechanisms in the brain are designed to maintain cerebral blood flow constant over a range of CPP ranging between 50 and 150 mm Hg. This highly adaptive capacity allows the brain to see constant blood supply, despite changes in position and activity. In the severely injured brain, cerebral blood flow passively follows CPP. In the extreme case, with cerebral autoregulation disabled, cerebral ischemia results as patients are maintained in a hypovolemic state with low mean arterial pressure to reduce cerebral blood volume and thereby ICP. In this practice, CPP was maintained below the autoregulatory threshold. Seemingly paradoxically, the best way to reduce ICP is to increase CPP into the autoregulatory range. This practice avoids hypotension and the ischemic damage that almost certainly attended the old practice of keeping patients with severe head injury "dry" and their arterial pressure low. At present, it is unclear what an adequate CPP is. Based on available data, including stepwise regression analysis, a CPP of 70 mm Hg has been suggested as a desirable level. Most head injury research protocols maintain this level.

Cerebral edema was thought to be aggravated by overzealous fluid administration, leading to increased intracranial pressure, brain ischemia and, ultimately, a poor outcome. However, in the patient with multiple injuries without head injury, aggressive volume resuscitation is a widely accepted method to maintain end-organ perfusion and adequate oxygen delivery. Traditional management strategies of the patient with severe head injury have changed with the knowledge of adverse effects of secondary brain insults. Much like the treatment of myocardial infarction for which the original zone of injury cannot be restored to normal, emphasis in the management of brain injury must be placed on avoidance of secondary insults to prevent extension of injury resulting from ischemia. An analysis of the Traumatic Coma Data Bank demonstrated that hypoxia and hypotension in the immediate period after head injury resulted in mortality rates of 28% and 50%, respectively. When the combined effect of hypoxia and hypotension during resuscitation was analyzed, the mortality rate increased to 57%. Later studies by other workers, using an algorithm guided by optimization of cerebral perfusion pressure, demonstrated a lower mortality in a cohort of patients thought to be similar to those enrolled in the Traumatic Coma Data Bank.

The second important consideration after avoidance of hypotension during resuscitation of the head-injured patient is the prevention of hypoxia. Hypoxia is one of the five top predictors of poor outcome in the National Traumatic Coma Data Bank with 30 to 60% of severely head-injured patients presenting with hypoxia. While the optimal Pao_2 level in the head-injured patient has not been determined, available data suggest that a level of <60 mm Hg (<8.0 kPa) is associated with poor outcome.

ICP is controlled with a variety of modalities. Our views on the use of these modalities and the management of head injury continue to evolve. Hyperventilation reduces ICP by reducing cerebral blood volume with increased cerebral vascular tone and induction of hypocapnia. Reduction in cerebral blood volume leads to intracranial blood volume loss and lower ICP. For many years, hyperventilation has been a primary means of reducing ICP. Hyperventilation can cause vasoconstriction independent of the metabolic demands of the brain. Hyperventilation may, therefore, reduce blood flow to the brain even if that reduction results in an ischemic injury. Recent studies, using jugular venous oximetry, have indicated that hyperventilation may produce cerebral ischemia. Other studies demonstrated that desaturation found in jugular venous blood is more common with hyperventilation than with other means employed for reduction in ICP. One prospective, randomized trial evaluated severely head-injured patients managed with hypocapnia vs normocapnia. The normocapnic group had better outcome at 3- and 6-mo follow-up. Increasing evidence indicates that hyperventilation is an ICP treatment with high cost, the threat of ischemia. Current management, therefore, includes use of less toxic means of reducing ICP, if available, rather than the use of hyperventilation. For example, drainage of cerebrospinal fluid (CSF) through ventricular drains should be started early with aggressive use of sedation, muscle relaxants, and administration of mannitol before resorting to hyperventilation.

Drainage of CSF and use of mannitol may be employed to control ICP and to optimize CPP. Some medical centers are facilitating drainage of CSF by placing ventriculotomy catheters when possible, as opposed to subarachnoid monitors which do not allow for CSF removal. Drainage of

CSF may be the first choice for the treatment of increased ICP. Mannitol is an osmotic diuretic given as a bolus that develops an osmotic gradient between the blood and the brain. Mannitol may also act by improving cerebral blood flow through reduction in hematocrit and viscosity. Mannitol, however, cannot be given to hypotensive patients as it will magnify shock states. In large doses, mannitol may lead to acute renal failure. If given as a constant infusion, mannitol may also open the blood-brain barrier and result in rebound cerebral edema. Mannitol drips, therefore, are not recommended. Serum osmolarity must be monitored in individuals who receive mannitol for control of ICP and optimization of CPP.

Recent developments in the care of the head-injured patient focus on the recognition of the importance of secondary brain injury as a determinant of prognosis. In studies of long-term outcome, the key elements of secondary brain injury, hypoxia and hypotension with secondary ischemia, are recognized to occur with increasing frequency. Optimal modalities to control secondary brain injury focus on maintenance of optimal CPP with the lowest possible ICP consistent with avoidance of cerebral ischemia. To control ICP, hyperventilation is now employed as an emergency tool rather than as a primary therapy.

Injury to Thoracic Aorta

Injury to the thoracic aorta is common among victims of high-speed motor vehicle crashes with an acute deceleration mechanism. Many victims of this injury are dead at the scene. An estimated 20% of the persons who sustain deceleration injury to the thoracic aorta live to reach the hospital due to containment of aortic rupture by connective tissue covering the aorta. Without recognition and treatment of this injury, 30% of these individuals will die within 12 hours and 50% within 1 week. The mechanism of injury is a combination of differential deceleration of the mediastinal contents and force provided by the steering wheel or dash board impacting the chest. Falls may also produce this injury. Most often, disruption occurs at the aortic isthmus, just distal to the origin of the left subclavian artery at the ligamentum arteriosum.

The initial anteroposterior chest radiograph is the single most important screening tool for injury to the thoracic aorta. Arteriography is the gold standard diagnostic study because of its ability to demonstrate the specific injury and reveal unsuspected vascular anomalies. Unfortunately, intimal flaps are being reported in up to 10% of studies. Most of these lesions resolve spontaneously and may be managed nonoperatively. In the emergency setting, newer spiral CT scans have become useful at rapidly diagnosing thoracic aortic injuries (particularly to the descending aorta) because of their greater speed and resolution. With a suspicious mechanism of injury, a clear chest radiograph is inadequate to rule out aortic injury. While mediastinal widening warrants aortography, 80% of the time the angiogram does not show injury to the thoracic aorta as the cause of mediastinal widening. Thus, latest-generation CT imaging is becoming an acceptable method for evaluation of the widened mediastinum with aortography in cases requiring further definition.

Patients who are unstable at the scene of a crash or during the first 4 hours of hospitalization have a mortality rate of >90%. Hemodynamically stable patients whose systolic blood pressure does not exceed 120 mm Hg, during the first to 6 to 8 hours after injury, have a survival rate of >90%. Of the operative procedures for repairing injuries to the descending aorta, the most dreaded complication is paraplegia. Unfortunately, no one causative or preventative factor has been identified.

Various reports have suggested that operative management of injury to the descending aorta may be delayed in stable patients for a period that can range from hours to months. These individuals should receive an afterload-reducing agent or a drug to alter dP/dT (change in pressure over time), have their blood pressure maintained at or <120/80 mm Hg, and have a stable mediastinal hematoma. Delayed reconstruction of chronic posttraumatic aneurysm of the descending aorta, using endovascular stented grafts, is also being reported. At this time, expeditious repair of injury to the descending aorta remains the most cost-effective approach with no additional risk of complications in adequately resuscitated patients.

Esophageal Perforation

Esophageal perforation is a true emergency and therapeutic challenge as delay affects survival.

Broad-spectrum antibiotics, improved nutrition and improved critical care have led to better results. Iatrogenic esophageal disruption (60%), spontaneous perforation (15%), and external trauma (20%) are responsible for the majority of esophageal ruptures. Perforation from penetrating or blunt trauma is often obscured by associated injuries and has a poor prognosis if diagnosis is delayed. Self-induced esophageal injury by acid or alkali may cause extensive necrosis and esophageal destruction.

Symptoms and signs vary with the cause and location of perforation as well as the time delay between perforation and diagnosis. Pain is the most consistent symptom, present in 70 to 90% of patients, and it is usually related to the site of disruption. Neck ache and stiffness suggest perforation after endoscopy. In the abdomen, dull epigastric pain radiating to the back may occur if the disruption is posterior and communicates with the lesser sac. Severe chest pain suggests thoracic perforation. Misdiagnosis of dissecting thoracic aneurysm, spontaneous pneumothorax or myocardial infarction is common. Acute pain in the epigastrium often suggests perforated peptic ulcer disease or acute pancreatitis. Dysphasia appears late and is generally related to thoracic perforation. Tachycardia and tachypnea are documented in 50 to 70% of patients. Hypotension and shock are present when sepsis or significant inflammatory third spacing occurs. Subcutaneous emphysema is seen frequently when perforation is cervical and less often with thoracic or abdominal injury.

Plain chest radiograph suggests the diagnosis in 90% of patients with esophageal perforation. However, immediately after disruption, the chest film may be normal. Pneumomediastinum, subcutaneous emphysema, mediastinal widening, or a mediastinal air fluid level must prompt investigation to rule out esophageal perforation. Perforation of the distal third of the esophagus leads to hydropneumothorax on the left. Contrast esophagogram with water-soluble material followed by dilute barium reveals primary sites or areas of leakage and determines whether perforation is confined to the mediastinum or communicates freely with the pleural or peritoneal cavities. Unfortunately, the rate of false negative esophagograms may be as high as 10%. CT of the chest can often show the site of perforation and is used when presentation is atypical, when signs or symptoms are vague or misleading, or when perforation involves the lesser sac. Mediastinal fluid and air on CT of the chest are strongly suggestive of esophageal perforation. Esophagoscopy can easily miss a perforation or enlarge a hole. This test is usually *not* performed to identify perforation.

Three factors affect management of esophageal perforation: origin, location, and delay between rupture and treatment. For example, postemetic perforation with massive contamination is the most morbid whereas pharyngeal perforation rarely ends in fatality because of relative ease of diagnosis, drainage, and repair. Morbidity and mortality increase as perforation extends into the thorax. Patients with perforations of the cervical esophagus have an 85% survival whereas thoracic disruption is associated with survival rates of 65 to 75%. Abdominal esophageal perforation is associated with 90% survival.

Conservative management is associated with a 22 to 38% mortality. The difficulty with non-operative management is determination that perforation will remain contained and not cause continued contamination with subsequent uncontrolled infection. Surgery remains the mainstay of treatment. Early surgical reinforced repair with drainage of contaminated spaces provides the best chance of survival after esophageal perforation. Before repair, all nonviable and grossly contaminated tissue in the mediastinum and around the esophagus is debrided. Decortication of trapped lung tissue may be necessary.

Sepsis, shock, pneumothorax, pneumoperitoneum, mediastinal emphysema, and respiratory failure are absolute indications for rapid surgical intervention. Preoperative preparation includes nasogastric intubation for gastric decompression, broad-spectrum antibiotics and intravenous fluid resuscitation. Cervical perforation is best treated by direct suture closure and drainage of the neck. Thoracic esophageal perforation requires right thoracotomy for exposure of the upper two thirds and left thoracotomy for control of the lower third. Lesions at the esophagogastric junction are approached by left thoracotomy or upper midline laparotomy and repairs may be buttressed by gastric fundoplication. Late perforations usually can be repaired primarily with muscle or pleural reinforcement. If repair is not possible, most operators favor esophageal resection, cervical esophagostomy and enteral feeding tube placement with later reconstruction. Perforations encountered late may initially be treated by wide drainage of the mediastinum by opening the pleura along the length of the esophagus. Patients with complex perforations should preferably be given a jejunostomy, enteral nutrition or parenteral hyperalimentation because gastrostomy should be avoided for later reconstruction. Alternative procedures (esophageal exclusion, T-tube drainage and esophageal resection) have been proposed for patients with late esophageal disruption. Exclusion of the perforated esophagus by division of the esophagus adjacent to the stomach and at the neck allows partial or total exclusion of the perforation. One of the major disadvantages of this approach is the obligation to perform a second major reconstructive procedure. T-tube drainage of the perforation creates a controlled esophagocutaneous fistula but continued leakage may progress to mediastinal and pulmonary sepsis. If extensive mediastinitis and sepsis are present with continued contamination, resection of the esophagus with delayed reconstruction is preferable.

In summary, treatment of esophageal perforation is directed toward fluid resuscitation, control of sepsis, operative drainage of the mediastinum and pleural cavity, suture repair of the esophagus if possible, and reinforcement of the suture line with vascularized tissue particularly muscle. Delay in diagnosis makes repair more difficult because of friability and necrotic tissue at the site of the tear. Primary repair may be possible but cervical diversion with esophageal exclusion and long-term tube feeding may be necessary. Postoperative care emphasizes control of infection and nutrition support until healing of an esophageal injury is demonstrated.

Blunt Cardiac Injury

Cardiac injuries from blunt chest trauma are usually the result of high-speed motor vehicle crashes. Falls from heights, crushing injuries from motor vehicle crashes and falling objects, blast injuries, and direct violent trauma from assault are less common causes of blunt cardiac injury. Blunt trauma to the heart ranges from minor injuries to frank cardiac rupture. Minor injury is a nonspecific condition frequently termed cardiac contusion, or myocardial contusion. Moderately severe lesions may include injury to the pericardium, valves, papillary muscles, and coronary vessels. The most severe of blunt cardiac injuries is the dramatic and often fatal condition of cardiac rupture.

The reported incidence of blunt cardiac injury depends on the modality and criteria used for diagnosis. The occurrence rate ranges from 8 to 71% in patients sustaining blunt chest trauma. The true occurrence rate remains unknown as there is no diagnostic gold standard. The lack of such a standard leads to confusion with respect to making the diagnosis, thereby making the available literature difficult to interpret. Key issues involve identification of a patient population at risk for adverse events from blunt cardiac injury and then appropriately monitoring and treating these individuals. Conversely, patients who are not at risk for complications could be discharged from the hospital with appropriate follow-up.

The Eastern Association for the Surgery of Trauma (EAST) has recently reviewed studies that focused on the identification of blunt cardiac injury. Based on randomized, prospective data, they recommended that an admission ECG should be performed in all patients in whom blunt cardiac injury was suspected. Additional recommendations included continuous ECG monitoring for 24 to 48 hours in patients where the initial ECG was abnormal. Similarly, if patients are hemodynamically unstable, evaluation should proceed with transthoracic echocardiography followed by transesophageal echocardiography, if an optimal study cannot be obtained. Finally, patients with coexisting cardiac disease and those with an abnormal admission ECG may undergo surgery if they are appropriately monitored. These individuals may require placement of a pulmonary artery catheter. The presence of sternal fracture does not predict the presence of blunt cardiac injury. To date, enzyme analysis is inadequate to identify patients with blunt cardiac injury.

Pelvic Fracture

Substantial blunt force is required to disrupt the pelvic ring. The extent of injury is related to the direction and magnitude of the force. Associated abdominal, thoracic, and head injuries are common. Forces applied to the pelvis can cause rotational displacement with opening or compression of the pelvic ring. The other type of displacement seen with pelvic fractures is vertical with complete disruption of the pelvic ring and the posterior sacroiliac complex.

Patients with pelvic ring injuries are easily subdivided into two groups on the basis of clinical presentation: (1) those who are hemodynamically stable; and (2) those who are hemodynamically unstable. There is a dramatic difference in the mortality rates between pelvic fracture patients who are hypotensive (38%) and those who are hemodynamically stable (3%). Hemodynamic instability and biomechanical pelvic instability are separate though related issues, which tend to confuse the clinical picture. The source of bleeding may be multifactorial and not directly related to the pelvic fracture itself. However, pelvic fracture blood loss that contributes to hemodynamic instability is a significant risk factor. Early fracture diagnosis and stabilization, using external skeletal fixation, are extremely important in the acute phase of patient management. Treatment of the patient is also directed by response to initial fluid resuscitation. It is essential to examine for other sources of hemorrhage (intrathoracic, intraperitoneal, external) in patients with evidence of ongoing bleeding. Retroperitoneal bleeding in a pelvic fracture patient usually arises from a low pressure source, the cancellous bone at the fracture site or adjacent venous injury. Significant retroperitoneal arterial bleeding occurs in only ~10% of patients. Clinical evidence has suggested that provisional fracture stabilization, using a simple anterior external fixator or even "wrapping" in a bed sheet can control low pressure bleeding. Continued unexplained bleeding after provisional fracture stabilization suggests an arterial source. Angiography with embolization of the involved vessel is then indicated. Therapeutic angiography may also be required after abdominal exploration if a rapidly expanding or pulsatile retroperitoneal hematoma is encountered. In general, definitive operative stabilization of pelvic fractures is delayed 3 to 5 days to allow the patient to recover from acute injury.

Deep Venous Thrombosis and Thromboembolism

That deep venous thrombosis and thromboembolism occur after trauma is incontrovertible. The optimal mode of prophylaxis has yet to be determined. Low-dose heparin (5000 units subcutaneously two or three times daily) represents one pharmacologic treatment modality used for prophylaxis against deep venous thrombosis and pulmonary embolism. A metaanalysis of 29 trials and >8,000 surgical patients demonstrated that low-dose heparin significantly decreased the frequency of deep venous thrombosis from 25.2% in patients with no prophylaxis to 8.7% in treated individuals. Similarly, pulmonary embolism was halved by low-dose heparin treatment (0.5% with treatment compared with 1.2% in controls). In double-blind trials, the occurrence rate of major hemorrhage was higher in patients treated with anticoagulation than in controls but the difference in incidence was not significant. Minor bleeding complications, such as wound hematomas, were more frequent in low-dose heparin treatment patients (6.3%) than in controls (4.1%).

Unfractionated low-dose heparin has not been shown to be particularly effective in preventing venous thromboembolism in trauma patients. Two recent prospective trials demonstrated that low-dose heparin was not better in preventing deep venous thrombosis than no prophylaxis in patients with an Injury Severity Score of >9. Sample sizes in these studies were small and statistical error could not be excluded. The results of low-dose heparin administration after injury with regard to pulmonary embolism were even more vague.

Defining the trauma patient at risk for venous thromboembolism is subjective and variable in the literature. The following injury patterns appear to differentiate high-risk patients for venous thromboembolism: closed-head injury (GCS score <8); pelvis plus long-bone fractures (multiple long-bone fractures) and spinal cord injury. Greenfield and associates have developed a risk factor assessment tool for venous thromboembolism; preliminary evidence supported this risk factor assessment tool as a valid indicator of the development of venous thromboembolism. In this scale, risk factors are weighted; scores of <3 represent low risk, scores of 3 to 5 represent moderate risk, and scores of >5 represent high risk (Table 6).

When EAST reviewed the literature regarding the effectiveness of low-dose heparin for trauma patients, a clear recommendation could not be produced. Most studies showed no effect of low-dose heparin on venous thromboembolism. However, many of the studies examined suffered from methodologic errors or poor study design. Similarly, the use of sequential compression devices on the lower extremities in patients at risk for deep venous thrombosis is widely accepted; however, clinical studies demonstrating efficacy in trauma patients are few. The mechanism of these devices is believed to be based on a combination of factors addressing venous stasis and hypercoagulability. These mechanisms are poorly understood at this time. The role of multimodality therapy to provide additional protection from venous thromboembolism in the setting of injury needs to be ascertained.

There is a wealth of randomized, prospective data supporting the use of low-molecular-weight heparin as venous thromboembolism prophylaxis in orthopedic surgery. This literature is derived primarily from total hip replacement and knee replacement patients. We now have data suggesting that low-molecular-weight heparin is superior to unfractionated heparin for prophylaxis in moderate- to high-risk trauma patients. Most data in many different types of patients confirm improved efficacy of low-molecular-weight heparin with the same or even less bleeding risk compared with prophylaxis with unfractionated heparin. Low-molecular heparin should be the standard form of venous thromboembolism prophylaxis in trauma patients with complex pelvic and lower extremity injuries as well as in those patients with spinal cord injuries. This agent is also safe for patients receiving craniotomy or nonoperative management of solid organ injury if started 24 or 72 hours after injury respectively. Finally, the literature is beginning to support the use of inferior vena cava filters in high-risk trauma patients without a documented occurrence of deep venous thrombosis or pulmonary embolism and who cannot receive prophylactic therapy.

For established deep venous thrombosis or pulmonary embolism, anticoagulation is a well-established treatment. Current evidence suggests that a 3- to 6-month period provides adequate treatment for the first episode of deep venous thrombosis or pulmonary embolism in a patient without clotting abnormality. Patients in whom the risk of recurrent venous thromboembolism extends >6 months may have anticoagulation extended indefinitely. In addition, patients whose injuries preclude the use of anticoagulants because bleeding would exacerbate their injury should have consideration given to placement of a vena cava filter. Recent evidence also supported initial treatment of venous thromboembolism with low-molecular-weight heparin.

Evaluation for deep venous thrombosis in the setting of injury receives continued study. Early identification of this complication would allow treatment to be initiated, thus decreasing the frequency and severity of complications. Studies in the nontrauma literature support the accuracy of both Doppler and duplex ultrasonography in the detection of deep venous thrombosis in the symptomatic patient. The overall accuracy of screening ultrasonography in the asymptomatic patient is less clear. Similarly, impedance plethysmography has high sensitivity and specificity in the detection of proximal deep venous thrombosis in symptomatic

Table 6. *Risk Factors Associated With Thromboembolism (VTE) in Trauma**

Underlying Condition
   Obesity
   Malignancy
   Abnormal coagulation factors on hospital admission
   History of VTE
Iatrogenic Factors
   Central femoral line >24 h
   ≥4 transfusions in first 24 h
   Surgical procedure ≥2 h
   Repair or ligation of major vascular injury
Injury-Related Factors
   AIS score of >2 for chest
   AIS score of >2 for abdomen
   AIS score of >2 for head
   Coma (GCS score of <8 for >4 h)
   Complex lower-extremity fracture
   Pelvic fracture
   Spinal cord injury with paraplegia or quadriplegia
Age (sequential increased risk with age)
   ≥40 but <60 yr
   ≥70 but <75 yr
   ≥75 yr

*Greenfield LJ, Proctor MC, Rodriguez LJ, et al. Posttrauma thromboembolism porphyraxis. J Trauma 1997; 42: 100–103

patients. Its low sensitivity in detecting deep venous thrombosis in asymptomatic patients precludes use as a surveillance technique in trauma patients at high risk for deep venous thrombosis. Logistical problems and complications associated with venography make the procedure less appealing than other noninvasive diagnostic measures. Venography still has a role in confirming deep venous thrombosis in trauma patients if diagnostic studies are equivocal. At present, it appears that future investigational efforts are best directed at developing the role of duplex ultrasonography in screening for deep venous thrombosis in the setting of injury.

Antibiotic Management

Much of the data surrounding antibiotic utilization in patients following injury comes from studies of patients with penetrating abdominal trauma. There are a wide variety of randomized prospective data available, which support clear recommendations regarding the use of antibiotics in this patient group. While antibiotic therapy must be initiated prior to operation or in the emergency department, the intensivist should be aware of available recommendations regarding appropriate agents, duration of therapy, and the impact of shock and resuscitation.

In a clinical management update produced by the Practice Management Guidelines Workgroup of EAST, evidence regarding antibiotic utilization in penetrating abdominal trauma was reviewed. These writers suggest that there are sufficient randomized prospective data to recommend the use of only a single preoperative dose of prophylactic antibiotics with broad-spectrum aerobic and anaerobic coverage as a standard of care for trauma patients sustaining penetrating abdominal wounds. If no hollow viscus injury is noted subsequently, no further antibiotic administration is warranted. The second issue addressed is the duration of therapy in the presence of injury to any hollow viscus. Based on available prospective randomized data, there is sufficient evidence to recommend continuation of prophylactic antibiotics for only 24 hours even in the presence of injury to any hollow viscus. Unfortunately, there are insufficient data to provide meaningful guidelines for reducing infection risks in trauma patients with hemorrhagic shock. Vasoconstriction alters the normal distribution of antibiotics, resulting in reduced tissue penetration. To alleviate this problem, administered antibiotic doses may be increased two- to three-fold and repeated after every tenth unit of blood transfusion until there is no further blood loss. As the patient is resuscitated, antibiotics with activity against obligate and facultative anaerobic bacteria should be continued for periods dependent on the degree of identified wound contamination. Notably, aminoglycosides have been demonstrated to exhibit suboptimal activity in patients with serious injury, probably due to altered pharmacokinetics of drug distribution. Finally, a metaanalysis has examined studies assessing effectiveness of a single agent versus combination therapy containing aminoglycosides for penetrating wounds. This report concludes that single β-lactam agents were as effective as combination therapy in the setting of penetrating abdominal trauma.

Fewer data are available regarding the utilization of antibiotics in the patient following blunt injury. In the absence of monitoring device placement or the use of tube thoracostomy, antibiotics are not warranted. Many practitioners, however, believe Gram-positive antibiotic coverage is appropriate in the patient with tube thoracostomy or with invasive monitors of intracranial pressure. There are no randomized prospective data or multidisciplinary guidelines available to address this issue.

Thermal Injury

Thermal injury is a major public health problem for 2 to 2.5 million people who seek medical treatment in the United States each year. Thermal injury results in 100,000 to 150,000 hospitalizations and 6,000 to 12,000 fatalities. Death rates are highest in the very young and the very old. Thirty-eight percent of the victims are <15 years of age. An equal number of thermal injury victims are 15 to 44 years of age. Only 7% of thermal injury patients are >65 years old, but the mortality in this age group is significant. Scalds are the most common form of childhood thermal trauma while electrical and chemical injuries affect adults in the workplace. Factors shown to relate to mortality in thermal injury include the size of cutaneous involvement, age, and the presence or absence of inhalation injury. A discussion, based on available evidence, of optimal burn care, "Practice Guidelines for Burn Care," is slated for publication in the next several months. When available, appropriate care options will be available to all practitioners treating the burn patient.

Wound

Characteristics of skin affect patterns of cutaneous injury. Skin is very thin in infants and increases in thickness until 30 to 40 years of age. After this, skin progressively thins. Males have thicker skin than females. Average skin thickness is 1 to 2 mm. In general, dermis is ten times thicker than associated epidermis. Cell types in the epidermis are predominately keratinocytes and melanocytes. The latter cells provide pigment generation against ultraviolet radiation. The predominant cell type in the underlying dermis, which is derived from the mesoderm, is the fibroblast which produces collagen and elastin, ground substance of glycosaminoglycans and proteoglycans. The dermis itself consists of a superficial papillary dermis and a thicker reticular dermis.

The skin serves a number of critical functions. Unfortunately, all of these functions may be lost with thermal injury. Most importantly, the skin is a principal barrier against infection. Sebum (discussed in reference 8) has noted antibacterial properties. Skin also helps to maintain antigen presentation to immune cells and protects our fluid, protein, and electrolyte homeostasis. Skin has various sensory functions, affects heat preservation, and is associated with vitamin production.

In thermal injury, damage to the skin results from temperature of the thermal source and the duration of exposure. At 40° to 44°C, enzymatic failure occurs within the cell with rising intracellular sodium concentration and swelling due to failure of the membrane sodium pump. At exposure to 60°C, necrosis occurs in one hour with release of oxygen free radicals. Three cutaneous zones of injury have been described:

- The *zone of coagulation* is the site of irreversible cell death with new eschar formation from local degradation of protein.

- The *zone of stasis* is the site of local circulatory impairment with initial cell viability. If ischemia follows in this zone, cell death will occur. Impaired circulation is thought to be secondary to platelet and neutrophil aggregates, fibrin deposition, endothelial cell swelling, and loss of erythrocyte deformability. These tissues are susceptible to secondary insults such as dehydration, pressure, overresuscitation, and infection. Measures implemented to minimize further tissue loss include nondesiccating dressings, careful fluid resuscitation, and topical antimicrobials.

- The *zone of hyperemia* is characterized by minimal cellular injury but prominent vasodilation and increased blood flow. Cell recovery generally occurs in this zone.

Vasoactive mediators, including thromboxane A_2 with platelet adherence and vasoconstriction, are seen in the burn wound. Beyond the vasoconstricting effects seen in the zone of stasis, the predominant effect and resuscitation issue are significant vasodilation and increased vascular permeability. The initial increase in vascular permeability may be related to short-term histamine release occurring soon after injury. The second longer period of vasodilation and increased vascular permeability is related to the release of a variety of vasoactive and oxidative products.

Wound Care

The degree of injury is assessed by the well-known rule of nines (Fig 2). Anatomical criteria can also be employed to recognize the depth of injury and coincident likelihood of healing (Table 7). Partial-thickness injuries should heal within 3 weeks and leave the stratum germinosum intact. Third-degree or full-thickness injuries involve all layers of epidermis and dermis. Some authors speak also of fourth-degree injuries, which involve deep structures, such as tendon, muscle, and bone.

Local care begins with serial debridement of nonviable tissue and blisters. Topical antimicrobials, one of the major advances in burn wound care, are applied once or twice daily after washes with antiseptic solutions (Table 8). These topical antimicrobials are applied in occlusive dressings

Trauma and Thermal Injury

AREA	0 to 1	1 to 4	5 to 9	10 to 15	ADULT	% TOTAL
Head	19	17	13	10	7	
Neck	2	2	2	2	2	
Anterior Trunk	13	17	13	13	13	
Posterior Trunk	13	13	13	13	13	
Right Buttock	2.5	2.5	2.5	2.5	2.5	
Left Buttock	2.5	2.5	2.5	2.5	2.5	
Genitalia	1	1	1	1	1	
Right Upper Arm	4	4	4	4	4	
Left Upper Arm	4	4	4	4	4	
Right Lower Arm	3	3	3	3	3	
Left Lower Arm	3	3	3	3	3	
Right Hand	2.5	2.5	2.5	2.5	2.5	
Left Hand	2.5	2.5	2.5	2.5	2.5	
Right Thigh	5.5	5.5	8.5	8.5	9.5	
Left Thigh	5.5	5.5	8.5	8.5	9.5	
Right Leg	5	5	5.5	6	7	
Left Leg	5	5	5.5	6	7	
Right Foot	3.5	3.5	3.5	3.5	3.5	
Left Foot	3.5	3.5	3.5	3.5	3.5	
LUND & BROWDER CHART					**TOTAL**	

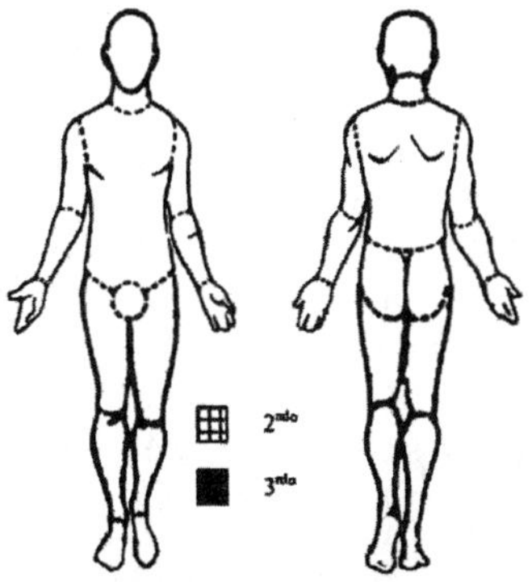

Figure 2.

which also help maintain fluid balance. The burn wound affords a warm, moist, protein-laden growth medium to Gram-positive and later Gram-negative bacteria. In general, systemic antibiotics are not employed in the initial days after injury.

Biologic dressings (cadaver allograft, porcine xenograft) are used for relatively clean wounds to reduce pain, bacterial colony counts, and fluid and protein loss. Rate of epithelialization is also increased, more so than with topical antimicrobials which tend to cause relative inhibition of wound epithelialization.

- Biologic dressings may be placed on newly debrided partial-thickness wounds in anticipation of healing without surgery.
- Biologic dressings cover granulating excised wounds awaiting autografts.
- Biologic dressings gauge readiness of a wound for autografting (via early "take").
- Biologic dressings may facilitate removal of necrotic tissue from granulating wounds.

Wound Excision

Excision of burned tissue which will clearly not heal (determined by clinical assessment) is generally performed within 3 to 5 days of injury. Generally, we do not excise >20% total body surface area (TBSA) at a time. If possible, wounds are covered with sheet or meshed autograft, harvested 3/ to 10/1000-inch thickness with a power

Table 7. *Classification of Burn Depth**

Degree of Burn	Depth of Tissue	Penetration Characteristics
First-degree	Partial thickness	Injury to the superficial epidermis, usually caused by overexposure to sunlight or brief heat flashes; classically described as sunburn.
Second-degree	Superficial partial thickness	Injury is to the epidermis and upper layers of the dermis. Wounds characteristically appear red, wet, or blistered, blanchable, and extremely painful. Will heal within 3 wk from epidermal regeneration from remaining remnants found in the tracts of hair follicles.
	Deep partial thickness	Injury is through the epidermis and may affect isolated areas of the deep thermal strata from which cells arise. This wound may appear red and wet or white and dry, depending on the extent of deep dermal damage. It heals without grafting but requires >3 wk with suboptimal cosmesis. Excision and split-thickness skin grafting are recommended.
Third-degree	Full thickness	Injury has destroyed both the epidermis and the dermis. The wound appears white, will not blanch, and is anesthetic. Tough, nonelastic, and tenacious coagulated protein (eschar) tissue may be present on the surface. This wound will not heal without surgical intervention.

*Reproduced with permission from the Society of Critical Care Medicine.

Table 8. *Topical Antimicrobial Agents**

Agent	Advantages	Disadvantages
Silver sulfadiazine	Painless application Broad spectrum Easy application Rare sensitivities	May produce transient leukopenia Minimal penetration of eschar Some Gram-negative species resistant
Mafenide acetate	Broad spectrum Easy application Penetrates eschar	Painful application Promotes acid-base imbalance Frequent sensitivity
Bacitracin, Polysporin	Painless application Nonirritating Transparent May be used on nonburn wounds	No eschar penetration
Silver nitrate (0.5% solution)	Painless application Broad spectrum Rare sensitivity Must be kept moist	No eschar penetration Electrolyte imbalances Discolors the wound and environment
Povidone-iodine	Broad spectrum	Painful application Systemically absorbed Requires frequent reapplication Discolors wounds
Gentamicin	Painless application Broad spectrum	Oto/nephrotoxic Encourages development of resistant organisms

*Reproduced with permission from the Society of Critical Care Medicine.

dermatome from unburned sites. Good harvest sites are the thighs, back, and scalp. Grafts can be meshed onto the burn area in a ratio from 1:1 to 1:9 to increase coverage with the assumption that the wound will reepithelialize within the mesh network. We generally do not use meshing >1:3 due to increased incidence of contractures and graft shear. Cadaveric allograft can be used to cover excised areas where donor skin is unavailable.

Sequential layered tangential excision of burned tissue is employed to reach viable tissue with visible punctate bleeding. While blood loss is greater with this method, cosmetic outcome is improved and the maximum amount of viable tissue is preserved. Excision to fascia is limited to large, full-thickness injuries, where the risks of blood loss and potential graft compromise from a suboptimal recipient bed may cause increased mortality.

Management of deeper thermal injury has always been complicated by loss of dermal tissue. Because the body does not naturally regenerate dermal tissue, surgeons are often left with few choices for wound coverage that will eventually result in minimal contraction and scarring. In addition, open wounds lead to fluid loss and an increase in metabolic rate which may impact overall physiologic condition of the patient.

Over the past decade, burn treatment has evolved to include early excision of necrotic tissue and immediate coverage of excised open wounds. A recent option for permanent wound coverage is a commercially available crosslinked collagen and chondronitin sulfate dermal replacement covered by a temporary silicone epidermal substitute. Within two to three weeks of application of this material, a new dermis forms and ultrathin autografts may then be placed over the neodermis. After healing, the synthetic dermis-supported skin graft appears to have histological structure and physical properties similar to those of normal skin.

A large postapproval study of this material was performed involving over 200 burn patients at 13 burn care centers. These patients had large injuries (average 36.5% TBSA). A low incidence of invasive infection or early application of the dermal substitute was noted (3.1%). Excellent mean rate of take for the dermal substitute was noted at an excess of 75%. Median take rate was 95%. Mean rate of healing for epidermal overlying autografts was 87% with a median healing rate of 98%. This large study supports the role of dermal substitutes as a standard of care for reconstruction of deep, large thermal injuries.

Burn Shock Resuscitation

Burn shock has both hypovolemic and cellular components. Mediator cascades and resuscitation strategies are based on fundamental observations of patients and animals following burn injury. The variety of resuscitation approaches available suggests the value of careful observation and adjustment of treatment based on patient clinical response.

Increased capillary permeability is one of the key components of the burn shock response. In small burns, maximal edema is seen in as little as 8 to 12 hours after injury, while larger burns manifest edema in a period of 12 to 24 hours post injury. The initial mediators seen after burn injury are histamine and bradykinin. Histamine release from mast cells in skin is seen early after injury but appears to be transient. The chief site of histamine action appears to be the venules. Blocker studies suggested that histamine explains only part of the early changes in burn wound permeability. Other mediators for vascular changes in burns include complement, prostaglandins, leukotrienes, stress hormones, and vasoactive amines.

- Prostaglandin (PG) E_2 and PGI_2 cause arterial dilation in burned tissue with increased blood and hydrostatic pressure favoring edema formation.
- Serotonin is released by platelet aggregation and serves to amplify the vasoconstrictive effect of norepinephrine and angiotensin II.
- Proteolytic cascades including coagulation, fibrinolysis, complement, and the kinin family have been found in activated states after burn injury.
- The end result of these changes is disruption of normal capillary barriers between interstitial and intravascular compartments with rapid equilibration between them.
- Plasma volume loss, manifested as hypovolemia, coincides with increased extracellular fluid.

Cellular Changes

Baxter (reviewed in references 14 and 15) described the cellular changes which provide the foundation of our present resuscitation strategies. He noted a decrease in cell membrane potential involving burned *and unburned* tissues. This potential change is associated with increased intracellular sodium, probably due to a decrease in sodium-ATP activity. Resuscitation only partly restores normal intracellular sodium and membrane potentials. Inadequate resuscitation leads to further decline in cell membrane potential and cell death. Later work on burn shock concluded that this phenomenon is due not only to intravascular hypovolemia but also extracellular sodium depletion.

Hemodynamic Response

Global hemodynamic changes include a decrease in extracellular fluid of as much as 30% to 50% in unresuscitated animal models by 18 hours after burn. In one study, cardiac output decreased to 25% of control at 4 hours after injury and increased to only 40% of control at 18 hours after a 30% TBSA injury. The principal site of volume loss was the functional extracellular intravascular fluid.

- Subsequent studies with salt solutions confirmed a variety of approaches to minimize extracellular fluid loss and maximize hemodynamic response in the first 24 hours after burn.
- During the first 24 hours, the work of Baxter showed that plasma volume changes were independent of the fluid type employed. Thus, colloids should not be used in the first 24 hours of burn resuscitation.
- After 24 hours, infused colloids can increase plasma volume by anticipated amounts as capillary integrity is restored.
- Peripheral vascular resistance was actually very high in the initial 24 hours after burn but decreased as cardiac output improved to supranormal levels coincident with the end of plasma and blood volume losses.

Burn wound edema is caused by dilation of precapillary arterioles and increased extravascular osmotic activity due to various products of thermal injury. All elements in the vascular space except red blood cells can escape from this site during the initial period of increased permeability.

Burn Resuscitation Strategies

In burn injury, intracellular and interstitial volume increase at the expense of plasma and blood volume. Edema formation is affected by resuscitation fluid administration. Thus, two principles are agreed upon:

- Give the least amount of fluid necessary to maintain adequate organ perfusion (as determined by vital signs, urine output, or function studies).
- Replace extracellular salt lost into cells and burned tissue with crystalloids and lactated Ringer's solution.

Probably the most popular resuscitation approach utilizes a modified Parkland formula, giving 4 mL/kg/% TBSA burn of fluid (lactated Ringer's solution) with half of the 24-hour volume required given in the first 8 hours. A variety of other formulas have been described (Table 9). All represent guidelines for the initiation of resuscitation. Continuation of this process requires perfusion as indicated by a urine output of 30 to 50 mL/hr in the adult. Hypoproteinemia and edema formation complicate the use of isotonic crystalloids for resuscitation. Hypertonic resuscitation solutions have the theoretical advantages of improved hemodynamic response and diminished overall fluid needs as intracellular water is shifted into the extracellular space by the hyperosmolar solution. A clear role for hypertonic resuscitation has not yet been defined. Some groups add colloid to resuscitation fluids as protein formulations or dextran after the first 8 hours when much of the capillary leak has subsided. Groups most likely to benefit from supplemental colloid are the elderly, those patients with large burns (>50% TBSA), and/or patients who have inhalation injury. Inhalation injury increases the overall fluid requirement of the burned patient from volume and total salt requirement standpoints.

Table 9. Resuscitation Formulas*†

Formula	Calculation: First 24 Hours	Calculation: Thereafter
Parkland	4 L/kg/% TBSA burn lactated Ringer's solution Give 50% total volume during first 8 h after burn and the remaining 50% over the subsequent 16 h	% dextrose in water, K, plasma to maintain normal serum sodium and K levels and colloid oncotic pressure
Brooke	2 mL/kg/% TBSA burn lactated Ringer's solution Give 50% total volume during the first 8 h after burn and the remaining 50% over the subsequent 16 h	Maintain urine output 0.5 to 1.0 mL/kg/h
Shrine	5000 mL/m² TBSA burn + 2000 mL/m² BSA lactated Ringer's solution Give 50% total volume during the first 8 h after burn and the remaining 50% over the subsequent 16 h	3750 mL/m² TBSA burn + 1500 mL/m² BSA May replace intravenous fluid with enteral feedings if GI function is normal

*TBSA = total body surface area; K = potassium; BSA = body surface area; GI = gastrointestinal.
†Reproduced with permission from the Society of Critical Care Medicine.

Overall, patients in good health with burns of <40% TBSA can be resuscitated with crystalloids alone. Where coexistent injury, comorbid conditions, limited cardiac reserve, and inhalation injury complicate burn trauma, a combination of crystalloid and colloids may be optimally employed. The resuscitation target is generally 30 to 50 mL/h of urine output with acceptable vital signs. In the patient with complicated trauma or thermal injury management, a pulmonary artery catheter may be needed.

Patients receiving crystalloid resuscitation will frequently require supplemental colloid during the second 24 hours after burn injury. Maintenance fluids must include allowance for evaporative losses. This fluid may come from intravenous repletion or enteral feeding. Evaporative losses = (25 + % TBSA burn) × BSA (in m²) × 24 hours. Potassium, calcium, magnesium, and phosphorus losses should be monitored and aggressively replaced. After 24 to 48 hours, a urine output of 30 to 50 mL/h is an inadequate guide to perfusion, due to relative osmotic diuresis with the metabolite loss of burns and deranged antidiuretic hormone metabolism. Adults require 1500 to 2000 mL/24 hours of urine output to excrete the osmolar products of large burns. Serum sodium concentration, weight change, intake and output records, and physical examination also guide ongoing fluid administration.

Inhalation Injury

Inhalation injury has emerged as a persisting cause of increased mortality in burn victims. Upper airway injury is frequently due to direct heat exposure, while laryngeal reflexes protect the lung from thermal injury in all cases except possibly high-pressure steam exposure. The upper airway is also an extremely efficient heat sink. Lower airway injury is predominantly due to chemical products of combustion carried to the lung on particles of soot (particle size 5-μm).

To a degree that varies unpredictably among affected patients, inhalation injury causes several physiologic derangements including:

- Loss of airway patency secondar to mucosal edema
- Bronchospasm secondary to inhaled irritants
- Intrapulmonary shunting from small airway occlusion caused by mucosal edema and sloughed endobronchial debris
- Diminished compliance secondary to alveolar flooding and collapse with mismatching of ventilation and perfusion
- Pneumonia and tracheobronchitis secondary to loss of ciliary clearance endotracheal bronchial epithelium
- Respiratory failure secondary to a combination of the above factors.

Injuries evolve over time and parenchymal lung dysfunction is often minimal for 24 to 72 hours.

- Aldehydes, oxides of sulfur and hydrochloric acid, combine with water in the lung to yield corrosive acids and oxygen radicals. Degradation of polyvinyl chloride, for example, yields up to 75 toxic compounds.
- Carbon monoxide exposure is also associated with inhalation injury but does *not* define this process as the true degree of exposure to carbon monoxide is frequently not detected. The half-life of carboxyhemoglobin in room air is 4 hours, 30 minutes at 100% oxygen. Therefore, increased carboxyhemoglobin levels are not often found.
- Diagnosis of inhalation injury is most commonly made with bronchoscopy which reveals airway edema, erythema, soot accumulation, and sometimes mucosal sloughing. This test picks up far more injuries than standard clinical criteria including history of closed-space burn injury, facial burns *with* nasal hair singeing, wheezing, and soot in the sputum. Chest radiography is frequently normal on hospital admission and hypoxia on blood gases is not frequently seen.

Chemical injury to the lung stimulates release of substances including histamine, serotonin, and kallikreins with recruitment of leukocytes to airways and lung parenchyma. Edema of airway mucosa and sloughing can combine with formation of plugs of fibrin and purulent material to create casts, which obstruct small airways. Neutrophils and other activated inflammatory cells also release oxygen radicals and lytic enzymes, which magnify tissue change. Pulmonary edema is also seen due to increased capillary permeability, which is magnified by cutaneous burns if present. Patients with cutaneous injury alone do not increase extravascular lung water.

Three stages of clinical inhalation injury have been identified. Acute hypoxia with asphyxia typically occurs at the fire scene, sometimes in association with high carbon monoxide exposure, and is followed by acute upper airway and pulmonary edema. Pulmonary edema with acute airway swelling usually resolves by the passage of the first several days after injury. Later complications are infections with the morbidity of pneumonia complicating that of inhalation exposure to heat and chemical irritants.

Optimal initial management of inhalation injury requires directed assessment and assurance of airway patency. Prophylactic intubation is not indicated for a diagnosis of inhalation injury alone. However, if there is concern over progressive edema, intubation should be strongly considered. Intubation is indicated if upper airway patency is threatened, gas exchange or compliance mandate mechanical ventilatory support, or mental status is inadequate for airway protection. Prophylactic use of steroids and antibiotics is not indicated in the initial management of inhalation injury. In patients requiring mechanical ventilatory support, transpulmonary inflating pressures over 40 cm H_2O should be avoided except in exceptional circumstances (*eg*, pH < 7.2 or Pao_2 < 60 mm Hg), or if impaired chest wall compliance suggests that inflating pressures measured at the endotracheal tube did not reflect transpulmonary pressures. Any mode of mechanical ventilation consistent with these limits is appropriate. Survivors of inhalation injury may have permanent pulmonary dysfunction, late endobronchial bleeding from granulation tissue, and upper airway stenosis. While there is no specific therapy for inhalation injury, proper initial management can have a favorable influence on outcome. Management goals during the first 24 hours are to prevent suffocation by assuring airway patency, to assure adequate oxygenation and ventilation, to forego the use of agents that may complicate subsequent care, and to avoid ventilator-induced lung injury.

In any situation where carbon monoxide exposure is possible, 100% oxygen should be provided to eliminate carbon monoxide. Resuscitation fluid administration should not be delayed or withheld in inhalation injury patients. These individuals may, in fact, require additional fluid. Humidification of inhaled gases may help to reduce desiccation injury. The role of early hyperbaric oxygen is minimized in the burn care community but remains popular among pulmonologists; prospective randomized clinical data are limited. Heparin nebulization is now employed in some centers over the initial days after inhalation injury due to presumed mucolytic and anti-inflammatory effects. This process may stimulate expectoration of accumulated proteinaceous material.

Carbon Monoxide Poisoning

Carbon monoxide poisoning is a serious health problem resulting in approximately 40,000 visits to emergency departments annually in the United States. In thermal injury, it may be a significant source of additional morbidity. Cognitive sequelae (memory, attention span or concentration, and affect) may occur immediately after exposure and persist or can be delayed. In general, neurologic changes occur within 20 days after carbon monoxide exposure. Cognitive sequelae lasting one month or more appear to occur in 25 to 50% of patients with loss of consciousness or carboxyhemoglobin levels greater than 25%. Recommended treatment for acute carbon monoxide intoxication is 100% normobaric oxygen. This is commonly delivered through a face mask or endotracheal tube. Hyperbaric oxygen therapy is sometimes recommended for patients with acute carbon monoxide poisoning, particularly if they have lost consciousness or have high carboxyhemoglobin levels.

Carbon monoxide is a colorless, odorless and nonirritant gas, which is easily absorbed through the lungs. The amount of gas absorbed is dependent on minute ventilation, duration of exposure, and relative concentrations of carbon monoxide and oxygen in the environment. Carbon monoxide is principally eliminated by the lungs as an unchanged gas. Less than 1% is oxidized to carbon dioxide. Ten to fifteen percent of carbon monoxide is bound to proteins including myoglobin and cytochrome C oxidase. Less than 1% of carbon monoxide exists in solution. Carbon monoxide toxicity appears to result from a combination of tissue hypoxia and direct carbon monoxide-mediated damage at the cellular level. Carbon monoxide competes with oxygen for binding to hemoglobin. The affinity of hemoglobin for carbon monoxide is 200 to 250 times greater than its affinity for oxygen. The consequences of this competitive binding are a shift in the oxygen hemoglobin dissociation curve to the left and its alteration to a hyperbolic shape. These alterations result in impaired release of oxygen at the tissue level and cellular hypoxia.

Notably, binding of carbon monoxide to hemoglobin alone does not account for all of the pathophysiologic consequences noted. In animal studies, transfusion of blood with highly saturated carboxyhemoglobin but minimal free carbon monoxide does not reproducibly result in clinical symptoms. Perhaps, the small fraction of free carbon monoxide in plasma has an important role. Other studies suggest that carbon monoxide-induced tissue hypoxia may be followed by reoxygenation injury, particularly to the central nervous system. Hyperoxygenation facilitates the production of partially reduced oxygen species, which in turn may oxidize essential protein and nucleic acids resulting in classic reperfusion injury. In addition, carbon monoxide exposure has been shown to cause degradation of unsaturated fatty acids culminating in reversible demyelination of central nervous system lipids. Carbon monoxide exposure creates oxidative stress with production of oxygen radicals resulting from the conversion of xanthene dehydrogenase to xanthene oxidase.

In the setting of pregnancy, greater sensitivity of the fetus to harmful effects of carbon monoxide has been noted. Data from animal studies suggest a lag time in carbon monoxide uptake between the mother and the fetus. Fetal studies state that carbon monoxide levels occur up to 40 hours after maternal steady-state levels are achieved. Final carboxyhemoglobin levels in the fetus may significantly exceed levels in the mother. Exaggerated leftward shift of the fetal carboxyhemoglobin dissociation curve makes tissue hypoxia more severe by causing even less oxygen to be released to fetal tissues.

Hyperbaric oxygen has been proposed as a treatment for acute carbon monoxide exposure. Reported advantages include increased dissolved oxygen content in the blood and accelerated elimination of carbon monoxide. Potential benefits of hyperbaric oxygen treatment include prevention of lipid peroxidation in the central nervous system and preservation of ATP levels in tissue exposed to carbon monoxide. Significant disadvantages of hyperbaric oxygen therapy include the risks associated with transport of patients and maintenance of critically ill individuals in the hyperbaric setting. Recent work with patients experiencing significant carbon monoxide exposure in the absence of significant thermal injury suggests that neurologic outcome measured at six weeks and twelve months after acute exposure will improve with acute hyperbaric oxygen administration. Notably, the patient sustaining significant thermal cutaneous injury is not represented in these studies. The optimal management of carbon monoxide exposure in the setting of significant thermal cutaneous injury remains unclear and the challenges of early administration of hyperbaric oxygen in the setting of multisystem trauma remain daunting.

Outcome

Currently, three papers have detailed the outcome for burn-injured patients. The first paper is from the American Burn Association Patient Registry, the largest and best organized body of data on burn-injured patients. Between 1991 and 1993, >6,000 patients were registered at 28 burn centers. The mean burn size was 14% of the TBSA. The overall survival rate was 95.9%. However, the mortality rate among patients with inhalation injury was 29.4%. In young adults, the size of burn that was felt to be lethal to 50% of these patients was 81% of TBSA. In the total population studied, mean length of hospital stay was 13.5 days.

A second review of >1,600 patients admitted to Massachusetts General Hospital and the Schriners' Burn Institute in Boston was published in early 1998. Logistic progression analysis was employed to develop probability estimates for mortality based on a small set of well-defined variables. Mean burn size and survival were similar to the larger report above. The following three risk factors for death were identified:

- Age >60 years
- TBSA burned, >40%
- Inhalation injury

The mortality formula developed from these data predicts 0.3%, 3%, 33%, or 90% mortality depending on whether 0, 1, 2, or 3 risk factors are present.

Case Fatality Rates

Trends in mortality according to age among adult burn patients have recently been examined over a 25-year period. In this important study, patients admitted to a regional burn center between 1973 and 1997 were divided into three age groups (18 to 34, 35 to 54 and 55 and older) and mortality rates were examined over time (Table 10).

Table 10. *Case Fatality Rates**

Age (yr)	Mid 1970s	Mid 1990s
18–34	11.6	3.9
35–54	22.9	6.6
≥ 55	51.0	20.8

*McGwin G Jr, Cross JM, Ford JW, et al. Long-term trends morality according to age among adult burn patients. J Burn Care Rehabil 2003; 24:21–25

Examination of relative rates of mortality suggests a reduction in death among adult burn patients across the age spectrum over the 25-year study. Reduction in mortality is greatest for young patients at approximately 3%/year while the middle-aged group saw an annual change in mortality of approximately 2%/year and the older patients saw a decline in mortality of approximately 1%/year.

Suggested Reading

General Trauma Management

1. Trunkey DD, Lewis FR, eds. Current therapy of trauma. 4th ed. St Louis, MO: Mosby, 1999
2. Moore EE, Feliciano DV, Mattox KL, eds. Trauma. 5th ed. New York, NY: McGraw-Hill, 2004

Chest Trauma

3. Sheridan R, Peralta R, Rhea J, et al. Reformatted visceral protocol helical computed tomographic scanning allows conventional radiographs of the thoracic and lumbar spine to be eliminated in the evaluation of blunt trauma patients. J Trauma 2003; 55:665–669
4. Miller PR, Croce MA, Bee TK, et al. ARDS after pulmonary contusion: accurate measurement of contusion volume identifies high risk patients. J Trauma 2001; 51:223–230
5. Malhotra AK, Fabian TC, Croce DS, et al. Minimal aortic injury: a lesion associated with advancing diagnostic techniques. J Trauma 2001; 51:1042–1048
6. Cohn SM. Pulmonary contusion: review of the clinical entity. J Trauma 1997; 42:973–979
7. Richardson JD: Outcome of tracheobronchial injuries: a long-term perspective. J Trauma 2004; 56:30–36

8. Mayberry JC, Terhes JT, Ellis TJ, et al. Absorbable plates for rib fracture repair: preliminary experience. J Trauma 2003; 55:835–839

ICU Resuscitation

9. McKinley BA, Kozar RA, Cocanour CS, et al. Normal versus supranormal oxygen delivery goals in shock resuscitation: the response is the same. J Trauma 2002; 53:825–832
10. McKinley BA, Kozar RA, Cocanour CS, et al. Standardized trauma resuscitation: female hearts respond better. Arch Surg 2002; 137:578–584
11. Balogh Z, McKinley BA, Cocanour CS, et al. Supranormal trauma resuscitation causes more cases of abdominal compartment syndrome. Arch Surg 2003; 138:637–643
12. McKinley BA, Marvin RG, Cocanour CS, et al. Blunt trauma resuscitation: the old can respond. Arch Surg 2000; 135:688–695

Damage Control

13. Shapiro MB, Jenkins DH, Schwab CW, et al. Damage control: collective review. J Trauma 2000; 49:969–978
14. Johnson JW, Gracias VH, Schwab CW, et al. Evolution in damage control for exsanguinating penetrating abdominal injury. J Trauma 2001; 51:261–271
15. Rotondo MF, Schwab CW, McGonigal MD, et al. "Damage control:" an approach for improved survival in exsanguination penetrating abdominal injury. J Trama 1993; 35:375–383

Abdominal Compartment Syndrome

16. Schein M, Wittmann DH, Aprahamian C, et al. The abdominal compartment syndrome: the physiological and clinical consequences of elevated intra-abdominal pressure. J Am Coll Surg 1995; 180:745–753
17. Chang MM, Miller PR, D'Agostino R Jr, et al. Effect of abdominal decompression on cardiopulmonary function and visceral perfusion in patients with intra-abdominal hypertension. J Trauma 1998; 44:440–445
18. Cheatham ML, White MW, Sagraves SG, et al. Abdominal perfusion pressure: a superior parameter in the assessment of intra-abdominal hypertension. J Trauma 2000; 49:621–627

Abdominal Organ Injury

19. Bee TK, Croce MA, Miller PR, et al. Failures of splenic nonoperative management: is the glass half empty or half full? J Trauma 2001; 50:230–236
20. Peitzman AB, Heil B, Rivera L, et al. Blunt splenic injury in adults: Multi-institutional study. J Trauma 2000; 49:177–189
21. Richardson JD, Franklin GA, Lukan JK, et al. Evolution in the management of hepatic trauma: a 25-year perspective. Ann Surg 2000; 232:324–330
22. Malhotra AK, Fabian TC, Katsis SB, et al. Blunt bowel and mesenteric injuries: the role of screening computed tomography. J Trauma 2000; 49:991–1000
23. Killeen KL, Shanmuganathan K, Poletti PA, et al. Helical computed tomography of bowel and mesenteric injuries. J Trauma 2001; 51:26–36
24. Velmahos GC, Toutouzas K, Radin R, et al. High success with nonoperative management of blunt hepatic trauma. Arch Surg 2003; 138:475–481
25. Omert LA, Salyer D, Dunham M, et al. Implications of the "contrast blush" finding on computed tomographic scan of the spleen in trauma. J Trauma 2001; 51:272–278
26. Ochsner MG, Knudson MM, Pachter L, et al. Significance of minimal or no intraperitoneal fluid visible on CT scan associated with blunt liver and splenic injuries: a multicenter analysis. J Trauma 2000; 49:505–510
27. Haan J, Ilahi ON, Kramer M, et al. Protocol-driven nonoperative management in patients with blunt splenic trauma and minimal associated injury decreases length of stay. J Trauma 2003; 55:317–322
28. Mohr AM, Lavery RF, Barone A, et al. Angiographic embolization for liver injuries: low mortality, high morbidity. J Trauma 2003; 55:1077–1082
29. Harbrecht BG, Zenati MS, Ochoa JB, et al. Management of adult blunt splenic injuries: comparison between level I and level II trauma centers. J Am Coll Surg 2004; 198:232–239

Management Guidelines for Common Problems in the Initial Care of Injury

30. Pasqulae M, Fabian TC. Practice management guidelines for trauma from Eastern Association for the Surgery of Trauma. J Trauma 1998; 44:941–956

31. Luchette FA, Borzotta AP, Croce MA, et al. Practice management guidelines for prophylactic antibiotic use in penetrating abdominal trauma: the EAST practice management guidelines workgroup. J Trauma 2000; 48:508–518

Head Injury

32. Letarte P. Brain and spinal cord injury. In: Roberts PR, ed. Multidisciplinary critical care board review course. Anaheim, CA: Society of Critical Care Medicine, 1998, 613–630
33. Gress DR, Diringer MN, Green DM, Mayer SA, et al, eds. Neurological and neurosurgical intensive care. Philadelphia, PA: Lippincott Williams & Wilkins, 2004
34. Brain Trauma Foundation. Management and prognosis of severe traumatic brain injury. J Neurotrauma 2000; 17:449–627
35. Rosner MJ, Daughton S. Cerebral perfusion pressure in the management of head injury. J Trauma 1996; 30:933–941
36. Marion DW, ed. Traumatic brain injury. New York, NY: Thieme, 1999
37. Sarrafzadeh AS, Peltonen EE, Kaisers U, et al. Secondary insults in severe head injury-do multiply injured patients do worse? Crit Care Med 2001; 29:1116–1123

General Burn Management

38. Herndon DN, ed. Total burn care, 2nd ed. London, England: WB Saunders, 2002
39. Monafo WW. Initial management of burns. N Engl J Med 1996; 335:1581–1586

Burn Outcome

40. Saffle JR, Davis B, Williams P. Recent outcomes in the treatment of burn injury in the United States: a report from the American Burn Association Patient Registry. J Burn Care Rehabil 1995; 16:219–232
41. Ryan CM, Schoenfield DA, Thorpe WP, et al. Objective estimates of the probability of death from burn injuries. N Engl J Med 1998; 338:362–366
42. McGwin G, Cross JM, Ford JW, et al. Long-term trends in mortality according to age among adult burn patients. J Burn Care Rehabil 2003; 24:21–25
43. Heimbach DM, Warden GD, Luterman A, et al. Multicenter postapproval clinical trial of Integra® dermal regeneration template for burn treatment. J Burn Care Rehabil 2003; 24:42–48

Hyperbaric Oxygen/Carbon Monoxide

44. Tibbles PM, Edelsberg JS. Hyperbaric oxygen therapy. N Engl J Med 1996; 334:1642–1648
45. Ernst A, Zibrak JD. Carbon monoxide poisoning. N Engl J Med 1998; 339:1603–1608
46. Weaver LK, Hopkins RO, Chan KJ, et al. Hyperbaric oxygen for acute carbon monoxide poisoning. N Engl J Med 2002; 347:1057–1067
47. Wang C, Schwaitzberg S, Berliner E, et al. Hyperbaric oxygen for treating wounds: a systematic review of the literature. Arch Surg 2003; 138:272–279

Notes

Notes

Mechanical Ventilation

Gregory A. Schmidt, MD, FCCP

Objectives:

- To describe the role of the ventilator in determining respiratory mechanics
- To recommend disease-specific ventilator strategies aimed at reducing the adverse consequences of mechanical ventilation
- To review new information regarding ventilation in ARDS
- To address the role of noninvasive ventilation
- To discuss the complications of mechanical ventilation

Key words: ARDS; assist-control ventilation; COPD; inverse ratio ventilation; mechanical ventilation; noninvasive ventilation; pressure control; pressure support; status asthmaticus; synchronized intermittent mandatory ventilation; tidal volume

---

This lecture offers an approach in which the ventilator is used as a probe of the patient's respiratory system mechanical derangements, and then the ventilator settings are tailored to the patient's mechanical and gas exchange abnormalities. This facilitates early stabilization of the patient on the ventilator in such a way as to optimize carbon dioxide removal and oxygen delivery within the limits of abnormal neuromuscular function, lung mechanics, and gas exchange.

The fundamental purpose of mechanical ventilation is to assist in elimination of carbon dioxide and uptake of adequate oxygen while the patient is unable to do so or should not be allowed to do so. Such patients fall into two main groups: (1) those in whom full rest of the respiratory muscles is indicated (such as during shock; severe, acute pulmonary derangement; or deep sedation or anesthesia), and (2) those in whom some degree of respiratory muscle use is desired (*eg*, to strengthen or improve the coordination of the respiratory muscles; to assess the ability of the patient to sustain the work of breathing; or to begin spontaneous ventilation). It is important for the intensivist to be explicit about whether the respiratory muscles should be rested or exercised because the details of ventilation (mode, settings) usually follow logically from this fundamental point.

If full rest of the respiratory muscles is desired, it is incumbent on the physician to assure that this is indeed achieved. Although some patients are fully passive while being ventilated (those with deep sedation, some forms of coma, metabolic alkalosis, sleep-disordered breathing), most patients will make active respiratory efforts, even on assist-control ventilation (ACV), at times performing extraordinary amounts of work. Unintended patient effort can be difficult to recognize but, aside from obvious patient effort, may be signaled by an inspiratory fall in intrathoracic pressure (as noted on a central venous or pulmonary artery pressure tracing, or with an esophageal balloon) or by triggering of the ventilator. Recognizing patient effort has been greatly aided by the provision of real-time displays of flow and pressure waveforms, now commonly available on modern ventilators.

Choosing a ventilatory mode and settings appropriate for each individual patient depends not only on the physician's goals (rest vs exercise), but also on knowledge of the mechanical properties of the patient's respiratory system. Most ventilators now have the capability of displaying waveforms of pressure, flow, and volume vs time, as well as flow vs volume. Using waveforms, it is easiest to gather information regarding the patient-ventilator interaction when patients are ventilated with a volume-preset mode (ACV or synchronized intermittent mandatory ventilation [SIMV]). Still, some useful information can be gleaned from waveforms during pressure-preset ventilation (pressure-support ventilation [PSV] and pressure-control ventilation [PCV]).

The first step is to seek signs of inspiratory effort in the pressure tracing. Respiratory muscle contraction does not cease in most patients receiving mechanical ventilation, even in the ACV mode. Thus, it is possible that a weak patient will remain weak, through continued breathing effort, despite the institution of mechanical support. In volume-preset modes, the signs of persistent effort include the presence of triggering, concavity during inspiration, and a variable peak airway opening pressure (Ppeak). When the goal of ventilation is to rest the respiratory muscles, ventilator adjustments, psychological measures, and pharmacologic sedation. Ventilator strategies to reduce the patient's work of breathing include increasing the minute ventilation to reduce Pco_2 (although this may run counter to other goals of ventilation, especially in patients with ARDS or severe obstruction), increasing the inspiratory flow rate, and changing the mode to pressure-preset ventilation (PSV or PCV). Only rarely is therapeutic paralysis required to achieve ventilatory goals.

The next step is to determine whether the patient has significant airflow obstruction. This can be inferred by inserting a brief end-inspiratory pause, then determining the difference between Ppeak and plateau airway pressure (Pplat). Alternatively, one can examine the expiratory flow waveform, seeking low flow and prolonged expiration, signs that are present regardless of the mode of ventilation (ACV, SIMV, PSV, PCV). Bronchodilator therapy can be assessed by noting whether expiratory flow increases, the expiratory time (TE) shortens, or there is a reduction in Ppeak, Pplat, or auto-positive end-expiratory pressure (autoPEEP).

Finally, one should assure that the patient and ventilator are synchronized, ie, that each attempt by the patient to trigger the ventilator generates a breath. The most common situation in which the patient fails to trigger breaths occurs in severe obstruction when autoPEEP is present. This is recognized at the bedside when the patient makes obvious efforts that fail to produce a breath. Using waveforms, these ineffective efforts cause a temporary slowing of expiratory flow, sometimes halting it completely.

Modes of Mechanical Ventilation

Technologic innovations have provided a plethora of differing modes by which a patient can be mechanically ventilated.[1] Various modes have been developed with the hope of improving gas exchange, patient comfort, or speed of return to spontaneous ventilation. Aside from minor subtleties, however, nearly all modes allow full rest of the patient, on the one hand, or substantial exercise on the other. Thus, in the great majority of patients, choice of mode is merely a matter of patient or physician preference. Noninvasive ventilation should be considered before intubation and ventilation in many patients who are hemodynamically stable and do not require an artificial airway, especially those with acute-on-chronic respiratory failure, postoperative respiratory failure, and cardiogenic pulmonary edema.

During volume-preset ventilation (and assuming a passive patient), Pplat is determined by the tidal volume (VT) and the static compliance of the respiratory system (Crs):

$$Pplat = V_T/Crs + PEEP$$

where PEEP (positive end-expiratory pressure) also includes autoPEEP.

On the other hand, in pressure-preset modes, a fixed inspiratory pressure (Pinsp) is applied to the respiratory system, whatever the resulting VT. However, the VT is predictable (again, assuming a passive patient) when the Crs is known:

$$V_T = (Pinsp - PEEP) \times Crs$$

assuming time for equilibration between Pinsp and alveolar pressure. Thus, a patient with static Crs of 50 mL/cm H_2O ventilated on ACV at a VT of 500 mL with no PEEP (or autoPEEP) will have a Pplat of about 10 cm H_2O, while the same patient ventilated on PCV at 10 cm H_2O will have a VT of about 500 mL. Thus, while physicians' comfort level with volume-preset and pressure-preset modes may be very different, the modes can be similar as they are tied to each other through the patient's Crs.

A potential advantage of pressure-preset ventilation is greater physician control over the Ppeak (since Ppeak = Pinsp) and the peak alveolar pressure, which could lessen the incidence of ventilator-induced lung injury. However, this same reduction in volutrauma risk should be attainable during volume-preset ventilation if a VT appropriate to the lung derangement is chosen. Indeed, the ARDSNet trial, which demonstrated a mortality reduction in the low-VT group, used ACV and a VT of 6 mL/kg. Nevertheless, pressure-preset modes make such a lung-protection strategy easier to carry out by dispensing with the need to repeatedly determine Pplat and periodically adjust the V_T. During use of pressure-preset modes, the patient also has greater control over inspiratory flow rate, and therefore potentially increased comfort. A disadvantage of pressure-preset modes is that changes in respiratory system mechanics (eg, increased airflow resistance or lung stiffness) or patient effort may decrease the minute ventilation, necessitating alarms for adequate ventilation. Also, the mechanics cannot be readily determined.

In the following descriptions, each mode is first illustrated for a passive patient, such as following muscle paralysis, then for the more common situation in which the patient plays an active role in ventilation. On some ventilators, V_T can be selected by the physician or respiratory therapist, while on others a minute ventilation and respiratory rate (f) are chosen, secondarily determining the V_T. Similarly, on some machines an inspiratory flow rate is selected, while on others flow depends on the ratio of inspiratory time (T_I) to total respiratory cycle time and f, or an inspiratory to expiratory (I:E) ratio and f.

Conventional Modes of Ventilation

Assist-Control Ventilation: Passive Patient—The set parameters of the assist-control mode are the inspiratory flow rate, frequency (f), and V_T. The ventilator delivers f equal breaths per minute, each of V_T volume. V_T and flow determine the T_I, T_E, and the I:E ratio. Pplat is related to the V_T and the compliance of the respiratory system, while the difference between Ppeak and Pplat includes contributions from flow and inspiratory resistance.

Active Patient—The patient has the ability to trigger extra breaths by exerting an inspiratory effort exceeding the preset trigger sensitivity, each at the set V_T and flow, and to thereby change T_I, T_E, and I:E ratio, and to potentially create or increase autoPEEP. Typically, each patient will display a preferred rate for a given V_T and will trigger all breaths when the controlled ventilator frequency is set a few breaths/min below the patient's rate; in this way, the control rate serves as an adequate support should the patient stop initiating breaths. When high inspiratory effort continues during the ventilator-delivered breath, the patient may trigger a second, superimposed ("stacked") breath (rarely a third as well). Patient effort can be increased (if the goal is to exercise the patient) by increasing the magnitude of the trigger or by lowering V_T (which increases the rate of assisting). Lowering f at the same V_T generally has no effect on work of breathing when the patient is initiating all breaths.

Synchronized Intermittent Mandatory Ventilation: In the passive patient, SIMV cannot be distinguished from controlled ventilation in the ACV mode. Ventilation is determined by the mandatory f and V_T. However, if the patient is not truly passive, he may perform respiratory work during the mandatory breaths. More to the point of the SIMV mode, he can trigger additional breaths by lowering the airway opening pressure below the trigger threshold. If this triggering effort comes in a brief, defined interval before the next mandatory breath is due, the ventilator will deliver the mandatory breath ahead of schedule in order to synchronize with the patient's inspiratory effort. If a breath is initiated outside of the synchronization window, V_T, flow, and I:E ratio are determined by patient effort and respiratory system mechanics, not by ventilator settings. The spontaneous breaths tend to be of small volume and are highly variable from breath to breath. The SIMV mode is often used to gradually augment the patient's work of breathing by lowering the mandatory breath f (or V_T), driving the patient to breathe more rapidly in order to maintain adequate ventilation, but this approach appears to prolong weaning.[2,3] Although this mode continues to be used widely, there is little rationale for it and SIMV is falling out of favor.

Pressure-Control Ventilation: In the passive patient, ventilation is determined by f, the inspiratory pressure increment (Pinsp − PEEP), I:E ratio, and the time constant of the patient's respiratory system. In patients without severe obstruction (ie, time constant not elevated) given a sufficiently long T_I, there is equilibration between the ventilator-determined Pinsp and alveolar pressure (Palv) so that inspiratory flow ceases. In this situation, V_T is highly predictable, based on Pinsp (= Palv), and the mechanical properties of the respiratory system (Crs). In the presence of severe obstruction or if T_I is too short to allow equilibration between ventilator and alveoli, V_T will fall below that predicted based on Pinsp and Crs.

The active patient can trigger additional breaths by reducing the airway opening pressure (Pao) below the triggering threshold, raising the I:E ratio. The inspiratory reduction in pleural pressure combines with the ventilator Pinsp to augment the transpulmonary pressure and the VT. Because TI is generally set by the physician, care must be taken to discern the patient's neural TI (from the waveforms display) and adjust the ventilator accordingly; otherwise, additional sedation might be necessary.

Pressure-Support Ventilation: The patient must trigger the ventilator in order to activate this mode, so pressure support is not applied to passive patients. Ventilation is determined by Pinsp, patient-determined f, and patient effort. Once a breath is triggered, the ventilator attempts to maintain Pao at the physician-determined Pinsp, using whatever flow is necessary to achieve this. Eventually flow begins to fall as a result of either cessation of the patient's inspiratory effort or increasing elastic recoil of the respiratory system as VT rises. The ventilator will maintain a constant Pinsp until inspiratory flow falls an arbitrary amount (*eg*, to 20% of initial flow) or below an absolute flow rate. The patient's work of breathing can be increased by lowering Pinsp or making the trigger less sensitive, and can inadvertently increase if respiratory system mechanics change, despite no change in ventilator settings. Respiratory system mechanical parameters cannot be determined readily on this mode because the ventilator and patient contributions to VT and flow are not represented by Pao; accordingly, these important measurements of Pplat, Ppeak – Pplat, and autoPEEP are measured during a brief, daily switch from PSV to volume-preset ventilation. A potential advantage of PSV is improved patient comfort and, for patients with very high drive, reduced work of breathing compared with volume-preset modes.

Mixed Modes: Some ventilators allow combinations of modes, most commonly SIMV plus PSV. There is little reason to use such a hybrid mode, although some physicians use the SIMV as a means to add sighs to PSV, an option not otherwise generally available. Because SIMV plus PSV guarantees some backup minute ventilation (which PSV does not), this mode combination may have value in occasional patients at high risk for abrupt deterioration in central drive.

Triggered Sensitivity: In the assist-control, SIMV, and pressure-support modes, the patient must lower the Pao below a preset threshold in order to "trigger" the ventilator. In most situations, this is straightforward: The more negative the sensitivity, the greater the effort demanded of the patient. This can be used intentionally to increase the work of breathing when the goal is to strengthen the inspiratory muscles. When autoPEEP is present, however, the patient must lower Palv by the autoPEEP amount in order to have any impact on Pao, then further by the trigger amount to initiate a breath. This can dramatically increase the required effort for breath initiation.

Flow-triggering systems ("flow-by") have been used to further reduce the work of triggering the ventilator. In contrast to the usual approach in which the patient must open a demand valve in order to receive ventilatory assistance, continuous-flow systems maintain a continuous high flow, then further augment flow when the patient initiates a breath. These systems can reduce the work of breathing slightly below that present when using conventional demand valves, but do not solve the problem of triggering when autoPEEP is present.

Unconventional Ventilatory Modes

Inverse-Ratio Ventilation: Inverse-ratio ventilation (IRV) is defined as a mode in which the I:E ratio is >1. There are two general ways to apply IRV: pressure-controlled IRV (PC-IRV), in which a preset airway pressure is delivered for a fixed period of time at an I:E ratio >1, or volume-controlled IRV (VC-IRV), in which a VT is delivered at a slow (or decelerating) inspiratory flow rate (or an end-inspiratory pause is inserted) to yield an I:E > 1. For PC-IRV, the physician must specify the inspiratory airway pressure, f, and I:E ratio, while VT and flow profile are determined by respiratory system impedance as discussed for PCV above. Commonly, the initial Pinsp is 20 to 40 cm H_2O (or 10 to 30 cm H_2O above the PEEP), f is 20/min, and the I:E is 2:1 to 4:1. For VC-IRV, the operator selects a VT, f, flow (typically a low value), flow profile, and, possibly, an end-inspiratory pause. The chosen values result in an I:E > 1:1 and as high as 5:1.

Compared with conventional modes of ventilation, lung oxygen exchange is often improved with IRV, owing to increased mean alveolar pressure and volume consequent to the longer time above functional residual capacity, or due to creation of autoPEEP. It is remotely possible that IRV causes better ventilation of lung units with long time constants, but these are so short in normal lungs (and shorter in acute hypoxemic respiratory failure) that such redistribution is unlikely to occur with slower flow, and could not reduce shunt even if it did. Because autoPEEP is a common consequence of IRV, serial determination of its magnitude is essential for safe use of this mode. Both PC-IRV and VC-IRV generally require heavy sedation with or without muscle paralysis.

Airway Pressure Release Ventilation: Airway pressure release ventilation consists of continuous positive airway pressure (CPAP) which is intermittently released to allow a brief expiratory interval. Conceptually, this mode is pressure-controlled IRV during which the patient is allowed to initiate spontaneous breaths. A potential advantage of airway pressure release ventilation is that mean alveolar pressure is lower than it would be during positive-pressure ventilation from the same amount of CPAP, possibly reducing the risks of barotrauma and hemodynamic compromise. Whether this mode provides any benefit over modern low-V_T ventilation remains to be shown.

Dual-Control Ventilation (Pressure-Regulated Volume-Control, Volume-Assured Pressure-Support): Some modes attempt to derive the benefits of volume- and pressure-preset modes at the same time. For example, pressure-regulated volume-control mode applies a time-limited pressure and adjusts the pressure of subsequent breaths, as needed, to assure a set V_T. The purported advantages of this mode are prevention of overdistention (by limiting pressure) and high initial inspiratory flows, while guaranteeing a V_T. A down side is that as patient effort increases, the ventilator reduces support. In the volume-assured pressure-support mode, volume is monitored during each pressure-support breath and, if a preset V_T is not achieved, additional volume is given at constant flow to augment that breath. The primary down side of this mode, compared with PSV, is that the extra volume may cause overdistention (and volutrauma).

The greatest problem with such newer modes is that they are very complex, the algorithm describing their function is not usually understood by practitioners, and they change during a breath, or from breath to breath, depending on patient effort, sometimes in ways that can provoke unanticipated effects.

Proportional-Assist Ventilation: Proportional-assist ventilation is intended only for spontaneously breathing patients. The goal of this novel mode is to attempt to normalize the relationship between patient effort and the resulting ventilatory consequences.[4] The ventilator adjusts Pinsp in proportion to patient effort both throughout any given breath and from breath to breath. This allows the patient to modulate his breathing pattern and total ventilation. This is implemented by monitoring instantaneous flow and volume (V) of gas from the ventilator to the patient and varying the Pinsp as follows:

$$\text{Pinsp} = f1 \times V + f2 \times \text{flow}$$

where f1 and f2 are selectable functions of volume (elastic assist) and flow (resistive assist), values for which can be estimated from the patient's respiratory mechanics. Potential advantages of this method are greater patient comfort, lower Ppeak, and enhancement of the patient's reflex and behavioral respiratory control mechanisms.

High-Frequency Ventilation: Several modes of ventilation have in common the use of V_T smaller than the dead space volume.[5] Gas exchange does not occur through convection as during conventional ventilation, but through bulk flow, Taylor diffusion, molecular diffusion, nonconvective mixing, and possibly other mechanisms. These modes include high-frequency oscillatory ventilation and high-frequency jet ventilation. Theoretical benefits of high-frequency ventilation (HFV) include lower risk of barotrauma as a result of smaller tidal excursions, improved gas exchange through a more uniform distribution of ventilation, and improved healing of bronchopleural fistulas. A substantial risk is that dynamic hyperinflation is the rule and alveolar pressure is greatly underestimated by monitoring pressure at the airway opening. HFV holds promise as the natural extension of lowering the V_T as a means to prevent volutrauma, and there is renewed interest in this old technique. In a recent controlled trial in patients with ARDS, HFV showed no advantage in terms of gas exchange or of short- or long-term mortality but did appear to be safe, at least during the performance of a clinical trial.[6] A nonsignificant trend toward a short-term mortality benefit for HFV has been interpreted as a reason to pursue additional clinical studies. It is worth mentioning, however, that the control arm ventilation strategy was not lung-protective, potentially biasing the study in favor of HFV.

Noninvasive Ventilation

Mechanical ventilation for acute respiratory failure carries a high morbidity and mortality due, in part, to violation of the glottis by the endotracheal tube. In patients with acute-on-chronic respiratory failure, numerous studies have demonstrated that noninvasive ventilation (NIV) effectively relieves symptoms, improves gas exchange, reduces the work of breathing, lessens complications, shortens the ICU length of stay, and improves survival.[7,8]

Both nasal and oronasal masks have been used successfully. Nasal masks are especially difficult to use in edentulous patients who are unable to control mouth leak. Careful attention to mask leaks and adjusting air flow and pressure-support levels are important considerations. Inflatable cuffs, nasal bridge protection, and the availability of a range of mask sizes to ensure proper fit can minimize mask complications. I find it useful to initiate ventilation by briefly holding the mask (already connected to the ventilator) onto the patient's face, rather than first strapping the mask on and then initiating ventilatory assistance. Sedative medications are occasionally appropriate and can improve tolerance of NIV, but carry some risk of respiratory depression and aspiration.

Patient-ventilator asynchrony (PVA) describes a patient's breathing efforts that are not coupled to machine output. During NIV, two mechanisms of PVA are common. The first is failure of the patient to lower sufficiently the proximal airway pressure (mask pressure) due to the presence of autoPEEP. As during invasive ventilation, counterbalancing the autoPEEP with externally applied PEEP provides a means by which to lower the work of triggering. The second common mechanism for PVA is failure of the ventilator to detect end inspiration because the patient's subsiding effort is cloaked by a mask leak. Most pressure-support ventilators terminate inspiration when inspiratory flow falls to a preset threshold, often at an arbitrary low value of flow or at a fixed percent of the peak inspiratory flow. Mask leaks prevent the flow from falling to this threshold, so the ventilator fails to switch off the inspiratory pressure even while the patient is making active expiratory efforts. This serves to increase patient discomfort and the work of breathing. Using other methods for terminating inspiration, such as time-cycled pressure-support or volume assist-control, can minimize this problem.

Either conventional ICU ventilators or one of many portable bilevel pressure-targeted ventilators, initially designed for home ventilation, can be used. Limitations of portable pressure-targeted ventilators include the lack of waveform displays, the inability to deliver a high fraction of inspired oxygen (FIO_2) [greater than about 40%; some new machines allow an FIO_2 as high as 1.0], and the potential for rebreathing of exhaled gas. Whether volume-preset ventilation (such as assist-control) or pressure-preset ventilation is superior for NIV remains debated. Both modes have been used successfully, but direct comparisons between modes are few.

I believe the following points will minimize the chances that NIV will fail:

1. Develop an individual and institutional commitment to NIV.
2. Select patients carefully, excluding those with hemodynamic instability, inadequate airway protective reflexes, or little prospect of improvement within the next several days.
3. Have available a selection of oronasal and nasal masks to increase the probability of a good fit.
4. Use the pressure-support mode, beginning with modest settings, such as PEEP = 3 cm H_2O, PSV = 5 cm H_2O, and the most sensitive trigger, periodically removing the mask to allow the patient to sense its effect.
5. Education, reassurance, and modest sedation (when required) may improve tolerance to the mask and ventilator.
6. Increase the PEEP to ease the work of triggering with a goal of (typically) 4 to 6 cm H_2O; raise

the level of PSV until the patient is subjectively improved, the VT is sufficient, and the rate begins to fall, with goal of 10 to 15 cm H$_2$O.
7. Detect and correct mask leaks by repositioning, achieving a better fit, changing the type of mask, removing nasogastric tubes (gastric decompression is not recommended during NIV), or adjusting the ventilator to reduce peak airway pressure.
8. Pay particular attention in the first hour to patient-ventilator synchrony, using waveform displays as a guide.

Management of the Patient

Initial Ventilator Settings

Initial ventilator settings depend on the goals of ventilation (eg, full respiratory muscle rest vs partial exercise), the patient's respiratory system mechanics, and minute ventilation needs. Although each critically ill patient presents myriad challenges, it is possible to identify five subsets of ventilated patients (1) the patient with normal lung mechanics and gas exchange; (2) the patient with severe airflow obstruction; (3) the patient with acute-on-chronic respiratory failure; (4) the patient with acute hypoxemic respiratory failure, and (5) the patient with restrictive lung or chest wall disease.[9]

In all patients, the initial FIO$_2$ should usually be 0.5 to 1.0 to assure adequate oxygenation, although it can usually be lowered within minutes when guided by pulse oximetry and, in the appropriate setting, applying PEEP. In the first minutes following institution of mechanical ventilation, the physician should remain alert for several common problems. These include, most notably, airway malposition, aspiration, and hypotension. Positive-pressure ventilation may reduce venous return and so cardiac output, especially in patients with a low mean systemic pressure (eg, hypovolemia, venodilating drugs, decreased sympathetic tone from sedating drugs, neuromuscular disease) or a very high ventilation-related pleural pressure (eg, chest wall restriction, large amounts of PEEP, or obstruction causing autoPEEP). If hypotension occurs, intravascular volume should be rapidly expanded while steps are taken to lower the pleural pressure (smaller VT, less minute ventilation).

The Patient With Normal Respiratory Mechanics and Gas Exchange

Patients with normal lung mechanics and gas exchange can require mechanical ventilation for several reasons: (1) because of loss of central drive to breathe (eg, drug overdose or structural injury to the brainstem); (2) because of neuromuscular weakness (eg, high cervical cord injury, acute idiopathic myelitis, myasthenia gravis); (3) as an adjunctive therapy in the treatment of shock; or (4) in order to achieve hyperventilation (eg, in the treatment of elevated intracranial pressure following head trauma). Following intubation, initial ventilator orders should be an FIO$_2$ of 0.5 to 1.0, VT of 8 to 15 mL/kg, rate of 8 to 12, and inspiratory flow rate of 40 to 60 L/min. Alternatively, if the patient has sufficient drive and is not profoundly weak, PSV can be used. The level of pressure support is adjusted (usually to the range of 10 to 20 cm H$_2$O above PEEP) to bring the respiratory rate down into the low 20s, usually corresponding to a VT of about 400 mL. If gas exchange is entirely normal, the FIO$_2$ can likely be lowered further based on pulse oximetry or arterial blood gas determinations. In patients who do not have lung injury or ARDS but are at risk of developing them, it may be prudent to use a low tidal volume since there is some evidence that mechanical ventilation at tidal volumes of roughly 11 mL/kg predicted body weight can induce lung injury.[10]

Soon after the initiation of ventilation, airway pressure and flow waveforms should be inspected for evidence of patient-ventilator dyssynchrony or undesired patient effort. If the goal of ventilation is full rest, the patient's drive can often be suppressed by increasing the inspiratory flow rate, frequency, or VT; of course, the latter two changes may induce respiratory alkalemia. If such adjustments do not diminish breathing effort (despite normal blood gases) to an undetectable level, sedation may be necessary. If this does not abolish inspiratory efforts and full rest is essential (as in shock), muscle paralysis should be considered. Measures to prevent atelectasis should include sighs (6 to 12/h at 1.5 to 2 times the VT) or small amounts of PEEP (5 to 7.5 cm H$_2$O).

Patients With Severe Airflow Obstruction

Severe obstruction is seen most commonly in patients with status asthmaticus, but also rarely in those with inhalation injury or central airway lesions, such as tumor or foreign body, that are not bypassed with the endotracheal tube. Some of these patients may benefit from NIV, but most will require invasive ventilation. These patients are usually extremely anxious and distressed. Deep sedation should be provided in such instances, supplemented in some patients by therapeutic paralysis, although the use of paralytic drugs occasionally causes long-lasting weakness. These interventions help to reduce oxygen consumption (and hence carbon dioxide production), to lower airway pressures, and to reduce the risk of self-extubation.

Because the gas exchange abnormalities of airflow obstruction are largely limited to ventilation-perfusion mismatch, an FiO_2 of 0.5 suffices in the vast majority of patients. Ventilation should be initiated using the ACV mode (or SIMV), the V_T should be small (5 to 7 mL/kg), and the respiratory rate 12 to 15 breaths/min. A peak flow of 60 L/min is recommended and higher flow rates do little to increase T_E. For example, if the V_T is 500, the respiratory rate 15, and the flow is 60 L/min, the T_E is 3.5 s. Raising flow (dramatically) to 120 L/min increases the expiratory time to only 3.75 s, a trivial improvement. In contrast, a small reduction in respiratory rate to 14/min increases the T_E to 3.8 s. This example serves to emphasize not only the relative lack of benefit of raising the flow rate but also the importance of minimizing minute ventilation when the goal is to reduce autoPEEP. Some patients who remain agitated during ACV can be made more comfortable by using PSV (or PCV) with a total inspiratory pressure of around 30 cm H_2O. Finally, if the patient is triggering the ventilator, some PEEP should be added to reduce the work of triggering.[11] Although this occasionally compounds the dynamic hyperinflation, potentially compromising cardiac output, usually autoPEEP increases little as long as PEEP is not set higher than about 85% of the autoPEEP. The goals are (1) to minimize alveolar overdistention (Pplat < 30) and (2) to minimize dynamic hyperinflation (autoPEEP < 15 cm H_2O or end-inspiratory lung volume < 20 mL/kg), a strategy that largely prevents barotrauma.[12,13] Reducing minute ventilation to achieve these goals generally causes the P_{CO_2} to rise above 40 mm Hg, often to 70 mm Hg or higher. Although this requires sedation, such permissive hypercapnia is tolerated quite well, except in patients with increased intracranial pressure, and perhaps in those with ventricular dysfunction or critical pulmonary hypertension.[14]

Patients With Acute-on-Chronic Respiratory Failure

Acute-on-chronic respiratory failure is a term used to describe the exacerbations of chronic ventilatory failure, often requiring ICU admission, usually occurring in patients with COPD. Unlike patients with status asthmaticus, patients in this population tend to have relatively smaller increases in inspiratory resistance, their expiratory flow limitation arising largely from loss of elastic recoil. As a consequence, in the patient with COPD and minimally reversible airway disease, peak airway pressures on the ventilator tend not to be extraordinarily high, yet autoPEEP and its consequences are common. At the time of intubation, hypoperfusion is common, as manifested by tachycardia and relative hypotension, and typically responds to briefly ceasing ventilation combined with fluid loading.

Because the majority of these patients are ventilated after days to weeks of progressive deterioration, the goal is to rest the patient (and respiratory muscles) for 24 to 48 h. Also, because the patient typically has an underlying compensated respiratory acidosis, excessive ventilation risks severe respiratory alkalosis and, over time, bicarbonate wasting by the kidney. Many such patients can be ventilated effectively with NIV, as described above. For those who require intubation, the goals of rest and appropriate hypoventilation can usually be achieved with initial ventilator settings of a V_T of 5 to 7 mL/kg and a respiratory rate of 20 to 24 breaths/min, with either an SIMV or an ACV mode set on minimal sensitivity. Because gas exchange abnormalities are primarily those of ventilation-perfusion mismatch, supplemental oxygen in the range of an FiO_2 of 0.4 should achieve better than 90% saturation of arterial hemoglobin.

The majority of patients with COPD will appear exhausted at the time when mechanical support is instituted and will sleep with minimal sedation. To the extent that muscle fatigue has played a role in a patient's functional decline, rest and sleep are desirable. Two to 3 days of such rest presumably will restore biochemical and functional changes associated with muscle fatigue, but 24 h may not be sufficient. Small numbers of patients are difficult to rest on the ventilator, continuing to demonstrate a high work of breathing. Examination of airway pressure and flow waveforms can be very helpful in identifying this extra work, and in suggesting strategies for improving the ventilator settings. In many patients, this is the result of autoPEEP-induced triggering difficulty. Adding extrinsic PEEP to nearly counterbalance the auto PEEP dramatically improves the patient's comfort.

Patients With Acute Hypoxemic Respiratory Failure

Acute hypoxemic respiratory failure is caused by alveolar filling with blood, pus, or edema, the end results of which are impaired lung mechanics and gas exchange. The gas exchange impairment results from intrapulmonary shunt that is largely refractory to oxygen therapy. In ARDS, the significantly reduced functional residual capacity arising from alveolar flooding and collapse leaves many fewer alveoli to accept the VT, making the lung appear stiff and dramatically increasing the work of breathing. The ARDS lung should be viewed as a small lung, however, rather than a stiff lung. In line with this current conception of ARDS, it is now clearly established that excessive distention of the ARDS lung compounds lung injury and may induce systemic inflammation.[15,16] Ventilatory strategies have evolved markedly in the past decade, changing clinical practice and generating tremendous excitement.

The goals of ventilation are to reduce shunt, avoid toxic concentrations of oxygen, and choose ventilator settings that do not amplify lung damage. The initial FIO_2 should be 1.0 in view of the typically extreme hypoxemia. PEEP is indicated in patients with diffuse lung lesions, but may not be helpful in patients with focal infiltrates, such as lobar pneumonia. In patients with ARDS, PEEP should be instituted immediately, then rapidly adjusted to the lowest PEEP necessary to produce an arterial saturation of 90% on an FIO_2 no higher than 0.6 ("least-PEEP approach"). An alternative approach is to set the PEEP at a value 2 cm H_2O higher than the lower inflection point of the inflation pressure-volume curve ("open-lung approach"), but this approach has not been validated, is rather complex, and is not recommended. Recruitment maneuvers have not been shown to be useful or necessary. The VT should be 6 mL/kg on ACV; a higher VT is associated with higher mortality. Presumably, PCV could be used as well, but the parameters that assure lung-protective ventilation are not known. In either mode, the respiratory rate should be set at 24 to 36/min. An occasional consequence of lung-protective ventilation is hypercapnia. This approach of preferring hypercapnia to alveolar overdistention, termed "permissive hypercapnia," is very well tolerated.

The Patient With Restriction of the Lungs or Chest Wall

A small VT (5 to 7 mL/kg) and rapid rate (18 to 24/min) are especially important in order to minimize the hemodynamic consequences of positive-pressure ventilation and to reduce the likelihood of barotrauma. The FIO_2 is usually determined by the degree of alveolar filling or collapse, if any. When the restrictive abnormality involves the chest wall (including the abdomen), the large ventilation-induced rise in pleural pressure has the potential to compromise cardiac output. This in turn will lower the mixed venous Po_2 and, in the setting of ventilation/perfusion mismatch or shunt, the Pao_2 as well. If the physician responds to this falling Pao_2 by augmenting PEEP or increasing the minute ventilation, further circulatory compromise ensues. A potentially catastrophic cycle of worsening gas exchange, increasing ventilator settings, and progressive shock is begun. This circumstance must be recognized because the treatment is to reduce dead space (eg, by lowering minute ventilation or correcting hypovolemia).

The Airway During Split-Lung Ventilation

The lungs may be separated for purposes of differential ventilation by two major means: (1) blocking the bronchus of a lobe or whole lung while ventilating with a standard endotracheal tube, or (2) passing a double-lumen tube (DLT). A number of different devices have been used to obstruct a bronchus, but experience is largest with the Fogarty embolectomy catheter. DLTs carry the advantages of allowing each lung to be ventilated, collapsed, re-expanded, or inspected independently.

Split-lung ventilation is only rarely useful in the critical care unit, but occasionally its benefits are dramatic. Large bronchopleural fistulas severely compromise ventilation and may not respond to HFV. A DLT will maintain ventilation of the healthy lung while facilitating closure of the bronchopleural fistula. During massive hemoptysis, lung separation may be lifesaving by minimizing blood aspiration, maintaining airway patency, and tamponading the bleeding site while awaiting definitive therapy. Finally, patients with focal causes of acute hypoxemic respiratory failure, such as lobar pneumonia or acute total atelectasis, may benefit from differential ventilation and application of PEEP.

References

1. Slutsky A. Mechanical ventilation. Chest 1993; 104:1833–1859
   A comprehensive review of many aspects of mechanical ventilation.
2. Brochard L, Rauss A, Benito S, et al. Comparison of three methods of gradual withdrawal from ventilatory support during weaning from mechanical ventilation. Am J Respir Crit Care Med 1994; 150:896–903
   One of two large, multicenter trials comparing weaning modes. SIMV was shown to be clearly inferior.
3. Esteban A, Alía I, Gordo F, et al. Extubation outcome after spontaneous breathing trials with T-tube or pressure support ventilation. Am J Respir Crit Care Med 1997; 156:459–465
   The other major weaning trial.
4. Younes M, Puddy A, Roberts D, et al. Proportional assist ventilation: results of an initial clinical trial. Am Rev Respir Dis 1992; 145:121–129
   A mode that adjusts pressure to meet patient demand.
5. Drazen JM, Kamm RD, Slutsky AS, et al. High-frequency ventilation. Physiol Rev 1984; 64:505–543
   Description of ventilation using tidal volumes less than the dead space volume.
6. Derdak S, Mehta S, Stewart TE, et al. High-frequency oscillatory ventilation for acute respiratory distress syndrome in adults: a randomized, controlled trial. Am J Respir Crit Care Med 2002; 166:801–808
   Randomized trial showing that HFV can be performed safely, but failing to demonstrate any significant clinical benefits compared with PCV in patients with ARDS.
7. Brochard L, Mancebo J, Wysocki M, et al. Noninvasive ventilation for acute exacerbations of chronic obstructive pulmonary disease. N Engl J Med 1995; 333:817–822
   The first trial to show convincingly the benefits of NIV.
8. Kramer N, Meyer TJ, Meharg J, et al. Randomized, prospective trial of noninvasive positive pressure ventilation in acute respiratory failure. Am J Respir Crit Care Med 1995; 151:1799–1806
   This trial confirmed the Brochard trial.[7]
9. Schmidt GA, Hall JB. Management of the ventilated patient. In: Hall JB, Schmidt GA, Wood LDH. Principles of critical care. 2nd ed. New York, NY: McGraw-Hill, 1998
   Describes ventilation based on individual patient physiology.
10. Gajic O, Dara SI, Mendez JL, et al. Ventilator-associated lung injury in patients without acute lung injury at the onset of mechanical ventilation. Crit Care Med 2004; 32:1817–1824
    This retrospective study found an association between the initial tidal volume and subsequent development of acute lung injury, suggesting that tidal volumes of 11 mL/kg may be injurious even before lung injury is established.
11. Ranieri VM, Giuliani R, Cinnella G, et al. Physiologic effects of positive end-expiratory pressure in patients with chronic obstructive pulmonary disease during acute ventilatory failure and controlled mechanical ventilation. Am Rev Respir Dis 1993; 147:5–13
    Demonstrates the impact of externally applied PEEP in patients with autoPEEP, showing reduced work of breathing.
12. Tuxen DV, Lane S. The effects of ventilatory pattern on hyperinflation, airway pressures, and circulation in mechanical ventilation of patients with severe air-flow obstruction. Am Rev Respir Dis 1987; 136:872–879
    This key paper demonstrated the link between minute ventilation and potentially detrimental consequences, such as barotraumas and hypotension.

13. Tuxen DV, Williams TJ, Scheinkestel CD, et al. Use of a measurement of pulmonary hyperinflation to control the level of mechanical ventilation in patients with acute severe asthma. Am Rev Respir Dis 1992; 146:1136–1142

    Demonstrated improved outcome by limiting minute ventilation.

14. Feihl F, Perret C. Permissive hypercapnia: how permissive should we be? Am J Respir Crit Care Med 1994; 150:1722–1737

    A comprehensive review of the risks and benefits of hypercapnic ventilation.

15. Ranieri VM, Suter PM, Tortoella C, et al. Effects of mechanical ventilation on inflammatory mediators in patients with acute respiratory distress syndrome: a randomized controlled trial. JAMA 1999; 282:54–61

    Demonstrated that large tidal volumes elaborate potentially damaging cytokines in patients.

16. Ventilation with lower tidal volumes as compared with traditional tidal volumes for acute lung injury and the acute respiratory distress syndrome: The Acute Respiratory Distress Syndrome Network. N Engl J Med 2000; 342:1301–1308

    Signal study establishing that V_T is an important determinant of outcome in patients with acute lung injury and ARDS.

Notes

Abdominal Problems in the ICU

David J. Dries, MD, MSE, FCCP

Objectives:

- Discuss the presentation, causes, diagnosis, and treatment of acute abdomen in the critically ill patient.
- Discuss the presentation, diagnosis, and treatment of acute pancreatitis in the ICU setting.
- Discuss the presentation, diagnosis, and treatment of biliary tract diseases, specifically acute cholecystitis and cholangitis, in the ICU patient.

Key words: abdominal pain; bowel obstruction; cholangitis; choleystitis; colitis; ileus; pancreatitis; ulcer disease

The Acute Abdomen

The development of acute abdomen can result in a patient entering the ICU. Alternatively, acute abdominal pain can develop in a patient who is in the ICU for another reason. Both of these situations can present a diagnostic dilemma. In particular, patients who are already critically ill may not be able to manifest typical physical findings of peritonitis. This chapter will focus on the presentation, diagnosis, and management of patients with acute abdominal problems coincident with or resulting in ICU care.

Pain

In 1986, Zoltie and Cust described a group of inpatients with acute abdominal pain treated with a semisynthetic opiate or placebo to determine whether analgesia could alleviate discomfort without reducing diagnostic accuracy. Before the publication of this article, clinicians followed the surgical dictum in the classic monograph of Sir Zachary Cope on acute abdominal pain: avoid early analgesic administration in patients presenting with severe, acute undifferentiated abdominal pain because it would impair diagnostic accuracy. Despite moderation of this position over the subsequent 10 to 20 years, the surgical and emergency medicine literature reflect widespread reluctance to administer analgesia for patients presenting with undiagnosed acute abdominal pain.

As this issue has moved largely to the emergency medicine literature, multiple studies have demonstrated that diagnostic accuracy and outcome are not affected by administration of analgesia. Nonetheless, contemporary publications indicate the continued reluctance of many surgeons to accept analgesia administration during evaluation of acute abdominal pain.

Despite methodologic limitations, all published clinical studies indicate that early administration of analgesia does not appear to impair clinical diagnostic accuracy in patients with acute undifferentiated abdominal pain. Studies have appeared in the emergency medicine, surgical, and pediatric literature. More recent editions of Cope's monograph on abdominal pain changes initial recommendations concerning withholding analgesia in these patients: Silen, the current author of Cope's monograph, condemns withholding analgesia for patients who are in pain and suffering. Recent work in the surgical literature supports early provision of analgesia to patients with undifferentiated abdominal pain.

Available literature has focused primarily on evaluation of acute undifferentiated abdominal pain in the uncompromised adult capable of participating in a clinical trial. The role of analgesia in infants, children <5 years old, and vulnerable adults, in whom a comparable pattern of more sophisticated interaction is not possible, continues to be controversial.

Presentation

Patients with acute abdominal pain present with sudden or gradual onset of discomfort. Sudden abdominal pain may develop as a consequence of rupture of a hollow viscus, acute bleeding into the abdomen as with aortic or visceral artery aneurysm, or progressive expansion of a structure in the abdomen. Gradual or nonspecific abdominal pain may begin with an inflammatory process such as appendicitis or diverticulitis. Associated symptoms of fever, tachycardia, tachypnea, nausea, and vomiting may be associated with any of these processes. However, the critical care patient may not manifest these changes. I have frequently received surgical consultation for patients with abdominal pain culminating in respiratory failure and admission to the pulmonary service. Thus, acute abdominal conditions may frequently be reflected by remote organ dysfunction.

Peritonitis is caused by irritation of the lining of the abdominal cavity. The peritoneum has visceral and parietal surfaces. Pain is said to be better localized when a portion of the parietal rather than visceral peritoneum is involved in the intra-abdominal process. Thus, the classic presentation of appendicitis is periumbilical abdominal pain (visceral localization of the mid gut), which progresses to right lower quadrant discomfort (parietal innervation, which is more localized). Generalized peritonitis is caused by irritation of the entire abdominal lining. Localized peritonitis reflects focal irritation of the peritoneum. Generalized peritonitis is more likely to result in a surgical emergency.

Patients with generalized peritonitis may lie quietly on the bed, as motion leads to peritoneal irritation and pain. A second type of patient is writhing in discomfort with nonspecific visceral but not parietal peritoneal irritation. These patients are classically described as having pain out of proportion to examination. Patients with an acute abdomen may have rapid shallow breathing, as diaphragmatic excursion is associated with pain. Thus, respiratory dysfunction may be a prominent presenting symptom if the location and the severity of the inciting process are not apparent. Physical findings of peritonitis include hypoactive or absent bowel sounds, rebound tenderness, and percussion tenderness.

Diagnostic Approach to the Patient With Acute Abdominal Pain

If the physical findings of an acute abdomen (diffuse peritonitis) are elicited, little other diagnostic testing is necessary. Routine laboratory tests are sent with an upright chest radiograph to enhance preoperative preparation and as a rapid screen to determine if there is free air in the abdomen. In some cases, additional plain radiographs including supine and upright abdominal films as well as lateral decubitus views are also obtained as part of a routine abdominal pain workup.

A CT scan is often obtained prior to or with a surgical consult. However, with the clinical diagnosis of generalized peritonitis, operative therapy is generally required and is delayed for additional imaging only with the consent of the surgeon. Patients with significant comorbidities may be candidates for further imaging, as the morbidity associated with negative laparotomy is significant. If the patient is otherwise stable, a CT scan may be obtained to corroborate a clinical diagnosis. A nondiagnostic CT scan in a patient with generalized peritonitis, however, should not deter operation.

Before operation in a patient with generalized peritonitis, a Foley catheter is placed and abnormalities of electrolytes, blood counts, and coagulation factors are corrected. Critical care admission may be required in those patients with comorbid conditions that require monitoring or additional treatment and those individuals whose volume status is inadequate to immediately tolerate the vasodilating effects of anesthetics and blood loss associated with anticipated surgery. Aggressive volume resuscitation is frequently required, and the arterial blood gas with base deficit can be useful in determining adequacy of resuscitation. However, in patients who are bleeding into the abdomen (the patient with a visceral artery laceration), adequate resuscitation cannot be attempted prior to achieving control of bleeding; in fact, these patients are better treated without aggressive fluid administration prior to surgery. General principles of surgical intervention are to control perforation of the GI tract and the leakage of bowel content, manage bleeding, drain purulence, resect bowel, and divert the fecal stream if necessary to permit treatment of an area of enteric leakage.

GI Conditions Resulting in Acute Abdominal Pain

Postoperative Ileus (Stomach, Small Bowel, Colon)

Ileus has been defined as the functional inhibition of propulsive bowel activity irrespective of pathogenic mechanisms. Postoperative ileus resolves spontaneously within 2 to 3 days, while paralytic postoperative ileus is defined as that form of ileus lasting >3 days after surgery. In postoperative ileus, inhibition of small-bowel motility is transient and the stomach recovers within 24 to 48 h, whereas colonic function takes 48 to 72 h to return. Determination of the end of postoperative ileus is controversial. Bowel sounds are sometimes used as an end point, but they require frequent auscultation and their presence does not indicate propulsive activity. Bowel sounds may be the result of small-bowel activity and not colonic function. Flatus also is not an ideal end point, as careful reporting is required and there is some question as to the correlation between flatus and bowel movements. Bowel movements are a reliable end point, but may be too nonspecific or representative of distal bowel evacuation as opposed to global function.

A variety of factors contribute to postoperative ileus. In the stomach and small intestine, normal basal electrical activity is impaired after surgical procedures. The colonic electrical activity is also affected and is the last to return to normal (approximately 72 h after surgery). Sympathetic nervous system input, which is increased during the postoperative period, is an inhibitory factor for bowel activity. Neurotransmitters including nitric oxide, calcitonin gene-related peptide, and corticotropin releasing factor may play a role. Finally, manipulation of the bowel and inflammation contribute to delayed return of postoperative bowel function.

Management of postoperative ileus begins with the choice of anesthetic. Anesthetic agents exert their strongest effects on regions of the bowel depending on neural integration. The large intestine is devoid of intercellular gap junctions, which makes the colon most susceptible to inhibitory actions of anesthetics. In theory, epidural anesthetics, which utilize local anesthesia, can block afferent and efferent inhibitory reflexes, increase splanchnic blood flow, and have antiinflammatory effects. Epidural anesthetics have the added benefit of blocking the afferent stimuli that trigger the endocrine metabolic response to surgery and thus inhibit catabolic hormones released during this process. Thoracic epidurals with local anesthetics significantly reduce ileus as opposed to systemic opioid therapy in patients undergoing abdominal surgical procedures. Other traditional therapies such as early postoperative feeding and the nasogastric tube are not supported by a consistent body of literature. In fact, inappropriate use of nasogastric tubes may contribute to postoperative complications such as fever, pneumonia, and atelectasis.

A number of additional drug strategies have been evaluated to improve outcomes with postoperative ileus. The most widely used are nonsteroidal antiinflammatory drugs, which can reduce the amount of opioid administered by 20 to 30%. An additional benefit in bowel motility may be derived from antiinflammatory properties of these agents. In both clinical and experimental studies, nonsteroidal antiinflammatory drugs resulted in decreasing nausea and vomiting and improved GI transit. Other stimulants including laxatives, prostaglandins, sympathetic inhibitors (edrophonium chloride) neostigmine, metaclopramide, and erythromycin have also been evaluated in small numbers of studies. Finally, hormone antagonists including cisapride (seratonin antagonist), cerulatide (cholecystokinin antagonist), and octreotide have been evaluated without consensus regarding their use.

The best treatment currently available is a multimodal regimen. Included in contemporary reports are utilization of epidural analgesia, early oral nutrition and mobilization, cisapride, and laxative stimulation. Perhaps it is best to recommend an approach that decreases factors contributing to postoperative ileus. Thus, limitation of narcotic administration and increased use of nonsteroidal antiinflammatory drugs with thoracic epidural catheter placement using local anesthetics should be employed. Nasogastric decompression is used selectively, and correction of electrolyte imbalances is also important.

Stomach

Early understanding of gastric physiology led to logical and time-tested surgical procedures aimed at acid reduction and lowering of ulcer recurrence rates. A shift in treatment occurred with the recognition and knowledge of *Helicobacter pylori*. Whereas surgery once dominated therapy for ulcer diathesis, medical therapy has now superseded. Despite a shrinking role for the surgeon in the management of this problem, several comments can be made.

Classic indications for surgery—perforation, bleeding, and gastric outlet obstruction—remain important. However, recent innovations in therapy have changed the natural history of ulcer disease. Acute perforations of the duodenum are estimated to occur in 2 to 10% of patients with ulcers. At present, simple patch closure is recommended for this patient population, and the importance of *H pylori* as a pathogen and therapeutic target has been emphasized. In addition to *H pylori* as a source of gastroduodenal perforation, cocaine ingestion has recently been reported by the Emory group. Feliciano and coworkers reported 50 patients with cocaine-related perforations in their series representing approximately 40% of patients with juxtapyloric gastroduodenal perforations in an inner-city hospital. Omental patch closure again was most often used. More extensive ulcer surgery should be reserved for patients with an ongoing history of gastroduodenal ulceration or due to compliance issues. If *H pylori* is effectively treated, a simple patch approach should be adequate.

The incidence of gastroduodenal bleeding secondary to peptic ulcer disease and hospital admission for this complication have not changed in recent decades. Despite improvements in nonsurgical modalities such as proton-pump inhibitors and therapeutic endoscopy, operation for bleeding peptic ulcer disease has remained constant; such operations are performed on 10 to 20% of all patients hospitalized for upper GI tract hemorrhage. Bleeding is more common as age increases. Mortality rates following ulcer bleeding have remained at approximately 10%. In general, when surgery is required, this occurs within 48 h of initial presentation with bleeding. The role of serial endoscopic procedures in reducing the need for emergency surgery continues to be discussed. At issue are delays to definitive therapy with increasing complication rates, as opposed to the reduced morbidity of early acid control operations. Factors associated with failure of repeat endoscopy for control of bleeding peptic ulcer disease include hypotension prior to the second endoscopic procedure or an ulcer known to be >2 cm in size. Of interest is a reported lower incidence of *H pylori* infection in those patients with significant upper GI tract bleeding secondary to peptic ulcer disease than in those individuals with uncomplicated ulcers or minor degrees of hemorrhage. At this time, no role for empiric treatment of *H pylori* in this bleeding cohort is believed to be present. Thus, surgical procedures for bleeding should be more aggressive due to the lower incidence of *H pylori* infection. A minimal surgical approach would therefore leave up to 50% of the population presenting with bleeding at risk for further hemorrhage.

Benign gastric outlet obstruction secondary to peptic ulcer disease represents 5 to 8% of ulcer-related complications. Approximately 2,000 patients per year in the United States are operated on for this problem. Pyloric channel stenosis leads to stasis raising the gastric pH and resulting in gastrin release with excess acid production. Both surgical and nonsurgical approaches are available. Endoscopic pneumatic dilatation has been available since 1982 and continues to be used, often as primary therapy. Long-term data, however, are limited. Unfortunately, it is also unclear whether *H pylori* infection is prominent in this patient population. Case reports suggest resolution of symptomatic and endoscopic outlet obstruction with medical treatment directed at *H pylori* infection without concurrent pyloric manipulation. Large series as yet have not confirmed this mode of therapy. Surgical options include highly selective vagotomy with some form of pyloroplasty, truncal vagotomy with gastroenterostomy, or truncal vagotomy with resection of the gastric antrum. Good results have been reported for all of these procedures.

Small Bowel

Obstruction: Obstruction of the small bowel due to adhesive bands is a common problem presenting in the ICU in the setting of deranged GI or remote organ physiology. Adhesions will not develop overnight in patients with this problem. Rather, obstruction is a manifestation of a mismatch between the character and volume of succus for passage and the capability of the bowel. Both factors, succus and bowel performance, can be affected by critical illness, which in my opinion contributes to frequent consults for bowel obstruction in the ICU.

Adhesive obstruction is a frequent complication of abdominal surgery. While the likelihood of surgical intervention in adhesive small-bowel obstruction increases with the number of episodes, the majority of patients presenting for operative management have undergone only one abdominal procedure. While surgeons frequently prefer, due to technical concerns, to manage bowel obstruction nonoperatively, at least one large study suggests that the risk of recurrence is significantly lower when the last bowel obstruction episode was treated surgically rather than without operation. Perhaps the greatest concern is bowel loss due to strangulation and destruction of blood supply. A large series of operative procedures places the rate of strangulation in bowel obstruction from 20 to 30%, with bowel resection required in 20% of cases. Surgeons are frequently concerned about creating bowel injury. Accidental enterostomy requiring repair occurs in approximately 5% of operations. The requirement for creation of colostomy or enterostomy is 0.2% and 0.8%, respectively. In patients receiving operative therapy for small-bowel obstruction, the initial episode requiring surgery occurred within 1 year of the last abdominal operation in 40% of patients and between 1 and 5 years after the last abdominal operation in 25% of patients.

It is important to note that abdominal pain presentation varies in adhesive small-bowel obstruction. Forty percent of patients reported pain greater than normal in a large survey. This group of patients described pain as moderate to fairly strong. Bowel obstruction patients frequently report a history of abdominal pain, which can extend back months prior to the crisis precipitating ICU admission.

Malignant Bowel Obstruction: There are many primary cancers known to cause malignant bowel obstruction. Knowledge of primary disease and individual patient history are important because treatment can be affected. Bowel obstruction occurs in 5 to 43% of patients with a diagnosis of advanced malignancy or metastatic intra-abdominal malignancy. The most common causes are ovarian (5 to 50%) and colorectal (10 to 28%) cancers; nonabdominal cancers including lung, breast, and melanoma occasionally lead to obstruction. Long-term survival for these individuals is poor. Lower-grade tumors can have a better outlook warranting consideration of more invasive treatment approaches.

A "gold standard" for diagnosing bowel obstruction, both benign and malignant, is emerging with the use of CT. The American College of Radiology endorses CT as highly appropriate in the evaluation of bowel obstruction. Studies have demonstrated CT to be highly sensitive in identifying small-bowel obstruction with specificity >90%. Additionally, the greatest use of CT can be in identifying the cause of obstruction including metastases. CT can distinguish among pathologic processes resulting in bowel obstruction including tumor involvement of bowel wall, mesentery, mesenteric vessels, and peritoneum. Small- or large-bowel contrast studies can be used when patterns of motility are unclear or the CT suggests multiple potential levels of obstruction.

Malignant bowel obstructions are usually partial and rarely urgent situations. The rarity of intestinal gangrene in malignant obstruction gives all parties involved some breathing room for making difficult management decisions. It is important to note that operative mortality in this setting is frequent (5 to 32%) most often related to progression of neoplasm. Morbidity is also common (42%), and reobstruction after operation can be as high as 10 to 50%. Prognostic criteria that have been identified in patients less likely to benefit from surgery include the presence of ascites, carcinomatosis, palpable intraabdominal masses, multiple sites of obstruction, and advanced disease with poor overall clinical status.

Treatment options for malignant bowel obstruction include simple lysis of adhesions or bowel resection. However, in this setting, resection might not allow restoration of bowel continuity. Operation may leave the patient with multiple stomas. Intestinal bypass is also an option. Nonsurgical management of these patients frequently includes the use of opioids, which produce an ileus pattern and may alleviate pain and/or octreotide for control of intestinal secretions. The nasogastric tube should be considered only as a proximal means of temporary decompression. Percutaneous gastrostomy can provide significant relief as a vent in proximal small-bowel obstruction.

Short-Bowel Syndrome: Short-bowel syndrome is a potential postoperative complication after intra-abdominal procedures. One fourth of patients presenting at tertiary centers with short-bowel syndrome experience this complication from previous abdominal surgery. Gynecologic and colon procedures are most frequently associated with short-bowel syndrome. As a rough rule of thumb, 100 cm of small bowel is required for adequate enteral nutrition. Even if intestinal length greater than this is available, adequate tolerance of enteral feeding may come slowly and combinations of parenteral and enteral nutrition may be required for extended periods of time.

Colon

Obstruction: Colonic obstruction has three major etiologies: malignancy, diverticular disease, and torsion or volvulus. In each case, surgical resection is appropriate but resuscitation prior to operative intervention is essential. CT scanning can be invaluable in determining the site and characteristics of the obstructing lesion. CT is the key study for working through the differential diagnosis of large-bowel obstruction. Newly diagnosed malignancy is generally resected with either primary anastomosis or more commonly end proximal colostomy or ileostomy, as adequate bowel preparation may not be possible.

Endoscopic stent placement has successfully relieved obstruction in a high percentage of patients with lower colorectal lesions (64 to 100%). This approach may be considered if necessary equipment and expertise are available. Typically endoscopy is utilized in the high-risk patient with significant comorbidities. Risks of stent placement for colorectal disease include perforation (0 to 15%), stent migration requiring replacement (0 to 40%), or reocclusion (0 to 33%). Stents can frequently lead to adequate palliation for extended periods of time. Diverticular disease causing obstruction is typically treated with resection and reconstruction or proximal colostomy and later restoration of GI continuity.

Diverticulitis: A growing body of data suggest that early management of acute diverticulitis can be nonoperative. A recent large population study with acute diverticulitis noted a relatively low risk of recurrent diverticulitis after initial nonoperative management. The overall recurrence rate was approximately 13% and the annual recurrence rate was 2% per year. These data argue against routine elective colectomy after an initial episode of acute diverticulitis. A higher rate of recurrent diverticulitis is found in patients <50 years old. Patients with organ system dysfunction or requiring drainage procedures are often better served by resection and elective reconstruction of the GI tract.

Notably, a large recent trial found no association between higher recurrence rates for diverticulitis and percutaneous drainage procedures. This challenges conventional teaching including the standards of the American Society of Colon and Rectal Surgeons. The traditional view presumes that patients with a drainable percutaneous abscess (*ie*, complicated diverticulitis) have worse disease. The findings in a large trial conducted in the Kaiser System suggest that patients who have undergone successful percutaneous drainage during initial hospitalization do not require subsequent elective colectomy. For the intensivist, therefore, aggressive and immediate surgical intervention should not be the expectation or the norm in patients presenting with diverticulitis even if a drainage procedure is required.

Colitis: Colitis can be broken down into ischemic and infectious etiologies. Causes of ischemic colitis are many, but the ultimate result is intestinal shock or end-organ hypoperfusion. Cardiac failure, systemic shock states, drugs, and underlying mesenteric vascular disease contribute to colonic ischemia. Initial management of ischemic colitis is nonoperative. Patients are resuscitated and placed on broad-spectrum antibiotics. This strategy is continued even if pneumatosis is identified with small amounts of free air. Where patients go on to multiorgan system dysfunction, emergent colectomy is appropriate. Patients who improve may resume enteral intake, discontinue antibiotics, and should receive endoscopy ≥6 weeks after the ischemic insult.

Patients with megarectum or megacolon can frequently present with primary or secondary colon toxicity associated with other organ dysfunction. In some cases, resection of the involved colon is the optimal approach. In patients with megacolon and a nondilated functional rectum, subtotal colectomy with ileorectal anastomosis is the procedure of choice, as a segmental colon resection results in a higher incidence of postoperative dysmotility. There is a definite mortality with this procedure and 20% morbidity, and further surgical intervention is commonly secondary to bowel obstruction. Patients with dilatation involving the entire colon and rectum may require removal of the entire affected large bowel and creation of an ileal pouch. Success rates in limited studies appear to be 70 to 80%, although this procedure is complex and may require a series of procedures in patients with multiorgan dysfunction. A coloanal anastomosis may be recommended in patients with distal large intestine dilatation or dismotility. While patients with megabowel require complex surgical management, acute surgical intervention should be reserved for patients with intractable symptoms or acute organ dysfunction. Ideally, patients should be supported through acute illness and undergo multidisciplinary evaluation including clinical, psychologic, and physiologic assessment.

Approximately 3% of healthy adults and 20 to 40% of hospitalized patients have *Clostridium difficile* colonization, which in healthy persons is inactive in the spore form. Reduction of competing flora with antibiotic use promotes conversion to vegetative forms that replicate and produce toxins. The characteristic clinical expression is watery diarrhea and cramps, with the pathologic finding of pseudomembranous colitis. Recently, *C difficile* with greater virulence has been reported in multi-institutional studies. Identified risk factors include fluoroquinolone use and age >65 years. These recent reports document the presence of more virulent strains of *C difficile* causing epidemic disease associated with more frequent and more severe presentation as indicated by higher rates of toxic megacolon, leukemoid reaction, shock, requirement of colectomy, and death.

In most cases, management of infectious colitis begins with identification of the offending organism and appropriate infection control procedures. Implicated antimicrobials must be stopped and administration of oral metronidazole or vancomycin initiated. *C difficile* is the most prominent organism associated with toxic colitis, but toxic colitis can also be seen in the absence of this organism. Again, fluid resuscitation and antibiotic management are initial steps in care of these patients, but colectomy must be considered for the patient with progressive organ dysfunction or hemodynamic instability.

Appendix

More than 250,000 appendectomies are performed in the United States each year, making appendectomy the most common abdominal operation performed on an emergency basis. While the diagnosis of appendicitis in young men with abdominal pain is usually straightforward, diagnostic considerations are far broader for premenopausal women and patients at the extremes of age. The later group, which may be in the ICU, presents a diagnostic challenge because of delays in seeking medical care or difficulty in obtaining a history and performing accurate physical examination. As delayed diagnosis and treatment of appendicitis are associated with an increased rate of perforation with resulting increase in morbidity and mortality, timely intervention is crucial.

If laparotomy is performed on the basis of physical examination, the appendix is normal in approximately 20% of patients. When advanced age or female gender confounds the usual signs or symptoms of appendicitis, the error rate in managing pain in the right lower quadrant can approach 40%. To improve diagnostic accuracy, imaging is seeing increasing use. Nonetheless, physical examination and history remain the diagnostic cornerstone for evaluating the patient with right lower quadrant pain. No single aspect of clinical presentation predicts the presence of disease, but a combination of signs and symptoms support the diagnosis of appendicitis. Three signs and symptoms most predictive of acute appendicitis are right lower quadrant pain, abdominal rigidity, and migration of discomfort from the umbilical region to the right lower quadrant.

As plain radiographs and laboratory tests are marked by low sensitivity and specificity for the diagnosis of appendicitis, CT has become the cornerstone of diagnostic modalities. With improvements in CT, the entire abdomen can be scanned at high resolution in thin slices during a single period of breath holding. Such scanning virtually eliminates motion and misregistration artifacts and routinely results in high-quality, high-resolution images of the appendix and periappendiceal tissue. For patients with suspected appendicitis, spiral CT has sensitivity of 90 to 97%, with accuracy of 94 to 100%. CT also provides an opportunity to diagnose alternative disorders should the appendix be normal. The differential diagnosis of appendicitis is broad and includes colitis, diverticulitis, small-bowel obstruction, inflammatory bowel disease and ovarian cysts, cholecystitis, pancreatitis, and ureteral obstruction.

Treatment of appendicitis routinely involves right lower quadrant investigation through a transabdominal or laparoscopic approach. The patient with perforated appendicitis can be managed with antibiotics followed by interval appendectomy, although follow-up data suggest that antibiotic treatment may reduce the need for later removal of the appendix. In patients who are critically ill, with consultation by the surgeon, appendicitis can be managed with antibiotics when the operative risk is prohibitive. Late management of such patients is unclear, as clinical series following such individuals are small and infrequent.

Acute Pancreatitis

Acute pancreatitis frequently has rapid onset manifest by upper abdominal pain, vomiting, fever, tachycardia, leukocytosis, and elevated serum levels of pancreatic enzymes. Common causes in the United States are gallstones and alcohol use. The two common severity-of-illness classifications for acute pancreatitis are the time-honored Ranson score and the more commonly used ICU scale, APACHE (acute physiology and chronic health evaluation) II. Severe acute pancreatitis is diagnosed if three or more of the Ranson criteria are present, if the APACHE II score is ≥8, or if shock, renal insufficiency, or pulmonary failure are present.

Pancreatitis may also be classified histologically as interstitial edematous or necrotizing disease according to inflammatory changes in pancreatic parenchyma. An international symposium in 1992 defined pancreatic necrosis as the presence of one or more diffuse or focal areas of nonviable pancreatic parenchyma. Pancreatic necrosis is typically associated with peripancreatic fat necrosis. Pancreatic necrosis represents a severe form of acute pancreatitis and is present in approximately 20 to 30% of the 185,000 new cases of acute pancreatitis reported each year in the United States (Table 1).

Diagnosis

Initial evaluation reveals signs of peritonitis that are sometimes generalized. Laboratory testing is often consistent with volume contraction related to sequestration of fluid into the retroperitoneum, and vomiting. Correlating data include elevated hematocrit and bicarbonate levels, hypokalemia, and acidosis. Amylase and lipase levels are frequently sent to evaluate pancreatitis. Amylase

Table 1. *Etiologies of Acute Necrotizing Pancreatitis*

Most Common
    Choledocholithiasis
    Ethanol abuse
    Idiopathic

Less Common
    Endoscopic retrograde cholangiopancreatography
    Hyperlipidemia (types I, IV, and V)
    Drugs
    Pancreas divisum
    Abdominal trauma

Least Common
    Hereditary (familial)

N Engl J Med 1999; 340:1412–1417. Copyright © 1999 Massachusetts Medical Society. All rights reserved.

elevation is less specific than lipase, as the former can be released by salivary glands. Bowel obstruction and other forms of small-bowel pathology are also associated with mild elevation in amylase.

With suspicion of the diagnosis of acute pancreatitis, the cause of this problem is sought. As most cases correspond to alcohol use or gallstones, history and diagnostic testing initially are focused on these entities. Right upper quadrant ultrasound is the initial test for gallstones. Identification of gallstones in a patient with acute pancreatitis should lead to the presumptive diagnosis of biliary or gallstone pancreatitis. Occasionally, ultrasound will demonstrate choledocholithiasis, a stone in the common bile duct. Cholangitis is also possible in this setting. Where gallstones are absent and a history of alcohol use cannot be obtained, other etiologies of acute pancreatitis must be considered including hyperlipidemia, drugs (steroids and anti-convulsants), trauma, pancreas divisum, and other mechanical insults such as endoscopic retrograde cholangiopancreatography (ERCP).

In the presence of diagnostic uncertainty at the time of presentation, a CT scan of the abdomen with IV contrast (in the absence of contraindications) should be performed after fluid resuscitation to confirm the diagnosis. CT also allows alternative diagnoses to be ruled out. The admission CT scan may serve as a baseline for future studies. Some authors recommend delaying the initial CT to identify local complications for 48 to 72 h if possible as necrosis may not be visualized earlier.

While CT is the preferred imaging modality for the pancreas in the setting of acute pancreatitis, magnetic resonance cholangiopancreatography (MRCP) is gaining favor as a means to detect common bile duct stones with resolution of gallstone pancreatitis. Surgical authors are now suggesting that if MRCP is negative, ERCP is not required in patients with gallstone pancreatitis and cholecystectomy may be performed. In the majority of patients with mild gallstone pancreatitis, the common bile duct stones pass spontaneously into the duodenum. Thus, the morbidity of nontherapeutic ERCP may be avoided with MRCP. Only 20% of patients with resolving gallstone pancreatitis are found to have stones in the extrahepatic biliary tree.

Management

Patients with acute pancreatitis require aggressive resuscitation and are at risk for early development of organ dysfunction as a result of inadequate resuscitation as well as systemic and local complications of pancreatitis. Clinical monitoring should focus on intravascular volume assessment including urine output and acid base status along with pulmonary function. It is important to note that aggressive fluid resuscitation may result in accumulation of ascites, pleural effusions, and hypoxemia. In severe cases, abdominal compartment syndrome may complicate resuscitation of severe pancreatitis (Table 2).

Early antibiotic administration has received attention in recent years as a therapy in acute pancreatitis. Despite initial studies favoring administration of broad-spectrum antibiotics and selective gut decontamination, recent consensus reports debate the value of routine antibiotic prophylaxis or administration of antifungal agents in patients with acute pancreatitis and/or pancreatic necrosis in light of contradictory evidence. When patients are strongly suspected of having pancreatic infection, imipenem, meropenem, fluoroquinolones, and metronidazole may be considered. In general, infection of necrotic pancreas involves bacteria from the GI tract. Because of this observation, gut decontamination has been advocated by some authors. Current data do not support routine use of this practice.

Nasogastric tube suctioning is warranted in patients with acute pancreatitis who are intubated or vomiting. Acid-suppression therapy with proton-pump inhibitors is reasonable, as stress-related ulcers are a risk and proton-pump inhibitors decrease GI tract fluid production. Enteral nutrition is used in preference to parenteral nutrition in patients with acute pancreatitis. This therapy should be initiated when initial resuscitation is completed. Placement of the feeding tube into the jejunum should be accomplished if possible. Parenteral nutrition is associated with an increased risk of infection and is used only if attempts at enteral nutrition have failed despite trials of 5 to 7 days.

Surgical Therapy

Sonographic or CT-guided fine-needle aspiration with Gram stain and culture should be obtained of pancreatic or peripancreatic tissue to discriminate between sterile and infected tissue in patients with radiologic evidence of pancreatic necrosis and clinical features consistent with infection. In general, debridement or drainage of patients with sterile pancreatic necrosis is not recommended. Pancreatic debridement or drainage is recommended in patients in whom infected pancreatic necrosis is documented and/or the presence of abscess is confirmed by radiologic evidence of gas in pancreatic or peripancreatic tissue or by results of fine-needle aspiration. The "gold standard" for pancreatic debridement is

Table 2. *Recognition of Clinically Severe Acute Pancreatitis*

Ranson's score ≥3 – Criteria of Severity:
  At admission
    Age >55 years
    White cell count >16,000/mm³
    Blood glucose >200mg/dl [11.1 mmol/liter]
    Serum LDH >350 IU/liter
    Serum AST >250 IU/liter

  During initial 48 hours
    Absolute decrease in hematocrit >10%
    Increase in blood urea nitrogen >5 mg/dl [1.8 mmol/liter]
    Serum calcium <8 mg/dl [2 mmol/liter]
    Arterial PaO$_2$ <60 mmHg
    Base deficit >4 mmol/liter
    Fluid sequestration >6 liters

APACHE II score ≥8

Organ failure

Substantial pancreatic necrosis (at least 30% glandular necrosis according to contrast-enhanced CT)

N Engl J Med 1999; 340:1412–1417. Copyright © 1999 Massachusetts Medical Society. All rights reserved.

open operative debridement. Minimally invasive techniques including laparoscopy or percutaneous intervention are options in selected patients. Operative necrosectomy and/or drainage should be delayed 2 to 3 weeks to allow demarcation of necrotic pancreas. The clinical course of pancreatitis is the primary determinant of the timing of operative intervention.

Conventional surgical drainage involves removal of necrotic pancreas with placement of standard surgical drains and reoperation as required by the presence of fever, leukocytosis, or lack of improvement based on imaging studies. Open or semiopen management of the abdomen involves removal of necrotic pancreas and either scheduled repeated laparotomies or open abdominal packing allowing for frequent changes of dressing material. Closed management involves removal of necrotic pancreas with extensive intraoperative lavage of the pancreatic bed with closure of the abdomen over large-bore drains for continuous high-volume postoperative lavage of the lesser sac. Effective debridement of necrotic pancreas is important since inadequately removed necrotic tissue remains infected with mortality as high as 40%.

In general, frequent operations are required to remove necrotic pancreas and peripancreatic material. If the abdomen is left open, the need for repeated laparotomy is eliminated and packing may be changed in the ICU. Repeated debridement and manipulation of abdominal viscera with contemporary operative techniques results in a high rate of postoperative local complications including pancreatic fistula, small- and large-bowel injury, and bleeding from the pancreatic bed. Pancreatic or GI tract fistulas occur in up to 40% of patients after surgical removal of necrotic pancreas and often require additional surgery for closure.

ERCP

Where obstructive jaundice or other evidence of acute obstruction of the biliary or pancreatic duct is present and acute pancreatitis is due to suspected or confirmed gallstones, urgent ERCP should be performed within 72 h of the onset of symptoms. This intervention showed improved outcome in patients with severe acute pancreatitis. While benefit has been attributed to relief of pancreatic ductal obstruction by impacted gallstones at the ampulla of Vater, other recent work suggests that improved outcome after endoscopic retrograde cholangiopancreatography and sphincterotomy in gallstone pancreatitis results from reduced biliary sepsis. Another theoretical concern is introduction of infection by incidental pancreatography during ERCP transforming sterile to infected acute necrotizing pancreatitis. Therefore, ERCP is used judiciously in patients with severe acute gallstone pancreatitis and should be reserved for those individuals in whom biliary obstruction is identified. MRCP, as noted above, is valuable in identifying the need for ERCP.

Complications

A variety of systemic and local complications of severe acute pancreatitis may occur. Systemic complications include ARDS, acute renal failure, shock, coagulopathy, hyperglycemia, and hypercalcemia. Local complications include GI hemorrhage, infected pancreatic necrosis, and adjacent bowel necrosis. Later local complications include pancreatic abscess and pancreatic pseudocysts. Infected necrosis develops in 30 to 70% of patients with acute necrotizing pancreatitis and accounts for >80% of deaths from acute pancreatitis. The risk of infected necrosis increases with the volume of pancreatic glandular necrosis.

Overall mortality in severe pancreatitis is approximately 30%. Deaths occur in two phases. Early deaths occurring within 1 to 2 weeks are due to multisystem organ failure associated with release of inflammatory mediators and cytokines. Late deaths result from local or systemic infection. If acute necrotizing pancreatitis remains sterile, overall mortality is approximately 10%. The mortality rate triples if there is infected necrosis.

Late Complications

Long-term endocrine and exocrine consequences of severe acute pancreatitis depend on a variety of factors, including severity of necrosis, etiology, whether the patient continues to use alcohol, and the degree of surgical pancreatic debridement. Persistent functional insufficiency has been noted in the majority of patients up to 2 years after severe acute pancreatitis. Use of pancreatic enzymes is restricted to patients with symptoms of steatorrhea and weight loss due to fat malabsorption. While glucose intolerance is frequent, overt diabetes is relatively uncommon. Obstructive pancreatic ductal abnormalities may account for persistent symptoms of abdominal pain or recurrent pancreatitis.

Key Points in Management of Severe Pancreatitis*

- In the presence of diagnostic uncertainty at the time of presentation, CT scan of the abdomen (with IV contrast if possible) should be performed after fluid resuscitation to confirm the diagnosis and rule out alternative diagnoses.
- When CT is employed to identify local complications of pancreatitis, this study may be delayed for 48 to 72 h if possible, as necrosis might not be visualized earlier.
- Routine antibiotic prophylaxis for bacterial and fungal pathogens is not warranted (a controversial topic!).
- Routine use of selective decontamination of the digestive tract is not warranted.
- Enteral nutrition is preferred to parenteral nutrition.
- The jejunal route should be used as possible.
- If used (after a 5- to 7-day trial of enteral nutrition fails), parenteral nutrition should be enriched with glutamine.
- Routine use of immune-enhancing enteral feeds is not recommended at this time.
- CT-guided fine-needle aspiration with Gram stains and culture of pancreatic or peripancreatic tissue is used to discriminate between sterile and infected necrosis. Debridement or drainage of patients with sterile necrosis is not recommended.
- Debridement or drainage in patients with infected pancreatic necrosis or abscess is best accomplished by open operative procedures.
- Open operative debridement of the pancreas should be delayed 2 to 3 weeks if possible to allow demarcation of necrotic pancreas.
- Gallstone pancreatitis should be suspected in all patients with acute pancreatitis and sonography and biochemical tests performed.
- In the setting of obstructive jaundice or other findings consistent with gallstones, ERCP should be performed within 72 h of the onset of symptoms.
- In the absence of obstructive jaundice, but with acute pancreatitis due to suspected or confirmed gallstones, ERCP should be considered within 72 h of onset of symptoms.
- Aggressive, early resuscitation is important to address the inflammatory response in acute pancreatitis.
- When infection has been documented in the setting of acute pancreatitis, management according to current sepsis guidelines should be initiated.
- Immune modulating therapies are not recommended in management of acute pancreatitis.
- Routine use of markers such as C-reactive protein or procalcitonin should not be used to guide decision making or predict clinical course of pancreatitis.

*Adapted From Crit Care Med 2004; 32:2524–2536

Biliary Tract Problems

Acute Cholecystitis

Acute cholecystitis is caused by obstruction of the cystic duct by an impacted gallstone or by local edema and inflammation. Obstruction results in gallbladder distension, subserosal edema, mucosal sloughing, venous and lymphatic congestion, and localized ischemia. The role of bacteria is debated, although positive cultures of bile or gallbladder wall tissue are found in most patients. If bacteria infiltrate the gallbladder wall, gangrenous or emphysematous cholecystitis may follow. Other complications include perforation, bile peritonitis, abscess, sepsis, gallstone ileus, or enteric fistula with the gallbladder. Sixty-five percent of patients with acute cholecystitis will also have evidence of chronic cholecystitis characterized by gallbladder wall fibrosis and chronic inflammation. While acute cholecystitis is commonly a disease of women aged 30 to 60 years, the female to male ratio decreases from 3:1 after the age of 50 years to 1.5:1.

The classic presentation is right upper quadrant tenderness with fever and leukocytosis. Clinical diagnosis is verified by gallbladder wall thickening with stones. Ultrasound is most commonly used to assess patency of the biliary tree, identify stones or sludge in the gallbladder, determine whether the gallbladder wall is thickened, inflamed, gangrenous, scarred, or calcified and evaluate surrounding structures. Pericholecystic fluid or impacted stones with a distended, thickened gallbladder are consistent with the diagnosis. The hydroxy iminodiacetic acid (HIDA) scan (cholescintigraphy) can contribute to diagnostic accuracy in cases in which ultrasound is indeterminate or additional information is required regarding the patency of the cystic duct. In a positive HIDA scan, obstruction of the cystic duct is evident when the radionuclide does not outline the gallbladder and flow normally into the common bile duct. HIDA scanning has high sensitivity and specificity and diagnostic accuracy of approximately 98% in patients with signs and symptoms of acute calculus cholecystitis. This test is less helpful (false-positive rates of 40%) if the patient has fasted for >5 days. CT with oral and IV contrast evaluates late complications of undiagnosed or misdiagnosed acute cholecystitis such as perforation, abscess, or enteric fistula.

In general, initial management is surgical resection of the gallbladder. Cholecystectomy is associated with a low complication rate and mortality of <0.2% and a bile duct injury rate of 0.4%. Open or laparoscopic procedures may be used to remove the gallbladder. Antibiotic coverage should include aerobic Gram-negative and anaerobic organisms. Patients presenting with elevated liver function test results or dilated bile ducts (>7.0 mm on ultrasound) should be evaluated for the presence of common bile duct stones. ERCP is the traditional approach employed. In some cases, MRCP may be considered. Endoscopic sphincterotomy and stone extraction before cholecystectomy is the preferred approach, with operative intervention as a fallback position for patients with failed ERCP or retained common bile duct stones.

ICU patients with acute cholecystitis have historical mortality rates >40%. Patients with acute cholecystitis in the ICU often present with atypical or nonspecific findings of abdominal sepsis including fever, leukocytosis, distension, and acidosis. Standard diagnostic strategies including ultrasound, HIDA scanning, and CT are more difficult in this population and may be less accurate due to comorbidities or sepsis. Early operative intervention should be attempted if patients are stable enough to tolerate laparoscopic or open cholecystectomy. Percutaneous drainage is effective and less risky in the critical care population. Percutaneous approaches will be inadequate if emphysematous cholecystitis occurs.

Percutaneous transhepatic cholecystostomy is performed under CT or ultrasound guidance and has a reported success rate of 95 to 100%. Complications include bleeding, catheter dislodgement, bile peritonitis, bowel perforation, and respiratory distress. Use of percutaneous cholecystostomy in the critical care context facilitates delayed laparoscopic or open removal of the gallbladder in >50% of patients. Some writers never attempt removal of the gallbladder in high-risk patients after cholecystostomy if the cystic duct is patent. Another prospective, randomized trial suggested that percutaneous cholecystostomy did not decrease mortality in comparison to conservative management.

Acalculous Cholecystitis

Acalculous cholecystitis is identified in 4 to 8% of acute cholecystectomy cases. It is more common in male than female patients and has been associated with recent surgery, major trauma, burns, multiple transfusions, childbirth, sepsis, shock, total parenteral nutrition, narcotic administration, and rheumatologic disorders. Patients are typically critically ill and require advanced monitoring. Where cholecystitis occurs in the perioperative period, two thirds of the cases are acalculous. Fifteen percent of cholecystitis following major trauma is acalculous. Pathogenesis includes gallbladder ischemia, biliary stasis or sludge, and local or systemic infection.

Diagnosis is often delayed, as symptoms are difficult to appreciate in noncommunicative patients in the ICU setting. Patients with recent major surgery, multisystem trauma, or complicated clinical conditions will not show characteristic clinical findings. Signs and symptoms are generally similar to those of calculus cholecystitis with right upper quadrant tenderness, fever, abdominal distension, diminished bowel sounds, leukocytosis, and elevated hepatic enzymes. The reported accuracy of HIDA scanning in these patients is variable, with sensitivity as low as 70% and specificity of 90%. Ultrasound may show nonspecific signs of gallbladder wall thickening, sludge, or distention. Sensitivity and specificity of ultrasound are reduced in acalculous cholecystitis. These patients have a high risk of gallbladder wall gangrene and perforation as well as higher morbidity and mortality because of delayed diagnosis and comorbid conditions. Cholecystostomy or cholecystectomy are preferred interventions. If the patient has progressed to gallbladder wall gangrene, percutaneous drainage may be inadequate therapy.

Acute Cholangitis

Acute cholangitis is caused by proliferation of microorganisms in the bile ducts. Management of the patient with acute cholangitis requires restoration of bile flow from the liver and gallbladder into the GI tract. Constant unimpeded flow of bile into the GI tract and the presence of Igs in the biliary mucosa keep bile ducts almost sterile in the normal state. Cholangitis will not develop with a properly functioning sphincterotomy or biliary enteric anastomosis. Cholangitis occurs when bile stasis promotes the growth of sufficient microorganisms to damage tissue, produce systemic inflammation, and ultimately seed the circulation. Biliary stones most commonly cause cholangitis, which can have iatrogenic causes with inadvertent biliary tract injury. The classic diagnostic trial of Charcot (abdominal pain, fever, and jaundice) describes the most common presenting symptoms of acute cholangitis. The Reynold pentad includes these findings with the addition of hypotension and mental status changes.

Imaging of patients with suspected acute cholangitis begins with ultrasound to assess biliary tree dilatation, state of the gallbladder (presence or absence of stones), and occasionally identify foreign bodies in the bile ducts. Radionuclide studies are less useful in the management of patients with acute cholangitis. CT scanning is more sensitive than ultrasound in evaluation of nonbiliary causes of obstruction in cholangitis such as periportal malignancy. It is also high sensitive for early biliary dilatation. MRCP is becoming more common in the diagnosis of biliary pathology but may be less effective in the critically ill patient due to logistic challenges associated with obtaining this test. Percutaneous transhepatic cholangiography has a long track record of success but greater associated morbidity than ERCP, which is the present "gold standard" for the diagnosis of intraluminal biliary pathology.

Patients frequently require fluid resuscitation and antibiotic support. Typical pathogens include *Escherichia coli*, Klebsiella species, Enterobacter, and enterococcus. After stabilization, the type and timing of interventions are determined. The choice of interventions includes open operation, percutaneous transhepatic drainage, or ERCP. In general, surgical procedures are not preferred due to greater associated morbidity. ERCP successfully removes >90% of common duct stones. If stones cannot be safely removed at the initial procedure, a stent will allow relief of biliary obstruction and remaining stones can be removed by subsequent ERCP, lithotripsy, or surgical common bile duct exploration. Bile duct strictures causing cholangitis can be treated with balloon dilatation utilizing ERCP or percutaneous methods. Percutaneous approaches are excellent for rapid decompression of intrahepatic bile ducts but offer fewer options for definitive, intermediate, and long-term treatment of cholangitis. For example, larger stones can only be removed after serial dilatation of the tube tract, and multiple procedures may be required to address strictures and malignancies.

ERCP combines the relative benefits of minimally invasive diagnosis and treatment with a variety of therapeutic options. Emergent stents can be placed in unstable or coagulopathic patients, and sphincterotomy allows later stone removal if initial basket procedures are unsuccessful. While all of these interventions depend on the skill of the endoscopist, in experienced hands in-hospital mortality with cholangitis is now well <10%.

Biliary Tract Injury

Following open and laparoscopic cholecystectomy, rapid recovery is commonplace, with patients returning to normal activity within 7 to 10 days after laparoscopic procedures. Patients in the early postoperative period with persisting abdominal complaints such as pain, anorexia, nausea, vomiting, and jaundice or evidence of infection require careful evaluation to rule out complications of cholecystectomy. After history and physical examination, laboratory testing includes liver function tests, amylase, lipase, and complete blood count. Iatrogenic biliary tract injuries result in significant morbidity and require further intervention. Approximately 75% of these complications go unnoticed intraoperatively. Injuries include bile duct leaks, strictures, division, or ligation.

Postoperative bile leaks occur in up to 1% of patients undergoing laparoscopy and cholecystectomy. Patients complaining of upper abdominal pain in the postoperative period must be evaluated for a bile leak. A variety of imaging methods may be utilized beginning with ultrasound and CT scanning. Either of these modalities will identify a fluid collection adjacent to the liver. MRCP and ERCP provide greater anatomic detail but are more costly. Nuclear medicine studies of the hepatobiliary tree and percutaneous transhepatic cholangiography may also be employed. Studies demonstrating intra-abdominal fluid near the liver and bile duct dilatation (ultrasound or CT) should raise suspicion of bile leakage or obstruction. ERCP then can delineate bile duct anatomy, diagnose leaks, and identify retained common bile duct stones. ERCP not only helps diagnose the site of biliary leak after bile duct injury, as a therapeutic modality it allows interventional procedures such as sphincterotomy, nasobiliary drainage, or stent placement. For example, after laparoscopy and cholecystectomy, the cystic duct stump can be the site of bile leakage. In this case, endoscopic, sphincterotomy, and stent placement to occlude the cystic duct remnant are usually adequate therapy. MRCP is less invasive but effectively demonstrates biliary tree anatomy and the presence of retained stones in the cystic, hepatic, or common bile ducts. Hepatobiliary isotope imaging reveals hepatocellular function and flow of bile into the duodenum. Extrabiliary collections of radioisotope suggest duct injury with bile leakage.

Intra-abdominal fluid collections in the early postoperative period may be secondary to bile, blood, or enteric contents secondary to unrecognized bowel injury. These may be drained percutaneously under ultrasound or CT guidance. Morbidity and mortality rates in patients with undrained bile collections are high. Prompt drainage is crucial to prevent sepsis and multiorgan failure. After drains have evacuated a bile collection, ERCP or percutaneous transhepatic cholangiography should be performed to define the site of a bile leak and the anatomy of the biliary tree. When major ductal injury has occurred, an operative treatment plan can be devised with this information. Once bile collections are drained, the major potential for immediate serious illness is generally eliminated. Then injury can be fully investigated with operative treatment executed in a controlled manner.

Selected Reading

Pain

Silen W. Cope's early diagnosis of the acute abdomen: 21st ed. Oxford, UK: Oxford University Press, 2005

Tait IS, Ionescu MV, Cuschieri A. Do patients with acute abdominal pain wait unduly long for analgesia? J R Coll Surg Edinb 1999; 44:181–184

Thomas SH, Silen W, Cheema F, et al. Effects of morphine analgesia on diagnostic accuracy in emergency department patients with abdominal pain: a prospective randomized trial. J Am Coll Surg 2003; 196:18–31

Zoltie N, Cust MP. Analgesia in the acute abdomen. Ann R Coll Surg Engl 1986; 68:209–210

Ileus

Luckey A, Livingston E, Tache Y. Mechanisms and treatment of postoperative ileus. Arch Surg 2003; 138:206–214

Stomach

Behrman SW. Management of complicated peptic ulcer disease. Arch Surg 2005; 140:201–208

Callicutt CS, Behrman SW. Incidence of Helicobacter pylori in operatively managed acute nonvariceal upper gastrointestinal bleeding. J Gastrointest Surg 2001; 5:614–619

Feliciano DV, Ojukwu JC, Rozycki GS, et al. The epidemic of cocaine-related juxtapyloric perforations: with a comment on the importance of testing for Helicobacter pylori. Ann Surg 1999; 229:801–806

Lau JY, Sung JJ, Lam YH, et al. Endoscopic retreatment compared with surgery in patients with recurrent bleeding after initial endoscopic control of bleeding ulcers. N Engl J Med 1999; 340:751–756

Ohmann C, Imhof M, Roher HD. Trends in peptic ulcer bleeding and surgical treatment. World J Surg 2000; 24:284–293

Rockall TA, Logan RF, Devlin HB, et al. Incidence of and mortality from acute upper gastrointestinal haemorrhage in the United Kingdom. Steering Committee and members of the National Audit of Acute Upper Gastrointestinal Haemorrhage. BMJ 1995; 311:222–226

Tokunaga Y, Hata K, Ryo J, et al. Density of Helicobacter pylori infection in patients with peptic ulcer perforation. J Am Coll Surg 1998; 186:659–663

Small Bowel

Bickell NA, Federman AD, Aufses AH Jr. Influence of time on risk of bowel resection in complete small bowel obstruction. J Am Coll Surg 2005; 201:847–854

Fevang BT, Fevang J, Lie SA, et al. Long-term prognosis after operation for adhesive small bowel obstruction. Ann Surg 2004; 240:193–201

Krouse RS, McCahill LE, Easson AM, et al. When the sun can set on an unoperated bowel obstruction: management of malignant bowel obstruction. J Am Coll Surg 2002; 195:117–128

Sosa J, Gardner B. Management of patients diagnosed as acute intestinal obstruction secondary to adhesions. Am Surg 1993; 59:125–128

Thompson JS, DiBaise JK, Iyer KR, et al. Postoperative short bowel syndrome. J Am Coll Surg 2005; 201:85–89

Colon/Appendix

Bahadursingh AM, Virgo KS, Kaminski DL, et al. Spectrum of disease and outcome of complicated diverticular disease. Am J Surg 2003; 186:696–701

Bartlett JG, Perl TM. The new *Clostridium difficile*: what does it mean? N Engl J Med 2005; 353:2503–2505

Broderick-Villa G, Burchette RJ, Collins JC, et al. Hospitalization for acute diverticulitis does not mandate routine elective colectomy. Arch Surg 2005; 140:576–583

Christopher FL, Lane MJ, Ward JA, et al. Unenhanced helical CT scanning of the abdomen and pelvis changes disposition of patients presenting to the emergency department with possible acute appendicitis. J Emerg Med 2002; 23:1–7

Gladman MA, Scott SM, Lunniss PJ, et al. Systemic review of surgical options for idiopathic megarectum and megacolon. Ann Surg 2005; 241:562–574

Loo VG, Poirier L, Miller MA, et al. A predominantly clonal multi-institutional outbreak of *Clostridium difficile*-associated diarrhea with high morbidity and mortality. N Engl J Med 2005; 353:2442–2449

Mittal VK, Goliath J, Sabir M, et al. Advantages of focused helical computed tomographic scanning with rectal contrast only vs triple contrast in the diagnosis of clinically uncertain acute appendicitis: a prospective randomized study. Arch Surg 2004; 139:495–500

Preventza OA, Lazarides K, Sawyer MD. Ischemic colitis in young adults: a single-institution experience. J Gastrointest Surg 2001; 5:388–392

Reilly PM, Wilkins KB, Fuh KC, et al. The mesenteric hemodynamic response to circulatory shock: an overview. Shock 2001; 15:329–343

Wong WD, Wexner SD, Lowry A, et al. Practice parameters for the treatment of sigmoid diverticulitis: supporting documentation. The Standards Task Force. The American Society of Colon and Rectal Surgeons. Dis Colon Rectum 2000; 43:290–297

Pancreas

Acosta JM, Katkhouda N, Debian KA, et al. Early ductal decompression versus conservative management for gallstone pancreatitis with ampullary obstruction: a prospective randomized clinical trial. Ann Surg 2006; 243:33–40

Acosta JM, Pellegrini CA, Skinner DB. Etiology and pathogenesis of acute biliary pancreatitis. Surgery 1980; 88:118–125

Baron TH, Morgan DE. Acute necrotizing pancreatitis. N Engl J Med 1999; 340:1412–1417

Buchler MW, Gloor B, Muller CA, et al. Acute necrotizing pancreatitis: treatment strategy according to the status of infection. Ann Surg 2000; 232:619–626

Eachempati SR, Hydo LJ, Barie PS. Severity scoring for prognostication in patients with severe acute pancreatitis: comparative analysis of the Ranson score and the APACHE III score. Arch Surg 2002; 137:730–736

Fan ST, Lai EC, Mok FP, et al. Early treatment of acute biliary pancreatitis by endoscopic papillotomy. N Engl J Med 1993; 328:228–232

Folsch UR, Nitsche R, Ludtke R, et al. Early ERCP and papillotomy compared with conservative treatment for acute biliary pancreatitis. The German Study Group on Acute Biliary Pancreatitis. N Engl J Med 1997; 336:237–242

Guzman EA, Rudnicki M. Intricacies of host response in acute pancreatitis. J Am Coll Surg 2006; 202:509–519

Hallal AH, Amortegui JD, Jeroukhimov IM, et al. Magnetic resonance cholangiopancreatography accurately detects common bile duct stones in resolving gallstone pancreatitis. J Am Coll Surg 2005; 200:869–875

Heinrich S, Schäfer M, Rousson V, et al. Evidence-based treatment of acute pancreatitis: a look at established paradigms. Ann Surg 2006; 243:154–168

Nathens AB, Curtis JR, Beale RJ, et al. Management of the critically ill patient with severe acute pancreatitis. Crit Care Med 2004; 32:2524–2536

Ranson JH. Etiological and prognostic factors in human acute pancreatitis: a review. Am J Gastroenterol 1982; 77:633–638

Rau B, Pralle U, Mayer JM, et al. Role of ultrasonographically guided fine-needle aspiration cytology in the diagnosis of infected pancreatic necrosis. Br J Surg 1998; 85:179–184

Biliary Tree

Berber E, Engle KL, String A, et al. Selective use of tube cholecystostomy with interval laparoscopic cholecystectomy in acute cholecystitis. Arch Surg 2000; 135:341–346

Buell JF, Cronin DC, Funaki B, et al. Devastating and fatal complications associated with combined vascular and bile duct injuries during cholecystectomy. Arch Surg 2002; 137:703–710

Chang L, Moonka R, Stelzner M. Percutaneous cholecystostomy for acute cholecystitis in veteran patients. Am J Surg 2000; 180:198–202

Gupta N, Solomon H, Fairchild R, et al. Management and outcome of patients with combined bile duct and hepatic artery injuries. Arch Surg 1998; 133: 176–181

Lai EC, Mok FP, Tan ES, et al. Endoscopic biliary drainage for severe acute cholangitis. N Engl J Med 1992; 326:1582–1586

Lillemoe KD, Martin SA, Cameron JL, et al. Major bile duct injuries during laparoscopic cholecystectomy: follow-up after combined surgical and radiologic management. Ann Surg 1997; 225:459–471

Lo CM, Liu CL, Fan ST, et al. Prospective randomized study of early versus delayed laparoscopic cholecystectomy for acute cholecystitis. Ann Surg 1998; 227:461–467

Murr MM, Gigot JF, Nagorney DM, et al. Long-term results of biliary reconstruction after laparoscopic bile duct injuries. Arch Surg 1999; 134:604–610

Spira RM, Nissan A, Zamir O, et al. Percutaneous transhepatic cholecystostomy and delayed laparoscopic cholecystectomy in critically ill patients with acute calculus cholecystitis. Am J Surg 2002; 183:62–66

The Southern Surgeons Club. A prospective analysis of 1518 laparoscopic cholecystectomies. N Engl J Med 1991; 324:1073–1078

Notes

Notes

Coma and Delirium

Thomas P. Bleck, MD, FCCP

Objectives:

- Understand the anatomic and physiologic determinants of consciousness
- Recognize the need for common definitions of behavior in comatose and delirious patients
- Be able to perform a rapid coma examination
- Develop an initial management approach

Key words: coma; death; delirium; obtundation; stupor; vegetative state

Altered mental status belongs in the category of terms that are widely understood but lack a consensual definition. In modern multidisciplinary ICUs, the combination of the diseases being managed and the drugs employed for that management results in a large percentage of patients who develop at least a temporary impairment of awareness or behavior. This area has been obscured by the psychiatric redefinition of delirium into a very broad concept which no longer requires agitation for its diagnosis. Intensivists should be aware of this as they interact with their psychiatric and neurologic colleagues.

Definitions

The following definitions are derived from Plum and Posner,[1] except as noted.

Confusion

Confused patients are bewildered, and often have difficulty following commands. Disorientation to place and time is common ("except in rare instances of acute delirium, disorientation to self is confined to psychologic disturbances"[1]). Memory is disturbed. Drowsiness is prominent, and may alternate with nighttime agitation.

Delirium

Delirium is "a floridly abnormal mental state characterized by disorientation, fear, irritability, misperception of sensory stimuli, and, often, visual hallucinations."[1] This definition is diagnostically more specific than that in the Diagnostic and Statistical Manual of Mental Disorders IV[2] ("The essential feature of a delirium is a disturbance of consciousness that is accompanied by a change in cognition that cannot be better accounted for by a preexisting or evolving dementia. The disturbance develops over a short period of time, usually hours to days, and tends to fluctuate during the course of the day. There is evidence from the history, physical examination, or laboratory tests that the delirium is a direct physiologic consequence of a general medical condition, substance intoxication or withdrawal, use of a medication, or toxin exposure, or a combination of these factors."[2]). Delirium has also been termed "acute brain failure," which may be a foreign notion to localizationists but is a valuable tool for communication.

Obtundation

Obtundation is mental blunting, associated with slowed psychological responses to stimulation and an increase in drowsiness and in the number of hours slept.

Stupor

Stupor is "a condition of deep sleep or behaviorally similar unresponsiveness in which the patient can be aroused only by vigorous and repeated stimuli."[1] This is not sleep from an EEG perspective.

Coma

Coma is "a state of unarousable psychologic unresponsiveness in which the subjects lie with eyes closed. Subjects in coma show no psychologically understandable response to external stimuli or inner need. They neither utter understandable words nor accurately localize noxious stimuli with discrete defensive movements."[1]

Vegetative State

Vegetative state is "the subacute or chronic condition that sometimes emerges after severe brain injury and comprises a return of wakefulness accompanied by an apparent total lack of cognitive function. An operational definition is that the eyes open spontaneously in response to verbal stimuli. Sleep-wake cycles exist. The patients spontaneously maintain normal levels of blood pressure and respiratory control. They show no discrete localizing motor responses and neither offer comprehensible words nor obey any verbal commands. *Persistent or chronic vegetative state* refers to this condition in its permanent form and designates subjects who survive for prolonged periods (sometimes years) following a severe brain injury without ever recovering any outward manifestations of higher mental activity. In most instances the vegetative state follows upon a period of sleeplike coma. Nearly all patients in coma begin to awaken within 2 to 4 weeks no matter how severe the brain damage. Although many such patients are akinetic and mute, others with apparently similar degrees of brain damage may be restless, noisy, and hypermobile."[1] Synonyms include coma vigil, apallic syndrome, cerebral death, neocortical death, total dementia, and akinetic mutism. It is important to recognize that persistent vegetative state after trauma, especially in the younger patient, does not carry nearly as dismal a prognosis for recovery as does that following anoxia.[3]

ICU Psychosis

Considerable debate exists about the existence of a specific disorder of behavior or perception related solely to ICU confinement. Opinions vary (even in the same text) from:

When faced with a patient who is confused and perhaps agitated, the first question must be "Is the patient delirious?" *The clinician should not attribute the change in mental status to an "ICU psychosis."* The brain's response to a physiologic (sic) insult, whether metabolic, anoxic, toxic, or infectious, is delirium.[4]

to:

The incidence of abnormal behavior, perception, or cognition in adult patients admitted to an ICU is somewhat disputed, but every observational study has reported some incidence of such abnormalities with the highest estimates placed at 70 %. These aberrations typically occur after 5 to 7 days of ICU stay, and risk of their development increases with duration of stay. It is perhaps intuitively clear that life in the ICU is sufficiently stressful to result in overt psychiatric consequences for the patient. Physically, the patient often experiences substantial pain. Sleep is unlikely to even approximate the normal architecture, and sleep deprivation is common. Perception is grossly distorted with loss of day-night cycles, immobilization, technology's noise, and overwhelming monotony. Emotionally, the patient must contend with the fear of death, the loss of self-control, the total invasion of privacy, and the dependence on staff and machines to perform even basic bodily functions. This physical and emotional crisis occurs most commonly in conjunction with polypharmacy and neurologic consequences of underlying disease.

Some authors have objected to the use of the term "ICU psychosis," largely because it is a convenient catchall obscuring the identification of specific disorders. Nonetheless, it is our observation that when all organic causes of abnormal mentation described above have been excluded, many patients are encountered with persisting difficulties that do respond to modification of the ICU experience. *We emphasize, however, that this is a diagnosis of exclusion and that other possibilities must be rigorously considered and sought.*[5]

Death

Rather than using terms like brain death, I find it more useful to think of death as death, and as a consequence of either complete cardiopulmonary or complete brain failure. This helps counteract the notion that "brain death" is somehow less a form of death than cardiopulmonary death. The old distinction of "death" and "brain death" is a major stumbling block in the pursuit of organ donation, and to a lesser extent, in the withdrawal of support from dead patients whose bodies are being ventilated and kept perfused with vasopressors.

Diagnosing Death by Neurologic Criteria

Diagnosing death by neurologic criteria requires a permissive diagnosis and the absence of brainstem reflexes. In certain circumstances, additional testing is needed.

Permissive diagnosis is a reason sufficient to explain death; failure to meet this criterion explains almost all cases of recovery after the diagnosis of "brain death." Hypothermia and drug intoxication must be excluded or corrected before proceeding, and intact neuromuscular transmission should be demonstrated (spinal reflexes are adequate; in case of question, train-of-four stimulation may be used).

Absence of brainstem reflexes usually include (1) cervico-ocular reflex; (2) vestibulo-ocular reflex; (3) cough reflex; (4) gag reflex; (5) corneal reflex; (6) pupillary reflexes; and (7) absence of response to noxious stimuli applied to the face. (8) *Apnea testing* should be included here but is often listed as a separate criterion. The patient should not breathe when the $Paco_2$ is allowed to rise from 40 torr to 60 torr (the British use 50 torr as the target). The patient must be adequately preoxygenated and should receive supplemental oxygen during the test (either 10 cm H_2O of continuous positive airway pressure or a tracheal catheter supplying a 10-L/min flow).

Confirmatory tests are not required in most circumstances. The exceptions to this are primarily in circumstances where the examinations above cannot be completed (*eg*, patients who do not tolerate the apnea test from a cardiovascular standpoint, or whose faces are too swollen to examine their eye movements).

- The most useful confirmatory test is a nuclide angiogram.
- Contrast angiography may also be used.
- EEG is not required and is of limited utility; the conditions that render the physical examination unreliable (*eg*, hypothermia, hyp nosedative drug intoxication) also may make the EEG appear to show cerebral electrical silence.

Unconsciousness

Unconsciousness is produced in one of three ways: diffuse bilateral involvement of the cerebral hemispheres, injury to the brainstem reticular activating system (RAS), or a combination of focal injuries to the cortex and brainstem. Herniation is a special case of RAS insult, caused by a cerebral space-occupying lesion that produces a mechanical shift of brainstem structures.

Consciousness has two necessary components: arousal and content. Specific structures in the CNS modulate arousal; lesions in these areas render the patient unable to respond in spite of intact sensory afferents. Unconsciousness is the condition in which the patient makes no appropriate responses to stimuli, either external (*eg*, pain) or internal (*eg*, thirst). This state does not exclude posturing and other reflex movements.

Causes of Unconsciousness

There are a large number of causes of coma, and it is convenient to classify them as those producing diffuse bihemispheric dysfunction vs those with structural lesions producing mass effect. Some of the major causes are shown in shown in Table 1. Nonconvulsive status epilepticus may present as unresponsiveness. Subtle signs, such as eyelid fluttering, mild facial twitching, or nystagmus may be the only evidence that the patient is seizing. Similarly, a postictal state may show prolonged unresponsiveness, and include focal signs of hemiparesis (Todd's paralysis) or posturing.

Psychiatric conditions mimicking coma include catatonia, conversion reactions, and feigned coma. In these conditions, pupillary responses will be normal, as will ocular movements. The motor examination may demonstrate normal tone in supposedly paretic limbs, and when asleep, the patient will have normal movements.

The Anatomy of Consciousness

Two major neuroanatomic structures are necessary for consciousness: the RAS and the cerebral hemispheres. The RAS is primarily responsible for arousal mechanisms, and the hemispheres influence the content of consciousness.

The RAS receives input from all major afferent tracts, and projects widely to the thalamus, basal forebrain, and the cerebral hemispheres. The crucial segment of the RAS for arousal is between the rostral midbrain and the midpons.

Isolated lesions in this portion of the RAS produce coma, whereas lower lesions do not. Damage to the thalamus or hypothalamus can also alter consciousness, which is understandable given the large interconnection between these structures and the RAS, but bilateral involvement is usually required.

Focal lesions in the cerebral cortex tend not to alter arousal but instead affect the content of consciousness. To affect arousal, large areas of both hemispheres need to be involved, either on a structural or metabolic basis. Large focal processes, such as tumor or infarction, may alter the contralateral hemisphere by pressure effects, or by disrupting circulation or metabolism. Dominant-hemisphere lesions may be more significant in affecting arousal than ones in the nondominant hemisphere.

Herniation

Herniation is caused when pressure of a mass lesion forces brain tissue to shift from one intracerebral compartment to another, and it can cause unconsciousness when pressure on the brainstem disrupts the RAS.[6] The total volume contained in the cranial vault is limited and a mass lesion must cause some shift of the intracerebral contents. Initially, a mass lesion displaces cerebrospinal fluid, but eventually a limit is reached and intracranial pressure (ICP) increases. Brain tissue is highly inelastic so this pressure causes herniation.

Central herniation is presumed to be from a pressure cone forcing the brain out towards its only exit, the foramen magnum. Uncal herniation occurs when the medial temporal lobe is forced over the tentorial edge into the space beside the lateral midbrain. This compresses the third cranial nerve and particularly the parasympathetic fibers to the pupil traveling around the outside of the nerve, causing unilateral dilation of the pupil on the side of the lesion, the "blown pupil."

Ropper[7] has ascribed many of the signs of herniation to horizontal displacement of the brainstem. Acute pupillary dilation often corrects within minutes of initiating therapy for increased ICP, which is more consistent with lateral displacement than with irreversible uncal herniation.

Downward herniation can distract the basilar artery, which is tethered to the skull base, away from the brainstem and cause hemorrhage or infarction. Eventually, the downward movement increases subtentorial pressure and forces the cerebellar tonsils out the foramen magnum. Tonsillar herniation can also occur if a lumbar puncture is performed on a patient with elevated ICP, generating a large transforamenal pressure gradient. This is often catastrophic, as acute pressure on the medulla causes sudden respiratory arrest. Upward herniation of brainstem structures through the tentorium is possible in the setting of large posterior fossa masses that increase subtentorial pressure.

Table 1. *Causes of Coma*

Presentation as Diffuse Bihemispheric Process (Usually Symmetric, Often With Intact Brainstem Reflexes)

Drug intoxication
    Barbiturates
    Opiates
    Alcohol
    Antidepressants
    Benzodiazepines
    Sedatives/tranquilizers
    Drugs of abuse
    Antipsychotic agents
    Anticholinergics
    Salicylates
Metabolic
    Hypo- or hypernatremia
    Hypoglycemia
    Nonketotic hyperosmolar coma
    Diabetic ketoacidosis
    Hypo- or hypercalcemia
    Hypothyroidism
    Uremia
    Hepatic encephalopathy
    Hypo- or hyperthermia
    Hypercarbia
    Hypoxia
Other Causes
    Diffuse presentations
        Toxins, especially carbon monoxide, methanol
        Meningitis/encephalitis: viral or bacterial
        Sepsis
        Hypertensive encephalopathy
        Subarachnoid hemorrhage (low grade)
        Head trauma, mild
        Seizures/postictal
    Presentation as brainstem process (often asymmetric, impaired brainstem function)
        Brainstem infarction/hemorrhage
        Posterior fossa tumor
        Herniation: from any cerebral space-occupying lesion (tumor, stroke, hemorrhage)
        Subarachnoid hemorrhage (higher grades)
        Trauma, severe

Evaluation of Unconsciousness

Evaluation must be rapid because morbidity is often related to how quickly therapy is begun. Many of the diffuse metabolic or toxic causes of coma resolve without long-term CNS damage, where as acute structural disease, especially if causing herniation, may be rapidly fatal.

A key tenet of the care of the comatose patient is that initial treatment must proceed simultaneously with diagnosis. Acute (over seconds to minutes) coma suggests cerebrovascular disease, either hemorrhagic or ischemic, or cardiac arrest. A recent history of head injury may indicate a subdural or epidural hematoma. A subacute course (many minutes to hours), may suggest intoxication or infection, while a more prolonged period of altered mental status might occur from a CNS tumor or a systemic metabolic disturbance. Weakness or falling to one side suggests a focal lesion. A history of epilepsy may point to a postictal state. Witnesses should be carefully questioned about possible toxic ingestion.

Laboratory Studies: Laboratory studies may not aid in acute management, but frequently help with assessment later in the patient's course. Serum biochemistry will identify major metabolic derangements, including hypoglycemia, nonketotic hyperglycemia, and diabetic ketoacidosis.[8] A complete blood count should be obtained, as either CNS or systemic infections can cause coma. Urinalysis should be routine, as urosepsis may present first as altered mental status, and often occurs without fever in the elderly. Hypothyroidism can cause coma of unknown etiology, so the thyroid-stimulating hormone level needs to be measured.

A urine toxicologic screen for drugs of abuse is almost always needed because drug overdose is one of the most common causes of coma of unknown etiology (Plum and Posner, 1980[1]). Drug abuse is frequently implicated in cases of trauma. Mixed intoxication with combinations of alcohol, barbiturates, opiates, and benzodiazepines may be seen, and these agents should be screened for routinely. Finally, unconsciousness with focal signs can be caused by cocaine intoxication, which can cause cerebral vasculitis and stroke.

Blood gas analysis is necessary to assess hypoxia, hypercarbia, or abnormal pH. Hypoxia may be caused by drug intoxication. Particular acid-base abnormalities are often helpful in diagnosing metabolic encephalopathies. Respiratory acidosis, with hypoxia, occurs with hypoventilation from respiratory depressants. Metabolic acidosis may suggest particular toxic ingestions (*eg,* salicylates or alcohols), diabetic ketoacidosis, uremia, sepsis, or lactic acidosis. Compensatory respiratory alkalosis can be seen with many of the metabolic acidoses. Pure respiratory alkalosis, with hyperventilation, may suggest psychogenic coma.

Examination

The neurologic examination is directed at assessing the etiology of unconsciousness, the goal being to determine whether there is a bihemispheric process vs an RAS problem, looking particularly for signs of herniation. One neurologic cause of pseudocoma needs to be excluded immediately, the "locked-in" state.[9] In this condition, usually due to pontine infarction or hemorrhage, all cortical control except of vertical gaze is disconnected. Often the patient is only able to look upward, but may not even be capable of opening his eyelids. If the patient can, when his eyelids have been opened, follow the command to look up, the patient is not comatose but locked in, and needs studies directed towards identifying a pontine lesion.

Pupillary Responses

The pupils should be examined, preferably with a bright light and with the room darkened. The pupillary light reflex requires both intact sympathetic and parasympathetic systems to dilate and constrict, respectively. The key paradigm to remember is that damage to the midbrain affects the RAS, but also pupil reactivity, whereas metabolic disease produces coma, but usually leaves the light reflex intact.

Specific structural lesions produce particular pupillary patterns: *hypothalamic lesions,* either by direct involvement or secondary to increased pressure from above, interrupt the efferent sympathetic pathways, producing small, reactive pupils. *Unilateral diencephalic dysfunction* may cause a Horner's syndrome of unilateral pupillary constriction and ptosis, which may be a an early sign of herniation. *Dorsal midbrain damage* interrupts the parasympathetic efferents, and the pupils become slightly large and unreactive, but may spontaneously fluctuate in size (hippus). *Central midbrain lesions* damage both sympathetic and parasympathetic tracts, producing fixed, often irregular, midposition pupils. This is most frequently seen in the setting of true transtentorial herniation and generally implies a poor outcome. *Pontine lesions*, usually hemorrhagic, interrupt the descending sympathetic fibers and irritate the parasympathetic fibers, producing pinpoint pupils. More *caudal lesions* affect only the sympathetic system, again causing a Horner's syndrome. Finally, a unilateral fixed, dilated pupil suggests *third nerve dysfunction*.

Small, reactive pupils are the hallmark of drug intoxication (particularly opiate) and metabolic disease, but there are a few exceptions. The light reflex is usually resistant to metabolic disease, but it may be suppressed in the setting of severe drug overdose, especially from barbiturates. Severe opiate intoxication may mimic the pinpoint pupils of pontine hemorrhage. Anticholinergics may produce large, unreactive pupils associated with altered mental status, as can glutethimide intoxication. Anoxia may cause fixed dilated pupils, which become reactive if cerebral oxygen delivery is restored in time.

Eye Movements

If purposeful movements, such as visual tracking movements looking toward a loud noise, are absent, check for spontaneous roving eye movements. Roving movements are often seen with metabolic encephalopathies. All of these findings imply intact cortical control of the brainstem. A fixed deviation of eyes usually means there is a hemispheral lesion on the side toward which the eyes deviate, often associated with a contralateral hemiparesis. Isolated pontine lesions can cause eye deviation toward the damaged side, associated with an ipsilateral (*ie*, contralateral to the pontine lesion). A fixed downward gaze is seen with midbrain compression from above. Inability of one eye to move medially is seen with upper brainstem lesions to the medial longitudinal fasciculus, on the side of the abnormal eye, and is called an internuclear ophthalmoplegia.

If no spontaneous movement is found, the cervico-ocular reflex should be tested (doll's eyes maneuver); an important caveat is to be sure that there is no possibility of a cervical cord or spine lesion prior to testing. The reflex is tested by rapidly turning the head from midline to one side and observing the eye movements. In the intact brainstem, this produces a contralateral conjugate eye movement, the net effect of which is to keep the eyes seemingly fixed on a point in space. After a few moments the eyes should return to midposition. The head should then be turned in the opposite direction to check for symmetry of the response. Failure of the reflex in either direction implies brainstem dysfunction. The reflex also works in the vertical plane, and should be tested in a similar fashion. If this maneuver fails, or is untestable because of neck injury, the vestibular-ocular reflex may be assessed by caloric testing. This is done by elevating the patient's head to 30 degrees if possible, and rapidly instilling about 50 mL of iced water in the ear canal with a syringe. It is important to first check that the ear canal is clear and that the tympanic membrane is not damaged, a relative contraindication to the test. Cold water instilled against the tympanic membrane produces cooling of the adjacent semicircular canal, increasing the local density of the endolymph and creating a net flow towards the cooler side. This direction of flow mimics head turning away from the stimulated side, and therefore causes reflex slow eye movement towards the stimulus. In an intact brain, the frontal eye fields attempt to override this brainstem-driven tonic eye deviation, producing rapid saccades away from the stimulus (nystagmus), but with cortical damage, the eyes will maintain a fixed deviation. Cold caloric testing is a potent stimulus to the brainstem and may produce gaze deviation even when head turning fails to do so. The key observation is that whenever conjugate gaze occurs, regardless of the stimulus, it implies an intact brainstem in the region of the RAS. Eye deviation from hemispheral lesions can usually be overcome by these maneuvers, where as with pontine lesions, the eyes will not cross midline. Total lack of response can be seen with severe brainstem dysfunction, drug ingestion (especially barbiturates, narcotics, and phenytoin), neuromuscular blockade, or bilateral vestibular lesions.

Motor Responses

The patient is observed for spontaneous movement or, if none is present, response to stimulus. The type of motor response and its symmetry provides important clues in assessing the location and severity of focal deficits. Any asymmetry of the motor patterns suggests a contralateral focal cerebral lesion. Comatose patients may not show purposeful movements, such as reaching for their endotracheal tube or localizing painful stimuli, which require an intact sensory system, efferent motor system, and cortical processing. Patients who cannot localize pain may withdraw from focal stimuli, again requiring functioning afferent and efferent tracts.

Abnormal motor responses include decorticate and decerebrate posturing. Decorticate posturing consists of flexion of the arms and extension of the legs, while in decerebrate posturing both the arms and the legs extend. The important principle of localization is that both forms of abnormal posture can occur with hemispheral as well as brainstem lesions. Prognostically, decerebrate is worse than decorticate posturing. Any comatose patient who develops either form of abnormal posturing needs intervention for acute worsening.

Extension of the arms with weak flexion of the legs or absent leg movement implies severe structural damage of the pontine tegmentum. This finding indicates severe brainstem dysfunction and carries a grave prognosis.[10] Total loss of tone does not necessarily mean upper brainstem damage and can be associated with spinal cord or medullary transection (spinal shock), peripheral nerve injury, or disease or neuromuscular blockade.

Finally, one must be careful not to confuse reflex activity with other responses. In particular, triple flexion of the lower extremity is a reflex signaling upper motor neuron dysfunction. It may look like spontaneous movement of the leg away from painful stimuli, but it is a reflex; the important finding is that the reflex response is very rapid and stereotyped.

Respiration

Respiration is controlled by brainstem structures with mediation by cortical influences, and specific respiratory patterns have localizing value. Unfortunately, these patterns are often not noticed in patients receiving mechanical ventilatory support. The most common abnormal respiratory pattern is Cheyne-Stokes respiration, in which there is a sequential waxing and waning of tidal volume, including periods of apnea. It can be seen in noncomatose patients with congestive heart failure, hypoxia, or occasionally during normal sleep, and is associated with bihemispheric dysfunction in unconscious patients. Respiratory centers in the brainstem increase or decrease the respiratory rate in response to elevated or lowered $Paco_2$ levels, respectively. There is, however, frontal lobe control such that even with very low $Paco_2$ levels, respiration does not stop but only slows, with a reduced tidal volume, until the $Paco_2$ normalizes. When bihemispheric dysfunction is present on a structural or metabolic basis, the modulating influence of the cortex is lost and Cheyne-Stokes respiration is seen.

Damage to the upper brainstem reticular formation is reported to cause sustained hyperventilation, called central neurogenic hyperventilation or central reflex hyperpnea. Tachypnea is often seen in comatose patients, but other causes, particularly hypoxia, neurogenic pulmonary edema, or metabolic disarray, are more likely. To diagnose true central neurogenic hyperventilation requires an increased Pao_2 and decreased $Paco_2$, without other metabolic changes or drug intoxication.

Apneustic, cluster, and ataxic breathing are patterns associated with lesions of the mid-lower pons, upper medulla, and caudal medulla, respectively, and all provide inadequate ventilation so mechanical support is needed. With apneusis, a patient has a prolonged inspiratory pause, or respiration may consist of cycles of quick inhalation/pause/exhalation/pause. Cluster breathing consists of several rapid shallow breaths followed by a pause, while ataxic breathing is irregular brief respirations of small, random tidal volumes. Finally, apnea is of poor localizing value and may be seen secondary to cardiac arrest, multifocal brain lesions, drug overdose, spinal cord transection, or primary pulmonary process.

CT Scanning

Any unconscious patient with focal signs will need a CT scan, as many such patients will have potentially treatable problems. The differential diagnosis of coma with focal signs includes tumor, increased ICP, intracranial hemorrhage, CNS infection, and stroke. Unfortunately, some structural lesions may not produce focal signs but only brainstem dysfunction. Because of this, most comatose patients with coma of unknown etiology will need early CT scanning. Any comatose patient may also have fallen, and be at risk for a traumatic subdural or epidural hematoma, in addition to the primary problem. Traumatic hematomas may appear after the initial CT, so acute worsening of any patient is an indication for repeat scanning.

Lumbar Puncture and Antibiotics

Other than suspected bacterial meningitis, a lumbar puncture is needed in any patient for whom the cause of coma is still unknown after initial evaluation to look for nonbacterial meningitis or encephalitis, especially viral or fungal, or occult subarachnoid hemorrhage.

Initial Management

Resuscitation

Acute care must always start with basic life support: a patent airway, ventilation, and circulation. An easily reversible cause of coma, if treated sufficiently rapidly, is hypoxia secondary to airway obstruction or pulmonary disease. However, CNS lesions can cause abnormal respiratory patterns as well. Quickly observing the patient's respiratory pattern may help with localization as described above. Comatose patients are frequently intubated for one of two reasons: ventilatory failure or airway protection. Airway-protective reflexes of gagging and coughing may be lost in coma, increasing the risk of aspiration. Also, the tongue and oropharynx relax, increasing the chance of airway obstruction. The aspiration risk is increased if gastric lavage is used for suspected toxic ingestion without a cuffed endotracheal tube in place.

Prior to intubation, the stability of the cervical spine must be assessed, particularly in patients with trauma. Also, patients who lose consciousness acutely may fall and injure their cervical spine. Because patients with altered mental status may be unable to tell the examiner about neck pain, all comatose patients should be treated as if they have a neck injury unless a reliable witness can attest to the lack of a fall or other potential for neck injury.

A patient in a hard cervical collar may be difficult to intubate orally as neck extension cannot and should not be attempted, so nasotracheal intubation may be preferred. The one exception to nasal intubation would be if there is a suspected basilar skull fracture. If raised ICP is at all possible, 100 mg lidocaine or 300 mg thiopental should be administered IV 1 min prior to intubation to blunt the rise in ICP normally associated with intubation.

A key part of the immediate evaluation is the patient's vital signs, which may themselves help decide the cause of unconsciousness. Severe hypotension can be sufficient to cause symptomatic CNS hypoperfusion and should be corrected urgently with fluids and/or vasopressors. Conversely, a severely elevated blood pressure may cause hypertensive encephalopathy, a neurologic emergency requiring rapid treatment.

Urgent Corrective Measures

Hypoglycemia can be catastrophic to the CNS, with degree of injury determined by the length of time and level of the low blood glucose.[8] Finger-stick determinations are potentially unreliable, as the glucometers can be less accurate at low values; a measured serum glucose may in reality be much lower than that estimated by finger-stick methods. A finger-stick glucose reading <60 mg/dL should prompt urgent replacement of glucose. A dose of 50 mL of D50/W should be given immediately to any patient with coma of unknown etiology. This will produce no detrimental effect on other causes of coma (except Wernicke's encephalopathy, discussed below). Even in the case of hyperglycemic states producing coma, the marginal increase in total body glucose will not adversely affect treatment or generate CNS damage. In the case of hypoglycemia, glucose replacement may produce rapid reversal of unconsciousness.

Prior to giving glucose, thiamine 1 mg/kg IV must be administered to prevent precipitating acute Wernicke's encephalopathy (confusion, ataxia, and ophthalmoplegia) with associated necrosis of the midline gray structures leading to permanent memory loss. Alcoholics are at particular risk because of poor general nutrition. Although most patients will not be thiamine deficient, the potentially terrible result if missed makes thiamine administration before giving glucose imperative.

Narcotic overdose is a common cause of coma in emergency room patients, as well as in hospitalized and particularly ICU patients. The classic findings in narcotic intoxication are coma, small, reactive pupils, shallow respirations, and hypotension. Unfortunately, not all patients may display these findings. Pupillary responses in particular may be unreliable. Other drug ingestion (eg, anticholinergics) may mask pupil findings. Hypoxia, brainstem lesions, or barbiturates may also blunt the response. Because the physical signs can be unreliable and narcotic overdose is common, any patient with coma of unknown etiology should be given naloxone 0.2 to 0.4 mg by slow IV injection.

Management of Specific Causes

Elevated ICP

If increased ICP is suspected, treatment needs to be initiated immediately, particularly if herniation is identified.[11] The patient's head should be elevated to between 30 and 45 degrees and, if possible, the neck placed in a neutral position to facilitate venous return. Adequate ventilation and oxygenation are essential as hypoxia or hypercarbia will increase cerebral blood flow and ICP. Hyperventilation to lower the patient's $Paco_2$ to approximately 25 to 30 mm Hg will acutely reduce cerebral blood volume and ICP, but this effect is transient, and other interventions to control ICP will need to follow.

For severe rises in ICP, mannitol should be administered at a dose of 0.25 to 0.5 g/kg every 4 to 6 h, taking care to correct serum electrolytes, osmolality, and polemic status. The mechanism of action of this agent is uncertain (extracellular space dehydration vs intravascular volume expansion), but its utility is not. Administration of steroids is somewhat controversial, being useful for tumors and abscesses, possibly efficacious in meningitis, and of no benefit in stroke or anoxia. If the cause of coma is unknown, and the patient has evidence of increased ICP, an initial IV dose of 4 to 6 mg dexamethasone may be given empirically while diagnostic studies are undertaken.

Other factors that should be considered in the acute management of ICP include: (1) adequate sedation, with the addition of neuromuscular blockade, if necessary to stop excess muscle activity; (2) low ventilator pressure settings, which allow for good central venous return; and (3) suppression of fever, which accelerates cerebral metabolism and thereby raises oxygen consumption, resulting in increased cerebral blood flow and higher ICP. Fever also accelerates neuronal damage from other causes. Finally, care should be taken not to acutely lower blood pressure (unless hypertension is very severe) to maintain cerebral perfusion pressure.

Investigation of the patient with raised ICP requires a CT scan to exclude a space-occupying lesion and neurosurgical support if one is found. Alternative considerations requiring specific treatment include cerebrovascular accident, subarachnoid hemorrhage, and metabolic encephalopathy.

Drug Intoxication

When drug overdose or toxin ingestion is suspected, activated charcoal at a dose of 50 to 100 mg should be given to prevent system absorption. Gastric lavage may also be useful and is preferred over emesis. Use of both charcoal and lavage require airway protection, and in patients with mental status changes, this usually mandates intubation prior to treatment. For suspected benzodiazepine intoxication, flumazenil given in divided doses up to 1 mg total may produce dramatic arousal, but it is contraindicated in cases where tricyclic antidepressants may also have be consumed, as there is an increased risk of seizures and status epilepticus. Flumazenil is also reported to improve mental function transiently in patients with hepatic coma, probably by reversing the GABAergic effect of accumulating endogenous benzodiazepine receptor ligands.

Seizures

Status epilepticus is another cause of coma requiring emergent action. Clinical generalized convulsive status epilepticus is readily recognized, but nonconvulsive status epilepticus (NCSE) may be difficult to discern. Often the only indication of NCSE may be subtle twitching of individual muscles, particularly the face, rhythmic eye movements, or blinking. Status epilepticus of either type needs rapid treatment both to suppress the seizures and to prevent their recurrence. Lorazepam at 0.1 mg/kg is often effective at terminating seizures. At the same time, 20 mg/kg of phenytoin or fosphenytoin should usually be administered (at a rate no greater than 50 mg/min), with an additional 5 mg/kg to be given if the patient is still seizing. Further therapy may include midazolam, propofol, or high-dose pentobarbital. An emergent EEG is indicated for any patient with suspected NCSE, or a patient being put in drug-induced coma to control seizures.

Meningitis

Emergent antibiotic therapy is indicated for any patient with suspected bacterial meningitis. In this life-threatening illness, treatment should not be delayed to obtain a CT or a lumbar puncture. Lumbar puncture results will not be significantly compromised if obtained immediately after antibiotic administration.

Supportive Care

Fluid therapy and vital organ support must be ongoing. The unconscious patient is totally dependent on nursing care, with particular attention paid to eye, mouth, and pressure area care. Nutritional requirements will usually be provided enterally.

The unconscious patient may be capable of supporting respiration without mechanical ventilation. However, protection of the airway may not be possible after the cessation of respiratory support. For this reason, an early tracheotomy is useful to provide some airway protection from oropharyngeal secretions.

Monitoring Unconsciousness and Prognostication

The Glasgow Coma Scale is a common method for monitoring the progress of coma, producing a score between 15 (normal) and 3 (deep coma) and taking into account eye opening, motor responses, and verbal responses. Frequent assessment with the Glasgow Coma Scale gives an objective measure of progress. Otherwise, the prognosis deteriorates with the duration of coma; patients with postanoxic coma for 3 days rarely survive without severe disability.[12]

Poor prognostic features are listed in Table 2. Outcome from coma is primarily dependent on the cause, assuming that appropriate steps are taken to avoid secondary injury from hypoxia, hypotension, etc. In cases of severe head injury, recent data give an overall mortality of 37%, and good or moderate outcome occurs in 43%.[13] Coma from anoxia is associated with a poor prognosis, with 90% mortality at 1 year if coma lasts >6 h. Septic encephalopathy carries a 35 to 53% mortality dependent on severity.[14] Hepatic coma is associated with good recovery in only 27% of patients.[15] Outcome from drug ingestion, if the patient survives until hospitalization, is quite good.

As part of the SUPPORT study, Hamel and colleagues[16] identified day-3 prognostic variables associated with 2-month mortality in a cohort of 596 patients with "nontraumatic coma" (31% cardiac arrest, 36% ischemic stroke or intracerebral hemorrhage, 33% other causes). The variables included abnormal brainstem response (any of absent pupillary response, absent corneal response, or absent or dysconjugate roving eye movements), odds ratio (OR) = 3.2 (95% confidence interval [CI], 1.3 to 8.1); absent verbal response (OR, 4.6; 95% CI, 1.8 to 11.7); absent withdrawal response to pain (OR, 4.3; 95% CI, 1.7 to 10.8); creatinine >1.5 mg/dL (OR, 4.5; 95% CI, 1.8 to 11.0); and age ≥70 years (OR, 5.1; 95% CI, 2.2 to 12.2). Two-month mortality for patients with four or five risk factors was 97%. Brainstem and motor responses best predicted death or severe disability at 2 months; with either an abnormal brainstem response or absent motor response to pain, the rate of death or severe disability at 2 months was 96%.

Somatosensory evoked potentials (SEPs) are useful adjuncts for prognostication.[17] A systematic review showed that the positive likelihood ratio, positive predictive value, and sensitivity were

Table 2. *Features Associated With a Poor Prognosis After Cardiorespiratory Arrest*

Decerebrate posturing and rigidity for >24 h in nontrauma patients
Decerebrate posturing and rigidity for >2 wk in trauma patients
Absent vestibulo-ocular reflex for >24 h
Absent pupillary reflexes for >24 h in postanoxic brain injury
Absent pupillary reflexes for >3 d in trauma patients

4.04, 71.2%, and 59.0%, respectively, for normal SEPs (predicting favorable outcome) and 11.41, 98.5%, and 46.2%, respectively, for bilaterally absent SEPs (predicting unfavorable outcome). Twelve of 777 patients were identified with bilaterally absent SEPs who had favorable outcomes. These false positives were typically pediatric patients or patients who had suffered traumatic brain injuries. More exotic techniques hold the promise of greater precision,[18] but as of now no technique is completely correct.

Cooling After Cardiac Arrest

The major advance in the therapy of cardiac arrest patients of the past several years is the induction of hypothermia. Two studies of external cooling published in 2002[19,20] led to several international recommendations to institute hypothermia within 3 hours of resuscitation in comatose survivors of cardiac arrest.[21,22] The future of this area may also include tight glucose control and induced hypertension.

References

1. Plum F, Posner JB. The diagnosis of stupor and coma. 3rd ed. Philadelphia, PA: FA Davis, 1980
   The standard work and still a treasure trove.
2. Diagnostic and statistical manual of mental disorders. 4th ed. Washington, DC: American Psychiatric Association, 1994
3. Bleck TP. Vegetative state after closed-head injury. Neurol Chronicle 1992; 1:10–11
   Review of prognostic information.
4. Wise MG, Terrell CD. Delirium, psychotic disorders, and anxiety. In: Hall JB, Schmidt GA, Wood LDH, eds. Principles of critical care. New York, NY: McGraw-Hill, 1992; 1757–1769
5. Pingleton SK, Hall JB. Prevention and early detection of complications of critical care. In: Hall JB, Schmidt GA, Wood LDH, eds. Principles of critical care. New York, NY: McGraw-Hill, 1992; 587–611
6. Bleck TP, Webb AR. The unconscious patient: causes and diagnosis. In: Webb AR, Shapiro MJ, Singer M, et al, eds. The Oxford textbook of critical care. Oxford, UK: Oxford University Press, 1999; 440–444
7. Ropper AH. Lateral displacement of the brain and level of consciousness in patients with an acute hemispheral mass. N Engl J Med 1986; 314,953–958
8. Malouf R, Brust JC. Hypoglycemia: causes, neurological manifestations and outcome. Ann Neurol 1985; 17:421–438
9. Hawkes CH. "Locked-in" syndrome: report of seven cases. Br Med J 1974; 4:379–382
10. Turazzi S, Bricolo A. Acute pontine syndromes following head injury. Lancet 1977; 2:62–64
11. Bleck TP, Webb AR. The unconscious patient: management. In: Webb AR, Shapiro MJ, Singer M, et al, eds. The Oxford textbook of critical care. Oxford, UK: Oxford University Press, 1999; 444–446
12. Levy DE, Caronna JJ, Singer BH, et al. Predicting outcome from hypoxic-ischemic coma. JAMA 1985; 253:1420–1426
13. Chesnut RM, Marshall LF, Klauber MR, et al. The role of secondary brain injury in determining outcome from severe head injury. J Trauma 1993; 34:216–222
14. Bolton CF, Young GB, Zochodne DW. The neurological complications of sepsis. Ann Neurol 1993; 33:94–100
15. Levy DE, Bates D, Caronna JJ. Prognosis in nontraumatic coma. Ann Intern Med 1981; 94:293–301
16. Hamel MB, Goldman L, Teno J, et al. Identification of comatose patients at high risk for death or severe disability: SUPPORT investigators. JAMA 1995; 273:1842–1848
17. Carter BG, Butt W. Review of the use of somatosensory evoked potentials in the prediction of outcome after severe brain injury. Crit Care Med 2001; 29:178–186
18. Guerit JM. The usefulness of EEG, exogenous evoked potentials, and cognitive evoked potentials in the acute stage of post-anoxic and post-traumatic coma. Acta Neurol Belg 2000; 100:229–236.
19. Bernard SA, Gray TW, Buist MD, et al. Treatment of comatose survivors of out-of-hospital cardiac arrest with induced hypothermia. N Engl J Med 2002; 346:557–563
20. Hypothermia After Cardiac Arrest Study Group. Mild therapeutic hypothermia to improve the neurologic outcome after cardiac arrest. N Engl J Med 2002; 346:549–556
21. Smith TL, Bleck TP. Hypothermia and neurologic outcome in patients following cardiac arrest: should we be hot to cool off our patients? Crit Care 2002; 6:377–380
22. Nolan JP, Morley PT, Vanden Hoek TL, et al. Therapeutic hypothermia after cardiac arrest: an advisory statement by the advanced life support task force of the International Liaison Committee on Resuscitation. Circulation 2003; 108:118–121

Notes

Acid-Base Disorders

Gregory A. Schmidt, MD, FCCP

Objectives:

- To describe the effects of acidemia and alkalemia in critically ill patients
- To present a structured approach to analyzing acid-base disorders
- To discuss the differential diagnosis of the fundamental acid-base derangements
- To discuss treatment of acid-base disorders

Key words: acidemia; acidosis; alkalemia; alkalosis; bicarbonate; lactic acidosis; permissive hypercapnia

---

Disturbances of acid-base equilibrium occur in a wide variety of critical illnesses and are among the most commonly encountered disorders in the ICU. In addition to reflecting the seriousness of the underlying disease, disturbances in H^+ concentration have important physiologic effects.

A blood pH less than normal is called *acidemia*; the underlying process causing acidemia is called *acidosis*. Similarly, *alkalemia* and *alkalosis* refer to elevated pH and the underlying process, respectively. While an acidosis and an alkalosis may coexist, there can be only one resulting pH. Therefore, acidemia and alkalemia are mutually exclusive conditions.

The approach to acid-base derangements should emphasize a search for the cause, rather than an immediate attempt to normalize the pH. Many disorders are mild and do not require treatment. Furthermore, treatment may be more detrimental than the acid-base disorder itself. More important is a full consideration of the possible underlying pathologic states. This may facilitate a directed intervention that will benefit the patient more than normalization of the pH would.

Approach to Acid-Base Disturbances

This discussion will generally follow the more widely accepted "bicarbonate-based" approach to understanding acid-base disturbances, although a superior method, developed by Peter Stewart, is available.[1,2] The Stewart method identifies the true determinants of the pH: the strong ion difference, or [SID]; the total concentration of weak acids, or Atot; and the Pco_2. Using any method, diagnosing disorders of acid-base homeostasis in the ICU can be challenging. Many critically ill patients have combinations of disorders. In addition, patients admitted to the ICU often have pre-existing disturbances—such as respiratory acidosis in patients with COPD, and metabolic alkalosis in patients taking diuretics—that must be taken into account when one is evaluating subsequent changes.

A stepwise, conventional, approach follows:

- *Step 1:* Do the numbers make sense? Use the Henderson equation: $[H^+] = 24 \times Pco_2/HCO_3^-$.
- *Step 2:* Determine whether an acidemia (pH< 7.36) or an alkalemia (pH >7.44) is present. In mixed disorders, the pH may be in the normal range, but the bicarbonate level, the Pco_2, or the anion gap will signal the presence of an acid-base disturbance).
- *Step 3:* Is the primary disturbance metabolic or respiratory? That is, does any change in the Pco_2 account for the direction of the change in pH?
- *Step 4:* Is there appropriate compensation for the primary disturbance (Table 1)?
- *Step 5:* Is the anion gap elevated? If so, is the Δgap $\approx \Delta HCO_3^-$? If not, there is an additional nongap acidosis or a metabolic alkalosis.
- *Step 6:* Put it all together: What is the most likely diagnosis?

Table 1. *Appropriate Compensation in Simple Acid-Base Disorders*

Metabolic acidosis	$Pco_2 = (1.5 \times HCO_3^-) + 8 \pm 2$
Metabolic alkalosis	$Pco_2 = (0.7 \times HCO_3^-) + 21 \pm 1.5$*
Respiratory acidosis	Acute: $HCO_3^- = [(Pco_2 - 40)/10] + 24$
	Chronic: $HCO_3^- = [(Pco_2 - 40)/3] + 24$
Respiratory alkalosis	Acute: $HCO_3^- = [(40 - Pco_2)/5] + 24$
	Chronic: $HCO_3^- = [(40 - Pco_2)/2] + 24$

*For a bicarbonate (HCO_3^-) level > 40, the formula to be used is $Pco_2 = (0.75 \times HCO_3^-) + 19 \pm 7.5$.

Physiologic Effects of Acidemia and Alkalemia

The effects of acidemia and alkalemia are difficult to discern because any physiologic consequences in patients may be obscured or modified by the severe illness causing the acid-base disorder.

Acidemia causes stimulation of the sympathetic-adrenal axis. In severe acidemia, this effect is countered by a depressed responsiveness of adrenergic receptors to circulating catecholamines. The net effect on ventricular performance, heart rhythm, and vascular tone depends on the relative effects of these competing influences. For example, mild acidemia causes increased cardiac output, a response that can be prevented by β-adrenergic blockade. Severe acidemia typically causes a decrease in cardiac output and vasodilation despite sympathetic stimulation. Clinically, no increase in arrhythmias is seen in patients with respiratory acidemia during permissive hypercapnia, except that attributable to hypoxia. Once ventricular fibrillation is established, acidemia has little or no effect on the success of conversion to sinus rhythm.

Acute respiratory acidemia causes marked increases in cerebral blood flow. When P_{CO_2} is >70 mm Hg, loss of consciousness and seizures can occur. This is likely due to an abrupt lowering of intracellular pH rather than to any effect of CO_2 *per se*. The encephalopathy of acute-on-chronic respiratory failure is poorly understood, but may include elements of intracellular acidosis, hypoxia, and endogenous neuropeptide secretion. Thus the term *CO_2 narcosis*, which implies a direct effect of CO_2, is a misnomer.

Acute hypercapnia causes depression of diaphragmatic contractility and a decrease in endurance time. This effect may contribute to the downward spiral of respiratory failure in patients with acute CO_2 retention.

During intentional hypoventilation, as practiced in patients with status asthmaticus or ARDS, hypercapnia has been tolerated quite well. No significant impact on systemic vascular resistance, pulmonary vascular resistance, cardiac output, or systemic oxygen delivery has been seen.[3] There are several cautions, however. Patients are generally carefully chosen so as to have no increased intracranial pressure or cardiac ischemia; the inspired gas must be oxygen-enriched to prevent hypoxemia; and patients should be well-sedated.[4] Alkalinizing medications are generally not given during permissive hypercapnia.

Alkalemia appears to increase myocardial contractility, at least to a pH of 7.7. Some animals exhibit spontaneous ventricular fibrillation at pH levels >7.8. There are reports of alkalemic patients with atrial and ventricular arrhythmias who were refractory to treatment until the alkalemia was corrected. Respiratory alkalosis lowers blood pressure and calculated systemic vascular resistance. Most vascular beds demonstrate vasodilation, but vasoconstriction predominates in the cerebral circulation. Cerebral blood flow falls maximally, to 50% of basal flow, at a P_{CO_2} of 20 mm Hg; this effect has been utilized to acutely lower intracranial pressure, but the effect lasts only 6 h. Both respiratory and metabolic alkalemia can lead to seizures. Alkalemia can also cause coronary-artery spasm with ECG evidence of ischemia. The clinical effect of alkalemia-induced changes in oxygen delivery is small, but in patients with ongoing tissue hypoxia, the increased hemoglobin oxygen affinity may be detrimental and clinically significant.

Metabolic Acidosis

Metabolic acidosis is characterized by a primary decrease in bicarbonate concentration and a compensatory reduction in the P_{CO_2}. The etiologies of metabolic acidosis are divided into those that cause an increase in the anion gap and those associated with a normal anion gap (hyperchloremic acidosis). The *anion gap* is the difference between measured cations and measured anions, defined as $[Na^+] - [Cl^-] - [HCO_3^-]$, with a normal value traditionally defined as 8 to 14 mEq/L. The majority of unmeasured anion normally is accounted for by plasma proteins, primarily albumin. The remainder consists of phosphate, sulfates, lactate, and other organic anions. Seventy percent of patients with an anion gap >20 mEq/L will have an identifiable organic anion, as will virtually all of those with an anion gap >30 mEq/L. However, significant lactic acidosis can be present despite a normal measured anion gap, typically due to the hypoalbuminemia of critical illness.

Table 2. *Etiologies of Renal Tubular Acidosis (RTA) in the ICU*

Proximal RTA
    Primary renal disease
    Nephrotic syndrome
    Systemic diseases
        Amyloidosis
        Multiple myeloma
        Systemic lupus erythematosus
    Drugs and toxins
        Heavy metal toxicity
        Carbonic anhydrase inhibitors
Type I distal RTA
    Primary renal disease
        Obstructive uropathy
        Renal transplant rejection
        Nephrocalcinosis
        Pyelonephritis
        Allergic interstitial nephritis
    Systemic diseases
        Cirrhosis
        Multiple myeloma
        Sickle cell disease
        Amyloidosis
        Systemic lupus erythematosus
    Drugs and toxins
        Amphotericin
        Lithium
        Analgesic abuse
Type IV distal RTA
    Primary renal disease
        Obstructive uropathy
        Hyporeninemia
    Systemic diseases
        Diabetes mellitus
        Addison's disease
        Sickle cell disease
    Drugs and toxins
        Spironolactone
        Triamterene
        Amiloride
        Pentamidine

Table 3. *Etiologies of Normal-Anion-Gap Metabolic Acidosis*

Gastrointestinal loss of bicarbonate
    Diarrhea
    Urinary diversion
    Small bowel, pancreatic, or bile drainage
    (fistulas, surgical drains)
    Cholestyramine
Renal loss of bicarbonate (or bicarbonate equivalent)
    Renal tubular acidosis
    Recovery phase of diabetic ketoacidosis
    Renal insufficiency
    Posthypocapneic
Acidifying substances
    HCl
    NH_4Cl
    Arginine HCl
    Lysine HCl
    $CaCl_2$ or $MgCl_2$ (oral)
    Sulfur

Table 4. *Etiologies of Increased-Anion-Gap Metabolic Acidosis*

Etiology	Anion
Ketoacidosis (diabetic, alcoholic, starvation)	Acetoacetate, β-hydroxybutyrate
Lactic acidosis	Lactate
Uremia	Phosphates, sulfates, organic anions
Toxins	
Ethylene glycol	Glycolate, lactate
Methanol	Formate, lactate
Salicylate	Salicylate, lactate, organic anions
Paraldehyde	Unknown

Normal-anion-gap acidosis occurs from the loss of bicarbonate (through the kidneys or through the gut) or from the addition of an acid with chloride as the accompanying anion. The most common cause of normal-gap metabolic acidosis in the ICU is diarrhea; in the absence of diarrhea, a renal tubular acidosis is likely. The causes of renal tubular acidosis encountered in the ICU are listed in Table 2. The other causes of normal-anion-gap acidosis are usually obvious from the history and medication list. The etiologies of normal-anion-gap metabolic acidosis are listed in Table 3. The etiologies of increased-anion-gap metabolic acidosis are given in Table 4.

Ketoacidosis

Ketoacidosis occurs when free fatty acids are overproduced and preferentially shunted to form ketones, typically in states of low insulin and increased glucagon. Diabetic ketoacidosis is a common reason for ICU admission and is easily diagnosed from glucose and ketone measurement. Treatment involves rehydration, insulin administration, and attention to electrolyte disturbances. Alcoholic ketoacidosis (AKA) generally occurs after binge drinking in alcoholics who have no food intake and repeated vomiting. It is characterized by a normal or slightly elevated serum glucose level with increased ketones. Because of the altered redox state of the liver, much of the ketones in AKA occur in the form of β-hydroxybutyrate, which is not measured by the Ketostix (Bayer Diagnostics; Tarrytown, NY) or Acetest (Bayer Diagnostics; Tarrytown, NY). Specific enzymatic testing is necessary to detect β-hydroxybutyrate. Rehydration and provision of glucose is generally sufficient therapy for AKA, although insulin may be useful in some patients. Alkali therapy is not useful in ketoacidosis.

Toxins

Toxin ingestion is an uncommon but important cause of increased-anion-gap acidosis. Any patient who presents with an anion-gap acidosis that is not explained by tests for ketones and lactate should be suspected of having ingested a toxin. However, it should also be remembered that lactic acidosis can occur with toxin ingestion, so an increased lactate level does not rule out an acidosis from toxins. Often the laboratory diagnosis of toxin ingestion is slow; thus the diagnosis must be suspected, and clinical clues sought, prior to laboratory confirmation. Specific tests must be ordered, as methanol and ethylene glycol are not included in a routine toxicology screen. Salicylate intoxication is the most common of these ingestions and often presents with a mixed respiratory alkalosis and metabolic acidosis, which can be an important diagnostic clue.

The toxic effects of ethylene glycol and methanol are mediated by metabolites—glycolate in the case of ethylene glycol, and formaldehyde and formate in the case of methanol. The osmolal gap, which is the difference between measured osmolality and that calculated from the formula osm = 2[Na$^+$] + [glucose]/18 + [BUN]/2.8 + [ethanol]/4.6, is increased above its normal value of <10 milliosmoles/L. The osmolal gap may lack sensitivity, however, and its value as a screening test has been questioned. The loss of retinal sheen or even frank papilledema seen with methanol poisoning and the characteristic urinary oxalate crystals seen with methylene glycol poisoning can be helpful diagnostically. Fomepizole, an inhibitor of alcohol dehydrogenase, is safe and effective in the treatment of ethylene glycol and methanol poisoning.[5]

The identification of the anion associated with an increased-anion-gap acidosis in the ICU is not as precise as it might seem from the relatively short list of possibilities. In some cases of acidosis, either no anion is found or the rise in anions accounts for only a fraction of the rise in the anion gap; the identity of the offending anion, or anions, in these circumstances has not been determined.

Lactic Acidosis

Lactic acidosis, commonly defined as a lactate level >5 mmol/L with an arterial pH <7.35, is the most common and most important metabolic acidosis encountered in the ICU. The acidemia serves as a marker for a diverse group of serious underlying conditions and has important prognostic implications. The etiologies of lactic acidosis are numerous and are listed in Table 5. Most cases of lactic acidosis encountered in the ICU occur secondarily to a handful of processes; shock is the most common cause, with hypoxia, seizures, regional ischemia (*ie*, mesenteric or in an extremity), and toxin exposure accounting for a majority of the remaining cases.

Sepsis is a common cause of lactic acidosis in the ICU, but the mechanism is still debated. The belief that the lactic acidosis of sepsis is caused by anaerobic metabolism has come under question based on several lines of evidence. If cellular oxygen lack were the basis of lactic acid production, the lactate-to-pyruvate ratio should be elevated, a finding that is absent in resuscitated septic patients. Furthermore, when the adequacy of cellular oxygenation has been assayed by various methods, it has been found to be adequate. Pathologic supply dependence, a finding that was often interpreted to support tissue hypoxia, now appears to be an artifact of mathematical coupling, at least regarding this phenomenon at the whole-body level. No dependence of oxygen consumption on oxygen delivery can be found when each is measured by independent means. Additionally, various methods of boosting oxygen delivery fail to lower lactate levels in resuscitated septic patients. Finally, in an animal model of sepsis and lactic acidosis, hypoxic challenge failed to worsen lactic acidosis. Possible alternate mechanisms include hypermetabolism-induced protein catabolism, leading to increased circulating levels of alanine, pyruvate, and lactate (consistent with the normal lactate-to-pyruvate ratio); regional (*ie*, gut) production of lactate, possibly due to local hypoxia; mitochondrial dysfunction; and many others.

Bicarbonate had long been the standard therapy for lactic acidosis, although its safety and efficacy came under scrutiny in the early 1980s. The accumulated data has challenged the traditional arguments for bicarbonate use and questioned the safety and efficacy in patients with lactic acidosis. Increased Pco_2 after bicarbonate administration may translate into an acute decrease in intracellular pH, because CO_2 equilibrates across cell membranes more rapidly than bicarbonate. Indeed, several animal studies have demonstrated a fall in intracellular pH in the liver and in muscle after bicarbonate administration, although this effect has not been seen in all studies. The rationale for bicarbonate use is to mitigate the adverse hemodynamic consequences of acidemia. Animal studies in numerous models have shown bicarbonate to be no more effective than saline in improving cardiac output, mean arterial pressure, and left ventricular contractility. In patients with lactic acidosis, bicarbonate effectively increases bicarbonate levels and arterial pH, but does not improve cardiac output, mean arterial pressure, or any other relevant hemodynamic parameter.[6,7] In mechanically ventilated patients with acute lung injury being ventilated with a lung-protection strategy, bicarbonate lowers the pH, largely because carbon dioxide excretion cannot be augmented in the face of limited ventilation and Pco_2 rises significantly.[8] Alternative alkalinizing treatments [dialysis, tris-hydroxy-methyl-amino-methane (THAM)] are largely untested. THAM is effective in raising blood pH when bicarbonate is not,[8] but whether this is beneficial is unknown.

The decision whether to use bicarbonate is a difficult one. It is the choice between (1) a longstanding but unproven therapy with potential deleterious effects and (2) reliance on limited studies; neither is an entirely satisfactory choice. The debate will most likely continue until additional trials of bicarbonate therapy are conducted. With respect to the primary rationale for bicarbonate use—improvement in cardiovascular function—bicarbonate has shown no benefit. Because of the lack of data supporting bicarbonate use in human beings and the arguments reviewed above, I do not recommend the use of bicarbonate in lactic acidosis, *regardless of the pH*.[9] This recommendation has been supported recently by the Surviving Sepsis Campaign.[10]

Metabolic Alkalosis

Metabolic alkalosis is characterized by a primary increase in the bicarbonate concentration

Table 5. *Etiologies of Lactic Acidosis*

Increased oxygen consumption
    Strenuous exercise
    Grand mal seizure
    Neuroleptic malignant syndrome
    Severe asthma
    Pheochromocytoma
Decreased oxygen delivery
    Decreased cardiac output
        Hypovolemia
        Cardiogenic shock (including pericardial and pulmonary vascular disease)
    Decreased arterial oxygen content
        Profound anemia
        Severe hypoxemia
    Regional ischemia (mesentery or extremity)
Alterations in cellular metabolism
    Sepsis
    Diabetes mellitus, hypoglycemia
    Thiamine deficiency
    Severe alkalemia
    Malignancy
    Mitochondrial myopathies
    AIDS (?)
Toxins and drugs
    Carbon monoxide
    Ethanol, methanol
    Biguanides (*eg*, metformin)
    Ethylene glycol, propylene glycol
    Salicylates
    Isoniazid
    Streptozocin, nalidixic acid
    Cyanide, nitroprusside
    Papaverine
    Acetaminophen
    Ritodrine
    Terbutaline
    Fructose, sorbitol, xylitol
    Epinephrine, norepinephrine, cocaine
    Zidovudine and other highly active antiretroviral drugs
    Kombucha tea (?)
    Propofol (?)
Congenital
    Glucose-6-phosphatase deficiency
    Fructose-1,6-diphosphatase deficiency
    Pyruvate carboxylase deficiency
    Pyruvate-dehydrogenase deficiency
    Oxidative phosphorylation defects
Decreased lactate clearance
    Fulminant hepatic failure
D-Lactate
    Short gut syndrome
    Antibiotic-induced

and a compensatory increase in the Pco_2. The fact that patients will hypoventilate to compensate for metabolic alkalosis, even unto hypoxemia, is often not fully appreciated.[11] For a metabolic alkalosis to persist, there must be both a process that elevates serum bicarbonate concentration (generally gastric or renal loss) and a stimulus for renal bicarbonate reabsorption (typically hypovolemia, hypokalemia, or mineralocorticoid excess). The major causes of metabolic alkalosis in the ICU—vomiting, nasogastric suction, diuretics, corticosteroids, and overventilation of patients with chronically increased bicarbonate levels—are obvious, when present, from a patient's history and medication list. A careful search of all substances given to the patient is needed to disclose administration of compounds, such as citrate with blood products, and acetate in parenteral nutrition, that can raise the bicarbonate level. If the etiology is not clear, a trial of volume and chloride replacement, as well as correction of hypokalemia, can be attempted. If this does not effect an improvement in the alkalosis, a search for increased mineralocorticoids may be warranted. The etiologies of metabolic alkalosis are listed in Table 6.

Table 6. *Etiologies of Metabolic Alkalosis*

Chloride-responsive
    Renal H+ loss
        Diuretic therapy
        Posthypercapnia
        Penicillin, ampicillin, carbenicillin therapy
    Gastrointestinal H+ losses
        Vomiting, nasogastric suction
        Villous adenoma, congenital chloridorrhea
        Watery diarrhea-hypokalemia-achlorhydria syndrome (VIPoma, pancreatic cholera)
    Alkali administration
        Bicarbonate
        Citrate in blood products
        Acetate in total parenteral nutrition
        Nonabsorbable alkali [$Mg(OH)_2$, $Al(OH)_3$] and exchange resins
Chloride-resistant
    Increased mineralocorticoid activity
        Primary aldosteronism
        Cushing's syndrome
        Drugs with mineralocorticoid activity
    Profound hypokalemia
    Refeeding
    Bartter's syndrome
    Parathyroid disease
    Hypercalcemia

In patients who require continued diuresis but exhibit rising bicarbonate levels, acetazolamide can be used to reduce the bicarbonate level. When rapid correction of severe alkalosis is desired, hemodialysis can be performed or hydrochloric acid can be infused (0.1 to 0.2 molar infused into a central vein at 20 to 50 mEq/h with arterial pH monitored every hour).

Respiratory Acidosis

Respiratory acidosis is characterized by a primary increase in the arterial Pco_2 and a compensatory increase in the bicarbonate concentration. Respiratory acidosis represents ventilatory failure or disordered central control of ventilation, the pathophysiology, etiology, and treatment of which are described elsewhere. In mechanically ventilated patients with hypercapnia, it is important to consider the consequences of attempting to raise the minute ventilation. In many, normalizing the Pco_2 comes at the cost of alveolar overdistention (volutrauma) or exacerbation of auto-positive end-expiratory pressure. The point here is that normalizing the Pco_2 comes at a cost, that cost being volutrauma or frank barotrauma. The experience with permissive hypercapnia for patients with ARDS or status asthmaticus,[12] in which hypercapnia and acidemia are tolerated in order to avoid alveolar overdistention, has changed many clinicians' perspective about the adverse impact of acidemia. In sedated and ventilated patients with ARDS, rapid intentional hypoventilation (pH falling from 7.40 to 7.26 in 30 to 60 min) lowered systemic vascular resistance while cardiac output rose. Mean systemic arterial pressure and pulmonary vascular resistance were unchanged. Furthermore, in many studies of patients undergoing permissive hypercapnia, a pH of well below 7.2 was tolerated well. The feared consequences of acidemia, projected from the experience with patients having lactic acidosis (and, usually, concomitant sepsis), failed to materialize. With data now available for many patients permissively hypoventilated, the systemic hemodynamic effects are quite small even as the pH falls to 7.15, with the typical patient experiencing no change or small increases in cardiac output and blood pressure. Patients whose pH falls far below 7.0 are fewer in number, so firm conclusions cannot be drawn, but they similarly tolerate their acidemia. The current practice of permissive hypercapnia does not generally include an attempt to alkalinize the blood to compensate for respiratory acidosis. When the ventilator is used to correct respiratory acidosis, the end-inspiratory plateau pressure and auto-positive end-expiratory pressure should be monitored routinely to detect any adverse effects of ventilation.

Respiratory Alkalosis

Respiratory alkalosis is characterized by a primary reduction in the arterial P_{CO_2}. Respiratory alkalosis is very common in the ICU and its causes range from benign (simple anxiety) to life-threatening (sepsis or pulmonary embolism). Distinguishing those respiratory alkaloses that are manifestations of serious disease requires a thorough clinical review. The etiologies of respiratory alkalosis are listed in Table 7.

The primary treatment of respiratory alkalosis is treatment of the underlying cause of hyperventilation. The alkalemia itself generally does not require treatment. In cases where a severe alkalemia is present—generally, when a respiratory alkalosis is superimposed on a metabolic alkalosis—sedation may be necessary. In sepsis, where a significant portion of cardiac output can go to the respiratory muscles, intubation and muscle relaxation are occasionally used to control hyperventilation and redirect blood flow.

Annotated References

1. Stewart PA. How to understand acid-base: a quantitative acid-base primer for biology and medicine. New York, NY: Elsevier, 1981
   This outstanding text, now out of print, develops acid-base medicine from the ground up, replacing the unwieldy "bicarbonate-based" approach with a more accurate and computationally amenable method. Describes the determinants of the pH: the difference in the concentrations of strong ions (the [SID]); the total concentration of weak acids (Atot); and the P_{CO_2}.

2. Fencl V, Jabor A, Kazda A, et al. Diagnosis of metabolic acid-base disturbances in critically ill patients. Am J Respir Crit Care Med 2000; 162: 2246–2251
   Compared two commonly used diagnostic approaches, one relying on plasma bicarbonate concentration and "anion gap," the other on "base excess," with Peter Stewart's approach, for their value in detecting complex metabolic acid-base disturbances. Of 152 patients, one sixth had normal base excess and plasma bicarbonate. In a great majority of these apparently normal samples, the Stewart method detected the simultaneous presence of acidifying and alkalinizing disturbances, many of them grave. The almost ubiquitous hypoalbuminemia confounded the interpretation of acid-base data when the customary approaches were applied.

3. Thorens J-B, Jolliet P, Ritz M, et al. Effects of rapid permissive hypercapnia on hemodynamics, gas exchange, and oxygen transport and consumption during mechanical ventilation for the acute respiratory distress syndrome. Intensive Care Med 1996; 22:182–191
   Describes the hemodynamic effects of acute respiratory acidosis in patients with ARDS, showing that permissive hypercapnia is well-tolerated.

4. Feihl F, Perret C. Permissive hypercapnia: how permissive should we be? Am J Respir Crit Care Med 1994; 150:1722–1737
   Commentary regarding the potential risks of permissive hypercapnia.

Table 7. *Etiologies of Respiratory Alkalosis*

Hypoxia
    High altitude
    Pulmonary disease
    Decreased fraction of inspired oxygen
    Profound anemia
Increased CNS respiratory drive
    Anxiety, pain, and voluntary hyperventilation
    CNS disease (cerebrovascular accident, tumor, infection, trauma)
    Fever, sepsis, and endotoxin
    Drugs (salicylates, catecholamines, progesterone, analeptics, doxapram)
    Hyperthyroidism
    Liver disease
    Pregnancy, progesterone
    Epinephrine
    Exercise
Pulmonary disorders
    Pneumonia
    Pulmonary embolism
    Restrictive lung disease
    Pulmonary edema
    Bronchospasm
    Pleural effusion
    Pneumothorax
Mechanical ventilation

5. Brent J, McMartin K, Phillips S, et al. Fomepizole for the treatment of methanol poisoning. N Engl J Med 2001; 344:424–429

   Clinical trial confirming the efficacy of an inhibitor of alcohol dehydrogenase in patients with methanol poisoning.

6. Cooper DJ, Walley KR, Wiggs BR, et al. Bicarbonate does not improve hemodynamics in critically ill patients who have lactic acidosis: a prospective controlled clinical study. Ann Intern Med 1990; 112:492–498

   Well-controlled study in patients with septic lactic acidosis, almost all of whom were receiving catecholamines, directly addressing the role of bicarbonate in these patients. These investigators showed that bicarbonate was no different from control with respect to any relevant hemodynamic parameter, despite the known catecholamine unresponsiveness during acidemia.

7. Mathieu D, Neviere R, Billard V, et al. Effects of bicarbonate therapy on hemodynamics and tissue oxygenation in patients with lactic acidosis: a prospective, controlled clinical study. Crit Care Med 1991; 19:1352–1356

   Another study demonstrating the lack of efficacy of bicarbonate with regards to any hemodynamic benefit.

8. Kallet RH, Jasmer RM, Luce JM, et al. The treatment of acidosis in acute lung injury with tris-hydroxymethyl aminomethane (THAM). Am J Respir Crit Care Med 2000; 161:1149–1153

   Patients mechanically ventilated for acute lung injury who also had significant metabolic acidosis were given THAM. Arterial pH rose and P_{CO_2} fell, in contrast to the effects of sodium bicarbonate (which lowered the pH and raised the P_{CO_2}).

9. Forsythe SM, Schmidt GA. Sodium bicarbonate for the treatment of lactic acidosis. Chest 2000; 117:260–267

   Critically reviews the clinical and laboratory data regarding bicarbonate therapy for metabolic acidosis, concluding that bicarbonate should not be given routinely for lactic acidosis, no matter what the pH.

10. Cariou A, Vinsonneau C, Dhainaut JF. Adjunctive therapies in sepsis: an evidence-based review. Crit Care Med 2004; 32(11 suppl):S562–S570

    Critical literature review of adjunctive therapies for patients with sepsis carried out by critical care and infectious disease experts representing 11 international organizations. This paper reviews the evidence regarding glycemic control, renal replacement, and correction of metabolic acidosis. Bicarbonate should not be given (Grade C). For those with pH < 7.15, the recommendation is uncertain (Grade E).

11. Javaheri S, Kazemi H. Metabolic alkalosis and hypoventilation in humans. Am Rev Respir Dis 1987; 136:1011–1016

    Study of patients with metabolic alkalosis showing that compensatory respiratory acidosis is a predictable response, even when the P_{O_2} falls significantly.

12. Tuxen DV, Williams TJ, Scheinkestel CD, et al. Use of a measurement of pulmonary hyperinflation to control the level of mechanical ventilation in patients with acute severe asthma. Am Rev Respir Dis 1992; 146:1136–1142

    Key study validating the approach of intentionally hypoventilating patients with status asthmaticus to avoid the consequences of barotrauma.

Notes

Notes

Obstetric Issues in Critical Care

Mary E. Strek, MD

Objectives:

- To describe the cardiopulmonary adaptation to normal pregnancy.
- To discuss the causes, assessment and treatment of shock during pregnancy.
- To outline the diagnosis and treatment of preeclampsia.
- To discuss the differential diagnosis of respiratory failure during pregnancy and summarize recommendations for ventilatory support.

Key words: preeclampsia, pregnancy, respiratory failure, shock

Physiology of Pregnancy

When critical illness occurs in pregnancy, the assessment, monitoring, and treatment of the patient must take into account both maternal and fetal well-being. Knowledge of the normal changes in maternal respiratory, cardiac, and acid-base physiology in pregnancy is essential to distinguish between adaptive and pathologic changes so that recognition and treatment of critical illness is possible.

Adaptation of the Circulation

During pregnancy, numerous circulatory adjustments occur that ensure adequate oxygen delivery to the fetus (Table 1). Early in pregnancy maternal blood volume increases, reaching a level 40% above baseline by the 30th week. This is due both to an increase in the number of erythrocytes with an even greater increase in plasma volume. A mild dilutional anemia results, with a decrease in hematocrit of about 12%. The magnitude of the increase in blood volume is greater with multiple births. This extracellular volume expansion is associated with parallel decreases in colloid osmotic pressure and in serum albumin concentration from 4.0 to 3.4 g/dL. The extracellular volume expansion is caused by activation of the renin-angiotensin system with increased aldosterone production and results in mild peripheral edema in 50% to 80% of normal pregnancies.

Coincident with the change in maternal blood volume is a 30% to 50% increase in cardiac output, most of which occurs in the first trimester and continues throughout gestation. The augmented cardiac output results from an increase in heart rate and, to a lesser degree, stroke volume, with heart rate reaching a maximum of 15 to 20 beats/min above resting nonpregnant levels by weeks 32 to 36. The increase in stroke volume is due both to an increase in preload caused by augmented blood volume and to a decrease in afterload caused by a 20% to 30% fall in systemic vascular resistance (SVR). The fall in SVR is attributed both to arteriovenous shunting through the low-resistance uteroplacental bed and vasodilation that may result from decreased vascular responsiveness to endogenous pressors and/or increased synthesis of vasodilators. Since left ventricular end-diastolic pressure remains normal despite a rise in left ventricular end-diastolic volume, ventricular diastolic compliance may be increased. Alternatively, a decrease in ventricular compliance has been suggested by studies demonstrating increased left ventricular wall thickness and mass. There is no increase in ejection fraction as calculated from echocardiography. The exact contributions of increased heart rate and stroke volume, loading conditions, and ventricular performance to the increase in flow have not been conclusively determined.

During the course of pregnancy, cardiac output becomes more dependent upon body position,

Table 1. *Circulatory Changes in Pregnancy*

Parameter	Direction
Heart rate	Increases
Blood pressure	Decreases
Cardiac output	Increases
Stroke volume	Increases
Systemic vascular resistance	Decreases
Pulmonary vascular resistance	Decreases

since the gravid uterus can cause significant obstruction of the inferior vena cava with reduced venous return. This effect is most notable in the third trimester. Vena caval obstruction is maximal in the supine position and much less pronounced in the left lateral decubitus position. During labor, uterine contraction can increase cardiac output 10% to 15% over resting pregnant levels by increasing blood return from the contracting uterus. This effect on cardiac output, however, may be tempered by blood loss during delivery.

Blood pressure decreases early in pregnancy owing to peripheral vasodilation. The peak decreases in systolic and diastolic pressures average 5 to 9 and 6 to 17 mm Hg, respectively, and occur at 16 to 28 weeks. Blood pressure then increases gradually, returning to prepregnancy levels shortly after delivery. Diastolic pressures of 75 mm Hg in the second trimester and 85 mm Hg in the third trimester should be considered the upper limits of normal.

The normal adaptation of the circulatory system to pregnancy results in a physiologic third heart sound in the majority of pregnant patients. The chest radiograph reveals an enlarged cardiac silhouette. Right ventricular, pulmonary artery and pulmonary capillary wedge pressures (PCWP) are unchanged from prepartum values in the healthy pregnant woman.

Adaptation of the Respiratory System

Oxygen consumption increases 20% to 35% in normal pregnancy; during labor there is a further increase (Table 2). This occurs to meet fetal and placental needs, as well as maternal requirements resulting from increases in cardiac output and work of breathing. Increased oxygen consumption is associated with an increase in carbon dioxide production by the third trimester, necessitating an increase in minute ventilation that begins in the first trimester and peaks at 20% to 40% above baseline at term. Alveolar ventilation is increased above the level needed to eliminate carbon dioxide, and Pco_2 falls to a level of 27 to 32 mm Hg throughout pregnancy. The augmented alveolar ventilation is attributed to respiratory stimulation due to increased levels of progesterone and results from a 30% to 35% increase in tidal volume (V_T) (from 450 to 600 mL) while respiratory rate is unchanged. Renal compensation results in a maternal pH that is only slightly alkalemic, in the range of 7.40 to 7.45, with serum bicarbonate decreasing to 18 to 21 mEq/L (Table 3).

Maternal Pao_2 is increased throughout pregnancy, to greater than 100 mm Hg, by virtue of augmented minute ventilation, but this increase does not significantly increase oxygen delivery. Mild hypoxemia and an increased alveolar-to-arterial oxygen gradient may occur in the supine position (Table 3). This may result from ventilation-perfusion mismatch due to airway narrowing or closure with resultant further decrease in the already reduced difference between functional residual capacity (FRC) and closing capacity that occurs in gravid individuals during normal tidal breathing. Whenever possible, arterial blood gas samples should be obtained in the seated position to avoid confounding effects from the mild positional hypoxemia of pregnancy.

FRC decreases progressively (10% to 25% at term) as a result of increased abdominal pressure from the enlarged uterus, which results in

Table 2. *Respiratory Changes in Pregnancy**

Parameter	Direction
$\dot{V}o_2$	Increases
RR	Unchanged
V_T	Increases
TLC	Unchanged
FRC	Decreases
FVC	Unchanged
FEV_1	Unchanged

*$\dot{V}o_2$, oxygen consumption; RR, respiratory rate; V_T, tidal volume; TLC, total lung capacity; FRC, functional residual capacity; FVC, forced vital capacity; FEV_1, forced expiratory volume in 1 s.

Table 3. *Typical Arterial Blood Gas Values**

	Pao_2	$Paco_2$	pH	A-a Gradient
Nonpregnant	98	40	7.40	2
Term pregnancy, seated	101	28	7.45	14
Term pregnancy, supine	95	28	7.45	20

*A-a gradient, alveolar-arterial oxygen content difference (gradient). Pao_2 and $Paco_2$ are expressed in mm Hg. To convert mm Hg to kPa, multiply the value by 0.1333.

diaphragmatic elevation and decreased chest wall compliance (Table 2). Expiratory reserve volume and residual volume are decreased during the second half of pregnancy. Total lung capacity decreases minimally because the function of the diaphragm and thoracic muscles is unimpaired and widening of the thoracic cage results in an increased inspiratory capacity. Vital capacity remains unchanged during pregnancy. Diffusing capacity is unchanged or slightly increased early in pregnancy and then decreases to normal or slightly below normal after the first trimester. The decreased FRC, when combined with the increased oxygen consumption found in pregnancy, makes the pregnant woman and fetus more vulnerable to hypoxia in the event of hypoventilation or apnea. This is an important consideration during endotracheal intubation.

Despite increases in levels of many hormones known to affect smooth muscle, the function of large airways does not appear to be altered in pregnancy. Forced expiratory volume in 1 second (FEV_1), the ratio of FEV_1 to forced vital capacity, and specific airways conductance are unchanged during pregnancy. The fact that flow-volume loops are also unaffected by pregnancy is further evidence of normal airway function. Lung compliance is unchanged.

Renal and Gastrointestinal Adaptation

Renal blood flow increases greatly during the first and second trimesters and then declines during the third trimester. Glomerular filtration rate rises early in pregnancy to 50% above baseline at 12 to 16 weeks and remains increased during pregnancy. This change means that serum creatinine during pregnancy (0.5 to 0.7 mg/dL) is somewhat lower than baseline. Therefore, creatinine levels that would be normal in a nonpregnant patient can indicate renal dysfunction in pregnant patients.

Lower esophageal sphincter tone decreases during the first trimester of pregnancy and remains low until near term, perhaps as a result of increased plasma progesterone levels. The gravid uterus displaces the stomach, further reducing the effectiveness of the gastroesophageal sphincter. Basal gastric acid secretion and pH remain unchanged during pregnancy. Labor and narcotic analgesics given during labor delay gastric emptying time, significantly increasing the risk of aspiration.

Fetal Oxygen Delivery

Oxygen delivery to the fetal tissues depends on the oxygen content of uterine artery blood, as determined by maternal Po_2, hemoglobin concentration and saturation, and uterine artery blood flow which reflects maternal cardiac output. The anemia of pregnancy reduces the oxygen content significantly, and thus the critically ill gravid patient is more dependent than the nonpregnant individual on cardiac output for maintenance of oxygen delivery.

Numerous factors affect uterine artery blood flow. The uterine vasculature is maximally dilated under normal conditions and therefore is unable to adapt to stress by increasing flow through local vascular adjustment. Fetal oxygen delivery can be decreased by uterine artery vasoconstriction. Exogenous or endogenous sympathetic stimulation and maternal hypotension elicit uterine artery vasoconstriction. In addition, maternal alkalosis causes uterine artery vasoconstriction.

Despite low umbilical vein Po_2 (30 to 40 mm Hg) and fetal arterial Po_2 (20 to 25 mm Hg) values at baseline, compensatory mechanisms maintain fetal oxygen delivery, and fetal oxygen content is relatively high. At all levels of Po_2, fetal hemoglobin has a higher affinity for oxygen than maternal hemoglobin, being 80% to 90% saturated at a Po_2 of 30 to 35 mm Hg. In addition, the fetus has a high hemoglobin concentration (150 g/L) and a high systemic cardiac output, with both left and right ventricles delivering blood to the systemic circulation. Protective responses to hypoxic stress include a shift to anaerobic metabolism, redirection of the fetal cardiac output to the brain, heart, and adrenal glands and decreased oxygen consumption.

In summary, during pregnancy, oxygen delivery to maternal and fetoplacental tissue beds is highly dependent on adequate blood flow and maternal oxygen content. Maternal oxygen consumption increases progressively during gestation and rises further in labor. In late pregnancy or near term, the fetoplacental unit is unable to increase oxygen delivery by local vascular adjustment. The fetus, however, is protected from hypoxic insult by the avidity of fetal hemoglobin for oxygen relative to maternal hemoglobin, the high fetal hemoglobin content, the high fetal cardiac output, and the autoregulatory responses of the fetal circulation in response to hypoxic insult. These general physiologic characteristics of pregnancy have the following implications for management of critical illness:

1. Assessment of blood flow must be done with an understanding that baseline flow is substantially increased, with further increases during active labor or with fever, infection, or pain.
2. Decreased placental blood flow represents a threat to fetal well-being and viability, especially if superimposed on maternal anemia, hypoxemia, or both. Maternal hypoxemia can be particularly damaging if it elicits vasodilation of nonplacental beds, as this results in redistribution of blood flow from the fetoplacental unit.
3. Oxygen delivery to the fetoplacental unit should be maximized by maintaining or restoring adequate circulating volume and cardiac function, blood transfusions to increase oxygen carrying capacity, placing the mother in the left lateral decubitus position to improve maternal cardiac output, and supplemental oxygen to increase maternal oxygenation.
4. If gestational age permits, delivery of the fetus may be the best option. Labor represents a tremendous "aerobic load" for the mother, thus the clinician must judge whether labor should be avoided or postponed during periods of critical illness in which oxygen delivery is marginal.
5. Early elective intubation and mechanical ventilation may be beneficial in selected patients to reduce aerobic requirements if the critically ill gravid patient is to assume the work of breathing in evolving respiratory failure.
6. Fetal monitoring is at present an inexact and evolving science and should be performed in conjunction with the obstetrical team. Measurement of fetal heart rate is a useful but nonspecific indicator of well-being and a late sign of inadequate oxygen delivery. It is most accurate after 32 weeks of gestation and is best used as a screening tool. Although continuous transcutaneous Po_2 measurement is feasible in the fetus, the results are difficult to interpret, and the low baseline value does not provide a wide margin for identifying worsening hypoxia. Fetal acid-base status can be measured by means of scalp blood sampling if membrane rupture and cervical dilation have occurred. A pH less than 7.2 suggests physiologic depression of the fetus. In general, the routinely obtained parameters of oxygen delivery and acid-base status in the mother are the best measures of the adequacy of oxygen delivery for both the fetus and the mother.

Circulatory Disorders of Pregnancy

In pregnancy, circulatory impairment may be life-threatening since mother and fetus depend on cardiac output for oxygen delivery. Common causes of hypoperfusion include hemorrhage, cardiac dysfunction, aortic dissection, trauma, and sepsis. Preeclampsia may occur as a result of uteroplacental hypoperfusion. These disorders account for a significant percentage of maternal deaths related to pregnancy.

The initial approach to the critically ill hypoperfused gravida is to distinguish between low-flow states, caused by inadequate circulating volume, cardiac dysfunction, or trauma, and high-flow states such as septic shock, while taking into account the physiologic alterations associated with pregnancy. Most often the state of perfusion of the critically ill gravid patient can be determined by bedside assessment. Occasionally, the adequacy of intravascular volume remains unclear despite a careful history, physical examination, and review of routine laboratory data. Other patients have obvious ventricular failure requiring the use of vasoactive drugs or respiratory failure requiring careful fluid management. In these instances, right heart catheterization should be considered although a survival benefit from this invasive procedure has not been documented in obstetric patients. When this procedure is necessary in a pregnant patient, a subclavian or internal jugular approach should be used. Femoral vein catheterization is relatively contraindicated because of the obstruction of the vena cava by the uterus and the possible need for emergent delivery. In the healthy pregnant woman, right ventricular, pulmonary artery, and PCWPs are unchanged from prepartum values. Cardiac output is increased, and SVR and pulmonary vascular resistance are decreased during pregnancy. Assessment of left and right ventricular hemodynamics by echocardiography has been shown to correlate with pulmonary artery catheter results in a heterogeneous group of critically ill obstetric patients. Thus in centers with sophisticated echocardiography techniques this may provide an alternative to invasive monitoring.

Hemorrhagic Shock

The common causes of hemorrhagic shock in pregnancy are listed in Table 4. When hemorrhage occurs in pregnancy, it can be massive and swift, necessitating immediate intervention. It is the second leading cause of both maternal death and admission to the ICU. Antepartum hemorrhage is most often caused by premature separation of the normal placental attachment site (placental abruption), disruption of an abnormal placental attachment (placenta previa), and spontaneous uterine rupture.

Placental Abruption: Placental abruption occurs in 1 of every 77 to 250 pregnancies, with an increased incidence in patients with hypertension (half from chronic hypertension, half from preeclampsia), high parity, cigarette smoking, cocaine use, and previous abruption. Maternal mortality, usually from postpartum hemorrhage, ranges from 0% to 5.2%, while fetal mortality is higher. The severity of maternal blood loss is correlated with the extent and duration of abruption and fetal demise. Blood loss averages 2 to 3 L when abruption results in fetal death, and much of this blood may remain concealed within the uterus. Maternal complications include acute renal failure and disseminated intravascular coagulation (DIC), which occurs in up to 30% of patients with fetal death. Patients may initially present with painful vaginal bleeding and be misdiagnosed as having premature labor. The diagnosis is made using a combination of clinical information and ultrasound.

Placenta Previa: Placenta previa occurs in approximately 1 of 200 pregnancies and only infrequently causes massive hemorrhage because near universal ultrasound examination during pregnancy leads to identification prior to delivery. Nonetheless, if vaginal examination results in disruption of the placenta over the cervical os, or if trophoblastic tissue invades the myometrium (placenta previa et accreta), the patient is at risk for massive hemorrhage at delivery. Placenta previa, is more common in multiparas patients with prior cesarean delivery and in cigarette smokers. Fetal mortality is low, but it can be much higher if maternal shock occurs.

Uterine Rupture: Uterine rupture occurs in approximately 1 of 2000 pregnancies. The most common setting in which rupture occurs spontaneously is the multipara with protracted labor. Other risk factors include prior cesarean section, operative (assisted) vaginal delivery, and use of uterotonic agents. In overt rupture, peritoneal signs may be observed. Nonetheless, substantial blood loss can occur in the absence of significant physical findings.

Common causes of postpartum hemorrhage include uterine atony, surgical obstetrical trauma, uterine inversion, retained placental tissue and coagulopathies due to DIC from amniotic fluid embolism, fetal death and saline solution abortion. Uterine atony occurs after prolonged labor, overdistention of the uterus from multiple gestation or hydramnios, abruptio placentae, oxytocin administration, or cesarean section, or as a result of retained intrauterine contents or chorioamnionitis. Hemorrhage from surgical obstetrical trauma may be due to cervical or vaginal lacerations or uterine incision for cesarean section.

Table 4. *Etiology of Hemorrhagic Shock in Pregnancy*

Early	Late (Third Trimester)	Postpartum
Trauma	Trauma	Uterine atony
Ectopic or abdominal pregnancy	Placenta previa or abruption	Surgical trauma
Abortion	Uterine rupture	Uterine inversion
DIC*	DIC	DIC
Hydatidiform mole	Marginal sinus rupture	Retained placenta

*DIC, disseminated intravascular coagulation.

Trauma: Trauma is a leading cause of nonobstetric maternal mortality. Hypoperfusion and shock may occur as a result of injury from motor vehicle accidents, falls, and assaults. The gravid woman is at greater risk of hemorrhage after trauma, as blood flow to the entire pelvis is increased. Some injuries are unique to pregnancy, including amniotic membrane rupture, placental abruption, uterine rupture, premature labor, and fetal trauma. Rapid deceleration injury can cause placental abruption (20% to 40% of major injuries) as a result of deformation of the elastic uterus around the less elastic placenta. In most cases, vaginal bleeding will be present when abruption has occurred. Abruption may be complicated by DIC, therefore coagulation profiles should be monitored. The cephalad displacement of abdominal contents in pregnancy increases the risk of visceral injury from penetrating trauma of the upper abdomen including splenic rupture. The urinary bladder is a target for injury, because it is displaced into the abdominal cavity beyond 12 weeks of gestation.

Management: Patients at increased risk of bleeding should be identified early, so that intravenous access and blood typing can be done. The physiologic changes of pregnancy make evaluation and treatment of the gravid patient more difficult. Borderline tachycardia and supine hypotension (from obstruction of the vena cava by the uterus in late pregnancy) may be caused by pregnancy itself and thus vital signs may not indicate significant blood loss. Clinical signs of hypovolemia are not observed in trauma victims until intravascular volume is reduced by 15% to 20%. When hypovolemia is clinically evident in gravid patients, it signifies enormous blood loss because of the expanded blood volume associated with pregnancy. When massive hemorrhage occurs, the initial management of the patient is similar to that of the nonpregnant patient, and two or three large-bore (16 gauge or larger) venous catheters should be inserted. Immediate volume replacement with crystalloid is instituted until blood is available, along with supplemental oxygen. Position the patient in the left lateral decubitus position to prevent vena caval obstruction from worsening the reduction in venous return that results from massive hemorrhage. Fetal monitoring is important, as fetal distress in the setting of obstetric hemorrhage indicates hemodynamic compromise.

If shock is not immediately reversed by volume resuscitation or is accompanied by respiratory dysfunction, elective intubation and mechanical ventilation is indicated. Blood replacement with packed red blood cells should begin immediately. Massive obstetric hemorrhage is one setting in which initial resuscitation may require the use of unmatched type-specific blood until more complete cross-matching can be accomplished. Because critical illness in pregnancy is frequently associated with DIC, massive bleeding should prompt an evaluation for a coagulopathy. If the peripheral blood smear, platelet count, prothrombin time, partial thromboplastin time, or fibrinogen level suggests excessive factor consumption (DIC), measurement of plasma levels of fibrin degradation products and specific factors should be performed. Measurement of factor VIII levels is inexpensive and can be accomplished more quickly than a full DIC screen. Massive blood loss can result in a dilutional coagulopathy with secondary thrombocytopenia, which needs to be corrected with appropriate blood product replacement.

Uterine atony is routinely treated with uterine massage, draining the bladder, and IV oxytocin. Oxytocin can cause hyponatremia by virtue of its antidiuretic effect. Alternatively, prostaglandin analogues such as carboprost tromethamine can be used to improve uterine contraction and decrease bleeding. Side effects include hypertension, bronchoconstriction and intrapulmonary shunt with arterial oxygen desaturation. Ergot preparations such as methylergonovine have been associated with cerebral hemorrhage and are contraindicated if the patient is hypertensive. Ultrasonography is used to diagnose retained intrauterine products of conception that require curettage. Embolization of the hypogastric, internal pudendal, or uterine artery can sometimes control hemorrhage and allow subsequent recanalization of the embolized vessel. Surgical exploration to repair lacerations, ligate arteries, or remove the uterus is necessary in some cases.

Cardiogenic Shock

Shock from cardiac dysfunction is most often caused by congestive heart failure due to either preexisting myocardial or valvular heart disease or to a cardiomyopathy arising de novo. The prevalence of heart disease during pregnancy is low, however, its presence increases the likelihood of maternal and fetal morbidity and mortality. Prior subclinical heart disease may manifest itself for the first time during pregnancy owing to the physiologic changes of pregnancy described earlier.

Etiologies: Patients with Eisenmenger syndrome, cyanotic congenital heart disease, or pulmonary hypertension have a high mortality rate (33% to 40%) during pregnancy. Predictors of maternal cardiac complications include prior cardiac events, poor functional class (New York Heart Association Class III or IV) or cyanosis, left heart obstruction (aortic or mitral stenosis), and left ventricular systolic dysfunction. Neonatal complications are associated with poor functional class or cyanosis, left heart obstruction, anticoagulation, smoking and multiple gestation. In one of every 1300 to 4000 deliveries, peripartum cardiomyopathy presents in the last month of pregnancy or the first 6 months after parturition. Postulated risk factors include black race, older age, twin gestations, multiparity, anemia, preeclampsia, and postpartum hypertension. Bacterial endocarditis rarely complicates pregnancy, most often occurring in patients with preexisting cardiac abnormalities, although infection of previously normal valves has been reported in pregnancy, particularly in patients with a history of intravenous drug use. Myocardial infarction is extremely uncommon during pregnancy but should be considered in the hypoperfused patient with chest pain. Maternal mortality is high in patients delivering within 2 weeks of infarction. There is an increased incidence of aortic dissection during pregnancy, perhaps related to the increase in shear stress on the aorta from the increased heart rate and stroke volume associated with pregnancy and hormonal factors. Aortic dissection presents most commonly during the third trimester, often as a tearing interscapular pain. Pulse asymmetry or aortic insufficiency may be noted on examination.

Management: It is essential to determine the cause of the underlying cardiac dysfunction and hypoperfusion. The chest radiograph may suggest the diagnosis; mediastinal widening is often noted in patients with aortic dissection. Echocardiography can help determine the volume status and detect valvular abnormalities, myocardial dysfunction or ischemia. Transesophageal echocardiography and magnetic resonance imaging are the most sensitive and specific tests for detecting aortic dissection although CT scan of the chest is often done first given its ready availability. Once the cause of cardiac dysfunction is determined, the initial management of the hypoperfused cardiac patient should focus on volume status, and hypovolemia should be excluded. Right heart catheterization may be helpful in this regard as well as in the further management of cardiogenic shock. Metabolic disturbances can worsen ventricular function in patients with a cardiomyopathy; therefore, hypocalcemia, hypophosphatemia, acidosis, and hypoxemia should be avoided. Vasoactive drugs are reserved for situations in which hypovolemia has been corrected and maternal perfusion remains inadequate. If cardiogenic shock persists despite an adequate preload, dobutamine is the drug of choice. It should be reserved for life-threatening conditions, however, because, at least in animal models, it reduces placental blood flow. When cardiogenic shock is complicated by pulmonary edema, parenteral furosemide should be given.

When cardiogenic shock persists despite inotropic drug support, afterload reduction with nicardipine should be considered. IV sodium nitroprusside or nitroglycerin are second-line agents and when used the dose and duration of therapy should be minimized, and oral agents, such as hydralazine or labetalol, should be substituted as soon as possible to avoid nitroprusside toxicity. Angiotensin-converting enzyme inhibitors are absolutely contraindicated during pregnancy, because they have been found to cause fetal growth retardation, oligohydramnios, congenital malformations and anuric renal failure in human neonates exposed in utero, as well as neonatal death.

Labor and delivery is an especially dangerous time for women with cardiac disease. The optimal method of delivery is an assisted vaginal delivery in the left lateral decubitus position. Epidural anesthesia will ameliorate tachycardia in response to pain, and its vasodilatory actions may be of benefit in patients with congestive heart failure. Since decreased SVR may lead to further decompensation in patients with aortic stenosis, hypertrophic cardiomyopathy, or pulmonary hypertension, general anesthesia may be preferred in these patients. Cesarean section should be reserved for cases with obstetric complications or fetal distress, although with improved surgical techniques and close hemodynamic monitoring, cesarean sections may be safer than in the past. Invasive monitoring may be required to follow shifts in volume status that occur from the tremendous "autotransfusions" produced by each uterine contraction during labor and the blood loss that occurs with delivery.

Septic Shock

Sepsis is another important cause of hypoperfusion in pregnancy, accounting for 13% of maternal deaths in the United States in the 1990s. The diagnosis of sepsis in the febrile gravid patient can be obscured by the normal hemodynamic changes of pregnancy (ie, increased cardiac output, decreased SVR). An awareness of the usual settings and patients at risk for sepsis will increase the chance of recognizing this life-threatening state. Animal data suggest pregnancy may cause increased vulnerability to the systemic effects of bacteremia and endotoxemia. In addition, pregnant patients have an increased susceptibility to infection with *Listeria monocytogenes* and disseminated herpesvirus, varicella, and coccidioidomycosis infections, perhaps owing to a decreased cell-mediated immune response during pregnancy.

Causes: The common causes of sepsis in pregnancy include septic abortions, antepartum pyelonephritis, chorioamnionitis, and postpartum infections (puerperal sepsis) (Table 5). Septic abortion is more often seen in countries where access to abortion is limited. Chorioamnionitis or intraamniotic infection complicates up to 1% of all pregnancies. It occurs most commonly after prolonged rupture of membranes or prolonged labor or after invasive procedures such as amniocentesis or cervical cerclage, but occasionally it reflects hematogenous spread from maternal bacteremia. Patients present with fever, tachycardia (both maternal and fetal), uterine tenderness, and foul-smelling amniotic fluid.

Sepsis in obstetric patients usually occurs postpartum. Clinical settings that increase the risk of postpartum sepsis include cesarean section, prolonged rupture of membranes, and prior instrumentation of the genitourinary tract. Infection usually occurs at the placental site, resulting in endometritis. Patients with endometritis may present with fever, abdominal pain and tenderness, and purulent lochia. Episiotomy sites and cesarean section incisions are less common sources of postpartum infection. Rarely, life-threatening wound infection with group A streptococci results in necrotizing fasciitis, while Clostridium spp may cause gas gangrene of the uterus. The bacteria that must be considered include a wide range of Gram-positive, Gram-negative and anaerobic bacterial organisms. Rarely, toxic streptococcal syndrome may occur as a result of infection with pyrogenic exotoxin A–producing group A streptococci in patients with necrotizing fasciitis or may unexpectedly follow an uncomplicated pregnancy and delivery. If a patient deteriorates while receiving appropriate antibiotic therapy, surgical exploration with possible hysterectomy is indicated.

The hemodynamic profile in septic shock is similar to that of the nonpregnant septic patient. While evidence of myocardial depression is often present, the predominant abnormality is high output hypotension with a decreased SVR. Complications of sepsis in pregnancy include pulmonary capillary leak with subsequent acute respiratory distress syndrome (ARDS) and DIC.

Table 5. *Bacterial Infections Associated With Sepsis in Pregnancy and Postpartum**

Obstetric
    Postpartum endometritis
    Chorioamnionitis (intra-amniotic infection)
    Septic abortion
    Septic pelvic thrombophlebitis
    Antepartum pyelonephritis
Nonobstetric
    Appendicitis
    Cholecystitis
    Pyelonephritis
    Pneumonia
Invasive procedures
    Abdominal wall or perineal incisions (necrotizing fasciitis)
    Amniocentesis/chorionic villus sampling (septic abortion)
Infected cerclage (chorioamnionitis)

*Reprinted with permission from Fein AM and Duvivier R. Sepsis in pregnancy. Clin Chest Med 1992; 13:709.

Management: The septic gravid patient requires thorough culturing and evaluation of pelvic sites. Empiric antibiotic therapy, designed to cover what is typically a polymicrobial infection involving Gram-positive, Gram-negative, and anaerobic organisms, should be given until specific bacteriologic cultures are available. Reasonable regimens to cover the above organisms should include at least two antibiotics such as clindamycin and a third-generation cephalosporin; in certain patients it is necessary to expand the initial regimen to include a semisynthetic penicillin, an aminoglycoside, or another broad-spectrum agent. If possible, however, it is best to avoid aminoglycosides in patients with sepsis antepartum, because these agents can be ototoxic and nephrotoxic to the fetus. Chorioamnionitis associated with sepsis is unlikely to respond to antibiotic therapy alone, and delivery of the fetus is required. Postpartum deterioration in septic patients receiving adequate antibiotic coverage suggests a localized abscess, a resistant organism, or septic pelvic thrombophlebitis. Surgical drainage of appropriate pelvic and abdominal sources, with possible hysterectomy, may be required, particularly in patients with myometrial microabscesses or gas gangrene from clostridial species.

Patients who have evidence of adequate tissue perfusion and oxygen delivery may not require fluid or vasoactive drugs for the treatment of tachycardia and moderate hypotension. Lactic acidosis or end-organ dysfunction is an indication for volume resuscitation. Mechanical ventilatory support should be instituted if needed. If hypoperfusion persists despite volume replacement, the use of vasoactive agents, such as dobutamine, to increase forward flow may be of value. The role that vasopressin might play in the pregnant patient with septic shock remains undefined, but institution of an infusion at 40 milliunits/hour is reasonable in the patient with refractory shock.

As in the nonpregnant septic patient, corticosteroids should be given if adrenal insufficiency is documented. The corticotropin stimulation test may be difficult to interpret in the pregnant woman because baseline cortisol may be elevated in pregnancy and stimulation tests have not been studied in this population. Recombinant protein C has not been systematically evaluated in pregnant patients and it is impossible to make informed commentary on its risk/benefit profile in this setting. At present, the essentials of treatment are early appropriate antibiotics, surgical treatment if necessary, and meticulous supportive care.

Preeclampsia

Preeclampsia is a unique disorder of pregnancy that complicates 5% to 10% of all pregnancies, accounting for a substantial proportion of obstetric ICU admissions (38% in a recent series in the United States) and 10% to 15% of maternal deaths. It occurs most often in nulliparous women after the 20th week of gestation, typically near term, and may even occur postpartum. It is characterized by hypertension, proteinuria, and generalized edema; however, these features may be mild and may not occur simultaneously, making the diagnosis of early disease difficult in some cases. Hyperuricemia is also present in almost all cases of preeclampsia and may be useful in differentiating preeclampsia from both preexisting chronic hypertension and gestational hypertension. Multiple other organ systems may be involved. Risk factors for the development of preeclampsia, besides the primigravid state, include both preexisting and gestational hypertension, maternal or paternal family history of preeclampsia, preexisting renal disease, diabetes mellitus, multiple gestation, hydatidiform mole, and antiphospholipid antibody syndrome. Preeclampsia may progress to a convulsive and potentially lethal phase, termed eclampsia, without warning. An especially fulminant complication of preeclampsia is the HELLP syndrome (hemolysis, elevated liver enzymes, low platelets), which occurred in 0.3% of deliveries in one large clinical series. Maternal and fetal morbidity and mortality are significant if eclampsia or the HELLP syndrome develops or if preeclampsia develops prior to 34 weeks gestation.

Cardiac output and plasma volume are reduced in preeclampsia, while SVR is increased. Right heart catheterization reveals low normal right atrial pressure and PCWP. Cardiac output may be reduced, normal or high.

Maternal complications of severe preeclampsia include seizures (eclampsia), cerebral hemorrhage or edema, renal dysfunction, pulmonary edema, placental abruption with DIC, the HELLP syndrome, and hepatic infarction, failure, subcapsular hemorrhage, or rupture. Although the risks of eclampsia are higher when the above markers of disease severity are present, in one large clinical series 20% of eclamptic patients had a blood pressure below 90 mm Hg or no proteinuria prior to experiencing convulsions. Renal dysfunction may result from intravascular volume depletion, renal ischemia, and glomerular disease characterized by swollen glomerular endothelial cells known as glomeruloendotheliosis. Acute renal failure is rare and most often is seen in patients with the HELLP syndrome, placental abruption, massive hemorrhage, or coagulopathy. Pulmonary edema is uncommon, having an incidence of 2.9% in patients with severe preeclampsia. Contributing factors include increased left ventricular afterload, myocardial dysfunction, decreased colloid osmotic pressure, vigorous fluid therapy and, in some cases, increased capillary permeability. It most commonly occurs after parturition. In a subgroup of patients, antepartum pulmonary edema develops. These patients are typically obese and chronically hypertensive with secondary left ventricular hypertrophy. The increased intravascular volume of pregnancy and the hemodynamic derangements of preeclampsia cause diastolic dysfunction with an elevated PCWP and pulmonary edema in these patients.

The HELLP Syndrome: The HELLP syndrome is characterized by multiorgan dysfunction arising from an endothelial abnormality with secondary fibrin deposition and organ hypoperfusion. A microangiopathic hemolytic anemia and consumptive coagulopathy develop. When DIC occurs, it is often in the setting of placental abruption, sepsis, or fetal demise. The liver involvement is characterized by periportal or focal parenchymal necrosis with elevated liver function tests. Intrahepatic hemorrage or subcapsular hematoma occurs in 2% of patients and may progress to hepatic rupture.

The HELLP syndrome occurs in 4% to 20% of patients with preeclampsia. There is an increased incidence in white women and in one series 45% of the patients were multiparous. Patients are more often preterm than those with uncomplicated eclampsia. In up to 30% of patients, the HELLP syndrome develops after parturition; typically it appears within 48 hours, but it has been reported up to 7 days postpartum. Presenting symptoms are usually nonspecific, the most common being malaise, epigastric or right upper quadrant pain, nausea, vomiting, and edema. Patients less frequently present with jaundice, GI bleeding, or hematuria. Signs and symptoms of preeclampsia may be mild or absent upon initial presentation. Complications include acute renal failure, ARDS, hemorrhage, hypoglycemia, hyponatremia, and nephrogenic diabetes insipidus. Fetal growth retardation and prematurity are the major causes of perinatal morbidity and mortality. Maternal mortality ranges from 0% to 24%, with higher perinatal mortality (8% to 60%).

Laboratory values that suggest the diagnosis include: (1) hemolysis demonstrated by an abnormal peripheral smear, (2) increased levels of bilirubin ($\geq$1.2 mg/dL) or lactate dehydrogenase ($\geq$600 U/L); (3) increased liver enzyme levels with an elevated serum level of glutamic oxaloacetic transaminase ($\geq$70 U/L); and (3) thrombocytopenia with a platelet count of <100,000/µL. Isolated thrombocytopenia that progresses may be one of the first clues to the diagnosis.

Management: The principles of management of preeclampsia include early diagnosis, close medical observation, and timely delivery. Delivery is curative in most cases. The differential diagnosis of preeclampsia includes thrombotic thrombocytopenic purpura (TTP), hemolytic uremic syndrome (HUS), acute fatty liver of pregnancy, and idiopathic postpartum renal failure. Once the diagnosis is made, further management is based on an evaluation of the mother and fetus. The presence of symptoms and proteinuria increases the risk of placental abruption and eclampsia. These patients and those with disease progression should be hospitalized and observed closely. In patients who have mild preeclampsia at term and have a favorable cervix, labor should be induced. There is no consensus regarding the utility of bed rest, antihypertensive therapy, or anticonvulsant prophylaxis in this group of patients. Based on a number of clinical trials, there is no clear benefit to antihypertensive drug treatment in women with mild gestational hypertension or preeclampsia.

Because severe eclampsia can progress rapidly, delivery is recommended in these patients. Immediate delivery is appropriate when there are signs of impending eclampsia, multiorgan involvement, or fetal distress, and in patients who are more than

34 weeks pregnant. Early in gestation, conservative management with close monitoring to improve neonatal survival and morbidity may be appropriate in selected cases at tertiary perinatal centers. The objective of antihypertensive therapy is to prevent cerebral complications such as encephalopathy and hemorrhage. A sustained diastolic blood pressure of 110 mm Hg or greater should be treated to keep the mean arterial pressure between 105 and 126 mm Hg and the diastolic pressure between 90 and 105 mm Hg. While hydralazine, 5 mg IV, every 20 min to a total dose of 20 mg has been the traditional treatment, blood pressure control in the ICU setting is best obtained with IV labetalol. A loading dose of labetalol 20 mg is recommended, followed by either repeated incremental doses of 20 to 80 mg at 20 to 30-min intervals or an infusion starting at 1 to 2 mg/min and titrated up until the target blood pressure is achieved. Nicardipine may be an acceptable alternative. Since calcium-channel blockers may be potentiated by magnesium infusion, care should be taken to avoid hypotension when the two medications are used together. Acute nicardipine infusion can induce severe maternal tachycardia. Nitroprusside is relatively contraindicated, and angiotensin-converting enzyme inhibitors are absolutely contraindicated, in pregnancy. Diuretics should be used with caution, as they may aggravate the reduction in intravascular volume that is often seen in preeclampsia. Antihypertensive therapy has no effect on the progression of disease and does not prevent complications such as HELLP.

Magnesium sulfate prophylaxis has been shown to be better than placebo, phenytoin, or nimodipine in the prevention of eclampsia. In a recent large study, magnesium sulfate was superior to both phenytoin and diazepam for the treatment and prevention of recurrent convulsions in women with eclampsia. Magnesium sulfate should be given to all women with either preeclampsia or eclampsia and for a minimum of 24 hours postpartum. Aspirin has no role in the treatment of preeclampsia.

The preeclamptic patient with oliguria may benefit from judicious volume loading and low-dose dopamine therapy. Invasive monitoring is recommended to prevent pulmonary and cerebral edema. Pulmonary edema is managed conventionally. Patients with delayed postpartum resolution of the HELLP syndrome with persistent thrombocytopenia, hemolysis, or organ dysfunction may benefit from plasma-pheresis with fresh frozen plasma. Many of these patients may actually have TTP or HUS, which can be difficult to distinguish from the HELLP syndrome. In two studies, administration of corticosteroids resulted in improved maternal platelet counts and liver function test results and in a trend toward better fetal outcome. No significant effect in delaying delivery was noted. Management of intrahepatic hemorrhage with subcapsular hematoma includes administration of blood products, delivery, and control of liver hemorrhage. Embolization of the hepatic artery is often successful, but evacuation of the hematoma and packing of the liver may be required.

Respiratory Disorders of Pregnancy

During pregnancy, ventilatory failure may occur as a result of a chronic lung disease such as cystic fibrosis or asthma and may require mechanical ventilation. A more common cause of respiratory compromise in pregnant women is venous thromboembolic disease or acute hypoxemic respiratory failure related to amniotic or venous air embolism, tocolytic-induced pulmonary edema, aspiration, or pneumonia. This section focuses on the diagnosis and management of both ventilatory and hypoxemic respiratory failure in the gravid patient. Asthma remains the most common pulmonary problem encountered in pregnancy, affecting 1% to 4% of all gravidas. When these conditions require mechanical support, ventilator management necessitates careful attention to the special needs of mother and fetus.

Mechanical Ventilation

If ventilatory failure is imminent, intubation and mechanical ventilation should be performed electively. The indications for intubation and mechanical ventilation are not significantly changed by pregnancy, although it is important to remember that the normal P_{CO_2} of 27 to 32 mm Hg during pregnancy should be considered when deciding on mechanical ventilation. Several difficulties in airway management should be anticipated in the

Table 6. Problems With Airway Management in Pregnancy

Upper airway edema
Diminished airway caliber
Propensity for hemorrhage
Increased risk of aspiration

critically ill pregnant patient (Table 6). Pharyngeal, laryngeal, and vocal cord edema are common, and the highly vascular upper airway may bleed from even minor intubation-related trauma. Relatively small endotracheal tubes (6- to 7-mm diameter) may be necessary, and nasotracheal intubation is best avoided because of this upper airway narrowing. There may be an increased risk of aspiration during pregnancy because of delayed gastric emptying, increased intraabdominal pressure from compression by the gravid uterus, and diminished competence of the gastro-esophageal sphincter. Use of cricoid pressure to minimize the risk of pulmonary aspiration is recommended. Control of the airway should be achieved in an early and elective fashion by a skilled individual. Noninvasive mask ventilation for acute respiratory failure has not been studied in pregnancy. In the awake patient needing temporary ventilatory assistance, noninvasive positive pressure ventilation is a reasonable first step. Theoretical limitations to this therapy include pregnancy-related upper airway edema and increased risk of aspiration.

The initial ventilator settings should be aimed at achieving eucapnea (P_{CO_2} of 28 to 35 mm Hg). Respiratory alkalosis should be avoided, since studies in animal models suggest that hyperventilation can reduce fetal oxygenation and decrease uteroplacental flow. In the asthmatic patient, the use of a lower V_T and respiratory rate minimizes the adverse effects of intrinsic positive end-expiratory pressure (PEEP).

The patient with acute pulmonary edema should be ventilated with a small V_T (4 to 6 mL/kg) and a high respiratory rate (24 to 30 per min). While recent studies of nonpregnant adults managed with mechanical ventilation for ARDS have shown improved survival when low (~6 mL/kg) V_T were used—even if this was associated with hypercapnia—the safety of this permissive hypercapnia in pregnancy remains to be determined.

During mechanical ventilation, continuous fetal monitoring should be conducted and if acute ventilatory changes are associated with evidence of fetal distress, they should be avoided. The third trimester of pregnancy can result in significant chest wall stiffness resulting from the gravid uterus, thus high airway pressures may not signal lung stiffness or overdistension per se. In summary, fetal monitoring, low V_T, avoiding acute rises in Pa_{CO_2} and increasing V_T if they result in fetal distress, and allowing plateau airway pressures to be somewhat higher than 30 cm H_2O are recommended in these patients.

When a diffuse lung lesion is present requiring toxic levels of oxygen, sufficient PEEP should be used to correct arterial hypoxemia at a nontoxic fraction of inspired oxygen (F_{IO_2} < 0.6). In the pregnant patient, the aim is to keep the Pa_{O_2} >90 mm Hg, a value higher than that used in the nonpregnant patient, to prevent fetal distress. To minimize the decrease in venous return that occurs with positive-pressure ventilation, it is important that the pregnant patient be managed in a lateral position whenever possible.

In patients with severe lung lesions requiring toxic concentrations of oxygen and high levels of PEEP and in patients with hemodynamic instability, muscle relaxation and sedation will decrease oxygen consumption and assist in stabilization. Nondepolarizing neuromuscular blocking agents, including cisatracurium, pancuronium, vecuronium, and atra-curium, produce no adverse fetal effects with short-term use. Of these, cisatracurium is preferred because it does not depend upon renal or hepatic function for elimination. Benzodiazepines may increase the risk of cleft palate when used early in pregnancy. Narcotic analgesics such as morphine sulfate and fentanyl may be used safely during pregnancy. These agents all cross the placenta; therefore, if given near the time of delivery, immediate intubation of the neonate may be required.

Asthma

The course of asthma during pregnancy is variable: In approximately one-third of pregnant asthmatic women the asthma does not change; in one-third it improves; and in one-third it worsens. Patients with more severe asthma are more likely to experience worsening of their asthma during pregnancy. Asthma typically worsens during the second and third trimester with improvement during the last month of pregnancy. Adverse maternal outcomes in pregnant woman with asthma have been noted including preterm labor, pregnancy induced hypertension and preeclampsia, chorioamnionitis and cesarean delivery. Adverse fetal outcomes include preterm birth and infants small for gestational age. Treatment of the gravid patient with asthma by a specialist reduces the likelihood of complications suggesting that control of asthma and prevention of acute exacerbations are crucial to a good outcome.

The management of the pregnant patient with status asthmaticus is similar to that of the nonpregnant patient, with a few exceptions. Mild hypoxemia should be treated aggressively because it is detrimental to the fetus. An arterial blood gas determination that shows a $PaCO_2$ of >35 mm Hg during status asthmaticus should alert the clinician to impending ventilatory failure. Experience with nonpregnant patients with status asthmaticus and mild hypercapnia, however, has suggested that many can be managed without mechanical ventilatory support.

Most drugs used to treat asthma are considered safe for use during pregnancy. Inhaled bronchodilators are standard therapy. Use of parenteral β-agonists is generally limited to the rare situations in which inhaled agents have been ineffective, since epinephrine causes vasoconstriction of the uteroplacental circulation in animal studies. Parenteral terbutaline is preferred but may inhibit labor and cause pulmonary edema if given near term. Inhaled corticosteroids have been shown to decrease the incidence of asthma attacks and hospital readmissions in studies of pregnant woman with asthma. Budesonide is the inhaled corticosteroid of choice during pregnancy, although other inhaled corticosteroids may be continued if the patient's asthma has been well controlled using these agents prior to pregnancy. Oral corticosteroids have been associated with a twofold increase in the incidence of preeclampsia and in one study an increased risk of cleft palate (0.4% absolute incidence). Systemic corticosteroids are recommended in the treatment of acute asthma exacerbations and patients with severe asthma. Although there is a risk of causing fetal adrenal insufficiency, this is a rare occurrence. Heliox, a low-density mixture of helium and oxygen, may decrease the work of breathing and preclude intubation and mechanical ventilation when given to subjects in status asthmaticus. Guidelines for managing asthma in pregnancy have just been updated.

Venous Thromboembolism

In the 1990s, venous thromboembolism (VTE) was the single greatest cause of mortality during pregnancy in the United States. The risk of VTE is increased fivefold during pregnancy. Hypercoagulability, venous stasis and endothelial damage to pelvic vessels during delivery or cesarean section all occur during normal pregnancy, thus all pregnant women are at increased risk of VTE (Table 7). Major risk factors include age greater than 35 years, operative vaginal delivery, cesarean section, obesity, previous VTE, thrombophilia and a family history of thrombosis. Thrombophilia

Table 7. *Challenging Problems in Management of Pregnant Patients vs Nonpregnant Patients With VTE**

Nonpregnant	Pregnant
1. Noninvasive leg studies helpful	1. Studies impaired
2. Fibrinogen studies to diagnose calf thrombosis	2. Contraindicated
3. Thrombolytic therapy—an option	3. Riskier and contraindicated at term
4. Filter below renal veins	4. Filter placed suprarenally
5. PTT monitoring	5. Heparin levels may be preferable
6. Warfarin conversion	6. Crosses placenta and contraindicated
7. Hypercoagulable states less common	7. Such states more common
8. 5000 U SC bid prophylactic	8. Higher doses may be required.

*PTT, partial thromboplastin time; SC, subcutaneous.

increases the risk even further and is noted in approximately 50% of woman with VTE during pregnancy. Deep venous thrombosis (DVT) and subsequent pulmonary embolism (PE) may occur in all three trimesters and the post partum period. The majority of DVTs in pregnancy are ileofemoral and thus more likely to embolize than the more common calf vein thrombosis in the nonpregnant individual. There is a disproportionate incidence of DVT of the left leg.

The diagnosis of VTE requires a high index of suspicion because dyspnea and mild lower extremity edema are often noted in normal pregnancy. Pregnant women occasionally present with lower abdominal pain, fever, and an elevated WBC count mimicking acute appendicitis. Table 7 summarizes the challenges in management of gravid patients with suspected VTE.

To evaluate suspected DVT real time or duplex ultrasound venography remains the diagnostic test of choice although the reliability of noninvasive leg studies as pregnancy progresses is not as certain. A positive study is considered sufficient to justify treatment and anticoagulation is begun. There is evidence to support the withholding of anticoagulant therapy in pregnant women with a clinical suspicion of DVT but negative results on *serial* noninvasive leg studies.

The initial diagnostic study in a pregnant woman with suspected PE is a perfusion lung scan. A normal perfusion lung scan rules out PE and avoids the extra radiation exposure from the ventilation scan which adds nothing in this setting. If the lung scan is abnormal, a ventilation scan and noninvasive leg studies should be performed. If either is positive, anticoagulation is started. In patients in whom the ventilation perfusion lung scan is nondiagnostic or with lung disease that may make interpretation of the lung scan difficult, a helical CT scan should be performed. Echocardiography may be useful to document right-sided clot or right heart strain. It is important to make a definitive diagnosis and the clinical presentation alone cannot be relied upon to rule in or out VTE.

Once a diagnosis of either DVT or PE is made, anticoagulation with heparin is begun. This is the treatment of choice since heparin does not cross the placenta. Either IV unfractionated heparin dosed by weight or subcutaneous low-molecular weight heparin should be given. For patients with heparin-induced thrombocytopenia either danaparoid (a low-molecular weight heparinoid, pregnancy category B) or lepirudin (recombinant hirudin, a direct thrombin inhibitor, pregnancy category B) may be given. Coumadin is absolutely contraindicated (category X) due to the high incidence of embryopathy in the fetus. Anticoagulation must be continued throughout the course of pregnancy with subcutaneous low-molecular weight heparin.

Amniotic Fluid Embolism

Amniotic fluid embolism is a rare occurrence but is estimated to account for over 10% of peripartum maternal deaths. The mortality rate is very high (80% to 90%) with many of the deaths occurring within 1 h of the onset of symptoms.

The two most important risk factors are advanced maternal age (mean, 32 years) and multiparity. It is important to note that, while most cases occur during labor and delivery, amniotic fluid embolism may be associated with uterine manipulation during first- and second-trimester abortions or trauma and has been reported to occur spontaneously at 20 weeks of gestation.

The classic presentation of amniotic fluid embolism, is the abrupt onset of severe dyspnea, tachypnea, and cyanosis during labor or soon after delivery, frequently in association with cardiovascular collapse, hypoxemia, and seizures. Shock and bleeding each are the initial presentation in 10% to 15% of cases. Bleeding secondary to DIC occurs in up to 50% of patients who survive the first 30 to 60 minutes. Most of the remaining patients will have evidence for DIC on laboratory tests. Amniotic fluid embolism is frequently complicated by pulmonary edema.

Treatment is supportive and is aimed at ensuring adequate oxygenation, stabilizing the circulation, and controlling bleeding. Initial management includes intubation, administration of 100% oxygen, and mechanical ventilation. Early sedation and muscle relaxation and PEEP are often necessary. Pulmonary artery catheterization may guide hemodynamic adjustments aimed at minimizing PCWP (to reduce vascular leak) while providing an adequate cardiac output. Pulmonary arterial blood can be examined cytologically for evidence of abnormal amniotic fluid components—fetal squamous cells, lanugo hairs, etc. Demonstration of these amniotic fluid elements in the maternal pulmonary circulation, however, is not sufficient to make this diagnosis, since small numbers of fetal squamous cells have been observed in patients without clinical evidence of amniotic fluid embolism. Vasoactive drugs are frequently necessary to reverse hypotension. Once DIC is established, factor replacement and heparin therapy, should be undertaken only in conjunction with a hematology consultant. IV corticosteroid therapy has been reported to be of benefit in limited case reports.

Tocolytic Therapy

Pulmonary edema associated with β-adrenergic agents given to inhibit preterm labor is seen in as many as 4.4% of patients receiving these drugs. Most of the reported cases have resulted from use of IV ß-mimetics such as ritodrine, terbutaline, isoxuprine, and salbutamol. There is an increased incidence in women with multiple gestations, concurrent infection and those receiving corticosteroid therapy. Most women have intact membranes at the time of presentation. Pulmonary edema typically develops during tocolytic therapy or within 24 hours after the discontinuation of these drugs. When pulmonary edema develops postpartum, the vast majority of cases are encountered within 12 hours of delivery.

Most patients complain of chest discomfort and dyspnea, manifest tachypnea, have tachycardia with crackles on lung auscultation, and have pulmonary edema on chest radiography. A positive fluid balance is often noted in the hours to days preceding the onset of symptoms. The history and clinical findings should help in distinguishing this disorder from acute thromboembolic disease, acid aspiration, and amniotic fluid embolism.

The course of this disease is usually benign, and invasive hemodynamic monitoring is usually not required. Treatment should consist of discontinuation of tocolytic therapy, oxygen administration, and diuresis. Response is usually rapid, with resolution of tachypnea and hypoxemia often occurring within hours.

Aspiration

Aspiration is an uncommon but well-described and ominous complication of the peripartum period. Factors that increase the risk of aspiration in the pregnant woman include the increased intragastric pressure that results from external compression by the enlarged uterus, relaxation of the lower esophageal sphincter due to progesterone, delayed gastric emptying during labor, and depressed mental status and vocal cord closure from analgesia. Injury due to aspiration of gastric contents is related to the volume of aspirated material, its acidity, the presence of particulate material, the bacterial burden of the aspirated material, and host resistance to subsequent infection. The early injury is a chemical pneumonitis, the severity of which is determined primarily by the acidity and volume of the aspirate. Diffuse lung injury with the development of ARDS may occur early in the course. A late complication of aspiration is the evolution to bacterial pneumonia.

Prevention of this dread complication should be the primary goal of all physicians assessing and managing the patient's airway. Once aspiration has occurred, treatment is supportive and is similar to that for the nonpregnant individual. Antibiotics should be given only if bacterial pneumonia develops.

Venous Air Embolism

Although a rare occurrence, venous air embolism may account for 1% of all maternal deaths. It occurs during normal labor, delivery of women with placenta previa, criminal abortions using air, orogenital sex, and insufflation of the vagina during gynecologic procedures. Symptoms include cough, dyspnea, dizziness, tachypnea, tachycardia, and diaphoresis. Sudden hypotension is usually followed by respiratory arrest. A "mill-wheel murmur" or bubbling sound is occasionally heard over the precordium. Right heart strain, ischemia, and arrhythmias have been noted on the electrocardiogram. Patients who survive the initial cardiopulmonary collapse may develop noncardiogenic pulmonary edema.

When venous air embolism is suspected, the patient should be placed immediately in the left lateral decubitus position to direct the air embolus away from the right ventricular outflow tract. The patient should be ventilated with 100% oxygen in an effort to decrease the size of the embolus by removing nitrogen. Hyperbaric therapy has been an effective way to treat air embolism in diving medicine. Anticoagulation with heparin to treat fibrin microemboli and administration of high-dose corticosteroids to decrease pulmonary edema formation have been proposed, but their usefulness in this disorder remains untested.

Pneumonia

The incidence of pneumonia in pregnancy may be increasing, reflecting a decline in the general health of a segment of the population of childbearing women and infection with HIV. Obstetric complications included preterm labor, preterm delivery and fetal mortality. Respiratory failure requiring mechanical ventilation and maternal mortality also occur. Underlying maternal disease, such as the AIDS and cystic fibrosis, are associated with maternal medical complications and preterm delivery. The spectrum of organisms that causes bacterial pneumonia is similar to that in the nonpregnant population. An increased incidence of influenza pneumonia was noted among pregnant patients during the 1918–1919 and 1957–1958 influenza pandemics. Autopsy reports noted the cause of death as respiratory insufficiency from fulminant influenza pneumonia, rather than from secondary bacterial infection as is usually the case in the nonpregnant population. Pregnancy has not been demonstrated to be a risk factor for severe influenza infection except during those pandemic years, however. Primary infection with varicella-zoster virus progresses to pneumonia more often in adults than in children. Some investigators have noted an increased rate of progression to pneumonia and an increased mortality in pregnant patients, but the validity of this claim has not been proved conclusively. Coccidioidomycosis is the fungal infection most commonly associated with increased risk of dissemination during pregnancy, especially if it is contracted in the third trimester or immediately postpartum. Infection with *Mycobacterium tuberculosis* during pregnancy occurs. Whether pregnancy adversely influences the course of active tuberculosis is a matter of debate. It is clear that with appropriate chemotherapy, the prognosis for pregnant women with tuberculosis is excellent. There is no evidence for increased activation of quiescent disease during pregnancy. In vivo studies suggest that pregnancy does not affect the response to tuberculin skin testing, and this test can be performed safely during pregnancy. Maternal and fetal mortality from advanced tuberculosis was high in the era before effective chemotherapy. At present, the outcome for mother and child is excellent except in rare cases of congenital or neonatal tuberculosis.

In the pregnant patient, HIV infection is complicated by the risk of perinatal transmission to the fetus, preterm delivery, and opportunistic infection, especially pneumonia. Testing for HIV infection and antiretroviral therapy to prevent vertical transmission are currently standard of care in the pregnant patient. *Pneumocystis carinii* pneumonia (PCP) may complicate pregnancy and may be especially virulent in this setting. It is the most common cause of AIDS-related death in pregnant woman in the United States with respiratory failure requiring mechanical ventilation occurring in 59% of patients and with a mortality rate of 50%. Fetal mortality is also high and appears to be worse if PCP occurs during the first or second trimester. The clinical presentation is not altered by pregnancy.

The choice of antibacterial agents to treat pneumonia during pregnancy should take into account potential fetal toxicity. The penicillins, cephalosporins, and erythromycin (except for the estolate, which increases the risk of cholestatic jaundice in pregnancy) are considered safe. Tetracycline and chloramphenicol are contraindicated, and sulfa-containing regimens should be avoided near term except for the treatment of PCP, as discussed below. Amantadine has been shown to be teratogenic at very high, but not at lower, doses in animals; its use has not been studied in pregnant women. Favorable results have been obtained using acyclovir to treat pregnant women with varicella pneumonia. No teratogenic effects have been noted in animal studies of acyclovir. It is important to initiate therapy with acyclovir early to affect outcome favorably. Thus, acyclovir should be started at the first sign of respiratory system involvement in pregnant patients with cutaneous varicella infection. Amphotericin B should be used to treat disseminated coccidioidal infections in pregnancy. Fluconazole and likely other azole antifungal agentss are teratogenic and best avoided. No adverse effects on the fetus have been reported for amphotericin. Active tuberculosis during pregnancy should be treated with isoniazid, rifampin, and ethambutol plus pyridoxine until drug susceptibility testing is complete. All three of these medications cross the placenta, but none has been shown to have teratogenic effects. In patients with sensitive organisms, isoniazid and rifampin should be continued for 9 months. Although pyrazinamide is recommended for routine use in pregnant woman by the World Health Organization, in which case the treatment duration is shortened to 6 months, the drug has not been routinely used in the United States due to lack of data regarding safety. Streptomycin is the only antituberculosis drug with documented harmful effects on the human fetus and it should not be used during pregnancy. PCP should be treated with trimethoprim-sulfamethoxazole. Treatment with trimethoprim-sulfamethoxazole, compared with other therapies, may result in improved outcome. Corticosteroids are added if clinically indicated as for the nonpregnant patient.

Other Disorders of Pregnancy

Acute Renal Failure

The incidence of acute renal failure associated with pregnancy is between 0.02 and 0.05%. Acute renal failure may complicate preeclampsia, the HELLP syndrome, and acute fatty liver of pregnancy. Acute tubular necrosis may occur from hemorrhage or sepsis. Acute cortical necrosis is associated with placental abruption, septic abortion, prolonged intrauterine retention of a dead fetus, hemorrhage, and amniotic fluid embolism. Acute oliguric renal failure necessitating dialysis typically results. Arteriography may demonstrate loss of the cortical circulation, and renal biopsy can confirm the diagnosis. While renal function often improves, end-stage renal failure is the eventual outcome. Idiopathic postpartum acute renal failure is an unusual complication of pregnancy and may occur days to weeks after a normal pregnancy and delivery. The etiology is unknown. The disorder may be a variant of HUS or TTP, since it is clinically and pathologically similar to these entities although without hemolysis or thrombocytopenia, and many patients respond to treatment with prednisone administration and plasmapheresis. In general, the treatment of acute renal failure in pregnancy is similar to that in the nonpregnant patient, with supportive care and dialysis as necessary. Renal dysfunction associated with preeclampsia and the HELLP syndrome should respond to delivery of the fetus, while TTP and HUS require plasmapheresis with fresh frozen plasma.

Acute Liver Failure

Acute liver failure is an uncommon complication of pregnancy. In pregnancy, de novo liver function test abnormalities are uncommon and occur in less than 5% of pregnancies in the United States. Serum alkaline phosphatase increases during the first seven months of pregnancy peaking at two to four times normal at term. Serum albumin concentrations decrease in pregnancy. Levels of serum aminotransferases and bilirubin are unchanged in normal pregnancy.

Liver failure rarely complicates preeclampsia and the HELLP syndrome; subcapsular hematoma and rupture are more common complications. Acute fatty liver of pregnancy is estimated to occur in 1 of 13,000 deliveries. Risk factors include male fetus, multiple gestations and a first pregnancy. Mean onset is at 36 weeks gestation, although the disorder can be seen as early as 26 weeks and postpartum. Patients present with nonspecific symptoms such as headache, nausea and vomiting, right upper quadrant or epigastric pain, malaise, and anorexia. The onset of acute fatty liver of pregnancy may be similar to the onset of preeclampsia with peripheral edema, hypertension and proteinuria. Jaundice may follow 1 to 2 weeks later. Cholestasis with mild-to-moderate elevations in serum aminotransferases is the rule. Ultrasound may show increased echogenicity. Computed tomographic abdominal scans are more sensitive and may demonstrate decreased attenuation, although this imaging exposes the fetus to significant radiation. Liver biopsy is sometimes necessary to make the diagnosis but must be undertaken with caution because these patients often have a coagulopathy. The biopsy is characterized by microvesicular fatty infiltration detected only on frozen sections. Acute fatty liver of pregnancy progresses to fulminant hepatic failure complicated by encephalopathy, renal failure, pancreatitis, hemorrhage, DIC, seizures, coma, and death. Because deterioration may occur rapidly, expectant management is generally not advised. The treatment is delivery of the fetus. Jaundice, liver dysfunction, and DIC may worsen for a few days after delivery but then should improve. Maternal and fetal mortality has improved with early delivery and is less than 20%. Full maternal recovery is to be expected. Because long-chain 3-hydroxyacyl-coenzyme dehydrogenase deficiency in the fetus has been reported to be associated with acute fatty liver of pregnancy in women in a recent study, infants may have hypoglycemia, hypotonia, acute or chronic skeletal and cardiac muscle dysfunction and sudden infant death syndrome.

FDA Drug Classification

Since pregnant patients being treated for critical illness may require multiple pharmacologic interventions, intensivists in the United States should be aware of the Federal Drug Administration use-in-pregnancy ratings. Commonly prescribed medications in the ICU are listed in Table 8. Category A drugs are those that have undergone adequate controlled studies in pregnant women and have not demonstrated a risk to the fetus. Category B drugs are those with no evidence of fetal risk in human beings (if animal studies demonstrate risk, human findings do not, or if human studies are inadequate, animal findings are negative). Category C agents are those in which risk cannot be ruled out (human studies are lacking, and animal studies are either positive for fetal risk or lacking; still, potential benefits may outweigh risk). Category D includes agents with positive evidence of fetal risk by virtue of investigational or postmarketing human data (still, in critical illness potential benefits may outweigh risks). Category X includes drugs contraindicated in pregnancy.

Bibliography

Ahmad H, Mehta NJ, Manikal VM, et al. *Pneumocystis carinii pneumonia* in pregnancy. Chest 2001; 120:666–671

American College of Obstetricians and Gynecologists, and American College of Allergy, Asthma and Immunology. The use of newer asthma and allergy medications during pregnancy. Ann Allergy Asthma Immunol 2000; 84:475–480

Assali NS. Dynamics of the uteroplacental circulation in health and disease. Am J Perinatol 1989; 6:105–109

Briggs GC, Freeman RK, Yaffe SJ. Drugs in pregnancy and lactation. 6th ed. Philadelphia, PA: Lippincott Williams & Wilkins, 2002; 390–535

Table 8. Safety of Drugs Used in the ICU, According to the Federal Drug Administration Classification of Drug Safety in Pregnancy*

Categories A & B	Category C		Categories D & X
Amphotericin	Acyclovir	Heparin	ACE inhibitors
Cephalosporins	Albuterol	Hydralazine	Acetylsalicylic acid
Cimetidine	Aminoglycosides	Labetalol	Aminoglycosides
Clindamycin	Atracurium	Merperidine	Benzodiazepines
Erythromycin	Atropine	Metronidazole	Coumadin
Glycopyrrolate	Bretylium	Nifedipine	Midazolam
Insulin	ß-blockers	Nitroglycerin	Tetracyclines
Lidocaine	Bupivacaine	Nitroprusside	
Magnesium sulfate	Dantrolene	Pancuronium	
Methyldopa	Digoxin	Phenytoin	
Naloxone	Haloperidol	Prednisone	
Penicillins	Inotropes	Procainamide	
Propofol	Flumazenil	Suxamethonium	
Ranitidine	Fluconazole	Thiopental	
Terbutaline	Furosemide	Vecuronium	
		Vancomycin	

*Reprinted with permission from Lapinsky SE, Kruczynski K, Slutsky AS: Critical care in the pregnant patient. Am J Respir Crit Care Med 1995; 152–427.

Elkus R, Popovich J. Respiratory physiology in pregnancy. Clin Chest Med 1992; 13:555–565

Fein AM, Duvivier R. Sepsis in pregnancy. Clin Chest Med 1992; 13:709–722

Fishburne JI, Meis PJ, Urban RB, et al. Vascular and uterine responses to dobutamine and dopamine in the gravid ewe. Am J Obstet Gynecol 1980; 137:944–952

Gilson G, Golden P, Izquierdo L, et al. Pregnancy-associated hemolysis, elevated liver functions, low platelets (HELLP) syndrome: An obstetric disease in the intensive care unit. J Intensive Care Med 1996; 11:173–178

Gluck JC, Gluck PA. Asthma and allergy during pregnancy. Immunol Allergy Clin North Am 2000; 20:729–743

Ginsberg JS, Greer I, Hirsh J. Use of antithrombotic agents during pregnancy. Chest 2001; 119:122S–131S

Greer IA. Prevention and management of venous thromboembolism in pregnancy. Clin Chest Med 2003; 24:123–137

Hayashi RH. Hemorrhagic shock in obstetrics. Clin Perinatal 1986; 13:755–763

Hollingsworth HM, Pratter MR, Irwin RS. Acute respiratory failure in pregnancy. J Intensive Care Med 1989; 4:11–34

Lapinsky SE, Kruczynski K, Slutsky AS. Critical care in the pregnant patient. Am J Respir Crit Care Med 1995; 152:427–455

Magee LA, Cham C, Waterman EJ, et al. Hydralazine for treatment of severe hypertension in pregnancy: meta-analysis. BMJ 2003; 327:1–10

Masson RG. Amniotic fluid embolism. Clin Chest Med 1992; 13:657–665

Moores L, Bilello KL, Murin S. Sex and gender issues in venous thromboembolism. Clin Chest Med 2004; 25:281–297

National Heart, Lung, and Blood Institute. NAEPP Expert Panel Report. Managing asthma during pregnancy: recommendations for pharmacologic treatment—2004 update. J Allergy Clin Immunol 2005; 115 36–46

Pereira A, Krieger BP. Pulmonary complications of pregnancy. Clin Chest Med 2004; 25:299–310

Clark SL. Asthma in Pregnancy. National Asthma Education Program Working Group on Asthma and Pregnancy. National Heart, Lung and Blood Institute, National Institutes of Health. Obstet Gynecol 1993; 86:1036–1040

Pisani RJ, Rosenow EC. Pulmonary edema associated with tocolytic therapy. Ann Intern Med 1989; 110:714–718

Ramsey P, Ramin KD. Pneumonia in pregnancy. Obstet Gynecol Clin North Am 2001; 28:553–569

Rizk NW, Kalassian KG, Gilligan T, et al. Obstetric complications in pulmonary and critical care medicine. Chest 1996; 110:791–809

Roberts WE. Emergent obstetric management of postpartum hemorrhage. Obstet Gynecol Clin North Am 1995; 22: 283–302

Rodrigues J, Niederman MS. Pneumonia complicating pregnancy. Clin Chest Med 1992; 13:679–691

Sibai BM. Treatment of hypertension in pregnant women. N Engl J Med 1996; 335:257–265

Strek ME, O'Connor M, Hall JB, Wood LDH. Critical illness in pregnancy. In: JB Hall, GA Schmidt, LD Wood, eds. Principles of Critical Care. 2nd ed. New York, NY: McGraw-Hill, 1998; 1571–1594

Varon J, Marik PE. The diagnosis and management of hypertensive crises. Chest 2000; 118:214–227

Weinberger SE, Weiss ST, Cohen WR, et al. Pregnancy and the lung. Am Rev Respir Dis 1980; 121:559–581

Notes

Severe Airflow Obstruction

Gregory A. Schmidt, MD, FCCP

Objectives:

- To review routine and innovative pharmacologic treatment of the nonintubated patient
- To delineate the principles of mechanical ventilation necessary to minimize lung hyperinflation
- To describe the appropriate use of inhaled β-agonists, sedatives, and paralytics in the intubated asthmatic

Key words: airflow obstruction; asthma; auto-positive end-expiratory pressure; bronchodilators; corticosteroids; heliox; mechanical ventilation; noninvasive ventilation; status asthmaticus

Management Prior to Intubation and Mechanical Ventilation

Patients with status asthmaticus (SA) usually have symptoms for several days before ICU admission, but a small subset has abrupt onset of profound bronchospasm. This second group, which may be biologically distinct, is at great risk for sudden death with subsequent attacks of asthma.[1] Characteristics of SA that correlate with near-fatal asthma include prior intubation, hypercapnia, barotrauma, hospitalization despite chronic steroid use, psychiatric illness, and medical noncompliance.[2] Some patients recovering from near-fatal asthma exhibit diminished ventilatory drive in the face of hypoxemic or mechanical stimuli.[3] Illicit drug and tobacco use and lower socioeconomic status have also been correlated with poor outcome.

Bedside findings that suggest extreme airflow obstruction and impending respiratory arrest in SA include diaphoresis, delirium, and inability to speak in full phrases or to lie flat. The magnitude of pulsus paradoxus corresponds to the work of breathing; small pulsus paradoxus indicates mild asthma or terminal fatigue, a difference that is readily apparent at the bedside. Objective measurement of airflow obstruction (peak expiratory flow rate or FEV_1) is more accurate than physician assessment (both overestimation and underestimation of the severity of obstruction are common errors) and is occasionally helpful when the diagnosis or response to treatment is in question. The sickest patients may not be able to cooperate adequately, however. Many physicians measure arterial blood gases upon ICU admission, but this is not often helpful or necessary. Severe hypoxemia is not typically present in SA,[4] and pulse oximetry ordinarily provides sufficient monitoring. Hypercapnia generally indicates an $FEV_1 < 25\%$ of predicted, but it is not an accurate predictor of the need for mechanical ventilation. Metabolic acidosis (generally lactic acidosis) is occasionally present and attributed to high work of breathing, decreased lactate clearance, or the effect of catecholamines. Lactic acidosis should resolve rapidly once the work of breathing falls, unless it is a consequence of high-dose catecholamines. Such patients may remain dyspneic until the dose of β-agonists is reduced substantially.

Pharmacologic Therapy

β-Agonists: Inhaled β-agonists are the drugs of choice to treat smooth muscle-mediated bronchoconstriction in acute asthma (Table 1). The onset of action is rapid and these agents are generally tolerated well. Larger and more frequent doses are needed in acute asthma because the dose-response curve and duration of activity of these drugs are affected adversely by the degree of bronchoconstriction. For patients with severe obstruction, β-agonists should be given continuously until an adequate clinical response is achieved or adverse side effects limit further administration (*eg*, excessive tachycardia, arrhythmias, tremor).[5] Prior use of an inhaled β-agonist at home should not limit its use in the emergency department or hospital unless adverse effects are identified.

In North America, albuterol and metaproterenol are the most frequently used agents in adults. They are generally similar in action, but albuterol may be slightly preferable because of a longer duration of action and more $β_2$ selectivity. For most patients, a metered-dose inhaler (MDI) with a spacer is as effective as a nebulizer as long as the patient can cooperate with an MDI. For patients too ill to use MDIs reliably, nebulized therapy is more appropriate. Patients too ill even for nebulized β-agonists (lethargy) or who fail to respond to inhalation therapy can be treated with subcutaneous epinephrine or terbutaline (preferred in pregnancy). IV infusion of β-agonists is not recommended other than under extreme circumstances such as cardiac arrest.[6]

In severe asthma treated in the emergency room, most asthmatics demonstrate an early and clear response to two treatments with albuterol. Those who do not may require admission to the hospital or ICU. After intubation, β-agonists remain a cornerstone of therapy (see below).

Corticosteroids: Corticosteroids are required for virtually all patients with SA and should be given immediately on presentation because the full benefits are not seen for hours. According to a recent metaanalysis, steroids given in the emergency department significantly reduce the rates of admission and the number of relapses in the next 7 to 10 days. Oral and IV steroids were effective as long as a minimum of 30 mg of prednisone (or its equivalent) was given every 6 h. Lower doses were less effective, and there was no obvious benefit to giving higher doses.[7] For patients sufficiently ill to require admission to the hospital (*eg*, SA) and certainly for those with incipient respiratory failure, higher doses (*eg*, solumedrol 125 mg q6h) are advisable because the pace of improvement is hastened (even though the ultimate degree of improvement is not). Somewhat lower doses are preferred in older patients taking multiple drugs who are at higher risk of developing steroid side effects. Oral steroids are usually given for the next 10 to 14 days as guided by peak expiratory flow readings. We no longer hold inhaled steroids during this period, hoping to gain additional benefit from treating the luminal side of the airway, as well as improved compliance.

Anticholinergics: The data supporting the use of anticholinergic agents in patients with acute asthma are rather weak, but the low side-effect profile makes them worth consideration as third-line therapy in the most severely ill (Table 1). They produce less bronchodilation at peak effect than β-agonists and achieve a somewhat more variable clinical response,[8] indicating that cholinergic mechanisms play a variable role in patients with acute asthma. Anticholinergics may be particularly useful in patients with bronchospasm induced by beta-blockade. Ipratropium bromide inhalation solution unit-dose vial (2.5 mL) may be used in conjunction with albuterol concentrate (0.5 mL). Alternatively, 2 mg of glycopyrrolate in 2.5 mL of normal saline solution may be administered by an updraft nebulizer over a 20-min period every 2 h. I would not advocate continued use of these agents unless there is a convincing clinical response. At least one theoretical adverse effect would be excessive drying of secretions, mucous plugging, and inspissated secretions.

Theophylline: Several studies have demonstrated that theophylline does not add to maximal doses of β-agonists in the first few hours of therapy and that theophylline increases the incidence of tremor, nausea, anxiety, and palpitations.

Table 1. *Drugs Used in the Treatment of Status Asthmaticus*

Standard Therapies

Albuterol	0.5 mL of 0.5% solution (2.5 mg) in 2.5 mL normal saline solution by nebulization or 4 puffs by MDI (with a spacer) every 20 min to start; for intubated patients, titrate to physiologic effect and side effects
Epinephrine	0.3 mL of a 1:1,000 solution subcutaneously every 20 min for 1 h in patients unable to cooperate with or not responding to inhaled therapy
Corticosteroids	Methylprednisolone, 60 to 125 mg IV q6h; or prednisone, 30 to 40 mg po q6h
Oxygen	1 to 3 L/min by nasal cannula; titrate using pulse oximeter

Controversial Therapies

Anticholinergics	Ipratropium bromide, 0.5 mg by nebulization or 4 to 10 puffs by MDI every 20 min; or glycopyrrolate, 2 mg by nebulization q2h times 3
Theophylline	6 mg/kg IV over 30 min loading dose in patients not taking theophylline, followed by 0.5 mg/kg/h IV maintenance dose; start with maintenance infusion in patients taking theophylline until serum levels are known
Magnesium sulfate	1 to 2 g IV over 20 min (total dose 2 g unless hypomagnesemic)
Heliox	80:20 or 70:30 helium:oxygen mix by face mask

In some studies, the addition of theophylline to β-agonists and corticosteroids in asthma managed in the emergency room has been associated with a decreased requirement for hospital admission. Nonbronchodilating effects of these compounds, such as improved neuromuscular function or enhanced mucociliary clearance, could confer such benefits. A simple recommendation for theophylline administration in SA is to use this agent when patients fail to respond initially to β-agonists and corticosteroids.

Magnesium Sulfate: Because a number of anecdotal reports suggested a benefit from magnesium administration in acute asthma, this relatively safe drug has been advocated by some (Table 1). However, prospective clinical studies have failed to confirm a clinically significant benefit.[9,10] In subset analysis, there was a trend toward greater response in women and individuals with more severe airflow obstruction. It is recommended that magnesium administration be restricted to either the context of clinical investigation or perhaps to patients in whom all other therapies have failed, who have progressed to respiratory failure, and who now require mechanical ventilation. A typical dose is 1 g of magnesium sulfate IV over 20 min, repeated every 30 to 60 min to reach a total dose of 2 to 4 g. Serum magnesium levels should be measured and kept below 5 mg/dL.

Heliox

In patients with upper airway obstruction, heliox (21% oxygen, 79% helium) improves symptoms of dyspnea, work of breathing, and arterial blood gas abnormalities. The mechanism for this beneficial effect resides in the density dependence of the flow-related pressure drop across the upper airway. The pressure needed to drive flow (and, therefore, the work of inspiration) is reduced threefold in accord with the reduced density of heliox. AutoPEEP may also be reduced, lowering the inspiratory threshold load of breath initiation.

In SA, data are limited. In a small, uncontrolled series of ventilated asthmatics, heliox reduced airway pressures and $Paco_2$. In prospective, controlled trials of spontaneously breathing asthmatic adults and children, peak flow rose and pulsus paradoxus fell with heliox.[11] The reduced work of breathing that heliox creates could buy time for bronchodilators to work, potentially preventing the need for intubation. Furthermore, there is some evidence that using heliox to drive nebulized β-agonists improves the delivery of drug to the airways. Heliox is quite safe (it is inert) and inexpensive. Using heliox during mechanical ventilation requires special measures to calibrate ventilator flows and volumes.

Mechanical Ventilation for Severe Airflow Obstruction

Mask Ventilation

Patients in whom the therapies delineated above fail should be considered for mechanical ventilatory support. Nasal continuous positive airway pressure between 5 and 7.5 cm H_2O has been shown to relieve tachypnea and improve dyspnea in severely obstructed asthmatics. In patients with severe obstruction and hypercapnia, pressure-support ventilation (expiratory positive airway pressure, 4 ± 2 cm H_2O; inspiratory positive airway pressure, 18 ± 5 cm H_2O) promptly lowered $Paco_2$, respiratory rate (RR), and heart rate.[12] While one might predict that the extreme dyspnea would make compliance with noninvasive ventilation low, and that the requirement for high inflating pressures would limit the efficacy of noninvasive ventilation, the uncontrolled published series report a compliance rate comparable to that seen in other forms of respiratory failure. In 30 patients treated in the emergency department for SA, those randomized to noninvasive ventilation (IPAP = 13/EPAP = 4) had faster resolution and fewer hospitalizations.[13] This mode of therapy deserves a trial in the individual patient and further formal study in larger patient populations.

Sedation and Paralysis

If adequate control of the patient's cardiopulmonary status cannot be achieved by mask ventilation, intubation and mechanical ventilation should be initiated. Because of the complications associated with paralytics in patients with SA (see below), aggressive use of sedatives (Table 2) and careful attention to patient-ventilator synchrony are advised.

Table 2. Sedatives Used in Status Asthmaticus

Agent	Dose	Cautions
Peri-intubation Period		
Midazolam	1 mg IV slow push; repeat every 2 to 3 min as needed	Hypotension; respiratory depression
Ketamine	1 to 2 mg/kg IV at a rate of 0.5 mg/kg/min	Sympathomimetic effects; respiratory depression; mood changes; delirium-type reactions
Propofol	60 to 80 mg/min up to 2.0 mg/kg	Respiratory depression
Sedation for Protracted Mechanical Ventilation		
Lorazepam	1 to 5 mg/h IV continuous infusion or IV bolus prn	Drug accumulation
Morphine sulfate	1 to 5 mg/h IV continuous infusion; avoid bolus	Ileus
Ketamine	3 µg/kg/min IV to start	Sympathomimetic effects; delirium
Propofol	1.5 mg/kg/h IV to start (titrate to desired level of sedation)	Seizures; hypertriglyceridemia

Preferred sedatives include benzodiazepines, opioids, propofol, and ketamine. Lorazepam or midazolam may be given by frequent bolus or continuous infusion, and the addition of morphine sulfate (1 to 5 mg/h IV infusion) provides analgesia and augments the sedating effect of the benzodiazepines. Midazolam and fentanyl may be the preferred benzodiazepine and opioid agents, respectively, for early bolus administration because of their rapid onset.

Ketamine has been used frequently as an aid to emergency intubation of patients with SA, and after such bolus administration it has been thought to provide bronchodilating effects. Improvement in bronchospasm after IV bolus administration is transient and generally does not persist beyond 20 to 30 min. Because this agent may increase heart rate and arterial pressure due to sympathomimetic effects, it is relatively contraindicated in patients with severe atherosclerotic vascular disease, increased intracranial pressure, or preeclampsia. Ketamine also lowers seizure threshold, alters mood, and may cause delirium in up to one third of adult patients. Ketamine is metabolized by the liver to norketamine, which also has anesthetic properties and has a half-life of 120 min. Thus, continuous infusions of ketamine may result in metabolite accumulation and protracted effects.

The benefits of sedatives include synchronization of the patient with the ventilator, avoidance of excessive hyperinflation, facilitation of permissive hypercapnia, and decrease in respiratory muscle activity (and hence muscle production of carbon dioxide). When sedation alone cannot achieve these end points, the ventilator settings should be re-examined for opportunities for improved patient comfort. Only in extreme cases should muscle paralytics be given (with concomitant sedation, of course). The preferred agents are vecuronium and atracurium,[14] both nondepolarizing agents virtually free of cardiovascular effects (large boluses of atracurium may cause histamine-induced hypotension). Vecuronium is largely cleared by the liver but two metabolites are renally excreted, making it a poor choice in patients with disease of either organ system. Atracurium is eliminated by esterase degradation in the serum. Pancuronium, which is metabolized in the liver and excreted by the kidney, is an acceptable alternative to vecuronium in most cases and is less expensive. However, its vagolytic properties are more likely to cause tachycardia and hypotension.

Paralytic drugs may be given intermittently by bolus injection or by continuous IV infusion. Ensuring adequate sedation is a challenge because the commonly used indicator of agitation—tachycardia—is unreliable in patients receiving high doses of adrenergic agents. Paralytic agents have fallen from favor because they appear to play a causative role in the development of myopathy in acute severe asthma.[15] This disorder can be devastating, resulting in quadriparesis and prolonged ventilator dependence. If a paralytic is continuously infused, a nerve stimulator should be available or the drug should be withheld every 4 to 6 h to avoid accumulation and prolonged paralysis. In any patient treated with a paralytic, the drug should be discontinued at the earliest opportunity. It is not clear whether anything other than complete avoidance of these agents will prevent this serious complication.

Hypotension Following Intubation

Postintubation hypotension in patients with severe airflow obstruction is extremely common. Causative factors are pulmonary hyperinflation, hypovolemia, and sedation. The degree of pulmonary hyperinflation is directly proportional to minute ventilation (VE). Dangerous levels of pulmonary hyperinflation can develop if patients are "bagged" excessively in a misguided attempt to stabilize or resuscitate. With severe airflow obstruction, delivery of even a normal VE may impair the circulation. Clinically, inspired breaths become difficult to deliver (as there is essentially no room for additional air), breath sounds are diminished, and neck veins are distended. Systemic blood pressure and pulse pressure fall and the pulse rate increases. In the same patients, hypovolemia related to previous dehydration, sedation, and muscle relaxation all act to decrease mean systemic vascular pressure, further decreasing venous return to the heart. This pathophysiology can be demonstrated by ceasing ventilation temporarily: mean intrathoracic pressure falls and, within 30 to 60 s, blood pressure rises and heart rate falls. The treatment is augmentation of intravascular volume combined with strategies to minimize lung hyperinflation (see below). Note that the clinical features of pulmonary hyperinflation mimic tension pneumothorax; and indeed, if cessation of ventilation doesn't remedy the hypotension, pneumothorax should be excluded or treated empirically (bilateral chest tubes). Just as important, chest tubes should not be inserted in unstable patients until there has been a trial of hypoventilation.

Ventilator Settings

The key principles of ventilator management in the severely obstructed patient are: (1) use modest VE to avoid severe dynamic hyperinflation; (2) monitor plateau airway pressure (Pplat) and auto-positive end-expiratory pressure (autoPEEP) as indicators of dynamic hyperinflation; (3) accept hypercapnia; and (4) use positive end-expiratory pressure (PEEP) to ease the work of triggering.

Choose ventilator settings to minimize dynamic hyperinflation and its consequences (hypotension and pulmonary barotrauma). For example, each of the following reduces hyperinflation: low tidal volume (VT), low RR, and short inspiratory time. For an average-sized adult, an initial VE of roughly 8 L/min (achieved by a VT between 5 and 7 mL/kg and a RR of 14/min), combined with an inspiratory flow rate of 60 L/min, is a good starting point. After making these settings (and assuming the patient is adequately sedated), the degree of lung hyperinflation should be measured. In the research setting, one can measure the total exhaled volume during a period of apnea (usually about 60 s) following a tidal breath. When the ventilator is adjusted so that this volume (end-inspiratory lung volume) is below 20 mL/kg (1.4 L in an average-sized adult), complications such as hypotension and barotraumas are unlikely.[16-18] Reasonable (but untested) surrogate measures of the degree of lung hyperinflation in the clinical setting are the level of autoPEEP and Pplat. Reasonable targets are autoPEEP < 15 cm H_2O and Pplat < 30 cm H_2O. Occasional patients can be severely hyperinflated with low measured autoPEEP because of completely trapped, noncommunicating areas of obstructed gas.[19] Once the minute ventilation is set at a reasonable level, such as 8 L/min, further reductions in rate have only a very small impact on autoPEEP.

AutoPEEP can be estimated by performing an end-expiratory pause maneuver, now readily available on most ICU ventilators. If autoPEEP > 15 cm H_2O or Pplat > 30 cm H_2O, VE should be reduced. As long as inspiratory flow is not unusually low (or decelerating), there is little to be gained by increasing it further. To illustrate this point, consider the consequences of the following ventilator settings: VT, 500 mL; RR, 15/min; and peak inspiratory flow rate, 60 L/min. These settings result in an inspiratory time of 0.5 s and an expiratory time of 3.5 s. Raising the inspiratory flow rate dramatically (and unrealistically) to

120 L/min shortens inspiratory time to 0.25 s, but increases expiratory time only from 3.5 to 3.75 s, a trivial gain. On the other hand, simply lowering the RR from 15 to 14 (without changing the flow rate or VT) increases expiratory time to 3.8 s. When the goal is to reduce hyperinflation, it is generally more effective to reduce VE than to change any other ventilator setting.

Just as the degree of dynamic hyperinflation is linked to the VE, so is the $Paco_2$. Lowering VE to minimize hyperinflation causes the $Paco_2$ to rise. Similarly, raising the VE to normalize $Paco_2$ causes the degree of dynamic hyperinflation to rise. Before the 1980s, the approach to this unavoidable tradeoff was to attempt to bring the $Paco_2$ into the normal range. During that decade, however, it became clear that outcomes could be improved by sacrificing normocapnia for safer ventilation targets. Hypercapnia and the consequent acidemia appear to be well tolerated in SA, as long as patients are sufficiently sedated. Most intensivists make no attempt to alkalinize the blood, especially because bicarbonate raises the $Paco_2$.

It is worth noting that lowering the VE causes less hypercapnia than one might predict from the equation $Paco_2 \propto 1/V_E$. This can be seen by referring to a more complete description of the determinants of the $Paco_2$ ($Paco_2 \propto Vco_2 \times k/V_T \times RR \times [1 - V_D/V_T]$) where Vco_2 = carbon dioxide production and V_D/V_T = physiologic dead space ventilation. The lower VE tends to raise $Paco_2$, but at the same time the reduced hyperinflation often lowers dead space (V_D/V_T). The net result of reducing excessive VE is often a very small change in $Paco_2$.

A major component of the work of breathing in the severely obstructed patient is the inspiratory threshold load presented by autoPEEP. This load can be counterbalanced by externally applied PEEP, explaining the dramatic benefit of continuous positive airway pressure in patients with severe airflow obstruction. It is also appropriate to use PEEP in the intubated and ventilated patient with SA (or COPD) for the same reason. As long as the PEEP is set at less than about 85% of the autoPEEP, there is little to fear from further hyperinflation. Because most ventilated patients tend to trigger the ventilator, PEEP should always be used. This is especially true when sedation (or paralysis) is reduced.

Even when flow rate and PEEP are optimally adjusted and high doses of sedative are given, some patients cannot be made comfortable on volume-preset modes of ventilation such as volume assist-control. Some intensivists have had good results by using pressure-support ventilation (eg, pressure-support ventilation 25 cm H_2O and PEEP 5 cm H_2O), a mode that allows for inspiratory flow patterns that are more responsive to the patient's need. These patients tend to breathe with a rather large VT (eg, 1.5 L) and very slow rate (eg, 3 to 5/min). This approach may reduce the need for paralytic drugs.

Inhaled Bronchodilators During Mechanical Ventilation

Many questions remain unanswered regarding optimal drug administration during mechanical ventilation, because aspects of the ventilator circuit, ventilator settings, connectors and circuitry for nebulizers or MDIs, endotracheal tube, and intrinsic properties of the patient's airways may influence drug delivery and efficacy (Table 3).

Whether nebulizers or MDIs are used, higher doses are required to achieve physiologic effect than in nonintubated patients. In studies with radioactively labeled drug, only small quantities (often < 5%) are delivered to distal airways by either MDI or nebulizer. Various routes of administration may be totally ineffective during mechanical ventilation, such as use of an in-line MDI *without* spacer. Whether drug is delivered by nebulizer or MDI, dosage should be titrated to a physiologic end point such as peak-to-pause airway pressure gradient.[21]

Adjunctive Therapies During Mechanical Ventilation

Rarely, the above strategies do not allow for adequate ventilation at a safe level of dynamic hyperinflation and other therapies are considered. Both halothane and enflurane are bronchodilators that can acutely reduce peak airway opening pressure (Ppeak) and $Paco_2$, but the effects do not last after drugs are stopped.

Heliox may also be administered during mechanical ventilation, but many practical problems arise. The flow meters on the ventilator that

Table 3. *Potential Determinants of Aerosol Delivery in Intubated, Mechanically Ventilated Patients*

Ventilator/Circuit-Related Factors

Ventilator settings
I. Inspiratory flow rate
II. Respiratory rate
III. Tidal volume
IV. Flow waveform
V. Ventilator cycling: volume vs pressure
VI. Delivery by manual bag inflations

Circuit determinants
I. Characteristics of the delivery device
   A. Nebulizer
      1. Volume of fill
      2. Frequency selection for ultrasonic devices
      3. Specifications of the nebulizer device used
      4. Flow rates for jet nebulization
   B. MDI
      1. Timing of the actuation
      2. Spacer device
      3. Actuator
      4. Intraendotracheal tube catheters
II. Amount of drug administered
III. Humidification of inspired gases
IV. Where in circuit MDI/nebulizer is administered
V. Length and diameter of ventilator tubing
VI. Diameter and length of the endotracheal tube
VII. Use of low-density gas (heliox)

Patient-Determined Factors

Airway determinants
I. Bronchoconstriction
II. Secretions
III. Mucosal function

Patient's effects on gas flow
I. Spontaneous respiratory pattern
II. Generation of autoPEEP

---

measure V_T are dependent on gas density and will underestimate V_T during heliox administration unless recalibrated. Thus, the benefit of diminished airway resistance may be confounded by adjustments of V_E upward if this phenomenon is not appreciated. Before a heliox ventilator is used, it should be validated in a lung model by the respiratory therapists and physicians who will use it clinically. A useful device is a simple spirometer on the expiratory port of the ventilator to confirm V_T during adjustments of heliox.

One of the most striking findings noted in patients dying of SA is the degree of mucous impaction of both large and small airways. In refractory patients, retained secretions contribute to airflow limitation and lung hyperinflation. Unfortunately, other strategies to mobilize mucus, such as chest physiotherapy or treatment with mucolytics or expectorants, have not proved efficacious in controlled trials. BAL has been recommended by some but it is not well studied, carries theoretical risks, and should be reserved for extraordinary circumstances of mucous impaction.

Extubation

Once airway resistance starts to fall (as determined by Ppeak, Ppeak - Pplat, and auto-PEEP) and $Paco_2$ normalizes, sedatives (and paralytic agents) should be withheld and the patient allowed to breathe. A quick return to spontaneous breathing and extubation is desirable, rather than the more prolonged spontaneous breathing trials used in most ventilated patients. This tempo minimizes endotracheal tube–induced bronchospasm and agitation.

References

1. Sur S, Crotty TB, Kephart GM, et al. Sudden-onset fatal asthma: a distinct clinical entity with few eosinophils and relatively more neutrophils in the airway submucosa? Am Rev Respir Dis 1993; 148:713–719
Suggests that a subset of patients with sudden-onset asthma may be different from other asthmatics.
2. Levenson T, Greenberger PA, Donoghue ER, et al. Asthma deaths confounded by substance abuse: an assessment of fatal asthma. Chest 1996; 110:604–610
3. Kikuchi Y, Okabe S, Tamura G, et al. Chemosensitivity and perception of dyspnea in patients with a history of near-fatal asthma. N Engl J Med 1994; 330:1329–1334
Patients with life-threatening asthma may have difficulty in perceiving the degree of airway obstruction, perhaps providing a mechanism for their greater risk of death.
4. Ferrer A, Roca J, Wagner PD, et al. Airway obstruction and ventilation-perfusion relationships in acute severe asthma. Am Rev Respir Dis 1993; 147:579–584
5. Newhouse MT, Chapman KR, McCallum AL, et al. Cardiovascular safety of high doses of inhaled fenoterol and albuterol in acute severe asthma. Chest 1996; 110:595–603

6. Salmeron S, Brochard L, Mal H, et al. Nebulized versus intravenous albuterol in hypercapnic acute asthma: a multicenter, double-blind, randomized study. Am J Respir Crit Care Med 1994; 149:1466–1470
7. McFadden ER Jr. Dosages of corticosteroids in asthma. Am Rev Respir Dis 1993; 147:1306–1310
8. Karpel JP, Schacter EN, Fanta C, et al. A comparison of ipratropium and albuterol vs albuterol alone for treatment of acute asthma. Chest 1996; 110:611–616
9. Green SM, Rothrock SG. Intravenous magnesium for acute asthma: failure to decrease emergency treatment duration or need for hospitalization. Ann Emerg Med 1992; 21:260–265
10. Bloch H, Silverman R, Mancherje N, et al. Intravenous magnesium sulfate as an adjunct in the treatment of acute asthma. Chest 1995; 107:1576–1581
11. Manthous CA, Hall JB, Caputo MA, et al. Heliox improves pulsus paradoxus and peak expiratory flow in nonintubated patients with severe asthma. Am J Respir Crit Care Med 1995; 151:310–314
    Demonstrates that a helium-oxygen breathing mixture reduces the work of breathing and improves expiratory flow, perhaps leading to reduced autoPEEP.
12. Meduri GU, Cook TR, Turner RE, et al. Noninvasive positive pressure ventilation in status asthmaticus. Chest 1996; 110:767–774
13. Soroksky A, Stav D, Shpirer I. A pilot prospective, randomized, placebo-controlled trial of bilevel positive airway pressure in acute asthmatic attack. Chest 2003; 123:1018–1025
14. Caldwell JE, Lau M, Fisher DM. Atracurium versus vecuronium in asthmatic patients: a blinded, randomized comparison of adverse events. Anesthesiology 1995; 83:986–991
15. Leatherman JW, Fluegel WL, David WS, et al. Muscle weakness in mechanically ventilated patients with severe asthma. Am J Respir Crit Care Med 1996; 153:1686–1690
    Describes a severe syndrome of prolonged muscle weakness following mechanical ventilation for status asthmaticus facilitated by therapeutic paralysis.
16. Tuxen DV, Williams TJ, Scheinkestel CD, et al. Use of a measurement of pulmonary hyperinflation to control the level of mechanical ventilation in patients with acute severe asthma. Am Rev Respir Dis 1992; 146:1136–1142
17. Tuxen DV, Lane S. The effects of ventilatory pattern on hyperinflation, airway pressures, and circulation in mechanical ventilation of patients with severe air-flow obstruction. Am Rev Respir Dis 1987; 136:872–879
18. Williams TJ, Tuxen DV, Scheinkestel CD, et al. Risk factors for morbidity in mechanically ventilated patients with acute severe asthma. Am Rev Respir Dis 1992; 146:607–615
19. Leatherman JW, Ravenscraft SA. Low measured auto-positive end-expiratory pressure during mechanical ventilation of patients with severe asthma: hidden auto-positive end-expiratory pressure. Crit Care Med 1996; 24:541–546
20. Leatherman JW, McArthur C, Shapiro RS. Effect of prolongation of expiratory time on dynamic hyperinflation in mechanically ventilated patients with severe asthma. Crit Care Med 2004; 32:1542–1545
21. Manthous CA, Hall JB. Administration of therapeutic aerosols to mechanically ventilated patients. Chest 1994; 106:560–571

Notes

Notes

Issues in Sedation, Paralytic Agents, and Airway Management

Michael A. Gropper, MD, PhD, FCCP

Objectives:

- To review the indications for sedative and paralytic agents and methods of administration of these agents in the ICU
- To review the pharmacokinetics and pharmacodynamics of sedative and paralytic agents
- To review techniques of airway management

Key words: assessment; cisatracurium; etomidate; fentanyl; ketamine; morphine; propofol; rocuronium; sedation; vecuronium

Sedation of Critically Ill Patients

Publications from the late 1980s suggested that approximately half of all patients in the ICU described their period of mechanical ventilation as unpleasant and stressful, and that their time requiring mechanical ventilation was associated with fear, agony, and panic. In the late 1990s and more recently, publications have suggested that there is an association between the administration of large quantities of sedative agents in the ICU and the development of posttraumatic stress disorders and memory problems in the recipients.[1] Furthermore, there have now been investigations that have documented undesirable outcomes associated with the administration of large quantities of sedatives. These outcomes include delayed weaning from mechanical ventilation, significantly prolonged length of stays in the ICU and in the hospital,[2,3] significantly increased acquisition of CT scans for patients because of depressed mental function,[3] and an increased incidence of nosocomial pneumonia in patients receiving sedation and paralytic agents.[4] Therefore, the present-day conundrum is how to appropriately sedate patients in the ICU to prevent their fear and anxiety, and which agents to utilize.

Assessment of Sedation

There is no consensus as to what level of sedation is optimal for patients in the ICU; most likely, the optimal level of sedation will vary depending on the underlying physical and mental problems of each patient and the level of movement that is safe for the patient. A recent investigation documented that the more severely ill a patient is in the ICU, the less the patients remember about their ICU experience.[5] The more severely ill patients tend to receive more sedation, as they require mechanical ventilation for more prolonged periods, and there is some question whether their illness and their medicines may affect short-term memory.[5] More is being discovered about the effects of sedatives on cognition, memory, and learning; precise goals may eventually be possible (ie, anxiolysis without decreased cognition). Furthermore, we may be able to achieve some anxiolysis with nonpharmacologic interventions; relaxation tapes, warm milk, and herbal tea were shown to be useful in the treatment of hospitalized elderly patients as the administration of these adjunctive "therapies" decreased the need for sedation and decreased the incidence of delirium.[6]

Despite the lack of consensus and our incomplete knowledge, sedation should only be administered after an assessment of the patient is done. Thus, some quantitative assessment of a patient's anxiety should be made before the administration of medication; the patient then should be reassessed after receiving the drug. The most common assessment tool utilized is the Ramsay scale (Table 1).

Table 1. *Sedation-Agitation Scale*

Score	Description
1	Patient anxious and agitated, or restless, or both
2	Patient cooperative, oriented, and tranquil
3	Patient responds to commands only
4	Brisk response to a light glabellar tap or loud auditory stimulus
5	Sluggish response to a light glabellar tap or loud auditory stimulus
6	No response to a light glabellar tap or loud auditory stimulus

This is a 6-point scale that describes the patient as anxious and agitated (+3) to unresponsive (level −3). The scale includes an assessment of movement; thus, that the administration of neuromuscular blockade would preclude the use of this assessment tool. Titration of sedative agents to these scoring systems allows continuous assessment of the appropriate amount of sedative agent.

Narcotics and Sedative-Hypnotic Agents

All the sedative-hypnotic agents utilized for sedation or to optimize airway management have a depressant effect on blood pressure and cardiac function. The effects vary depending on the patient's age,[7] underlying medical problems, and cardiovascular stability. Furthermore, when drugs are used in combination, their effects are more than additive. This potentiation of effects can be beneficial, as when analgesic effects are intensified; however, combinations of drugs may also potentiate respiratory depression and cardiovascular instability. Therefore, the decision to administer a sedative-hypnotic agent must first address whether the patient is stable enough to tolerate such a medication and if so, what dose the patient will tolerate.

Patients who do not tolerate the cardiac depressant effects of sedative-hypnotics include patients who are in shock, bleeding, severely volume-depleted, or who have inadequate cardiac function. Patients who have suffered a cardiac arrest or are very hypotensive should not be given normal doses of sedative-hypnotic agents, as the drugs will hinder cardiac function. Conversely, analgesics should not be withheld if blood pressure can be supported with volume resuscitation and low doses of inotropes or vasopressors. Aging affects the pharmacokinetics and pharmacodynamics of the sedative-hypnotics; furthermore, the sensitivity of the elderly brain to sedative-hypnotic agents appears to be increased.[7] Sedative-hypnotics are also associated with confusion and delirium in the elderly (see the chapter titled "Pain, Delirium, and Ischemia in the Perioperative Period").

Liver disease affects the metabolism of drugs in many ways, and is hard to predict. In severe cirrhosis (associated with altered clotting times and encephalopathy), elimination half-lives of drugs are increased and drug clearance is reduced. These results suggest that smaller doses of drugs should be administered, and should be administered less frequently.[7-9] Metabolism of drugs that undergo glucuronidation (*ie*, lorazepam, oxazepam) appear to be relatively unaffected by liver disease. Drugs that are metabolized by phase I oxidative pathways (*ie*, diazepam and chlordiazepoxide) are affected by acute and chronic liver disease.[8] Nonetheless, morphine, which undergoes glucuronidation, is associated with an increased half-life and decreased clearance in patients with end-stage, decompensated liver disease.[8] Titration of sedatives to a scoring scale should simplify the complex pharmacology of drug administration in patients with hepatic and renal dysfunction.

A retrospective examination of the medical records of 28 patients who required more than 7 days of intensive care documented the occurrence of withdrawal symptoms and signs (restlessness, irritability, nausea, cramps, muscle aches, dysphoria, insomnia, myoclonus, delirium, sweating, tachycardia, vomiting, diarrhea, hypertension, fever, seizure, or tachypnea) in 9 of these patients.[10] The patients had to have three or more signs, or three or more symptoms, to be considered as having withdrawal. These patients received several-fold higher doses of analgesic and sedative hypnotic medications than the patients who did not experience withdrawal symptoms.[10] The patients who did not experience withdrawal received an average daily dose of fentanyl equivalent to 1.4 mg/d and lorazepam equivalent to 11.1 mg/d. The patients who experienced withdrawal were significantly more likely to have received neuromuscular blocking agents. Increased doses of narcotics and sedatives might have been given to ensure that patients were not paralyzed and awake. The patients who experienced withdrawal symptoms were also significantly younger than those that did not experience the symptoms; the younger patients may be more prone to tolerance of opioids and sedatives, or the younger patients may have been more likely to survive. The authors recommended: (1) weaning the doses of the drugs by 5% to 10% per day, (2) that drugs might be weaned even more slowly if both opioids and benzodiazepines are being weaned, and (3) that long-acting oral agents could be given, which can be weaned outside the ICU.[10] For example, oral methadone provides an efficient method for opiate weaning.

Continuous Infusions

The clearance of a sedative drug is affected by the duration of the infusion of the drug. Both midazolam and lorazepam become longer-acting drugs when they are administered as continuous infusions.[11] Patients also rapidly become tolerant to benzodiazepines when these agents are administered frequently.[11] Nevertheless, continuous infusion can minimize hemodynamic instability associated with analgesic and sedative administration. A reasonable target is for approximately 50% of the total analgesic or sedative dose to be administered as a continuous infusion, with the balance as needed.

Assessment of Pain

The treatment of pain is not only compassionate, but it is now mandated by the Joint Commission on Accreditation of Healthcare Organizations. Pain associated with procedures should be treated with analgesics. Chronic pain may require therapy other than opioids, as most patients who have been treated for chronic pain are tolerant to narcotics. They may also have a component of pain mediated by the sympathetic nervous system, which may respond to other agents such as nonsteroidal anti-inflammatory drugs (NSAIDs), antidepressants, and membrane-stabilizing agents. Patients with chronic pain may benefit from a multidisciplinary approach to their pain treatment.

A patient's pain should be quantified prior to and after treatment. The typical assessment tool is a visual analog scale (VAS), which has been validated and shown to have good inter-observer reproducibility.

Morphine Sulfate

Morphine is highly water soluble, and has a rapid initial redistribution phase of 1 to 1.5 min and an initial half-life of 10 to 20 min; the terminal elimination half-life is between 2 to 4.5 h.[8,9] Compared to fentanyl, morphine has low lipid solubility; this is important in that morphine slowly penetrates the blood-brain barrier. Therefore, morphine's peak effect is after 20 to 30 min, whereas the peak effect of the highly lipid-soluble fentanyl is within a few minutes. Fentanyl rapidly redistributes away from the brain and hence is short-acting; in contrast, morphine's low lipid solubility prevents rapid redistribution and causes a longer duration of action (Table 2). Morphine is primarily metabolized by the liver; however, the kidneys metabolize 40% of the drug. A major metabolite of morphine (morphine-3-glucuronide) has opiate activity and persists in the circulation of patients with renal failure, and can cause prolonged sedation.[3,8,9]

The sensitivity to pain decreases with age; opiate receptor density is decreased in the elderly, and there is evidence for reduced activity within the opiate receptor system with increasing age.[7,8] Elderly patients are found to develop increased concentrations of morphine when compared to younger patients given the same dose, and the morphine plasma concentration persists for longer intervals, suggesting decreased clearance. Therefore, smaller doses of morphine should be utilized in elderly patients.

Table 2. *Pharmacokinetics and Pharmacodynamics of Opioid Agents**

Drug	Lipid Solubility	Half-life (h)	Onset of Action (min)	Peak Effect (min)	Duration of Action (h)
Morphine	Low	2–3	5	20–30	2–7
Fentanyl	High	4–10	1–2	5–15	0.5–1
Meperidine	Moderate	5–8	5	20–60	2–4
Hydromorphone	Low	2.5–3	10–15	15–30	2–4

*Pharmacokinetic and pharmacodynamic parameters are based on single IV dosing in normal patients. Reproduced with permission from Volles DF, McGory R. Pharmacokinetic consideration. Crit Care Clin 1999; 15:64.

Morphine administration is associated with hypotension; doses of 1 to 4 mg/kg IV are commonly associated with hypotension, but hypotension has been reported with doses of 5 mg IV.[9] The faster the rate of administration, the more pronounced the hypotension seen; morphine can also be associated with histamine release, and morphine causes arterial and venous dilation that potentiates hypotension. Finally, morphine can slow the heart rate, probably by its stimulation of the vagus nerve and its depressant effects on the sinoatrial node. These hemodynamic effects are magnified when pain levels, and therefore circulating catecholamines, are increased. Continuous infusion, by preventing development of pain, may minimize hypotension.

Fentanyl

Fentanyl is 50 to 100 times more potent than morphine (fentanyl has greater affinity for the mu opiate receptor), so that the usual intravenous doses are 50 to 100 µg, depending on the condition of the patient. As fentanyl is very lipid-soluble (40 times more lipid-soluble than morphine), it penetrates the central nervous system quickly and leaves it quickly, and therefore has a very rapid onset of action and a short duration of action (Table 2). The onset of action of fentanyl is within 30 s, and its peak effect is within 5 to 15 min.[9,12] The liver metabolizes fentanyl and the kidney eliminates inactive metabolites. Decreased liver perfusion can decrease the clearance of fentanyl. When fentanyl is administered as a continuous infusion, the terminal half-life of the drug is 16 h; prolonged effects seen after infusions or repeated bolus injections of fentanyl occur due to the large amounts of the drug, which accumulate in the fatty tissues and then have to be metabolized by the liver.

Fentanyl is similar to morphine in that fentanyl concentrations are higher in elderly patients, apparently due to decreased clearance of the drug. Fentanyl is more potent in the elderly in that loss of consciousness occurs with smaller doses. Chest wall rigidity may occur with rapid administration of large doses of fentanyl.[7,12,13]

Fentanyl administration infrequently causes hypotension; however, it can cause hypotension by causing bradycardia and decreased sympathetic tone.[12,13] Patients who are maintaining their blood pressure by an increase in sympathetic tone can become hypotensive with the administration of fentanyl.[12-14] The rate of administration appears to affect the development of bradycardia; when fentanyl is administered rapidly, bradycardia more frequently develops.[12,14]

Remifentanil

Remifentanil is an ultrashort-acting narcotic with potency that is similar to fentanyl. Remifentanil penetrates the blood-brain barrier within 1 min, and its blood concentration decreases 50% by 6 min after a 1-min infusion and 80% by 15 min.[15] The novel aspect of remifentanil is its rapid hydrolysis by circulating and tissue nonspecific esterases (the beta adrenergic blocker esmolol is metabolized by similar enzymatic machinery). Unlike fentanyl, there does not appear to be a cumulative effect seen with longer infusions because of this unique metabolism. Organ dysfunction does not appear to alter the metabolism of this drug.[15] The clearance of remifentanil is reduced by about 25% in the elderly, according to the product information.

This drug produces respiratory depression, hypotension, bradycardia, and hypertonus of skeletal muscle; the rigidity produced by this drug can make ventilation by mask difficult or impossible. The administration of propofol or a paralytic agent prior to the administration of remifentanil can attenuate the skeletal rigidity seen with the drug. In studies where fentanyl, 1 µg/kg IV was compared to 0.5 to 1 µg/kg IV of remifentanil, hypotension occurred somewhat more often with fentanyl.[14-16] Peak hemodynamic effects of remifentanil are seen within 3 to 5 min after the administration of a single bolus, and hemodynamic effects are dose-dependent.

It has been shown that when large doses of remifentanil are administered intraoperatively, patients develop acute opioid tolerance. Tolerance occurs more quickly in response to shorter-acting narcotics such as remifentanil and alfentanil. In fact, profound tolerance can be documented after 90 min of remifentanil administration to volunteers. However, it also appears that the administration of large doses of opioids can also produce delayed hyperalgesia, suggesting a central sensitization that reduces the threshold to receptive fields. In support of this, the administration of N-methyl-D-aspartate receptor antagonists before the administration of large doses of opioids can block the hyperalgesia that can be induced by heroin or fentanyl. Because of its potency and short half-life, this agent is complex to use, and is usually reserved for intraoperative use.

Etomidate

Etomidate exists as 2 isomers, but only the + isomer is active; etomidate is R−(+)-ethyl-1-(α-methylbenzyl)-1H-imidazole-5-carboxylate. It is formulated as a 2-mg/mL solution in 35% propylene glycol. The propylene glycol is irritating to veins, and etomidate should not be mixed with other intravenous solutions. Etomidate had been utilized in critical care units throughout the world because of its characteristics, including its minimal hemodynamic effects, minimal respiratory depression, and cerebral protective effects. However, etomidate causes a dose-dependent, temporary, and reversible inhibition of steroid synthesis after a single dose or after an infusion. Other side effects that discourage its use include nausea and vomiting due to activation of the nausea center (concurrent administration of fentanyl increases the incidence), pain on injection, superficial thrombophlebitis 48 to 72 h after injection, and myoclonus. Etomidate appears to enhance the neuromuscular blockade of nondepolarizing paralytic agents[17]. Nonetheless, etomidate continues to be utilized as it causes minimal hemodynamic perturbations when small doses are administered.

The liver metabolizes etomidate, and its main metabolites are inactive. Doses of etomidate that have been utilized are 0.2 to 0.6 mg/kg; this dose can be decreased if narcotics and/or benzodiazepines are also administered. After 0.3 mg/kg, the effect is seen within the time that it takes the drug to circulate to the brain; redistribution is the mechanism that terminates the effects of a bolus of etomidate. Hepatic dysfunction does not appear to alter the rapid recovery from the hypnotic effects of etomidate.[17,18] The elimination half-life of the drug is 2.9 to 5.3 h.[17] In the elderly, the elimination clearance and volume of the central compartment are both decreased, causing a higher blood concentration from a given dose.[18]

Etomidate affects transmission at γ-aminobutyric acid-a receptors and may increase the number of γ-aminobutyric acid-a receptors.[12] Etomidate causes hypnosis and does not have analgesic activity. Etomidate has minimal effects on ventilation; in fact, etomidate can produce a brief period of hyperventilation, which can be followed by apnea.[17,18] Hiccups and coughing may also be seen after etomidate administration. After the administration of 0.3 mg/kg to patients, there is almost no change in heart rate, mean arterial pressure, mean pulmonary artery pressure, central venous pressure, stroke volume, or cardiac index.[17,18] Etomidate does not affect the sympathetic nervous system or baroreceptor function. Because of etomidate's potential for adrenal suppression, it should not be used in repeated doses or as a continuous infusion. It is, however, a desirable agent for brief procedures such as endotracheal intubation.

Propofol

Propofol is a short-acting sedative hypnotic widely used for sedation and general anesthesia. Propofol, 2,6,-diisopropylphenol, is formulated as a 1% aqueous emulsion, containing 10% soybean oil, 2.25% glycerol, and 1.2% egg phosphatide.[19] EDTA has recently been added to propofol in an attempt to discourage bacterial growth; propofol has been found to be the drug most frequently contaminated by bacteria. An ampule of the drug should only be utilized for one patient; great care should be taken when the drug is used for infusions so that bacterial contamination does not occur.

The effects of propofol 2.5 mg/kg are seen within the time it takes for the drug to circulate to the brain. The duration of the hypnosis is 5 to 10 min after a bolus injection; redistribution and elimination terminates the effects of propofol. Propofol has no analgesic activity but has some antiemetic properties. The clearance of propofol cannot be explained by hepatic clearance alone; there appear to be extra-hepatic sites of elimination. The clearance of propofol is extremely rapid, and the recovery from propofol remains rapid even after prolonged infusions.[17] The pharmacokinetics of propofol in patients age 65 years and older reveal that the elimination clearance is slower, but that plasma concentrations appeared similar to those of younger patients.[18]

Propofol causes dose-dependent hypotension that is very similar or somewhat greater than the hypotension produced by the administration of thiopental. Propofol causes vasodilation and myocardial depression.[19] The hypotensive effects of this drug can be exaggerated in elderly patients and in patients who have poor cardiac function or hypovolemia.[17-19] Propofol causes respiratory depression; initially, an increase in respiratory rate is seen for about 30 s and then apnea occurs. Airway reflexes are depressed; propofol prophylactically attenuates induced bronchoconstriction by depression of neurally induced bronchoconstriction.[17,20] Propofol does not affect resting airway tone, nor has it been utilized in asthmatics to treat acute bronchoconstriction.[19,20]

Side effects produced by propofol include intense dreams and disinhibition, dystonic or choreoform movements, pain at the injection site, phlebitis, hyperlipidemia, and pancreatitis.

Ketamine

Ketamine, a phencyclidine derivative, is unique among the intravenous agents in that it causes analgesia as well as amnesia. The drug does not necessarily cause a loss of consciousness, but the patient is not aware; the drug appears to cause a dissociative state by electrophysiologic inhibition of the thalamocortical pathways and stimulation of the limbic system.[20-22] The drug is a racemic mixture of two optical enantiomers; the S(+) ketamine has approximately fourfold greater affinity at phencyclidine binding sites on the N-methyl-D-aspartate receptor than does the R(−) ketamine. The S(+) ketamine appears to allow the use of significantly smaller doses, faster recovery, and possibly fewer side effects. The compound will be in use in Europe.[20-22]

Doses of 0.1 to 0.5 mg/kg of ketamine have analgesic action and can be utilized before the onset of pain for effective preemptive analgesia. Ketamine has an elimination half-life of 3 h. Recovery from an induction dose (0.5 to 1.5 mg/kg) is from redistribution from its receptor. Ketamine causes amnesia, altered short-term memory, decreased ability to concentrate, altered cognitive performance, nightmares, nausea, and vomiting. Thus, it is common practice to administer small doses of benzodiazepine with ketamine; this practice does prolong recovery from ketamine, but usually eliminates these adverse effects.

Ketamine directly stimulates the autonomic nervous system, releases catecholamines and steroids, and causes tachycardia and increases blood pressure. If a patient cannot release catecholamines (*ie*, is critically ill or has autonomic nervous system blockade), then ketamine administration can cause vasodilation and myocardial depression.[20-22] Data regarding ketamine in the elderly are lacking; the emergence phenomena and dysphoria ketamine causes may be difficult for the elderly, particularly if the baseline mental status is not normal.[20-22]

Ketamine is a useful agent for patients with reactive airway disease in that it attenuates neurally-induced bronchoconstriction.[20] It also has a small direct effect on smooth muscle activation; however, it is unclear whether it can be utilized to improve asthma attacks. Ketamine administration will decrease the neurally induced bronchoconstriction that occurs with airway manipulation during intubation.

Midazolam

Midazolam is a water-soluble benzodiazepine that has the notable property of causing antegrade amnesia in conscious patients. Midazolam has an elimination half-life of 2.7 h (compared to 46.6 h for diazepam).[17,18] In the elderly, the elimination half-life is longer and elimination clearance decreases.[17,18] Drug effects are terminated by redistribution, suggesting that pharmacodynamic changes in the elderly cause the prolonged effects seen in this age group.[17,18]

After doses of 0.05 to 0.2 mg/kg of midazolam IV, tidal volumes will decrease by 40%, but minute ventilation remains unchanged. However, after slightly larger doses, apnea is seen. When opioids and midazolam are administered together, respiratory depression is assured, as midazolam decreases the tidal volume and the opioids will decrease the respiratory rate. In patients with chronic obstructive airways disease and in patients with altered respiratory drives, more prolonged and more profound respiratory depression has been noted.[17,18]

Midazolam causes more hypotension than etomidate; when given to patients with normal cardiovascular function, small decreases in blood pressure and increases in heart rate are seen. When midazolam was given to patients who had valvular heart disease, some impairment of cardiac function was seen; when it was utilized for cardiac catheterization in patients with coronary artery disease, these patients experienced approximately a 15% decrease in their mean arterial pressures.[17,18] When patients have significant cardiac dysfunction or are hypovolemic, midazolam will depress cardiovascular function and has been associated with fatalities.

Unlike propofol, ketamine, or etomidate, midazolam will take longer for its peak effect on the central nervous system. The drug takes approximately 5 min to achieve its peak effect; recovery of normal central nervous function takes about 20 min after one dose.[17,18] However, in the elderly, prolonged amnesia even during the recovery period may occur.

Midazolam and the other benzodiazepines, except for lorazepam or temazepam, have been noted to interact with protease inhibitors including ritonavir, indinavir, nelfinavir, and saquinavir. The interaction involves the inhibition of P-450-3A enzyme that metabolizes many of the benzodiazepines. Therefore, the levels of the benzodiazepines can be increased and cause prolonged amnesia and sedation.[23] There is now a warning on the protease inhibitors to avoid the administration of the above benzodiazepines to patients who are taking protease inhibitors. The warning also exists for meperidine, fentanyl, codeine, and hydromorphone, levels of which are also increased by the protease inhibitors.[23]

Dexmedetomidine

Dexmedetomidine, an α_2-adrenoreceptor agonist, is a new class of sedative drug that is being introduced for use in the ICU. It binds α_2-agonist receptors eight times more avidly than clonidine and is shorter acting.[24] Beneficial properties include marked sedation with only mild reductions in minute ventilation, reduced hemodynamic response to intubation and extubation, attenuated stress response to surgery, and potentiation of analgesics.[25] A prospective, randomized study reported that ICU patients who received dexmedetomidine required significantly less additional sedative or analgesic medication than did the control patients.[26] In 1999, dexmedetomidine was approved by the US Food and Drug Administration for short-term (<24 h) infusion as a sedative agent in critically ill patients. It has not been approved for use in Europe. Patients sedated with dexmedetomidine appear tranquil while being readily arousable and interactive when stimulated.[24]

The adverse effects include hypertension, followed by hypotension and bradycardia from inhibition of sympathetic activity in the central nervous system.[27] Because of this, boluses may not be tolerated as well as maintenance infusions in critically ill patients. Elimination may be prolonged in the presence of hepatic dysfunction, but additional data will be necessary to determine whether this drug can be used in patients with renal or hepatic failure.[27]

Neuromuscular Alterations in Critically Ill Patients

A variety of neuromuscular alterations have now been described in critically ill patients. Critical illness polyneuropathy (CIP) is the most frequent acute polyneuropathy in this population. Risk factors for CIP include parenteral nutrition, autoimmune disorders, steroid use, use of muscle relaxants (pancuronium or vecuronium), hyperglycemia, hyperosmolality and catecholamine use.[28] Intensive insulin therapy in critically ill patients was found to reduce the incidence of CIP by 44%.[29] Mortality was found to be up to 3.5 times higher for patients with CIP versus patients without CIP.[28]

Data suggest 58% of patients who remain >1 week in the ICU will develop CIP and 82% of patients with sepsis and multiorgan failure will develop CIP. CIP is associated with persistent ataxia, muscle weakness and paralysis in survivors of critical illness.[30] CIP is an acute axonal polyneuropathy; affected nerves have a reduced number of fibers so that the amplitude of nerve action potentials are reduced while the nerve conduction velocity is normal. Latency and conduction velocity are unchanged. Sensory and motor nerves are typically involved but pure motor and pure sensory forms have been described. Deep tendon reflexes are decreased or absent. Creatine kinase levels can be normal or slightly increased. Diaphragmatic denervation may play a role in ventilator dependency.[31]

Critical illness myopathy (CIM) is a primary myopathy and it appears to be as frequent as CIP. To differentiate between CIP and CIM, the patient has to cooperate with the electromyogram diagnostic study. Muscle biopsies are usually required to confirm CIM. Muscle biopsies should be considered in patients with normal sensory neurography, low motor amplitudes and little spontaneous activity for the degree of weakness, findings typical of myopathies.[28] CIM encompasses a spectrum of disease, including acute necrotizing myopathy to evidence of intact muscle. Direct stimulation of muscle fibers is now being utilized, instead of and in addition to muscle biopsies, to confirm the diagnosis of CIM when there is an absolute reduction in direct response compound motor action potential below critical values.[32] In patients with sepsis and SIRS, patients frequently have both CIP and CIM.[28]

An algorithm has been created to simplify the differential diagnosis of weakness in critically ill patients. Steroids are associated with a thick-filament myopathy. The steroid components of the muscle relaxants pancuronium and vecuronium have been suggested as a cause of necrotizing myopathy.[28]

Introduction to Muscle Relaxants

Muscle relaxants are utilized for several reasons, including facilitating endotracheal intubation, facilitating mechanical ventilation, reducing elevated intracranial pressure, reducing work of breathing, reducing spasms associated with tetanus, and reducing movement associated with status epilepticus.[33] Short-term use is considered <2 d, because complications have rarely been reported with administration for <2 d.[33] Complications associated with muscle relaxants include anaphylaxis, hyperkalemia associated with succinylcholine administration (seen in patients with burns, neurologic injury, muscle trauma, long-term immobilization, or elevated serum potassium), inadequate ventilation of paralyzed patients, inadequate analgesia and sedation of paralyzed patients, and persistent weakness after long-term use.[33,34]

Most investigations have not found neuromuscular blocking agents to be associated with CIP.[28] Persistent weakness occurs in about 20% of patients who receive muscle relaxants for >6 d and in up to 70% of patients who are receiving steroids as well as receiving muscle relaxants.[33] Risk factors for prolonged weakness include vecuronium in female patients who have renal failure, high-dose steroids, and >2-d duration of relaxant administration and administration of high doses of muscle relaxants.

There appear to be several etiologies to the persistent weakness. The persistent weakness may be due to persistent paralysis. Vecuronium has an active metabolite, 3-desacetyl vecuronium, which persists particularly in female patients with renal failure. Pancuronium and pipecuronium also form these metabolites. Therefore, these drugs should not chronically be administered to patients who have renal failure.

Patients taking corticosteroids who receive long-term muscle relaxants appear to develop a myopathic syndrome characterized by flaccid paralysis, increased creatine kinase, and myonecrosis; these patients recover after many months. Plasma creatine kinase concentrations appear to increase when the myopathy develops; therefore, serum creatine kinase should be monitored in patients taking corticosteroids who are receiving muscle relaxants. All muscle relaxants have been associated with this syndrome.

A motor neuropathy has been reported after the administration of vecuronium, pancuronium, or atracurium. The neuropathy affects all extremities, is associated with absent tendon reflexes, and can be accompanied by muscle wasting. This syndrome also takes months to resolve. Another syndrome consisting of persistent motor weakness but with preservation of sensory function has been reported in patients receiving pancuronium, vecuronium, or metocurine. These patients do not have normal neuromuscular transmission, and their symptoms also took months to resolve.

Patients do become tolerant to the effects of the muscle relaxants. The tolerance can develop within 24 to 48 h and appears to be due to upregulation of acetylcholine receptors secondary to chronic denervation. One method to decrease the incidence of tolerance is to minimize the amount of muscle relaxant given; the drug should only be given for a defined clinical outcome. The only reason to monitor the train-of-four method is to document that complete block is not obtained, as the presence of a train-of-four response does not ensure that persistent weakness will not occur.

Comparison of Muscle Relaxants

For rapid tracheal intubation, either succinylcholine or rocuronium (Table 3) should be administered. Succinylcholine only lasts for 5 to 10 min, which may be helpful if there is concern that the patient's trachea cannot be intubated. Succinylcholine has several significant side effects, including hyperkalemia, bradycardia, junctional arrhythmias, ventricular arrhythmias, masseter spasm, and muscle pains. Rocuronium is the first nondepolarizing muscle relaxant that has a fast onset similar to succinylcholine; however, paralysis will persist for up to 90 min, thus mask ventilation and/or tracheal intubation must be successful. Succinylcholine should not be used in patients with hyperkalemia, or in patients with burns, massive trauma, or denervation injuries such as paraplegia or quadraplegia. In these patients, acetylcholine receptors are upregulated hyperkalemia will be exaggerated and may result in cardiac arrest.

Vecuronium has active metabolites that have been associated with persistent weakness, particularly in female patients with renal failure. Rocuronium does not have active metabolites. Atracurium and cisatracurium are utilized because their duration of action is not affected by liver or kidney disease. Cisatracurium's duration of action is as long as, if not longer than, that of rocuronium. All muscle relaxants have been associated with allergic reactions. In fact, muscle relaxants are the leading cause of perioperative anaphylaxis (succinylcholine is associated with 48% of the cases).[34] A recent report of cisatracurium-induced anaphylaxis documented that cardiovascular collapse can be the only sign of the allergic reaction.[34]

Airway Management

When one needs to emergently secure an airway, there are certain principles to remember: oxygenation even without removal of carbon dioxide

Table 3. *Properties of Muscle Relaxants Used in the ICU*

Drug	Initial Dose* (mg/kg)	Duration† (min)	Cost Factor‡	Advantages	Complications
Pancuronium	0.07–0.1	60–120	1	Inexpensive	Tachycardia; active metabolite
Pipecuronium	0.05–0.07	60–120	5	CVS stability	Active metabolite
Doxacurium	0.04–0.05	60–120	5	CVS stability	None
Vecuronium	0.1	30–45	20	CVS stability	Active metabolite
Atracurium	0.05	30–45	20	Reliable recovery	Histamine release; active metabolite
Rocuronium	0.6–1.2	30–90	20	Rapid onset	None
Cisatracurium	0.1–0.2	30–90	10	Reliable recovery	Slow onset; active metabolite
Mivacurium	0.2	10–20	N/A	Short duration	Histamine release; metabolites
Succinylcholine 1–2	5–10	N/A	Fast onset; fast recovery	Hyperkalemia; dysrhythmia	

CVS, cardiovascular system; N/A, not recommended for long-term use.
* For tracheal intubation.
† Time from intubation dose until first Train-of-Four response might return.
‡ Numbers are multiples of the cost of pancuronium, which is ~$10/day.
Reproduced with permission from Caldwell JE, Miller RD: Muscle relaxants in the intensive care unit. Hospital Physician 1996; 32:14

can be life-saving, and the complete inability to oxygenate will cause brain damage within 3 min. Therefore, as long as a needle can be placed in the trachea and oxygen can be given, the patient can be kept alive until a surgical airway can be obtained. Percutaneous kits are available to perform emergency cricothyroidotomies; the operator must be able to complete the procedure in <3 min, and preferably the procedure should be completed within 1 min.

If a patient is not actively vomiting or otherwise soiling the airway, then mask ventilation should be attempted. Successful mask ventilation can require two or more hands, and an oral and/or nasal airway. Mask ventilation is all that is required if aspiration is not a risk and the operator is not expert at tracheal intubation. The complications of mask ventilation include damage to the eyes, insufflation of the stomach, and possible regurgitation.

Intubation of the trachea can be done via conventional laryngoscopy; this procedure requires practice. A laryngeal mask can be placed at the patient's glottic opening by pushing it into the patient's mouth and down the pharynx; proper placement of the laryngeal mask may require less practice and training than conventional laryngoscopy. The laryngeal mask does not protect against aspiration, but has been utilized in patients whose tracheas cannot be intubated using conventional laryngoscopy. Operators with expertise in tracheal intubation may encounter patients where conventional laryngoscopy is unsuccessful. An algorithm is then to be followed; depending on the status of the patient, either the procedure is aborted or a surgical airway is obtained (Fig 1).[35]

Situations where conventional laryngoscopy may be difficult include restriction of the oral airway, reduced pharyngeal space, noncompliant

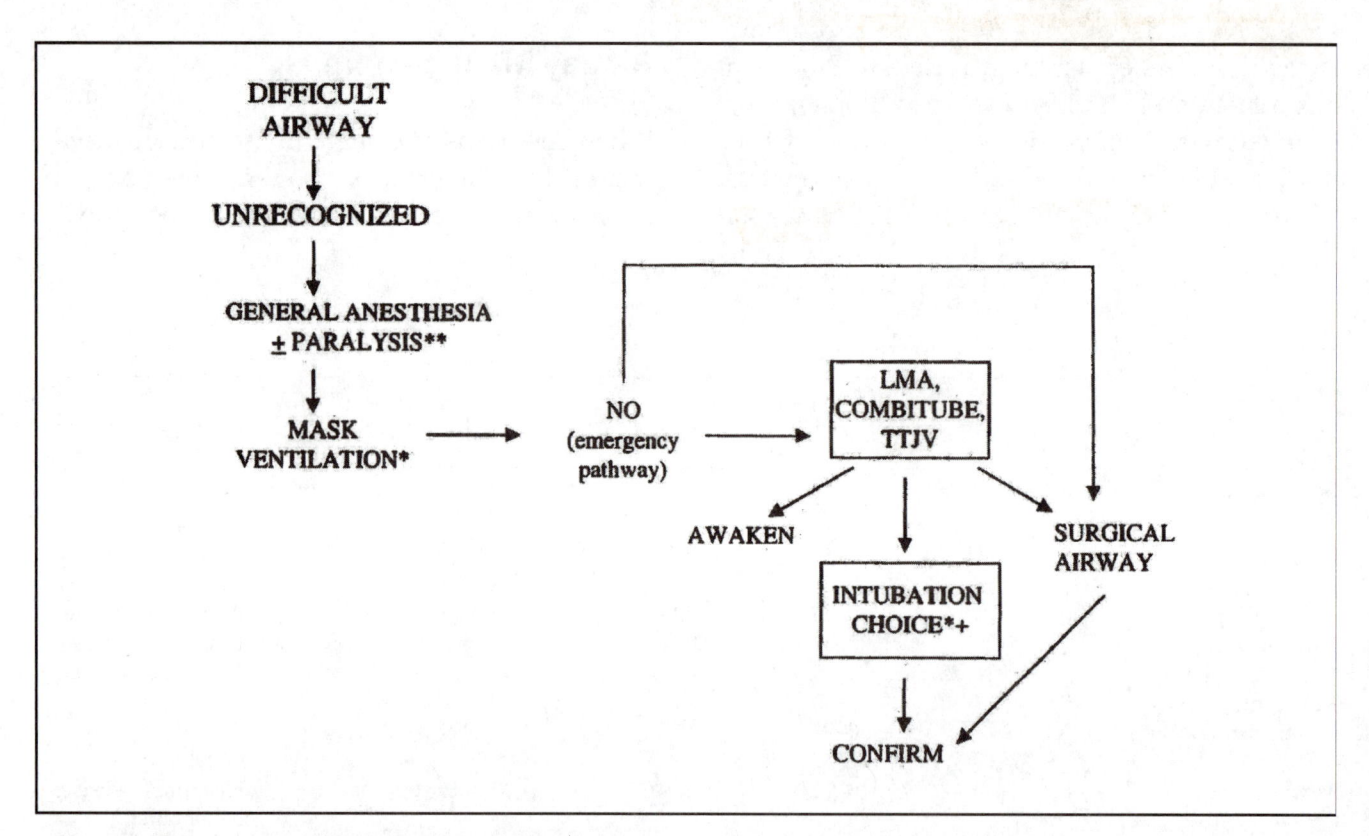

Figure 1. Difficult airway algorithm. Reproduced with permission from Benumof JL. Laryngeal mask airway and the ASA difficult airway algorithm. Anesthesiology 1996; 84:687.
*Always consider calling for help (eg, technical, medical, surgical, etc) when difficulty with mask ventilation and/or tracheal intubation is encountered.
**Consider the need to preserve spontaneous ventilation.
+ Nonsurgical tracheal intubation choices of laryngoscopy with a rigid laryngoscope blade (many types), blind orotracheal or nasotracheal technique, fiberoptic/stylet technique, retrograde technique, illuminating stylet, rigid bronchoscope, percutaneous dilational tracheal entry. See reference 3 for a complete discussion of these tracheal intubation choices.

submandibular tissue, limited atlanto-occipital extension, and partial airway obstruction. Small mouth openings are encountered in patients who have temporomandibular joint disease, scarring near the mouth, congenital and surgical deformities, large tongues, and diseased teeth. The pharyngeal space can be decreased by edema and by masses. The submandibular tissue can be altered by infection (Ludwig's angina), by scarring as from burns, by surgery, by radiation, and by cancer. Patients who cannot extend their necks include patients in a Halo-jacket, those with ankylosing spondylitis, cervical disc disease, or cervical spinal injuries. Airway obstruction occurs when there is epiglottitis, pedunculated tumors and cysts in the airways, large tonsils, mediastinal and subcutaneous emphysema, or edema is present. In these patients, the safest approach is nasal or oral fiberoptic bronchoscopic intubation while the patient maintains spontaneous ventilation.

References

1. Nelson BJ, Weinert CR, Bury CL, et al. Intensive care unit drug use and subsequent quality of life in acute lung injury patients. Crit Care Med 2000; 28:3626–3630
2. Brook AD, Ahrens TS, Schaiff R, et al. Effect of a nursing-implemented sedation protocol on the duration of mechanical ventilation. Crit Care Med 1999; 27:2609–2615
3. Kress JP, Pohlman AS, O'Connor MF, et al. Daily interruption of sedative infusions in critically ill patients undergoing mechanical ventilation. N Engl J Med 2000; 342:1471–1477
4. Cook DJ, Walter SD, Cook RJ, et al. Incidence of and risk factors for ventilator-associated pneumonia in critically ill patients. Ann Intern Med 1998; 129:433–440
5. Rotondi AJ, Chelluri L, Sirio C, et al. Patients' recollections of stressful experiences while receiving prolonged mechanical ventilation in an intensive care unit. Crit Care Med 2002; 30:746–752
6. Inouye SK, Bogardus ST, Jr., Charpentier PA, et al. A multicomponent intervention to prevent delirium in hospitalized older patients. N Engl J Med 1999; 340:669–676
7. Silverstein J, Bloom H, Cassel C. Geriatrics and anesthesia. Clin Anesthesiol 1999; 17:8–12
8. Volles DF, McGory R. Pharmacokinetic considerations. Crit Care Clin 1999; 15:55–75
9. Cammarano W, Wiener-Kronish J. Analgesics, tranquilizers, and sedatives. In: Brown D, ed. Cardiac intensive care. Philadelphia: WB Saunders, 1998; 591–602
10. Cammarano WB, Pittet JF, Weitz S, et al. Acute withdrawal syndrome related to the administration of analgesic and sedative medications in adult intensive care unit patients. Crit Care Med 1998; 26:676–684
11. Lowson SM, Sawh S. Adjuncts to analgesia. sedation and neuromuscular blockade. Crit Care Clin 1999; 15:119–141
12. Bailey P, Stanley T. Intravenous opioid anesthetics. In: Miller R, ed. Anesthesia. Vol. 1. New York: Churchill Livingstone, 1994; 291–388
13. Ornstein E, Matteo R. Effects of opioids. In: McLeskey C, ed. Geriatric anesthesiology. Baltimore: Williams and Wilkins, 1997; 249–260
14. Peng PW, Sandler AN. A review of the use of fentanyl analgesia in the management of acute pain in adults. Anesthesiology 1999; 90:576–599
15. Egan TD, Lemmens HJ, Fiset P, et al. The pharmacokinetics of the new short-acting opioid remifentanil (GI87084B) in healthy adult male volunteers. Anesthesiology 1993; 79:881–892
16. Song D, Whitten CW, White PF. Use of remifentanil during anesthetic induction: a comparison with fentanyl in the ambulatory setting. Anesth Analg 1999; 88:734–736
17. Reves J, Glass P, Lubarsky D. Nonbarbiturate intravenous anesthetics. In: Miller R, ed. Anesthesiology. Vol. 1. New York: Churchill Livingstone, 1994; 291–388
18. Fragen R. Effects of barbiturates, benzodiazpines, and other intravenous agents. In: McLeskey C, ed. Geriatric anesthesiology. Baltimore: Williams and Wilkins, 1997; 249–260
19. Smith I, White PF, Nathanson M, et al. Propofol. an update on its clinical use. Anesthesiology 1994; 81:1005–1043
20. Brown RH, Wagner EM. Mechanisms of bronchoprotection by anesthetic induction agents: propofol versus ketamine. Anesthesiology 1999; 90: 822–828
21. Eames WO, Rooke GA, Wu RS, et al. Comparison of the effects of etomidate, propofol, and thiopental on respiratory resistance after tracheal intubation. Anesthesiology 1996; 84:1307–1311

22. Kohrs R, Durieux ME. Ketamine: teaching an old drug new tricks. Anesth Analg 1998; 87:1186–1193
23. Flexner C. HIV-protease inhibitors. N Engl J Med 1998; 338:1281–1292
24. Coursin D, Coursin D, Maccioli G. Dexmedetomidine. Curr Opin Crit Care 2001; 7:221–226
25. Scheinin B, Lindgren L, Randell T, et al. Dexmedetomidine attenuates sympathoadrenal responses to tracheal intubation and reduces the need for thiopentone and peroperative fentanyl. Br J Anaesth 1992; 68:126–131
26. Venn R, Bradshaw C, Spencer R, et al. Preliminary UK experience of dexmedetomidine, a novel agent for postoperative sedation in the intensive care unit. Anesthesia 1999; 54: 1136–1142
27. Bhana N, Goa KL, McClellan KJ. Dexmedetomidine. Drugs 2000; 59:263–268
28. van Mook WN, Hulsewe-Evers RP. Critical illness polyneuropathy. Curr Opin Crit Care 2002; 8:302–310
29. van den Berghe G, Wouters P, Weekers F, et al. Intensive insulin therapy in the critically ill patients. N Engl J Med 2001; 345:1359–1367
30. Garnacho-Montero J, Madrazo-Osuna J, Garcia-Garmendia JL, et al. Critical illness polyneuropathy: risk factors and clinical consequences. a cohort study in septic patients. Intensive Care Med 2001; 27:1288–1296
31. Leijten FS, De Weerd AW, Poortvliet DC, et al. Critical illness polyneuropathy in multiple organ dysfunction syndrome and weaning from the ventilator. Intensive Care Med 1996; 22: 856–861
32. Bednarik J, Lukas Z, Vondracek P. Critical illness polyneuromyopathy: the electrophysiological components of a complex entity. Intensive Care Med 2003; 29:1505–1514
33. Caldwell J, Miller R. A review of muscle relaxants and their use in the intensive care unit. Hospital Physician 1996; 32:11–24
34. Toh KW, Deacock SJ, Fawcett WJ. Severe anaphylactic reaction to cisatracurium. Anesth Analg 1999; 88:462–464
35. Benumof JL. Laryngeal mask airway and the ASA difficult airway algorithm. Anesthesiology 1996; 84:686–699

Notes

Notes

Blood Products in the Critical Care Setting

Aryeh Shander, MD, FCCP

Objectives:

- List the available blood products currently in use
- Review the current recommendations for RBC transfusion
- Review the indications for platelet and plasma transfusions
- Review and understand the current risks and complications associated with allogeneic blood transfusions

Key words: allogeneic transfusions; component therapy; cryoprecipitate; fresh frozen plasma; transfusion-associated lung injury; transfusion reactions

Introduction

Transfusion medicine has evolved over the last hundred years to provide patients with blood products on demand. The discovery of the ABO system by Landsteiner in the early 1900s shaped what was at times a deadly therapy to a therapeutic intervention thought to save lives and improve the quality of those who survived hemorrhage. After World War II, the storage of blood and blood derivatives was perfected to the point that blood products are available on demand. Blood, a liquid tissue (organ), thought of as an acceptable therapeutic intervention, was taking on the characteristics of a pharmaceutical product and hence the term given to blood banks, *wet pharmacy*. It was not until the 1980s, the break of the HIV epidemic, when blood became a threat to its recipients. Prior to this deadly epidemic, the few patients who contracted hepatitis C from transfused blood were an acceptable risk compared to the perceived benefit of blood transfusions.

Transfusion medicine has undergone significant change since then. No longer thought of as a therapeutic intervention, blood transfusions are perceived as a negative outcome. Outcome data in critically ill patients favors a conservative rather than a liberal approach to RBC transfusion and questions the efficacy of plasma therapy as well. With no prospective trials available on the benefit of allogeneic blood transfusions, the treatment approach to the anemic patient in the ICU has changed dramatically. Large amounts of blood product transfusions and nondirected transfusion therapy are a thing of the past. In spite of this, transfusion of blood products remains an emotional behavior rather than rooted in evidence. The important issues of ethics, legal, and economic implications of transfusion therapy are beyond the scope of this article. In the ensuing sections, a discussion of blood products, risks and, complications and a rational approach to their use will be discussed.

Components Available From the Blood Bank

Whole Blood

Whole blood, generally stored in an acid citrate-dextrose medium, is available in few US hospitals. Its use is reserved for replacement during acute hemorrhage, when transfusion of RBCs and clotting factors are needed. Use of whole blood is not uncommon in the military setting, and its long-term implications are poorly understood. Because of the higher yield of products, whole blood is fractionated into RBCs and plasma. On average, the yield is approximately 1.4 U of product from a single unit of whole blood donated. Whole blood from autologous predeposit or from designated donors is tested and stored in similar fashion to banked blood from volunteer donors. Designated donor blood that carries infection is destroyed; many institutions also destroy autologous blood that is not infectious since this blood is not part of the "donor pool."

Packed RBCs

Packed red blood cells (PRBCs) are essentially all of the RBCs in a unit of blood, with plasma largely removed, so that the resulting cells are at a hematocrit of approximately 70%. They are stored for up to 42 days at 4°C (Table 1). This

Table 1. Blood Products: Volumes and Storage Time

Blood Products	Volume, mL	Storage Time Limit	Storage Temperature (Range), °C
PRBCs	280	42 d	4(1–6)
Random donor platelets	70	5 d	20–24
Apheresis platelets	300	5 d	20–24
FFP	250	1 yr	−18
Apheresis plasma	500	1 yr	−18
Cryoprecipitate	15	1 yr	−18
Predonated PRBCs (whole blood)	510	35 d	4(1–6)
Directed donors	280	42 d	4

"cold storage" results in significant changes to the morphology and the function of these cells. Within days of storage, 2,3-diphosphoglycerate (2,3-DPG) is reduced to <10% of normal and with more prolonged storage is absent completely. The repletion of 2,3-DPG may take up to ≥24 h. A fraction of stored cells also gradually lyse, releasing potassium, hemoglobin, and red cell stroma into the pack. These damaged cells, low to no 2,3-DPG, and the resulting debris have placed the efficacy of stored blood in question. The glaring absence of 2,3-DPG reduces or eliminates the ability of RBCs to unload oxygen in the periphery. In critically ill patients, data suggest that improving the patients' hemodynamics is favored over increasing the oxygen delivery through transfusions.

Heat and mechanical fragmentation can both disrupt stored RBCs. Blood warmers must be checked for temperature accuracy because exposure to temperatures >42°C can result in significant hemolysis of RBCs.

Specialized Red Cells

RBCs store well when frozen, usually in glycerol or dimethyl sulfoxide. Their shelf life is vastly extended, and they can be shipped with little risk of loss. PRBC units donated by persons with rare blood types may be stored and shipped to institutions with an acute need and no available donors. Frozen RBCs are no less likely to transmit most diseases than refrigerated stored RBCs. Unfreezing these cells and "deglycerating" them reduces their shelf life from 42 days to 24 h. Work done by civilian and military blood banks has rendered a longer shelf life for these defrosted cells. "Washed" RBCs are produced by recentrifugation in saline solution in order to remove plasma and contaminating WBCs. This procedure may reduce reactions to RBC transfusions in sensitized patients or those in need of receiving many transfusions over time.

Leukodepletion is a process that reduces the number of WBCs in a unit of PRBC. Generally, a unit of PRBC contains approximately 10^9 WBCs (referred to as *passenger leukocytes*). These WBCs are thought to generate an inflammatory reaction in the recipient of the PRBCs. Leukodepletion has been shown to do the following: (1) reduce the WBC count in PRBCs to 10^6; (2) reduce febrile reactions; and (3) in patients undergoing cardiac surgery, improve survival. In Western Europe and Canada, leukodepletion is mandatory but not in the United States, although >90% of hospitals in the United States deplete their blood of leukocytes.

Plasma and Plasma Fractions

Fresh frozen plasma (FFP) may be obtained from two sources: donated whole blood or apheresis donation. Each bag of plasma from donor and apheresis sources contains 250 mL and 500 mL of plasma, respectively. FFP can be kept frozen for 1 year, but one must keep in mind the different half-lives of the clotting factors in plasma. For example, the half-life of factors II and IX are 2 to 3 days, whereas factor VII is only 3 to 6 h. Cryoprecipitate is prepared from fresh plasma by freezing, then slow thawing to 15.5°C. What precipitates is factor VIII (including von Willebrand moiety), fibrinogen (approximately one third of that in the unit of blood), and fibronectin. When made into cryoprecipitate, a unit of plasma yields approximately 80 to 100 U of factor VIIIc/von Willebrand factor and approximately 150 mg of fibrinogen. Cryoprecipitate can be reconstituted in extremely small volumes, making it useful when volume overload is a concern. Both products have long shelf lives although shorter half-lives when transfused than their native counterparts.

Specific coagulation factors may be commercially manufactured from pooled plasma or as recombinant DNA products. Although they are expensive, they seem to have a broader function and fewer complications including disease transmission. Volunteer donors are screened individuals, so blood bank products are presumably slightly safer than pooled commercial plasma products, which may represent a pool of as few as 4 to 10 donors or hundreds to thousands of donors. However, the safety of commercial preparations of factor complexes, such as prothrombin complex and cryoprecipitate, compares favorably to that of blood bank products.

Platelets

Platelets are removed from fresh whole blood by sedimentation and are stored at 22°C under continuous agitation. They may also be obtained by pheresis of a single donor, which harvests about the same amount as 5 to 6 U of platelets. Stored platelets may be good for up to a week, although older units have a shorter survival: transfused platelets last up to 72 h in normal recipients. Transfusion of 1 U of platelets raises the recipient's platelet count by 6,000 to 10,000/μL, assuming average body size and no consumption.

Platelets pheresed from a single donor may be used prospectively to reduce the risk of immunization of recipients who will be repeatedly exposed to platelet transfusions. The routine use of single donor platelets in such individuals does reduce the risk of platelet sensitization and resultant immune destruction. Platelets may be cross-matched to specific platelet antigens, or human leukocyte antigen haplotype matching of donor to recipient may also be used to reduce the likelihood of sensitization. Both techniques have been used to successfully give platelet transfusions to recipients who have already become sensitized to random donor platelets.

WBCs

Granulocytes are obtained by pheresis of single donors and are collected either by centrifugation or by nylon filtration; donors are often treated with steroids to increase the peripheral WBC numbers or with hydroxyethyl starch to promote rapid RBC sedimentation. Granulocytes must be administered promptly, both because of the risk of contamination and because of spontaneous aggregation and degranulation. The only defined role for granulocyte transfusion is in the neutropenic patient with documented bacteremic infection in whom appropriate antibiotic therapy is failing; this may include immunosuppressed patients and neonates. The use of granulocyte transfusions is now largely supplanted by use of growth factors.

Lymphocytes are harvested from individual donors by pheresis, and are employed in transplantation to boost donor immune function and either increase engraftment or increase graft-vs-tumor effects in bone marrow transplantation. Their use is accompanied by a higher risk of graft-vs-host disease (GVHD).

Indications for Transfusion of Blood Products

Indications for RBC Transfusion

Critically ill patients are at risk for anemia and thus at high risk for being exposed to allogeneic blood transfusions. Anemia in this population can be attributed to a variety of causes including GI bleeding (subacute and acute GI bleed), postsurgical bleeding, and trauma. The repeated and large amounts of phlebotomy blood have been demonstrated to aggravate the anemia mentioned above. Critically ill patients have been shown to have reduced erythropoietin (EPO) production, reducing the available new RBCs. In spite of normal iron stores, anemia develops in these patients as a direct impact of the inflammatory response. This anemia, termed *anemia of chronic disease*, responds well to treatment with exogenous EPO.

Clear indications for RBC transfusion do not exist. Many professional societies and the

National Institutes of Health have had to resort to consensus formation since evidence-based transfusion indications are not available. Whatever recommendations are quoted, an argument based on preclinical or clinical data can refute those recommendations.

The controversy regarding the tolerable versus optimal hemoglobin has not been resolved. Transfusion trigger has always been related to a hemoglobin level, but this approach has changed over the last two decades.

Table 2 demonstrates the difficulty in obtaining a single number as a trigger for transfusion, and without clinical correlation a single hemoglobin determination should not be used as a trigger for transfusion. A range of hemoglobin from 6 to 8 g/dL is a trigger to consider PRBCs but not conclusive. The presence of hypovolemia with low hemoglobin needs to be corrected first before blood is administered.

Symptoms of tissue hypoxia that are considered standard indications for RBC transfusion of anemic individuals include chest pain, confusion, syncope, congestive heart failure, and arrhythmias. Many clinicians also regard headaches, lightheadedness or dizziness, and marked fatigue as standard indications of hypoxia, although these are less reliable. However, these symptoms may be difficult to ascertain in the ICU setting and may be late signs of oxygen depravation. A few factors complicate this intervention further. Assessment of oxygen depravation at the organ level is clinically impossible until it is too late. Noninvasive methods are not readily available yet, so it remains a judgment call. If oxygen depravation is suspected, then the use of banked allogeneic blood may actually compound the problem. These RBCs are devoid of 2,3-DPG, are adenosine triphosphate deficient, and promote poor survival altering the microcirculation by inducing vasoconstriction or occlusion of the microcirculation.

Moreover, outcome clinical data in critically ill patients do not favor transfusion over conservative approach, *ie*, withholding PRBCs and using other modalities to treat anemia. A prospective, Canadian, randomized study of a "liberal" hemoglobin target (10 to 12 g/dL) vs a "conservative" hemoglobin target (7 to 9 g/dL) for RBC transfusion in a variety of critically ill, nonbleeding patients, demonstrated no major outcome differences between the two strategies; and indeed there was suggestive evidence that for younger patients and perhaps those with significant vascular disease, clinical outcomes may be superior using a conservative transfusion strategy.

With all that, in the ICU setting, in the absence of reported symptoms, physiologic indicators of inadequate tissue oxygenation are often substituted. During anemia, peripheral oxygen extraction rises and mixed venous oxygen saturation falls. Experts have proposed the following measures as indicative of tissue hypoxia: (1) a mixed venous $P_{O_2} < 25$ mm Hg; (2) oxygen consumption falling to < 50% of the baseline value, assuming this value is known; and (3) oxygen extraction ratio > 50% [(oxygen consumed)/(oxygen delivered) ≥ 50%; or (arterial oxygen content–mixed venous oxygen content)/arterial oxygen content ≥ 0.5]. Although hypoxia is derived via the above calculations, no data are available on benefit of transfusions in this situation; in a few studies comparing improving hemodynamic status to transfusions, inotropic medication prevailed.

Judgments about the utility of an individual RBC transfusion are ultimately clinical choices. However, the clinician who has made the judgment to transfuse should do it 1 U at a time and document the effect of that transfusion.

Table 2. *Hemoglobin Thresholds for ABT: Published Guidelines*

Organizations	Year	Hb, g/dL
National Institutes of Health Consensus*	1988	8
American College of Physicians†	1992	7
American Society of Anesthesiologists‡	1996	6
Canadian Medical Association§	1997	Insufficient
Association of Anaesthetists‖	2001	8 (a)
Scottish Intercollegiate Guidelines¶	2001	7 (b)

*National Institutes of Health. *JAMA* 1988; 260:2700–2703.
†American College of Physicians. *Ann Intern Med* 1992; 116:403–406.
‡American Society of Anesthesiologists. *Anesthesiology.* 1996; 84:732–747.
§Canadian Medical Association. *Can Med Assoc J* 1997; 156(suppl 11):S1–S24.
‖Association of Anaesthetists of Great Britain and Ireland. *Blood Transfusion and the Anaesthetist: Red Cell Transfusion,* 2001.
¶Scottish Intercollegiate Guidelines Network, 2001.

Indications for Platelet Transfusion

Platelet transfusions are also subject to some controversy. The purpose of platelet transfusion is to either aid in correcting a coagulopathy when the patient is actively bleeding or to prevent spontaneous hemorrhage in a patient with profound thrombocytopenia. Platelet transfusion as prophylaxis is indicated in a very limited number of situations. In nonbleeding patients, the risk of spontaneous hemorrhage is low when platelet count is $>10 \times 10^9/L$.

Platelet counts $>50,000/\mu L$ are adequate for general surgical procedures and closed medical procedures, and transfusion over that amount generally applies only to major cardiovascular procedures and neurosurgery. The bleeding time is not useful in predicting which thrombocytopenic patients are at risk of bleeding. In the adult population, random donor platelets are usually transfused in groups of 5 U at a time. The relative contraindications to platelet transfusions are as follows: thrombotic thrombocytopenic purpura; heparin associated/induced thrombocytopenia; and posttransfusion purpura.

Guidelines for platelet transfusion vary to some extent, especially at low platelet levels without evidence of bleeding. In patients with cancer who have received chemotherapy, platelet counts of $5,000/\mu L$ are tolerated without bleeding. Yet, counts $\leq 30,000 \mu L$ with suggestion of cavity bleeding should be treated with platelet transfusions. The presence of "anti-platelet" medication (becoming more and more prevalent) is a controversial indication for transfusion. Platelet dysfunction secondary to medications is common in the ICU setting, and removal or discontinuation is recommended whenever possible. Transfusion of fresh donor platelets may not help in the presence of circulating antiplatelet drugs.

As a rule, in patients with bleeding or surgical intervention, the goal is to maintain platelets either at a level that will stop bleeding or at $>50,000/\mu L$. The risk of spontaneous life-threatening CNS hemorrhage becomes increased at platelet counts of approximately 10,000 to $20,000/\mu L$. If the patient has other risk factors for hemorrhage, transfuse at $20,000/\mu L$; if none, transfuse at $10,000/\mu L$.

Septic patients in the ICU who may receive drotrecogin alfa present a challenge because of increased risk of bleeding and increased mortality if platelet counts drop $>30,000/\mu L$. The judicious use of platelets under those circumstances remains a clinical judgment, and no clear guidelines are available.

Indications for FFP Transfusion

In a commentary published in *Transfusion* in 2005, W. Dzik refers to the fact that there are no established indications for the transfusion of FFP. Replacement of isolated factor deficiencies (factors II, V, VII, IX, X, XI) are considered indications, but the emergence of recombinant proteins may change these indications in the future. Clinicians need to be aware of the amount of plasma required to replace a given factor (for example, very little for factor X). One "indication" that is difficult to challenge is the presence of closed space bleeding in a patient receiving warfarin therapy. Common practice is to transfuse FFP to patients receiving warfarin therapy undergoing emergency surgery. However, it makes more sense to have FFP for transfusion if life-threatening bleeding occurs. The routine administration of FFP to patients with an elevated international normalized ratio (INR) has no scientific or clinical basis. In the past and current recommendations, plasma can be used for reversal of warfarin anticoagulation in patients with life-threatening bleeding.

When encountering heparin resistance due to antithrombin III deficiency, FFP can be used to replace antithrombin III when the commercial preparation is not available for those patients who require surgery or must have heparin for treatment of acute thrombosis. Plasma may be used in the course of treating coagulopathy due to massive blood transfusion, in which whole blood is not available and bleeding is demonstrably due to factor deficiency. Rarely, plasma is used for treatment of certain immunodeficiencies, *eg*, protein-losing enteropathy in infants not responding to parenteral nutrition. There are no other routine or prophylactic situations in which FFP should be used. It is not an appropriate volume expander or source of nutrition or albumin.

Summary of Relative Indications

Relative indications are as follows (1) correction of excessive microvascular bleeding (*ie*, coagulopathy) in the presence of a prothrombin time >1.5 times normal or INR >2.0, or an activated partial thromboplastin time >2 times normal; (2) correction of excessive microvascular bleeding secondary to coagulation factor deficiency in patients transfused with PRBCs only for more than one blood volume (approximately 70 mL/kg) and when activated prothrombin time or INR and activated partial thromboplastin time cannot be obtained in a timely fashion; (3) urgent reversal of warfarin therapy; (4) correction of known coagulation factor deficiencies for which specific concentrates are unavailable; and (5) heparin resistance (antithrombin III deficiency) in a patient requiring heparin.

FFP Is Not Indicated Solely for Augmentation of Plasma Volume or Albumin Concentration

FFP should be administered in doses calculated to achieve a minimum of 30% of plasma factor concentration (usually achieved with administration of 10 to 15 mL/kg of FFP), except for urgent reversal of warfarin anticoagulation, for which 5 to 8 mL/kg of FFP usually will suffice. Of note, four to five platelet concentrates, 1 U of single-donor apheresis platelets, or 1 U of fresh whole blood provide a quantity of coagulation factors similar to that contained in 1 U of FFP. The amount of factors present in a unit of FFP varies significantly from one unit to another.

Indications for Cryoprecipitate Transfusion

If possible, a fibrinogen concentration should be obtained prior to the administration of cryoprecipitate in a bleeding patient. Transfusion of cryoprecipitate is rarely indicated if fibrinogen concentration is >150 mg/dL. Transfusion of cryoprecipitate is usually indicated for the following: (1) when the fibrinogen concentration is <80 to 100 mg/dL in the presence of excessive microvascular bleeding; (2) to correct excessive microvascular bleeding in massively transfused patients when fibrinogen concentrations cannot be measured in a timely fashion; and (3) for patients with congenital fibrinogen deficiencies.

Whenever possible, decisions regarding patients with congenital fibrinogen deficiencies should be made in consultation with the patient's hematologist. The determination of whether patients with fibrinogen concentration from 100 to 150 mg/dL require therapy should be based on the potential for anticipated or ongoing bleeding, and the risk of bleeding into a confined space (eg, brain or eye). Bleeding patients with von Willebrand disease should be treated with specific concentrates if available. If concentrates are not available, cryoprecipitate is indicated. Each unit of cryoprecipitate contains 150 to 250 mg of fibrinogen. Each unit of FFP contains 2 to 4 mg of fibrinogen per milliliter. Therefore, it should be noted that each unit of FFP delivers the equivalent amount of fibrinogen as 2 U of cryoprecipitate.

Drugs to Treat Coagulopathy

Factor VIII and factor IX are available as recombinant DNA products for use in the treatment of hemophilia A and B. Prothrombin complex preparations are available from a variety of manufacturers for the treatment of a variety of acquired coagulopathies, including warfarin overdose and acquired autoimmune factor deficiencies, and for the treatment of hemophilia patients who have acquired antibodies to factor VIII. Activated factor VII was created to specifically address the treatment of hemophilia patients with bleeding and high levels of antibodies (inhibitors) to factor VIII. Both prothrombin complex and activated factor VII have been used (separately) in a variety of other off-label bleeding scenarios. Both may cause hypercoagulability and thrombosis as complications and should be used with great caution in situations in which thrombosis is a risk. Guidelines for the use of activated factor VII in a variety of these situations is referenced below. No clear safety data to the use of these agents are available, and they ought to be used with caution.

Risks and Complications of Blood Transfusions

Cross-Matching and Sensitization

RBCs are matched by reacting recipient serum with type-specific (ABO and Rh) donor cells at two different temperatures (major cross-match). Cross-matching may be difficult owing to a variety of problems. Nonspecific cold agglutinins are seen in a host of medical conditions, and they cause difficulty matching at room temperature and sometimes at 37°C. Cold agglutinins are usually not associated with hemolytic reactions *in vivo* unless complement is fixed in the cold (hence cold agglutinin disease). Not only do they make cross-matching difficult, but they may mask the presence of other antibodies. Warm antibodies, usually IgG, are associated with autoimmune disease and certain malignancies, and make conventional cross-matching of RBCs almost impossible. Certain blood banks have techniques for eluting out the warm antibodies so that a cross-match may be performed, but this service is not widespread. If antibody elution is not available, the consensus is that one arrives at the best possible match of type-specific blood and uses that blood, knowing that hemolysis will probably be no greater than it is endogenously. Surface antigens are weakly expressed in neonates, elderly persons, and massively transfused patients, making cross-matching difficult. Larger volumes of blood will be needed to cross-match these persons.

Platelets and plasma are not routinely cross-matched. Because the plasma they contain may have antibodies to the recipient's cells, they are generally type-specific, but in an emergency, even this is not done.

In spite of cross-matching, sensitization to homologous blood transfusion occurs (alloimmunization) and may become a clinical problem for individuals receiving repetitive transfusions, especially those who have rare blood types. The risk of sensitization to RBCs is estimated at 1% per transfusion episode; the risk of platelet sensitization is 5 to 10% per pooled random donor transfusion episode. Platelet cross-matching, either by human leukocyte antigen haplotype or by platelet antigens, is available when multiple platelet transfusions are likely to occur, usually in the course of treatment of acute leukemia and other hematologic disorders. Sensitization to leukocyte antigens is also common and may be the basis for some febrile reactions. Leukoagglutination reactions may rarely cause systemic reactions and ARDS.

Hemolytic Transfusion Reactions

Intravascular hemolysis of transfused RBCs is caused by ABO or Rh incompatibility, or by a strong, high-titer antibody such as anti-Kell, with complement fixation and rapid intravascular destruction. The syndrome that results from massive intravascular hemolysis is caused by the release of red cell stroma, which causes cytokine, bradykinin, and granulocyte mediator release. Hypotension, capillary leak, and oliguria are manifestations that follow very rapidly after the onset of intense intravascular hemolysis. The most feared complications are disseminated intravascular coagulation, acute renal failure, and ARDS. The majority of acute hemolytic transfusion reactions are caused by delivery errors; this is responsible for approximately 5 to 10 deaths per annum and significant morbidity (renal failure and other organ damage).

The treatment of hemolytic transfusion reactions is supportive. Recognizing the syndrome and stopping the offending transfusion are critical. Most clinicians believe that supporting high urine output with added base as bicarbonate is important, but diuretics should be used only if the patient shows intravascular volume overload. The use of mannitol is controversial. There is no role for steroids, antihistamines, heparin, colloid, or other specific pharmacologic intervention.

Delayed Transfusion Reactions

RBC sensitization may result in an antibody response that is initially weak and does not persist. The next exposure of a patient to that RBC antigen will arouse an anamnestic immune response and higher titers of antibody may occur within days after transfusion. This produces a response capable of fixing complement resulting in patients experiencing intravascular hemolysis of the transfused cells within a few days of transfusion. These rapid delayed transfusion reactions usually produce jaundice, elevated lactate dehydrogenase, and low haptoglobin levels, but they may occasionally be severe and result in oliguria. If the antibody does not fix complement, extravascular hemolysis of the transfused RBCs will occur. This type of delayed transfusion reaction is often subtle but results in elevations in lactate dehydrogenase and indirect bilirubin, occasionally the appearance of spirocytes in the peripheral blood smear, a positive Coomb test result, and falling hemoglobin levels. Documentation of such a reaction is important so that future transfusions are more carefully screened.

Other Transfusion Reactions

Febrile transfusion reactions are most often attributed to the presence of granulocytes in transfused blood, although they may also be caused by plasma protein factors such as exogenous Igs. They may be distinguished from the fever associated with hemolytic transfusion reactions by the lack of hypotension or their signs of hemolysis and by delayed onset of fever compared with hemolytic transfusion reactions. Febrile reactions are usually treated with acetaminophen or aspirin; use of these drugs for prophylaxis is also common. Patients who receive repetitive transfusions and who have febrile reactions should receive leukodepleted (WBC-filtered) blood.

Urticarial transfusion reactions are thought to be caused by plasma components. One rare subset of patients with congenital IgA deficiency may have anaphylaxis due to plasma exposure, but in general urticarial reactions are not accompanied by a risk of anaphylaxis. They are usually treated with antihistamines and may be treated prophylactically. Patients who have repetitive urticarial reactions in spite of prophylaxis may need to receive related donor blood products.

Leukoagglutination and pooling of granulocytes in the lungs may occur, although it is rare in settings other than granulocyte transfusions. Most of the time, leukoagglutination results in mild dyspnea and pulmonary infiltrates that spontaneously resolve, but occasionally acute lung injury and ARDS occur as a result of this phenomenon.

GVHD occurs when immunocompetent lymphocytes are transfused into a recipient whose immune system does not recognize and destroy them. The donor lymphocytes proliferate and respond to recipient human leukocyte antigen and other antigens. The GVHD syndrome develops as fever, skin rash, and liver function abnormalities occurring 2 to 6 weeks after transfusion. GVHD is highly lethal in reported cases outside of the transplantation situation; it is very morbid in transplant, leukemia, and other types of severely immunosuppressed patients, but it has been reported in cardiac surgery and neonates. GVHD has not been reported in AIDS. The correct diagnosis is made by recognizing the syndrome and obtaining a skin biopsy. Prevention in the non-bone marrow transplant setting is to irradiate blood products before use. Treatment of active GVHD involves further immunosuppression with cyclosporine and other T-cell–directed therapies, steroids, and cytotoxic drugs. When critically ill patients in the ICU are receiving blood transfusions from family members, those related-donor products should be irradiated.

Risks of Disease Transmission

Hepatitis transmission due to blood transfusion has become a low-frequency complication. Screening for hepatitis B virus is universal. The current-generation screening test for hepatitis C virus provides good protection: it detects approximately 90% of potentially infectious units of blood, and is thought to have reduced the rate of posttransfusion hepatitis to <5% nationwide. The vast majority of individuals with hepatitis C virus infection acquire antibodies within the first 6 months after transmission. Some hepatitis C carriers may lose their antibodies later on, hence the less-than-perfect screening test. Posttransfusion hepatitis may also be caused by other, as yet poorly characterized hepatitis viruses, but it is an uncommon event when donor screening by questionnaire and serology is performed.

AIDS transmission is also an unusual event. The enzyme-linked immunosorbent assay is an effective way to screen donor blood; some blood banks add viral load testing. The risk of AIDS transmission is less than 1 in 2,500,000 transfusions. Effective donor questionnaires in addition to serologic screening are critical to ending transfusion-related cases of AIDS.

Cytomegalovirus (CMV) transmission remains a clinical problem. The prevalence of prior exposure to CMV is high, and clinical studies have estimated that transmission occurs in 3 to 12 recipients per 100 U of blood transfused. Rises in antibody titers or seroconversion have been shown in up to 30% of transfused surgical patients. Chronic infection is often asymptomatic. More than 90% of seroconverters/titer increases are asymptomatic. Neonates, premature, or low-birth-weight infants are at highest risk: 25 to 30% acquire CMV, and up to one in four patients die of it. Bone marrow transplant recipients have a high rate of early deaths due to CMV pneumonitis, although most of this is thought to represent endogenous reactivation of virus replication. Seronegative bone marrow transplant recipients who receive marrow from a seropositive donor are at the highest risk, however. Other vulnerable patients include cancer patients, AIDS patients, and those who have undergone splenectomy. Adler has estimated that 20% of all transfused patients in the United States fall into the category of immunosuppressed, and that estimate was made before the AIDS epidemic. Symptomatic acute CMV infection results in a clinical syndrome that resembles infectious mononucleosis. Chronic infection is usually asymptomatic. Treatment of CMV diseases is marginally effective; antiviral drugs are useful in treating retinitis and enteritis in AIDS but are not very effective in the bone marrow transplant setting. Chemoprophylaxis appears to work better in the bone marrow transplant setting, and transmission is prevented in neonates by the use of seronegative donor blood products. Seropositive transplant recipients may also receive antiviral prophylaxis. Since the introduction of leukodepletion, CMV transmission has been reduced significantly.

Other transfusion transmissible diseases include parvovirus, Epstein-Barr virus, malaria, brucellosis, trypanosomiasis, Trypanosoma *cruzii*, syphilis, toxoplasmosis, West Nile virus, severe acute respiratory syndrome, and perhaps variant Creutzfeldt-Jakob disease. These events are rare in the United States, but vigilance is warranted since the threat of transmitted disease is always looming.

Other Competing Modalities to the Use of Blood Bank Products

Presurgical storage of patient blood is allowed in most blood banks nationally. Studies suggest that the use of autologous predonated blood is declining. Generally, practice has been to have patient donate a unit every 1 to 2 weeks prior to surgery, taking iron during that time. There is some evidence that more units may be predeposited with the concomitant use of erythropoietin; 50% of patients present for surgery anemic requiring their units back at outset of surgery. Although the Food and Drug Administration (FDA) permits the use of autologous units that are hepatitis or AIDS infected (for autologous use only); individual institutions may not wish to assume the risk of handling such units and may reject such autologous donors.

Designated donors, usually members of a patient's family, are often requested by physicians and patients as sources of blood products, usually with the idea that designated donors are less likely to have infectious diseases. Unfortunately, the data available suggest that in comparison with regular volunteer donors who have been screened, designated-donor blood is more likely to test positive for infectious diseases. Designated donor blood is most likely unsafe compared with volunteer-donor banked blood.

Blood substitutes or artificial oxygen carriers are still in clinical development. Perfluorocarbon products are chemically inert polyflourinated hydrocarbons. The oxygen delivery capability of these products is estimated to be three times that of encapsulated hemoglobin, but the use of perfluorocarbons is limited due to reduced oxygen dissociation. This requires a higher than normal inspired oxygen delivery. In addition, the drug has a relatively short half-life of approximately 18 to 24 h. There are two hemoglobin-based artificial oxygen carriers available for clinical research: a bovine preparation called Hemopure, (Biopure Corporation, Cambridge, MA; Northfield Laboratories, Inc., Evanston, IL) and one produced from expired human donor blood called Polyheme. These agents have had a rocky investigation coarse and are not FDA approved for clinical use. The concern of safety profile of either agents is still pending, and early experience with diaspirin-crosslinked agent has given these products an unfavorable profile. Hemopure is allowed restricted use in South Africa. Used predominantly in trauma and vascular insufficiency, data are still pending and are not available for synthesis. The major concern is the vasoactivity associated with these agents and its ultimate impact on physiology and survival.

Acute normovolemic hemodilution and intraoperative autologous blood salvage are used to avoid transfusion in surgery in which large blood loss is anticipated. Hemodilution is a process by which whole blood is removed and cellular fluids are administered to maintain the patient euvolemic. By reducing the RBC mass, any blood loss during surgery will lose few RBCs, and the blood removed can be replaced at the end of surgery or when a transfusion indication occurs. Studies in cardiac surgery, orthopedic surgery, and patients who are Jehovah Witnesses suggest that hemodilution techniques are safe and can eliminate or reduce blood transfusions.

Intraoperative scavenging and reuse of RBCs using cell-saver technology has become widespread practice in major blood loss surgeries such as cardiac, liver, and vascular procedures. It remains controversial in trauma or "dirty" operative fields; the few published data show no to little risk if systemic antibiotics are used. The advantage of cell-salvage blood in trauma setting is its rapid availability and ABO compatibility. Washing of RBCs as part of the process is thought to be the safest procedure in terms of contamination, hemolysis, and coagulopathy. A great number of nonrandomized, selected case reports attest to the relative safety of most "washing" cell savers now in use.

Other Modalities for Anemia Treatment

The use of EPO in the critical care unit has been advocated as a way to limit patients' exposure to RBC transfusions. In two large prospective, randomized, blinded placebo-controlled trials, EPO recipients had a significant reduction in allogeneic transfusions, and their ending hemoglobin was statistically higher than placebo groups. While EPO, usually administered in pharmacologic doses weekly, may reduce transfusions, the effect of hemoglobin rise takes 5 to 10 days to appear. Despite that, early (hours) release of reticulocytes improves the patient's oxygen delivery and utilization so that the impact of EPO use is felt early before the hemoglobin rise. EPO administration should have concomitant small-dose iron supplementation to overcome the functional iron deficiency associated with EPO therapy.

Additional Reading

Alvarez GG, Fergusson DA, Neilipovitz DT, et al. Cell salvage does not minimize perioperative allogeneic blood transfusion in abdominal vascular surgery: a systematic review. Can J Anaesth 2004; 51:425–431

American Society of Anesthesiologists Tasks Force on Perioperative Blood Transfusion and Adjuvant Therapies. Practice guidelines for perioperative blood transfusion and adjuvant therapies. Available at: www.asahq.org/publicationsAndservices/practiceparam.htm#blood

Bolton-Maggs PH, Perry DJ, Chalmers PW, et al. The rare coagulation disorders—review with guidelines for management from the United Kingdom Haemophilia Centre Doctors' organization. Haemophilia 2004 Sep; 10(5):593–628

Corwin HL, Hebert P. Blood transfusion in the critically ill. Crit Care Clin 2004; 20:179–186

Corwin HL, Surgenor SD, Gettinger A. Transfusion practice in the critically ill. Crit Care Med 2003; 31(12 suppl):S668–S671

Dzik WH, Anderson JK, O'Neill EM, et al. A prospective, randomized clinical trial of universal WBC reduction. Transfusion 2002; 42:1114–1122

Dzik W, Rao, A. Why do physicians request fresh frozen plasma? Transfusion 2004; 44:1393–1394

Fowler RA, Berenson M. Blood conservation in the intensive care unit. Crit Care Med 2003; 31(12 suppl): S715–S720

Goodnough LT, Despotis GJ. Transfusion medicine: support of patients undergoing cardiac surgery. Am J Cardiovasc Drugs 2001; 1:337–351

Goodnough, LT, Shander, A, Brechor, ME. Transfusion medicine: looking to the future. Lancet 2003; 361:161–169

Hebert PC, Fergusson D, Blajchman MA, et al. Clinical outcomes following institution of the Canadian universal leukoreduction program for red blood cell transfusions. JAMA 2003; 289:1941–1949

Hebert PC, Wells Gl, Blajchman MA, et al. A multicenter, randomized, controlled clinical trial of transfusion requirements in critical care. New Engl J Med 1999; 340:409–417

MacLaren R, Gasper J, Jung R, et al. Use of exogenous erythropoietin in critically ill patients. J Clin Pharm Ther 2004; 29;195–208

Practice Guidelines Development Task Force of the American College of American Pathologists: practice parameter for the use of fresh-frozen plasma, cryoprecipitate, and platelets. JAMA 1994; 271:777–781

Ramsey G. The pathophysiology and organ-specific consequences of severe transfusion reactions. New Horiz 1994; 2:575–581

Spiess BD, Spence RK, Shander A. Perioperative transfusion medicine, 2nd ed. New concepts in oxygen transport. Baltimore, MD: Lippincott, Williams & Wilkins, 2006; 117–127

Shander A. Surgery without blood. Crit Care Med. 2003; 31(12 Suppl):S708–S714

Shander A. Anemia in the critically ill. Crit Care Clin 2004; 20:159–178

Shander A. Emerging risks and outcomes of blood transfusion in surgery. Semin Hematol 2004 Jan; 41 (1 Suppl):117–124

Shander A, Goodnough LT, Ratko, T, et al. Consensus recommendations for the off-label use of recombinant human factor VIIa (Novo Seven) therapy. P&T. November 2005; 30:11

Notes

Notes

Issues in Postoperative Management: Postoperative Pain Management and Intensive Glycemic Control

Michael A. Gropper, MD, PhD, FCCP

Objectives:

- Understand the implications of pain management practices in critically ill patients
- Review the pharmacodynamics and pharmacokinetics of commonly used opiates
- Understand the use of intrathecal and epidural opiates and local anesthetics
- Understand the importance of the stress response and glycemic control in perioperative patients

Key words: epidural analgesia; insulin; glycemic control; opiates; pain; stress response

Introduction

As intensive care therapies have evolved, there is now greater understanding as to the importance of pain management. Failure to control pain may have deleterious effects. Fortunately, due to the development of better analgesics and sedatives and better methods of drug delivery, significant advances have been made in our ability to address these issues.

Consensus recommendations to guide analgesic and sedative therapy in the ICU were published in 1995 and then revised in 2002; however, substantial variability in practice still exists. The reasons for this disparity are multifold, but the most important reasons are that (1) no single depth of sedation or single sedative agent is appropriate for every patient and every situation encountered in the ICU, and (2) we still lack reliable methods for measuring pain and anxiety.

Theoretically, the choice of the ideal drug should be based on pharmacokinetic and pharmacodynamic properties, cost of therapy (including the drug and the required delivery apparatus), and the cost of treating side effects, but the critically ill often have systemic illnesses, multiple organ failure, and hemodynamic instability which limit drug choices. This syllabus will discuss complications from inadequate pain and sedation therapy, the assessment of pain and sedation, pharmacokinetic and pharmacodynamic properties of analgesics and sedatives used in today's critical care practice, and some recent practice guidelines on the use of analgesics and anxiolytics in the ICU.

Complications From Pain and Anxiety

Under-treated pain results in many physiologic responses that are associated with poor outcomes.[1] Stimulation of the autonomic nervous system and release of humoral factors such as catecholamines, cortisol, glucagon, leukotrienes, postaglandins, vasopressin and β-endorphins following injury, sepsis or surgery are known as the stress response. This activation of the sympathetic nervous system increases heart rate, blood pressure, and myocardial oxygen consumption, which can lead to myocardial ischemia or infarction.[2] The altered hormonal milieu can lead to hypercoagulability due to increased levels of factor VIII and fibrinogen-platelet activity and inhibition of fibrinolysis.[3] The stress hormones also produce insulin resistance, increased metabolic rate and protein catabolism. Immunosuppression is common due to the reduction in number and function of lymphocytes and granulocytes.[4] Previously, the stress response was considered a homeostatic mechanism that was beneficial, but more recent data have shown that this response may be detrimental in part. Many studies have shown that the adequate treatment of pain can decrease the magnitude of these changes that occur following surgery and thereby decrease some postoperative complications.[5-8]

The ICU environment can lead to psychological difficulties as well. Of patients discharged from the ICU, 40% recall having pain and 55% recall having anxiety during their stay in the ICU.[9] Patients who have been ventilated, sedated, and paralyzed have reported experiencing hallucinations, delusions, and altered sense of reality.[10] Although some procedures can be explained to the patient in order to relieve some anxiety, unfortunately not all patients who require procedures during the acute illness are in a state receptive to reasoning. These experiences lead some patients to develop posttraumatic stress syndromes after their stay in the ICU.[11] For these patients, effective therapy for anxiety and pain can reduce some of the emotional suffering and decrease the incidence of postoperative neurosis.[12]

Assessment of Pain and Anxiety

Pain and anxiety are intrinsically subjective. They are difficult to standardize and monitor from one care provider to another unless a standard is developed for assessing and monitoring these states. This is what makes management of sedation in critically ill patients one of the more challenging areas of ICU care.

For pain, the most widely used scale is the visual analog scale (VAS), where patients point to a point on a horizontal line that is a representation of the spectrum of pain from "no pain" to "the worst pain I've ever had." The scale is simplistic and has a high degree of reliability and validity,[13] but ignores other dimensions such as the qualitative aspects of pain. Not all critically ill patients can use this scale due to the severity of their illnesses. Sometimes, bedside nurses have to use behavioral signs such as facial expressions, movement, or posturing, or physiologic signs such as tachycardia, hypertension or tachypnea. Unfortunately, none of these methods are exact. They depend on cultural interpretation of pain, and often the type of illness and use of other drugs can alter the hemodynamic parameters.

Monitoring sedation is also inexact and a true gold standard has not been established. The Glasgow Coma Scale is widely used for the assessment of level of consciousness, but validity is established only in patients with neurologic deficits. A scale that may be more applicable to the medical-surgical ICU is the 6-point Ramsay Scale.[14] The Ramsay Scale is a numerical scale of motor responsiveness based on increasing depth of sedation. Most comparative studies have used the Ramsay Scale, but it also has drawbacks. Because it is based on motor response, the scale has to be modified for patients receiving muscle relaxants, and like the assessment of pain; there is no consensus as to what represents an adequate level of sedation in an individual patient. Other scales include the Sedation-Agitation Scale (SAS) and the Motor Activity Assessment Scale (MAAS), but all have similar drawbacks.

On the horizon, the bispectral index (BIS) of the electroencephalogram is known to provide information about the interaction between cortical and subcortical regions.[15,16] BIS, which is based on a score between 0 and 100 is an index of the level of consciousness.[17] It is more often used in the operating room as an index of the degree of the depth of general anesthesia, to prevent awareness. Recently, attempts have been made to extend the use of BIS into the ICU, but preliminary reports have been conflicting because of muscle-based electrical activity or metabolic or structural abnormalities of the brain in ICU patients.[18,19] Additional studies are required to validate this technique in ICU patients, but the theoretical benefits of a noninvasive monitor of cerebral function are plausible. To date, however, no data has been able to show that BIS monitoring when used to assess depth of sedation significantly alters patient outcomes in the ICU.[20] Because of the lack of evidence, routine use of this device was not recommended by the new clinical practice guidelines.[21]

Analgesics

Pain in the critically ill is best treated with a pure opioid agonist. The commonly available opiates all work at the mu-receptor, so the choice of which agent to use should be based on pharmacokinetic characteristics. In a recent clinical guideline,[21] the recommended choices have been narrowed to morphine, fentanyl, and hydromorphone. Since the use of meperidine, nonsteroidal anti-inflammatory drugs (NSAIDs), and mixed opioid agonist-antagonist agents are discouraged because of potential side effects, their use will not be discussed here. However, drugs such as methadone, a long-acting opioid that can be given parenterally or enterally, and ketamine, a sedative drug with analgesic qualities, will be discussed at the end of this section because they do have specific advantages in the ICU patient and can be used for the difficult to sedate patient.

Morphine

Recommended as the first-line opioid for use in the ICU, morphine, because of its water-solubility, has a delayed peak effect when compared with the more lipid soluble opioids such as fentanyl (30 min vs 4 min, respectively). Morphine administration leads to venodilation and decreases heart rate through sympatholysis and direct effects at the sinoatrial node.[22] The primary side effect is its propensity to cause respiratory depression. Other side effects include sedation, nausea, ileus, and spasm of the sphincter of Oddi. The primary non-receptor based side effect from morphine is histamine release, causing hypotension, tachycardia, and possibly bronchospasm in susceptible patients. Morphine has an elimination half-life of 2 to 4 h. It does have an active metabolite, morphine-6-glucuronide, that may accumulate and cause excessive sedation in patients with renal failure.[23]

Fentanyl

Fentanyl is the preferred analgesic agent for critically ill patients with hemodynamic instability or those with a morphine allergy. Fentanyl is a synthetic opioid that is 80 to 100 times more potent than morphine. Fentanyl has similar opioid receptor based side effects as morphine, but it does not release histamine. Fentanyl only causes minor hemodynamic changes and does not affect the inotropic state of the heart. Virtually all hemodynamic variables, including cardiac output and systemic and pulmonary vascular resistance are unchanged after large doses of fentanyl.[24] Rapid administration of large doses may be associated with bradycardia and chest wall rigidity.

Because of fentanyl's lipid-solubility, the duration of action with small doses is short due to redistribution from the brain to other tissues. Larger cumulative doses become dependent on elimination as opposed to redistribution. The duration of action lengthens and becomes similar to morphine since the drugs' elimination half-lives is similar. The pharmacokinetics of fentanyl are not significantly altered in the presence of liver or kidney dysfunction.[25] Fentanyl metabolites may accumulate, but they are largely inactive and nontoxic, and the terminal elimination half-life of fentanyl is based on release from tissue stores rather than hepatic elimination.[26] Only with severe hepatic dysfunction and high dose fentanyl will altered pharmacokinetics be observed.

Hydromorphone

Recommended as an acceptable alternative to morphine, hydromorphone is a semi-synthetic opioid that is 5 to 10 times more potent than morphine. Time to onset and duration of action are similar to morphine. It has minimal hemodynamic effects and does not result in histamine release. Studies have also shown that pruritis, sedation, and nausea and vomiting may occur less with hydromorphone than morphine,[27] so it can be a good alternative, especially in patients who are unable to tolerate morphine. Like morphine, hydromorphone is metabolized by conjugation with glucuronide, but it also undergoes reduction via a nicotinamide adenine dinucleotide phosphate reductase to two active metabolites. The metabolites have greater analgesic activity than the parent compound, but are in such small amounts that they are probably insignificant except in the presence of renal failure or large doses over a prolonged time, where their levels may accumulate to toxic levels.[28]

Methadone

Methadone is a synthetic opioid agent with morphine-like properties that can be given enterally and parenterally. It is much longer acting than morphine and has a similar receptor-associated side effect profile, but it is less sedating. The oral bioavailability is three times greater than the bioavailability of oral morphine.[29] Methadone has had a negative stigma given its association with drug abuse and opioid detoxification, and its long half-life makes titratability very difficult for most ICU patients. While methadone is not the drug of choice for an acutely ill patient whose hospital course is rapidly changing, it is a good alternative for the patient who has a long recovery ahead and an anticipated prolonged ventilatory wean. Often once things are stable, transition from fentanyl or morphine infusions to methadone via the feeding tube can help simplify care regimens and decrease dependence on infusions.

Methadone, unlike morphine, lacks active metabolites.[30] It is metabolized in the liver and a small portion of it is eliminated in the kidney. Nonrenal routes eliminate 60%, so it does not accumulate in patients with renal failure.[29]

Ketamine

Ketamine, a phencyclidine compound, is an intravenous anesthetic that has analgesic properties. It works via the N-methyl-D-aspartate receptor as well as the mu-receptor.[31] Traditionally, its primary use in the ICU has been during short procedures with intense pain such as dressing changes and wound debridement in burn patients. An advantage of ketamine is that it causes minimal respiratory depression.

Ketamine increases blood pressure, heart rate and cardiac output by causing the release of catecholamines.[32] Patients who have been critically ill for a prolonged period may have exhausted their catecholamine stores and may exhibit the myocardial depressant effects of ketamine.[33]

Sub-hypnotic doses of ketamine infusions have been used for patients that are very difficult to sedate with narcotic and benzodiazepine infusions.[34] These low-dose ketamine infusions (<5 µg/kg/min) do not seem to be associated with the usual side effects of ketamine such as hypertension, tachycardia, increased intracranial pressure, excessive secretions and vivid dreams and hallucinations (termed emergence reactions).[34] Tolerance is known to develop with prolonged use of larger bolus doses, but has not been observed at lower dosages due to limited experience. Because of its potential adverse side effects, ketamine is not recommended for routine sedation of the critically ill patient, but it can be helpful for more difficult situations. Ketamine also has bronchodilatory effects, which could be beneficial during intubation of asthmatic patients.[35]

Postoperative Pain and Pain Relief

Several investigations (although not all) in experimental animals and in patients have documented that preemptive analgesia improves the quality of postoperative pain management.[36] Preemptive analgesia can decrease the sensitization of the central nervous system that would ordinarily amplify subsequent nociceptive input; preemptive analgesia requires the administration of local anesthesia or other pain medication prior to the development of pain.[36] Patients who have more severe pain preoperatively will require larger quantities of pain medication perioperatively than patients who deny pain or have infrequent pain preoperatively.[37]

The choices for pharmacologic postoperative pain relief therapy for hospitalized patients include: the administration of nonsteroidal antiinflammatory medications including cyclooxygenase-2 inhibitors[38] and the administration of narcotic or narcotic-like medications parentally, into the epidural space or into the cerebrospinal fluid. The administration of NSAIDs can decrease the total dose of narcotic medication required for postoperative pain control; there is no significant data that cyclooxygenase-2 inhibitors provide a major advantage over traditional nonsteroidal anti-inflammatory medication.[38] Moreover, NSAIDs should not be administered to patients with renal insufficiency, or with a history of ulcer disease or with bleeding tendencies. Patients who have undergone craniotomies or major vascular surgery are therefore, not considered good candidates for these medications.

The intrathecal administration of narcotics is not as popular as the administration of these medications into the epidural space because of the duration of the analgesia and the respiratory depression and headaches that can be associated with this procedure.[39] Usually only one dose of intrathecal opioid is given, thus, the duration of pain relief is a problem for some patients. After the administration of 0.5 to 1.0 mg of intrathecal morphine, 15 to 22 h of analgesia has been reported.[39,40] Nonetheless, intrathecal opioids are now utilized for perioperative analgesia for cardiac surgeries, vascular surgeries and hip surgeries, and patients receive parenteral narcotics if the spinal narcotic is insufficient for pain relief. Another reason intrathecal opioids have been underutilized is the fear of respiratory depression. The incidence of this event in a recent report was 3% of 6000 patients (180 patients) who had received intrathecal preservative-free morphine, 0.2 to 0.8 mg, plus 25 µg of fentanyl; none of the patients required intubation and all of the patients responded to naloxone infusions without reversal of their analgesia.[41] Pruritis (37% incidence) and nausea and vomiting (25% incidence) occurred at the same frequency that is seen after the administration of parenteral or epidural opioids.[42] (Pruritis should be treated with naloxone, rather than benadryl, as it is not due to histamine release). Finally, there is a fear of severe postdural puncture headaches that can require an epidural blood patch for relief. This complication and therapy occurred in 0.37% of 6000 patients who received intrathecal opioids.[42] However, the investigators admitted that intrathecal opioids were not offered to patients who had a history of frequent headaches.

The administration of epidural opioids is associated with similar complications to those as the intrathecal administration of opioids. The incidence of dural puncture with epidurals ranges between 0.16 to 1.3% and the incidence of headache in the group of patients that had a puncture is between 16% and 86%.[43,44] A unique complication to the epidural approach is the formation of epidural hematomas. The incidence of epidural hematomas appears to be very rare unless the patient is anticoagulated or has a coagulation disorder.[45] There have been epidural hematomas reported in patients who have received low-molecular weight heparin and then had epidural catheters placed.[45] There have been three separate national advisory panels on this issue; there is now a warning in all packages of low-molecular weight heparins. Because of these reports, guidelines have been generated; our local practice is that epidural catheters not be placed for 12 h after the last dose of low-molecular heparin.[45]

Local anesthetics and narcotics are often administered in combination via epidural catheters, as investigations have documented improved perioperative outcomes with this technique, including improved pulmonary function, decreased pulmonary complications and decreased sedation.[40,44] Similarly, the administration of local anesthetics via an epidural catheter appears to reduce postoperative ileus, reduce the requirements of systemic opioids, and decrease the duration of hospitalization after abdominal surgeries.[40,44] The local anesthetic appears to be the important agent in achieving these outcome benefits. However, as local anesthetics have significant hemodynamic side effects that depend on the extent of the neural blockade and can cause motor blockade, which precludes postoperative ambulation, small doses of local anesthetic are administered in combination with opioids via the epidural catheters to obtain pain relief, minor nerve blockade and to produce minimal side-effects from both agents. For example, a solution of 0.05% ropivacaine (a new local anesthetic that causes less motor blockade than bupivicaine) and 1 μg/mL fentanyl has been administered at 8 mL/h via an epidural catheter and postoperative patients obtained optimal pain relief without motor blockade.[46] Note that patients are only allowed to ambulate with assistance when they are receiving these agents and specific orders are required regarding additional pain medication.

Perioperative Glycemic Control

Critically ill patients are frequently hyperglycemic. The metabolic response to critical illness includes stimulation of the hypothalamic-pituitary-adrenal (HPA) axis, resulting in increased growth hormone and prolactin levels. Growth hormone levels are high early in the course of critical illness, and then typically become quite low. Takala et al[47] demonstrated that growth hormone administered to patients with prolonged critical illness resulted in increased mortality when compared to placebo. Cortisol levels are usually increased, and these endocrine changes result in hyperglycemia. Catecholamines, both endogenous and exogenous, also contribute to the hyperglycemia of critical illness. Whereas previous practice had been to treat only marked hyperglycemia (eg, > 200 mg/dL), recent evidence suggests that control should be much more rigorous.

Van den Berghe and colleagues[48] performed a prospective, randomized trial of intensive insulin therapy in critically ill patients, most of whom had undergone cardiac surgery. The intervention group received an insulin infusion to maintain serum glucose concentration between 80 and 100 mg/dL, whereas control group blood glucose was maintained between 180 and 200 mg/dL. ICU mortality was decreased in the treatment group from 8% to 4.6% (p < 0.04). In addition to mortality reduction, the patients with insulin infusion had fewer infections, decreased transfusion requirements, and a shorter duration of mechanical ventilation. The mechanism for this outcome is unclear. Possibilities include both the avoidance of hyperglycemia and a therapeutic effect of insulin. Can the results of this study be extrapolated to other critically ill patients? Unlike the other studies discussed, the patients in this study did not require a diagnosis of sepsis to be enrolled. It is possible that because of a longer length of stay, these patients may obtain even greater benefit. This hypothesis, however, must be tested prospectively.

A recently published prospective, observational study examined the effects of glucose control in 523 patients admitted to a single surgical ICU.[42] In this trial, the primary determinant of a bad outcome was hyperglycemia, rather than hypoinsulinemia. That is, lower mortality was associated with glycemic control, rather than a protective effect of insulin administration. Indeed, increased insulin dosing was associated with increased mortality across all ranges of glycemia. These data suggest that keeping blood glucose below 140 mg/dL may provide similar survival benefit as the "tighter" range of 80 to 110 mg/dL used by van den Berghe.

Synthesis of these two studies is difficult. There is agreement that hyperglycemia is associated with increased mortality, but it remains unclear whether this is a function of insulin resistance, or if control of hyperglycemia with large doses of insulin is harmful. Implementation of strict glucose control protocols is difficult. For example, implementation of a similar protocol in our 24-bed medical-surgical ICU required extensive nurse and physician training. Whereas "tight" control may not be feasible in settings other than the ICU, more attention needs to be paid to perioperative glycemic control.

References

1. Lewis KS, Whipple JK, Michael KA, Quebbeman EJ. Effect of analgesic treatment on the physiological consequences of acute pain. Am J Hosp Pharm 1994; 51:1539-1554
2. Mangano DT, Siliciano D, Hollenberg M, et al. Postoperative myocardial ischemia: therapeutic trials using intensive analgesia following surgery. Anesthesiology 1992; 76:342-353
3. Britton BJ, Hawkey C, Wood WG, et al. Stress—a significant factor in venous thrombosis? Br J Surg 1974; 61:814-820
4. Slade MS, Greenberg LJ, Yunis EJ, et al. Integrated immune response to standard major surgical trauma in normal patients. Surgical Forum 1974; 25:425-427
5. Swinamer DL, Phang PT, Jones RL, et al. Effect of routine analgesia on energy expenditure (Ee) in critically ill patients. JPEN J Parenter Enteral Nutr 1987; 11:5S
6. Moller IW, Dinesen K, Sondergard S, et al. Effect of patient-controlled analgesia on plasma catecholamine, cortisol and glucose concentrations after cholecystectomy. Br J Anaesth 1988; 61:160-164
7. Modig J, Borg T, Bagge L, et al. Role of extradural and of general anesthesia in fibrinolysis and coagulation after total hip replacement. Br J Anaesth 1983; 55:625-629
8. Salomaki TE, Leppaluto J, Laitinen JO, et al. Epidural versus intravenous fentanyl for reducing hormonal, metabolic and physiologic responses after thoracotomy. Anesthesiology 1993; 79:672-679
9. Jones C, Macmillan RR, Griffiths RD. Providing psychological support for patients after critical illness. Clin Intensive Care 1994; 5:176-179
10. Parker M, Schubert W, Shelhamer J, et al. Perceptions of a critically ill patient experiencing therapeutic paralysis in an ICU. Crit Care Med 1984; 12:69-71
11. Stoll C, Haller M, Briegel J, et al. Health-related quality of life in long-term survivors after treatment with extracorporeal membrane oxygenation (ECMO) for the acute respiratory distress syndrome (ARDS). Anaesthesist 1998; 47:24-29
12. Bond M. Psychological and psychiatric aspects of pain. Anaesthesia 1978; 33:355-361
13. Chapman CR, Casey KL, Dubner R, et al. Pain measurement: an overview. Pain 1985; 22:1-31
14. Ramsay MA, Savege TM, Simpson BR, et al. Controlled sedation with alphaxalone-alphadolone. BMJ 1974; 2:656-659
15. Shapiro BA. Bispectral Index: better information for sedation in the intensive care unit? Crit Care Med 1999; 27:1663-1664
16. Glass PS, Bloom M, Kearse L, et al. Bispectral analysis measures sedation and memory effects of propofol, midazolam, isoflurane, and alfentanil in healthy volunteers. Anesthesiology 1997; 86:836-847
17. Liu J, Singh H, White PF. Electroencephalographic bispectral index correlates with intraoperative recall and depth of propofol-induced sedation. Anesth Analg 1997; 84:185-189
18. Shah N, Clack S, Chea F, et al. Does bispectral index of EEG correlate with Ramsay sedation score in ICU patients? Anesthesiology 1996; 85:A469
19. Frenzel D, Greim C, Sommer C, et al. Is the bispectral index appropriate for monitoring the sedation level of mechanically ventilated surgical ICU patients? Intensive Care Med 2002; 28:178-183
20. De Deyne C, Struys M, Decruyenaere J, et al. Use of continuous bispectral EEG monitoring to assess depth of sedation in ICU patients. Intensive Care Medicine 1998; 24:1294-1298
21. Jacobi J, Fraser G, Coursin D, et al. Clinical practice guidelines for the sustained use of sedatives and

analgesics in the critically ill adult. Crit Care Med 2002; 30:119-141
22. Hsu HO, Hickey RF, Forbes AR. Morphine decreases peripheral vascular resistance and increases capacitance in man. Anesthesiology 1979; 50:98-102
23. Osborne R, Joel S, Slevin M. Morphine intoxication in renal failure; the role of morphine-6-glucuronide. Br Med J (Clin Res Ed) 1986; 293:1101
24. Stanley T, Webster L. Anesthetic requirements and cardiovascular effects of fentanyl-oxygen and fentanyl-diazepam-oxygen anesthesia in man. Anesth Analg 1978; 57:411-416
25. Bodenham A, Shelly MP, Park GR. The altered pharmacokinetics and pharmacodynamics of drugs commonly used in critically ill patients. Clinical Pharmacokinet 1988; 14:347-373
26. Haberer J, Schoeffler P, Courderc E, et al. Fentanyl pharmacokinetics in anaesthetized patients with cirrhosis. Br J Anaesth 1982; 54:1267-1270
27. Sarhill N, Walsh D, Nelson KA. Hydromorphone: pharmacology and clinical applications in cancer patients. Support Care Cancer 2001; 9:84-96
28. Zheng M, McErlane KM, Ong MC. Hydromorphone metabolites: isolation and identification from pooled urine samples of a cancer patient. Xenobiotica 2002; 32:427-439
29. Davis MP, Walsh D. Methadone for relief of cancer pain: a review of pharmacokinetics, pharmacodynamics, drug interactions and protocols of administration. Support Care Cancer 2001; 9:73-83
30. Felder C, Uehlinger C, Baumann P, et al. Oral and intravenous methadone use: some clinical and pharmacokinetic aspects. Drug Alcohol Depend 1999; 55:137-143
31. Irifune M, Shimizu T, Nomoto M, et al. Ketamine-induced anesthesia involves the N-methyl-D-aspartate receptor-channel complex in mice. Brain Res 1992; 596:1-9
32. Gooding J, Dimick A, Tavakoli M, et al. A physiologic analysis of cardiopulmonary responses to ketamine anesthesia in noncardiac patients. Anesth Analg 1977; 56:813-816
33. Waxman K, Shoemaker W, Lippmann M. Cardiovascular effects of anesthetic induction with ketamine. Anesth Analg 1980; 59:355-358.
34. Joachimsson PO, Hedstrand U, Eklund A. Low-dose ketamine infusion for analgesia during postoperative ventilator treatment. Acta Anaesthesiol Scand 1986; 30:697-702

35. Corssen G, Gutierrez J, Reves J, et al. Ketamine in the anesthetic management of asthmatic patients. Anesth Analg 1972; 51:588-596
36. Gottschalk A, Smith DS, Jobes DR, et al. Preemptive epidural analgesia and recovery from radical prostatectomy: a randomized controlled trial. JAMA 1998; 279:1076-1082
37. Slappendel R, Weber EW, Bugter ML, et al. The intensity of preoperative pain is directly correlated with the amount of morphine needed for postoperative analgesia. Anesth Analg 1999; 88:146-148
38. Gilron I, Milne B, Hong M. Cyclooxygenase-2 inhibitors in postoperative pain management: current evidence and future directions. Anesthesiology 2003; 99: 1198-1208
39. Gwirtz KH, Young JV, Byers RS, et al. The safety and efficacy of intrathecal opioid analgesia for acute postoperative pain: seven years' experience with 5969 surgical patients at Indiana University Hospital. Anesth Analg 1999; 88:599-604
40. Peyton PJ, Myles PS, Silbert BS, et al. Perioperative epidural analgesia and outcome after major abdominal surgery in high-risk patients. Anesth Analg 2003; 96:548-554
41. Bates JJ, Foss JF, Murphy DB. Are peripheral opioid antagonists the solution to opioid side effects? Anesth Analg 2004; 98:116-122
42. Finney SJ, Zekveld C, Elia A, et al. Glucose control and mortality in critically ill patients. JAMA 2003; 290:2041-2047
43. Peyton PJ, Rigg JA, Jamrozik K, et al. The MASTER Trial has successfully addressed requirements of protocols for large trials. Anesth Analg 2003; 97:922-923
44. Rigg JR, Jamrozik K, Myles PS, et al. Epidural anaesthesia and analgesia and outcome of major surgery: a randomised trial. Lancet 2002; 359:1276-1282
45. Horlocker TT, Wedel DJ. Spinal and epidural blockade and perioperative low molecular weight heparin: smooth sailing on the Titanic. Anesth Analg 1998; 86:1153-1156
46. Liu SS, Moore JM, Luo AM, et al. Comparison of three solutions of ropivacaine/fentanyl for postoperative patient-controlled epidural analgesia. Anesthesiology 1999; 90:727-733
47. Takala J, Ruokonen E, Webster NR, et al. Increased mortality associated with growth hormone treatment in critically ill adults. N Engl J Med 1999; 341:7857-7892
48. van den Berghe G, Wouters P, Weekers F, et al. Intensive insulin therapy in the critically ill patients. N Engl J Med 2001; 345:1359-1367

Notes

Perioperative Evaluation and Management of Pulmonary Disease

Jeanine P. Wiener-Kronish, MD, FCCP

Objectives:

- To review which patients are at risk for perioperative pulmonary complications
- To review the perioperative risk patients face when they have COPD, asthma, pulmonary hypertension, or sleep apnea
- To review perioperative therapies that may prevent or treat perioperative pulmonary complications

Key words: prophylaxis for deep venous thrombosis; pulmonary disease; risk assessment; sleep apnea

Patients at Risk for Perioperative Pulmonary Complications

Noncardiac Surgery

A prospective cohort study was conducted in a preadmission clinic at the University of Alberta Hospital, a tertiary care university hospital. The investigators received consent from 1,055 consecutive adults scheduled for elective nonthoracic surgery. The investigation excluded patients who were hospitalized or mechanically ventilated, patients who were scheduled to enter the ICU postoperatively, or patients who were known to have sleep apnea or had cognitive impairment. One investigator performed physical exams on all the subjects, and spirometry was performed on all the subjects. Another investigator collected the data postoperatively regarding complications, including respiratory failure requiring mechanical ventilation, pneumonia, atelectasis that required bronchoscopy, pneumothorax, or pleural effusions that required percutaneous intervention[1].

Twenty-eight (2.6%) of these patients suffered one of the pulmonary complications within 7 days of surgery—13 (1.2%) developed respiratory failure, 9 (0.8%) developed postoperative pneumonia, and 5 had atelectasis requiring bronchoscopy. One patient had a pneumothorax. Four variables were found to independently be associated with an increased risk of these postoperative pulmonary complications. Age, perioperative nasogastric tube, duration of anesthesia, and a positive cough test (subject asked to inspire and cough; if coughs more than once, the test is positive). This investigation did find that FEV_1 less than 1 L was significantly associated with a pulmonary complication; however, it was not independently associated with complications, and the authors do not delineate how many of the 14 patients with decreased FEV_1 developed a pulmonary complication. Notably, this report confirms the low incidence of pulmonary complications (<3%) and the incidence of life-threatening pulmonary complications is closer to 2%. Whether these complications can be prevented was not investigated.[1]

The National Veterans Administration Surgical Quality Improvement Program has recently developed and validated a preoperative risk index for predicting postoperative respiratory failure.[2,3] An index was formulated based on data from 81,719 patients and then validated using 99,390 patients. Postoperative respiratory failure was defined as mechanical ventilation for >48 h after surgery or the need for reintubation and institution of mechanical ventilation after extubation. The investigation excluded female patients, ventilator-dependent patients, and comatose patients or patients who were not to be resuscitated. The investigation found that postoperative respiratory failure (PRF) developed in 3.4% of postoperative patients. The factors that were associated with PRF included abdominal aortic aneurysm repair, thoracic surgery, neurosurgery, upper abdominal surgery, peripheral vascular surgery, neck surgery, emergency surgery, albumin level <30 g/L, BUN level >30 mg/dL, dependent functional status, age, and COPD (Table 1).

Table 1. *Respiratory Failure Risk Index**

Preoperative Predictor	Point Value
Type of surgery	
• Abdominal aortic aneurysm	27
• Thoracic	21
• Neurosurgery, upper abdominal, or peripheral vascular	14
• Neck	11
Emergency surgery	11
Albumin (<30 g/L)	9
Blood urea nitrogen (>30 mg/dL)	8
Partially or fully dependent functional status	7
History of chronic obstructive pulmonary disease	6
Age (years)	
• ≥70	6
• 60–69	4

*Modified from Arozullah and colleagues.[2]

The type of surgery is of the utmost importance in determining a patient's risk for perioperative problems. The only factor that possibly might be altered preoperatively in the index is the BUN level. The same research group developed a multifactorial risk index for postoperative pneumonia after major noncardiac surgery (Table 2).[2] Using the same patients as discussed for the PRF index, patients were defined as having postoperative pneumonia when they met the Centers for Disease Control definition of nosocomial pneumonia. This definition includes rales or dullness to percussion on physical examination and either new purulent sputum, a positive blood culture, or isolation of a pathogen from a pulmonary sample. The definition also includes the patient with a new pulmonary infiltrate or pleural effusion and isolation of a pathogen from a pulmonary sample. However, this definition is not accepted worldwide for the diagnosis of nosocomial pneumonia.[4] The investigation did not include patients who had received preoperative assisted ventilation.

The investigators found that postoperative pneumonia developed in 2,466 of the patients investigated (1.5%).[2] The mean age of patients with postoperative pneumonia was about 69 years, whereas the patients without pneumonia averaged about 61 years. Patients in whom pneumonia developed also had respiratory failure, systemic sepsis, cardiac arrest requiring cardiopulmonary resuscitation, prolonged ileus, and myocardial infarctions. The patients in whom pneumonia developed had a 21% perioperative mortality rate, whereas those who did not have postoperative pneumonia had a 2% mortality rate.[2] The Risk Index that predicted postoperative pneumonia includes high-risk surgical procedures, age, poor functional status, and history of COPD. However, a history of cerebrovascular accident and transfusions (>4 units) also increased the risk of pneumonia. Chronic steroid use, smoking, and drinking alcohol also increased the risk of perioperative pneumonia. Patients may be able to decrease their risk of perioperative pneumonia by abstaining from alcohol and smoking and perhaps by postponing surgery until steroid treatment can be safely discontinued.

Cardiac Surgery

A retrospective investigation from Canada documented that in 1,829 sequential patients, prolonged ventilation after coronary artery bypass grafting (CABG) occurred more frequently when patients had COPD (twofold increased incidence of prolonged ventilation).[5] Other factors that increased the chances of postoperative ventilation included unstable angina, ejection fraction of <50%, preoperative renal failure, female sex, and age >70 years. This investigation found that the perioperative mortality rate increased to 18% when patients required prolonged mechanical ventilation.[5]

However, in a prospective investigation of 272 patients who underwent CABG in Greece, mild to moderate COPD did not appear to influence perioperative outcome significantly.[6]

Routine spirometry was performed to diagnose COPD. Among the patients with COPD who underwent CABG, the length of stay was 8 days and the perioperative mortality rate was 1.4%. In comparison, patients who did not have COPD had a 7.5-day hospital stay and a 0.7% perioperative mortality; thus, the results are similar.[6] Therefore, in patients with COPD, the risk of prolonged intubation or mortality from CABG procedures is not clear. However, if a patient with COPD also has significant cardiac disease, renal failure, or diabetes and is currently smoking,[7] he or she appears to have a significant risk for prolonged intubation and perioperative complications.

Patients With COPD—Lung Volume Reduction Surgery Investigation

Some of the most important data in the area of perioperative complications have come from the National Emphysema Treatment Trial Research Investigation.[8-9] The main goal of the investigation has been to determine the survival and exercise capacity of surgical patients years after lung volume reduction surgery and to compare these findings with those in a control group of similar patients who underwent medical therapy. No previous randomized, controlled investigations had included so many patients or included a medical treatment group. The results of these studies can be generalized when considering perioperative risks in COPD patients, as the data were generated in a trial of thoracic surgery in patients with severe COPD. Patients with severe COPD are often denied elective surgery; however, the results of the National Emphysema Treatment Trial are reassuring in that only the patients with the most severe COPD had a significant increase in their perioperative mortality.

Some of the results of the investigation were reported[8] when a subgroup of patients were found to exceed the guidelines for perioperative mortality

Table 2. *Postoperative Pneumonia Risk Index**

Preoperative Risk Factor	Point Value
Type of surgery	
• Abdominal aortic aneurysm repair	15
• Thoracic	14
• Upper abdominal	10
• Neck	8
• Neurosurgery	8
• Vascular	3
Age (years)	
• ≥80	17
• 70–79	13
• 60–69	9
• 50–59	4
Functional status	
• Totally dependent	10
• Partially dependent	6
Weight loss > 10% in past 6 months	7
History of chronic obstructive pulmonary disease	5
General anesthesia	4
Impaired sensorium	4
History of cerebrovascular accident	4
Blood urea nitrogen level	
• <2.86 mmol/L (<8 mg/dL)	4
• 7.85–10.7 mmol/L (22–30 mg/dL)	2
• ≥10.7 mmol/L (≥30 mg/dL)	3
Transfusion >4 units	3
Emergency surgery	3
Steroid use for chronic condition	3
Current smoker within 1 year	3
Alcohol intake >2 drinks/d in past 2 weeks	2

*Modified from Arozullah and colleagues.[3]

(a 30-day mortality cutoff of >8% had been adopted as unacceptable). Patients had been included in the investigation if they had an FEV_1 of ≤45% of their predicted value but ≥15% of the predicted value. The patients also had to have a total lung capacity ≥100% of the predicted value and a residual volume that was ≥150% of the predicted value, a Pco_2 of ≤60 mm Hg while breathing room air, a Pao_2 of ≥45 mm Hg while at rest and breathing room air, and an ability to walk >140 m (459 feet) in 6 min. In addition, patients had to complete a measurement of carbon monoxide diffusing capacity of the lung (DLCO) but were not excluded on the basis of the value. Cessation of smoking for 6 months was required before extensive preoperative testing that included physiologic tests and quality of well-being questionnaires. All patients completed 6 to 10 weeks of pulmonary rehabilitation, after which they were tested again and then randomly assigned to receive either surgery or medical treatment.

The data and safety monitoring board reviewed subgroups of patients every 3 months. In April 2001, these analyses suggested that a low FEV_1 (≤20% of the predicted value), a homogeneous pattern of emphysema, and a high perfusion ratio predicted an increased risk of mortality. Also, a low FEV_1 (≤20% of the predicted value) and a low DLCO were associated with an increased risk of 30-day mortality. Additional analyses led to the identification of a high-risk subgroup with a low FEV_1 (≤20% of the predicted value) and either a low DLCO (≤20% of the predicted value) or a pattern of homogeneous emphysema. These characteristics were associated with an increased risk of death after lung volume reduction surgery, as patients with all three characteristics had a 30-day mortality rate of 25%.[8] These patients most frequently died of respiratory complications (90% of the patients), and pneumonia was diagnosed in 30% of these high-risk patients within 30 days of their operations.

These important results suggest there are pulmonary function data that define a group of patients with COPD who should *not* undergo elective thoracic surgery, as their perioperative mortality is extremely high. These results were generated in a large, multicenter trial and so should be considered applicable to a similar population of patients with COPD. Patients with a low FEV_1 (≤20% of the predicted value) and a low DLCO (≤20% of the predicted value) might be at high risk for mortality after surgery in the upper abdomen, when perioperative pulmonary function can be compromised. Notably, no single pulmonary function test identified a group at high risk of increased mortality. Although advanced age, low values on the 6-min walk test, and hypercapnia were associated with a slightly increased mortality rate after lung volume reduction surgery, these variables did not identify patients who were at an increased risk when compared with similar patients who received medical treatment.

Asthma

Stable asthmatics have no significant increased perioperative risk from their disease; however, there are few data regarding perioperative risk in patients with poorly controlled asthma.[10,11] Asthmatics should be distinguished from patients who smoke and have increased airway reactivity as well as from patients with COPD, as their perioperative outcomes appear to be different.

Preoperative Assessment: Patient characteristics associated with poorly controlled asthma include diaphoresis, inability to talk, and silent respirations, as well as the usual symptoms of prolonged expiration, use of accessory muscles, and wheezing.[11] Consensus guidelines suggest a severe episode of asthma exists when one or more of the following features is present: accessory muscle activity, a paradoxical pulse >25 mm Hg, a heart rate >110 beats/min, a respiratory rate >25 to 30 breaths/min, a limited ability to speak, a peak expiratory flow rate (PEFR) or FEV_1 <50% of predicted, and an arterial oxygen saturation of <91%.[10]

The more objective way to quickly assess the functional status is to compare the patient's current PEFR to his or her personal best or predicted PEFR. A >50% reduction in PEFR is indicative of a severe asthma exacerbation. Arterial blood gas sampling is not necessary to determine whether a stable patient is acceptable for surgery. However, arterial blood gas sampling may be useful in the management of severe asthmatics who need emergency surgery.

Poorly Controlled Airway Reactivity: Airway Manipulations: Bronchodilators should be given just prior to airway manipulation (endotracheal intubation) regardless of the recent course of the disease, as airway manipulation stimulates airway reflexes. Metered-dose inhalers with spacers have been shown to be equally as effective as nebulizers and are, owing to their ease of use, the preferred choice for preventive preoperative treatment.[13,14]

For sedation during airway manipulation, drugs that have been shown to have bronchodilatory effects include propofol (1 to 2.5 mg/kg) and ketamine (1 to 2 mg/kg).

Eames and colleagues[15] demonstrated that respiratory resistance and wheezing were lower after induction with propofol than with thiopental or high-dose etomidate. There are no clinical trials that document the superiority of one drug over another in this group of patients.

Other measures that can help blunt airway reflexes stimulated by laryngoscopy include the administration of IV lidocaine, the administration of inhaled lidocaine and salbutamol, or salbutamol inhalation alone.[16,17] The use of the laryngeal mask airway (LMA), instead of laryngoscopy and endotracheal intubation, should be considered in patients undergoing minor surgery, as airway reflexes are stimulated less significantly. After induction of general anesthesia, the LMA is placed (without laryngoscopy) in the posterior pharynx above the vocal cords. Note that the LMA does not protect the airway from aspiration and is not effective in ventilating patients who have a significant elevation in airway pressure.

Maintenance of sedation can be achieved by either IV infusion of propofol (50 to 200 mg/kg/min). Fentanyl (1 to 3 mg/kg) and its derivatives do not release histamine and therefore are the preferred choices among opioids. Various muscle relaxants, including atracurium and mivacurium, have been associated with histamine release and should be avoided in patients with asthma. Vecuronium (0.08 to 0.12 mg/kg) and rocuronium (0.6 to 1.2 mg/kg) are devoid of histamine release and are the preferred choices for muscle relaxation.[18,19] Asthmatics who are steroid-dependent should be given additional therapy perioperatively in order to avoid adrenal insufficiency during surgery. In addition, these patients are at high risk for myopathy when they receive repeated administration of any muscle relaxants. Therefore, muscle relaxants should be administered only for the duration of surgery.[20]

Pulmonary Hypertension

Cardiovascular diseases, including pulmonary hypertension, are a major cause of perioperative morbidity and mortality. The adrenergic response to surgical stimulation and the circulatory effects of anesthetic agents, endotracheal intubation, positive pressure ventilation, blood loss, fluid shifts, and alterations in body temperature impose an additional burden on an already compromised cardiovascular system. Airway manipulation and mechanical ventilatory management of patients with pulmonary hypertension requires a thorough understanding of the condition's etiology and severity, the patient's functional status, and appropriate medical management.

Regardless of the etiology, pulmonary hypertension in perioperative patients has significant impact on postoperative morbidity and mortality. Preoperative pulmonary hypertension has been shown to be a significant and independent predictor of hospital mortality in elderly patients undergoing cardiac procedures.[21] Similarly, in pregnant women, pulmonary hypertension carries a high risk of maternal death, often shortly after the delivery of the newborn.[21-25] Finally, in a retrospective study, patients with moderate to severe portopulmonary hypertension (mean pulmonary artery pressure, >35 mm Hg) undergoing liver transplantation had a mortality rate of up to 50%.[25] Therefore, it is clear that surgery is associated with a greater mortality in these patients than in other groups of patients with lung diseases.

Preoperative Assessment: The goals of the preoperative assessment are (1) to identify undiagnosed patients at high risk for pulmonary hypertension and (2) to identify the etiology and evaluate the functional status of patients with known pulmonary hypertension. Unlike primary (idiopathic) pulmonary hypertension, which is characterized by progressive dyspnea and a rapid downhill course, secondary pulmonary hypertension can be difficult to recognize clinically when signs are nonspecific and symptoms are primarily those of the underlying disease (*ie*, dyspnea and fatigue). Dull retrosternal chest pain resembling angina pectoris may be present. Fatigue and syncope on exertion may also occur secondary to decreased cardiac output related to increased pulmonary pressure. The signs of pulmonary hypertension are narrow splitting of the second heart sound, accentuation of the pulmonic component of the second heart sound, and a systolic ejection click. In advanced pulmonary hypertension, tricuspid and pulmonary valve insufficiencies and signs of right ventricular failure are found. In any patient in whom pulmonary hypertension is suspected, appropriate laboratory tests and imaging studies should be performed.

The role of the ECG in pulmonary hypertension is somewhat controversial. While it was demonstrated in one study that ECG may have a prognostic role in primary pulmonary hypertension with regard to survival,[26] another study found ECG inadequate as a screening tool to rule out clinically relevant pulmonary hypertension.[27] However, ECG changes, when present, are those of right-axis deviation, right ventricular strain or hypertrophy, and right atrial enlargement. Echocardiography is particularly helpful in evaluating patients with underlying valvular disease and, despite potential limitations in patients with severe COPD, the procedure is a feasible, noninvasive tool that can identify patients who have cor pulmonale.[28,29] Doppler ultrasonography is a noninvasive means of estimating pulmonary systolic artery pressure, but precise hemodynamic measurements can be obtained only with right heart catherization. Routine pulmonary function tests reveal no findings diagnostic of pulmonary hypertension. In chronic disease, there is often dilation of the central pulmonary arteries radiographically. In advanced pulmonary hypertension, right ventricular and right atrial enlargement may be present.

Once the diagnosis of pulmonary hypertension is confirmed, its etiology should be sought. With the diagnosis confirmed and etiology (primary vs secondary hypertension) established,[30,31] the patient's functional status must be assessed and medical management optimized before the patient can be cleared for surgery.

Sleep Apnea and Morbidly Obese Patients

The number of bariatric surgeries performed in 2003 in the United States was 100,000. Despite the large numbers of surgeries, there are no reliable data as to the perioperative mortality or morbidity in this population. These morbidly obese patients are at risk for perioperative pulmonary complications. Problems include obtaining an airway prior to surgery. Endotracheal intubation is more difficult in patients with large neck circumferences.[32] Standard tracheotomy tubes are too short or too curved for proper positioning. Removal of cervical fat or use of larger tubes has been utilized.[32]

Mechanical ventilation of the morbidly obese patient cannot utilize tidal volumes based on the patient's actual body weight. A recommendation is that the tidal volume be calculated according to ideal body weight.[32] However, inflation pressures are difficult to interpret given the reduced compliance of the total respiratory system. One approach suggests limiting transpulmonary pressure to 35 cm H_2O; there have been no randomized, controlled trials to validate an approach in these patients. Thus, the optimal tidal volume in these patients is unknown.

Morbidly obese patients frequently have sleep apnea and are therefore at risk for prolonged apnea and airway obstruction, especially if they have severe sleep apnea or receive narcotics or sedatives.[33,34] A small investigation documented that the administration of pain medication to patients with sleep apnea who had undergone painful procedures led to a significant increase in perioperative pulmonary and cardiac complications. Peripheral surgeries that do not require pain medication or sedation can be performed in this population as outpatient surgery without an increase in complications.[35] Morbidly obese patients with sleep apnea should be evaluated for pulmonary hypertension.

Perioperative Analgesia

Perioperative epidural analgesia has been suggested to be important in decreasing pulmonary complications. A recent meta-analysis[2] suggested that a significant number of perioperative complications were decreased by the administration of epidural analgesia (epidurals that included local anesthetics alone or in combination with opioids). The incidence of perioperative deaths, myocardial infarctions, pulmonary emboli, and deep venous thromboses was shown to be significantly decreased in this meta-analysis. In a randomized, multicenter, controlled trial of 915 patients undergoing major abdominal surgery with epidural analgesia (utilizing narcotics and local anesthesia) for 72 h, the authors documented that there was no difference between the control group and experimental group in terms of mortality.[36] However, there was a significant decrease in the frequency of respiratory failure in the experimental group, who had received epidural analgesia; the authors found that 15 patients would need to have received epidural analgesia to prevent one episode of respiratory failure.[36] The investigation also found that pain scores were significantly lower in the epidural group.[36]

Another randomized, controlled trial of epidural analgesia was recently performed in the Veterans Hospitals.[37] This investigation involved 1,021 patients who underwent surgery for intraabdominal aortic, gastric biliary, or colon operations. The patients were elderly with a mean age of about 67 years. Approximately 33% of the patients had the diagnosis of COPD, and almost 40% of the patients were active smokers. In this study, epidural analgesia did not decrease mortality, except in patients who underwent aortic repairs.[37] The patients who underwent aortic vascular surgery and received epidural analgesia (that included local anesthesia) had a significant decrease in their incidence of myocardial infarctions, respiratory failure, and stroke compared with the group that was treated with parenteral analgesia. Again, the patients who received epidural analgesia had significantly better pain control. However, the length of intubation and length of ICU stay, although significantly shorter in patients who underwent aortic vascular surgery and had received epidural analgesia were only 13 h and 3.5 h, respectively, shorter than in the control group.[37] A very recent randomized, controlled trial also documented that the use of epidural analgesia led to only a few hours less of mechanical ventilation.[38] Therefore, perioperative epidural analgesia appears to consistently produce superior pain relief,[38] but does not significantly decrease pulmonary complications in all investigations.

References

1. McAlister FA, Bertsch K, Man J, et al. Incidence of and risk factors for pulmonary complications after nonthoracic surgery. Am J Respir Crit Care Med 2005; 171:514–517
2. Arozullah A, Khuri S, Henderson W, et al. Development and validation of a multifactorial risk index for predicting postoperative pneumonia after major noncardiac surgery. Ann Intern Med 2001; 135:847–857
3. Arozullah A, Daley J, Henderson W, et al. Multifactorial risk index for predicting postoperative respiratory failure in men after major noncardiac surgery. Ann Surg 2000; 232:242–253
4. Chastre J, Fagon J-Y. Ventilator-associated pneumonia. Am J Respir Crit Care Med 2002; 165:867–903
5. Legare JF, Hirsch GM, Buth KJ, et al. Preoperative prediction of prolonged mechanical ventilation following coronary artery bypass grafting. Eur J Cardiothoracic Surg 2001; 20:930–936
6. Michalopoulos A, Geroulanos S, Papadimitrious L, et al. Mild or moderate chronic obstructive pulmonary disease risk in elective coronary artery bypass grafting surgery. World J Surg 2001; 25:1507–1511
7. Yende S, Wunderink R. Validity of scoring systems to predict risk of prolonged mechanical ventilation after coronary artery bypass graft surgery. Chest 2002; 122:239–244
8. National Emphysema Treatment Trial Research Group. Patients at high risk of death after lung-volume reduction surgery. N Engl J Med 2001; 345:1075–1083
9. Fishman A, Martinez F, Naunheim K, et al. A randomized trial comparing lung-volume-reduction surgery with medical therapy for severe emphysema. N Engl J Med 2003; 348:2059–2073
10. McFadden ER. Acute severe asthma. Am J Respir Crit Care Med 2003; 168:740–759
11. Rodrigo GJ, Rodrigo C, Hall JB. Acute asthma in adults: a review. Chest 2004; 125:1081–1102
12. Gluckman TJ, Corbridge T. Management of respiratory failure in patients with asthma. Curr Opin Pulm Med 2000; 6:79–85
13. Idris AH, McDermott MF, Raucci JC, et al. Emergency department treatment of severe asthma: metered-dose inhaler plus holding chamber is equivalent in effectiveness to nebulizer. Chest 1993; 103:665–672
14. Turner JR, Corkery KJ, Eckman D, et al. Equivalence of continuous flow nebulizer and metered-dose inhaler with reservoir bag for treatment of acute airflow obstruction. Chest 1988; 93:476–481
15. Eames WO, Rooke GA, Wu RS, et al. Comparison of the effects of etomidate, propofol and thiopental

on respiratory resistance after tracheal intubation. Anesthesiology 1996; 84:1307–1311
16. Scalfaro P, Sly PD, Sims C, et al. Salbutamol prevents the increase of respiratory resistance caused by tracheal intubation during sevoflurane anesthesia in asthmatic children. Anesth Analg 2001; 93:898–902
17. Groeben H, Silvanus MT, Beste M, et al. Combined lidocaine and salbutamol inhalation for airway anesthesia markedly protects against reflex bronchoconstriction. Chest 2000; 118:509–515
18. Fisher DM. Clinical pharmacology of neuromuscular blocking agents. Am J Health Syst Pharm 1999; 56:S4–S9
19. Naguib M, Magboul MM. Adverse effects of neuromuscular blockers and their antagonists. Drug Saf 1998; 18:99–116
20. Behbehani NA, Al-Mane F, D'Yachkova Y, et al. Myopathy following mechanical ventilation for acute severe asthma: the role of muscle relaxants and corticosteroids. Chest 1999; 115:1627–1631
21. Kirsch M, Guesnier L, LeBesnerais P, et al. Cardiac operations in octogenarians: perioperative risk factors for death and impaired autonomy. Ann Thorac Surg 1998; 66:60–67
22. Weiss BM, Zemp L, Seifert B, et al. Outcome of pulmonary vascular disease in pregnancy: a systematic overview from 1978 through 1996. J Am Coll Cardiol 1998; 31:1650–1657
23. Weiss BM, Hess OM. Pulmonary vascular disease and pregnancy: current controversies, management strategies and perspectives. Eur Heart J 2000; 21:104–115
24. Lupton M, Oteng-Ntim E, Ayida G, et al. Cardiac disease in pregnancy. Curr Opin Obstet Gynecol 2002; 14:137–143
25. Krowka MJ, Plevak DJ, Findlay JY, et al. Pulmonary hemodynamics and perioperative cardiopulmonary-related mortality in patients with portopulmonary hypertension undergoing liver transplantation. Liver Transpl 2000; 6:443–450
26. Bossone E, Paciocco G, Iarussi D, et al. The prognostic role of the ECG in primary pulmonary hypertension. Chest 2002; 121:513–518
27. Ahearn GS, Tapson VF, Rebeiz A, et al. Electrocardiography to define clinical status in primary pulmonary hypertension and pulmonary arterial hypertension secondary to collagen vascular disease. Chest 2002; 122:524–527
28. Bach DS, Curtis JL, Christensen PJ, et al. Preoperative echocardiographic evaluation of patients referred for lung volume reduction surgery. Chest 1998; 114:972–980
29. Bossone E, Duong-Wagner TH, Paciocco G, et al. Echocardiographic features of primary pulmonary hypertension. J Am Soc Echocardiogr 1999; 12:655–662
30. Fishman AP. Clinical classification of pulmonary hypertension. Clin Chest Med 2001; 22:385–391
31. Humbert M, Nunes H, Sitbon O, et al. Risk factors for pulmonary arterial hypertension. Clin Chest Med 2001; 22:459–475
32. El-Solh AA. Clinical approach to the critically ill, morbidly obese patient. Am J Respir Crit Care Med 2004; 169:557–561
33. Gupta RM, Parvizi J, Hanssen AD, et al. Postoperative complications in patients with obstructive sleep apnea syndrome undergoing hip or knee replacement: a case-control study. Mayo Clin Proc 2001; 76:897–905
34. Brown KA, Morin I, Hickey C, et al. Urgent adenotonsillectomy. Anesthesiology 2003; 99:586–595
34. Sabers C, Plevak DJ, Schroeder DR, et al. The diagnosis of obstructive sleep apnea as a risk factor for unanticipated admissions in outpatient surgery. Anesth Analg 2003; 96:1328–1335
35. Rigg J, Jamrozik K, Myles P, et al. Epidural anaesthesia and analgesia and outcome of major surgery: a randomized trial. Lancet 2002; 359: 1276–1282
36. Park WY, Thompson JS, Lee KK, et al. Effect of epidural anesthesia and analgesia on perioperative outcome: a randomized, controlled Veterans Affairs cooperative study. Ann Surg 2001; 234: 560–569
37. Peyton PJ, Myles PS, Silbert BS, et al. Perioperative epidural analgesia and outcome after major abdominal surgery in high-risk patients. Anesth Analg 2003; 96:548–554
38. Block BM, Liu SS, Rowlingson AJ, et al. Efficacy of postoperative epidural analgesia: a meta-analysis. JAMA 2003; 290:2455–2463

Notes

Notes

Perioperative Evaluation and Management of Cardiovascular Disease

Jeanine P. Wiener-Kronish, MD, FCCP

Objectives:

- To review risk factors for cardiac events in perioperative patients
- To review evidence regarding perioperative treatment with β-blockade and/or α$_2$-agonists
- To review glycemic control and its importance in prevention of ischemia and infarction
- To review deep venous thrombosis (DVT) prophylaxis in high-risk patients
- To review the role of transfusions in patients with ischemia

Key words: cardiovascular disease; prevention of ischemia; risk assessment

In a recent investigation of 3,970 surgeries performed in a 4-year period that were associated with cardiac and pulmonary complications, orthopedic procedures had the highest incidence of these two types of complications (35%).[1] Eleven percent of perioperative pulmonary and cardiac complications occurred after intrathoracic procedures, 16% after abdominal procedures, and 19% after vascular procedures (7% after abdominal aortic aneurysm repairs).[1] Notably, patients who had cardiac complications or events (myocardial infarction [MI], ventricular fibrillation, pulmonary edema, or cardiac arrest) also had an increased incidence of pulmonary complications.[1]

Perioperative Risk Reduction for Cardiac Events

There have been many investigations into the significant risk factors for perioperative cardiac events.[2] Although there have been several guidelines published recently,[3,4] a simple index was validated that identified six factors that were predictive of cardiac events (death, MI, ventricular fibrillation, or tachycardia) in patients undergoing noncardiac surgery.[5] These factors were as follows: (1) the surgery (high-risk surgeries are intrathoracic, vascular procedures, procedures requiring large quantities of blood transfusions, or suprainguinal procedures); (2) a history of coronary artery disease (angina, MI); (3) a history of congestive heart failure (rales, paroxysmal nocturnal dyspnea, etc); (4) a history of cerebrovascular disease (transient ischemic attack or stroke); (5) the use of insulin; or (6) a creatinine level >2.0 mg/dL. When a patient has zero or one of these factors, the risk of perioperative cardiac events is 0.4 to 0.9% (Table 1). If a patient has two of these factors, the risk for perioperative cardiac events is 6.6%. Finally, if a patient has more than three of these factors, the risk for perioperative cardiac events is 11%.[5]

Patients who have two or more risk factors should be considered for β-blockade or α$_2$-agonist perioperative therapy, as their risk for cardiac events can be decreased with these treatments.[5,6] In fact, perioperative treatment with β-blockers decreased recurrent coronary events and all causes of mortality.[5,6] Patients with COPD generally do not respond to β-blockade with an increase in bronchoconstriction,[7] and also generally have heart disease secondary to smoking. Therefore, β-blockade should be considered for patients with COPD. However, patients with asthma should not be given β-blockers. (See Figure 1 for perioperative β-blockade orders.)

Table 1. *Six Factors Predictive of Cardiac Events**

No. of Factors Present	Risk of Cardiac Events, %
0–1	0.4–0.9
2	6.6
≥3	11

*The six factors are as follows: type of surgery, coronary artery disease, congestive heart failure, cerebrovascular accident, creatinine >2.0 mg/dL, and diabetes mellitus (use insulin). Modified from Lee et al.[5] See order sheet (Fig 1) for example of perioperative β-blockade.

		Nursing Noted
☐ **Ischemic Heart Disease:** History of MI, use of nitrates symptoms of ischemic CP, (+) stress test, Q waves on ECG ☐ **Higher-Risk Surgery:** intraperitoneal, intrathoracic or vascular procedures ☐ **Preoperative Use of Insulin To Treat DM**	☐ **History of CHF:** Pulmonary edema, symptoms of PND, S3 gallop, or CXR evidence of vascular redistribution ☐ **History of TIA or CVA** ☐ **Preoperative Serum Creatinine >2.0 mg/dL**	
The rate of occurrence of either cardiac arrest, MI, development of 3o heart block or pulmonary edema, and/or cardiac mortality during the surgical admission for other patients associated with this number of factors is 0–1 factors: 0.4–0.9% 2 factors: 6.6% 3 or more factors: ?11% The above cardiac complications are often attributed to perioperative cardiac ischemia. Reduce this patient's risk by continuing below if associated with 2 or more factors above. For patients associated with 0 to 1 factor, also continue if they exhibit 2 or more of the following: ☐ Age >65 yr ☐ HTN ☐ Current Smoking ☐ Total Cholesterol > 240 mg/dL		

☐ The patient does not exhibit any of the following exclusion criteria:
   Heart rate <55 bpm w/o pacemaker   2° or 3° AV block w/o pacemaker
   Systolic blood pressure <100 mmHg   Severe LV dysfunction (LVEF < 30%)
   Poorly controlled asthma or COPD
   *Use caution with concomitant use of calcium channel blockers or established b-blocker therapy		

☐ Record Baseline VS: HR_____ BP_____ RR_____ O2SAT_____% on _____		
☐ Notify H.O. and withhold b-blocker dose if prior to administration or at any time during therapy the patient exhibits: SBP <100 mm Hg and/or HR <55 bpm 2° or 3° AV block Wheezing, dyspnea, and/or O$_2$ saturation <92% on RA The appearance or worsening of CHF		
Implementation of therapy: **Outpatients seen prior to scheduled surgical day** ☐ SBP >100 and HR >65. Rx atenolol 100 mg po qam or metoprolol 50 mg po bid. ☐ SBP >100 and HR ? 55 but ?65. Rx atenolol 50 mg po qam or metoprolol 25 mg po bid. ***Be aware that clearance of atenolol is renal while metoprolol has primarily hepatic clearance. **Inpatients seen prior to scheduled surgical day** ☐ Establish and/or verify IV access. Notify H.O. if IV access is not obtained or is lost. ☐ Record HR, BP, RR, and O$_2$Sat q4h and prior to dosage during therapy. ☐ Enteral medication route can be used. The above indicated oral dosing regimen may be given via either po or NGT in a nonmonitored care area. ☐ IV route must be used. The patient must in a monitored care setting to receive IV metoprolol. ☐ Record HR, BP, RR, and O$_2$Sat just prior to and q5min x 3 after IV metoprolol. ☐ SBP >100 and HR ?55 but ?65. Give metoprolol 5 mg IV over 5 min. ☐ SBP >100 and HR >65. Give metoprolol 5 mg IV over 5 min, wait 15 min, and then repeat x 2 if SBP remains >100 and HR remains ?55. ☐ Repeat the above IV dosing regimen q12h as indicated.		
Name of Physician entering order set _____ Date ___/___/_____ Time ___:___ Signature of Physician entering order set_____ ID #_____		

Figure 1. Example of perioperative β-blockade orders. CP = chest pain; CHF = congestive heart failure; PND = paroxysmal nocturnal dyspnea; CXR = chest radiograph; TIA = transient ischemic attack; CVA = cerebrovascular accident; DM = diabetes mellitus; HTN = hypertension; AV = atrioventricular; LV = left ventricular; LVEF = left ventricular ejection fraction; VS = vital signs; RR = respiratory rate; H.O. = house officer; SBP = systolic blood pressure; RA = room air; qam = every morning; NGT = nasogastric tube; PACU = postanesthesia care unit; POD = postoperative day.

α_2-Adrenergic agonists have been shown to decrease cardiac complications after cardiac and noncardiac surgery.[8] α_2-Agonists dilate poststenotic coronary vessels and attenuate the severity of perioperative hemodynamic abnormalities.[8,9] The use of α_2-agonists has been associated with hypotension during cardiac surgery, but statistically significant increases in postoperative hypotension, bradycardia, or heart failure were not seen.[8] It is not known whether there is a synergistic or additive effect of combining α_2-agonists and β-blockers. α_2-Agonists also improve pain relief and lower the need for pain medications.[10]

Perioperative Issues Regarding Cardiac Surgery

An important recent investigation documented that having a patient undergo elective coronary-artery revascularization prior to elective vascular surgery did not improve the long-term outcome of the patients.[11] Interestingly, of 5,859 patients admitted to the 18 Veteran's Hospitals for elective vascular surgery, 4,669 (80%) were excluded due to insufficient cardiac risk or because they had already undergone CABG or percutaneous coronary intervention. Another 363 patients were excluded because they had nonobstructive coronary artery disease, and 215 had coronary artery disease not amenable to surgical correction. Therefore, 510 patients ultimately underwent randomization, 258 assigned to preoperative coronary-artery revascularization and 252 to medical treatment. Of the 258 assigned to CABG, 240 underwent CABG or percutaneous coronary intervention (141 patients). Nine of the patients assigned to medical treatment had to undergo CABG due to unstable changes in their cardiac status.[11]

Ultimately, 258 patients in the CABG group underwent their planned vascular surgery, as did 237 of 252 of the patients in the medical treatment group. Notably, 10 of 33 patients who had been assigned to the CABG group did not undergo vascular surgery because 10 died after the CABG or percutaneous coronary intervention, 5 developed serious conditions that prevented the surgery, and 18 decided not to undergo the vascular surgery. Of the 15 patients who had been assigned to the medical treatment who did not undergo the vascular surgery, 1 died after an emergently performed CABG, 9 decided not to undergo surgery, and 5 developed a serious condition preventing the surgery.[11]

Before vascular surgery there were 10 deaths in the revascularization group and 1 death in the medical treatment group. Within the 30-day postoperative interval after vascular surgery, there were seven more deaths in the revascularization group and eight deaths in the medical treatment group. Three months after vascular surgery, the left ventricular ejection fraction was about 54% in the revascularization group and 55% in the medical treatment group. After a median of 2.7 years after randomization, 22% of the patients in the revascularization group were dead and 23% were dead in the no-revascularization group. The groups used the same number of ß-blockers, antiplatelet agents, angiotensin converting enzyme inhibitors and statins. These results emphasize that perioperative infarcts involve more complex mechanisms than just the number of stenotic coronary vessels.[11]

Cardiac revascularization (CABG) is being done increasingly in older and more complex patients, while younger patients undergo interventional revascularization; for example, in 2000, 561,000 patients underwent percutaneous transluminal coronary angioplasty, while 314,000 patients underwent CABG.[12] Investigations have shown that postoperative elevations in creatine kinase-myocardial band (CK-MB) isoenzyme measurements are associated with an increased mortality rate. For example, mortality rates were 3.4% in patients with an increase of CK-MB of less than five times the upper limit of normal after CABGs. In contrast, the mortality rate was 20.2% in patients who had a postoperative peak of CK-MB of >20 times the upper limit of normal after their CABGs.[13] Similarly, elevated concentrations of cardiac troponin I (cTnI) measured 20 h after the end of surgery was found to be an independent predictor of in-hospital death after cardiac surgery.[14]

Preoperative assessments of patients undergoing cardiac surgery should, perhaps, include the measurement of B-type natriuretic peptide (BNP). Preoperative BNP levels >385 pg/mL predicted morbidity and mortality in men.[15] Preoperative BNP was found to be highly specific but had a low sensitivity and positive predictive value.[15] In another recent prospective observational cohort investigation in Scotland,[16] preoperative and postoperative BNP were also found to be predictive of the need for perioperative cardiovascular support and prolonged ICU stays. The implication of these investigations is that the patients with more elevated preoperative BNP levels may require more support and require prolonged ICU care. Perhaps increased medication preoperatively could improve outcomes in these patients; more investigation is warranted.

Perioperative Glucose Control in Diabetics

There is increasing evidence that tight control of glucose improves outcomes in diabetic patients during acute coronary syndromes. In the Diabetes and Insulin-Glucose Infusion in Acute Myocardial Infarction (DIGAMI) study,[17] mortality was reduced by 30% when the serum glucose level was kept at <200 mg/dL.

Of the 17 million diabetic patients in the United States, 25% will undergo coronary revascularization procedures. Investigations have documented that diabetics have a significant incidence of restenosis after vascularization procedures. One recent investigation found that diabetics had a higher body mass index than nondiabetic patients (32 vs 29 kg/m^2) undergoing percutaneous revascularization procedures. Furthermore, diabetics with a hemoglobin A1c value of ≤7% had an incidence of restenosis that was comparable to that in nondiabetic patients. Diabetic patients with a hemoglobin A1c value of >7% had an incidence of restenosis that was twofold higher than in the other patients. Finally, diabetic patients with a hemoglobin A1c level >7% had a higher incidence of recurrent angina and cardiac rehospitalizations.[18] This is just one of many investigations that has documented a significant increase in all-cause, cardiac, and ischemic mortality with increasing levels of hemoglobin A1c.[19]

Patients with diabetes mellitus who undergo coronary bypass graft surgery have increased perioperative mortality and morbidity, significantly reduced long-term survival, and less freedom from recurrent episodes of angina.[20] Investigations utilizing insulin infusions to keep serum glucose values below 200 mg/dL have documented significant improvements in wound infections, respiratory failure, and decreased length of stay in the ICU and in the hospital.[20] Cardiac indices and long-term survival were significantly improved in patients whose serum glucose values remained below 200 mg/dL.

There is an association between increased levels of hemoglobin A1c levels and the incidence of heart failure.[21] Each 1% increase in the level of the hemoglobin A1c was associated with an 8% increase in the risk of heart failure hospitalization or death. Only 7.3% of patients with type II diabetes achieve the optimal goal of a hemoglobin A1c of <7%;[22] a recent investigation suggests that patients treated with carvedilol achieved better glycemic control than patients given metoprolol as an antihypertensive.[23] Carvedilol appears to reduce insulin resistance.[24] Analysis of four previous randomized trials suggests that cardiovascular outcomes correlated with baseline level of glycemia; those patients with greater degrees of hyperglycemia had more benefit from rennin angiotensin system blockade, which is known to decrease insulin resistance.[24-25]

It is clear that serum glucose level must be kept below 200 mg/dL in diabetic patients, but the optimal serum glucose level may even be lower given the data from the ICU investigations.[21] As in the investigation in the ICU,[26] serum glucose may need to be monitored and managed in both diabetic and nondiabetic patients, but more investigations are needed. Other treatments that may also improve outcomes for diabetics include tighter blood pressure control[27] and treatment with angiotensin-converting enzyme inhibitors, which may prevent the development of major cardiovascular events and heart failure in patients with diabetes, even if they do not have hypertension.[28]

Perioperative Concerns of Obese Patients

About 100,000 surgeries were done for obesity management in 2003.[29] The major complications of bariatric surgery include pulmonary embolism, respiratory failure, gastrointestinal leaks from the breakdown of the staple or suture line, stomal obstruction, and bleeding.[29] The risk appears to be related to the specific procedure, the patient's age, and the degree of obesity. As there is no registry, accurate data are not available; statements regarding perioperative mortality range from 0.1 to 2%, but the risk depends on the patient's comorbid conditions.[29] Morbidly obese patients often have other conditions that increase their risk for surgery. They need to be evaluated for sleep apnea (see "Perioperative Evaluation and Management of Pulmonary Diseases" chapter), pulmonary hypertension, cirrhosis, diabetes, hypertension, coronary disease, and heart failure; pulmonary hypertension and cirrhosis can increase the perioperative mortality to 50%.[30]

Deep Venous Thrombosis Prophylaxis for Morbidly Obese Patients

There is no consensus regarding deep venous thrombosis (DVT) prophylaxis for this population because there are inadequate data. Generally accepted DVT prophylaxis includes a combination of compression devices and subcutaneous unfractionated heparin or low-molecular-weight heparin (LMWH). Compression stockings appear to function more by preventing distention of veins and require patient compliance.[31] As routine doses may be inadequate, larger doses should be considered, and assessment of factor Xa should be considered when LMWH is utilized.

Diagnosis of pulmonary embolism may be difficult given the weight restrictions of CT scanners. Echocardiography or pulmonary angiography may be helpful.

DVT Prophylaxis for Perioperative Patients

For an example of treatment guidelines, see the UCSF recommendations at the end of this chapter. For more than 25 years, clinical research has investigated the optimal practice for perioperative prophylaxis to prevent venous thromboembolism. Pulmonary embolism is the most common cause of preventable death in patients hospitalized for surgical procedures.[32] Patients who undergo general surgery without prophylaxis have rates of DVT and fatal PE from 15 to 30% and 0.2 to 0.9% respectively.[32] These rates were derived from studies performed in the 1970s and 1980s, utilizing radioactive fibrinogen.[32] Graduated compression stockings effectively reduce the risk for VTE in patients undergoing general surgery; the stockings provide a 52% relative risk reduction compared to no prophylaxis.[33] Low-dose unfractionated heparin (LDUH or UFH) and low-molecular-weight heparin (LMWH) are the most effective therapies in reducing the incidence of DVT, providing a 68% and 76% risk reduction, respectively.[34] Patients are at higher risk when there is a diagnosis of cancer, the procedure takes a long time, the patient has had previous thromboembolic disease (VTE), or is of advanced age or is obese.[33,34] At least nine metaanalyses and systemic reviews have compared LMWH regimens with UFH for the prevention of thromboembolism after general surgery.[33] The analyses show that LMWH and UFH have comparable efficacy and safety in preventing VTE. Patients who are undergoing surgery for cancer should receive prophylactic doses of >3400 anti-Xa units of LMWH, as these doses provide greater protection than lower doses.[32]

It has become the standard practice to use oral warfarin or fixed doses of LMWH after major orthopedic surgery. Controversies that still exist include the optimal time for the administration of the first dose of prophylaxis after surgery. Data from the North American Fragmin Trial document that the administration of LMWH (dalteparin) beginning 6 h after surgery was more effective than warfarin for preventing DVT and did not increase clinically important bleeding.[35] In clinical trials comparing fondaparinux (a synthetic factor Xa inhibitor) given subcutaneously 4 to 8 h postoperatively with enoxaparin 30 mg given bid subcutaneously starting 12 to 24 h postoperatively, a >50% reduction in DVT was documented with fondaparinux.[35] A recent summary suggests that the first dose of LMWH should be given about 6 h postoperatively and not later than 12 h after surgery. Clinically important bleeding is seen if too large a dose of LMWH is given 6 h after surgery, or if the dose is given earlier than 6 h postoperatively.[35]

Investigations of direct thrombin inhibitors (oral ximelagatran and subcutaneous melagatran) suggest that their administration may decrease the rates of DVT even further without increasing bleeding.[36] However, a recent investigation compared the direct thrombin inhibitors with preoperative administration of LMWH,[35] a practice not found to be optimal (see above discussion).

The benefit of VTE after laparoscopic and arthroscopic surgery is unclear. Pharmacologic prophylaxis with UFH or LMWH should be used in patients with additional risk factors for VTE.[32,37] The benefit of screening patients after orthopedic or other high risk surgeries has not been shown. However, several studies have shown benefit of extended prophylaxis after discharge in high risk patients.[32-34] For example, prophylaxis should be extended for 4 weeks in patients undergoing elective hip replacement and undergoing surgery for cancer.[34,37]

Transfusions in Patients With Heart Disease

A recent investigation reported the results of an observational study examining the relationship between anemia, blood transfusion, and survival based on combined data from three large randomized trials involving 24,111 patients who had sustained acute MIs.[38,39] The investigation by Rao and colleagues only had 2,400 patients receiving transfusions or 10% of the population, and their mortality rate was about 4%. This investigation found that transfusions were not associated with improved survival when nadir hematocrit values were in the range of 20 to 25% and were clearly associated with worsened outcomes when values were greater than 30%.[38,39]

In contrast, earlier retrospective data from nearly 79,000 patients documented that lower hematocrit values were associated with increased mortality in patients with MIs.[40] Blood transfusions were found to reduce the short-term mortality among elderly patients with anemia who had acute MI if the hematocrit was ≤30% on admission. In fact, transfusion may have been effective for patients with hematocrit levels as high as 33%.[41] The retrospective study by Wu and colleagues[40] evaluated a wide population of elderly patients, whereas the most recent investigation by Rao and colleagues[38] included younger individuals. Therefore, it may be that more elderly patients would benefit from a higher hematocrit value.[39] Furthermore, there is evidence that treatment with epoetin may be beneficial in patients with heart failure, ischemic heart disease, or both, when it is used to achieve hematocrit values of >30%.[41] However, there is consensus that patients who receive transfusions when they have higher hematocrit values appear to be harmed by the transfusions.[38,39]

In contrast, patients who are normovolemic and have no major comorbid disease can tolerate a hemoglobin level of 7 g/dL. Critically ill patients who do not have coronary artery disease will also tolerate a hemoglobin level of 7 g/dL or higher, so transfusions should be given when a hemoglobin level of 7 g/dL is reached.[42] Until randomized controlled trials of transfusions are done in patients with acute MIs, we will not be certain of the optimal hemoglobin trigger for this group of patients.

References

1. Fleischmann KE, Goldman L, Young B, et al. Association between cardiac and noncardiac complications in patients undergoing noncardiac surgery: outcomes and effects on length of stay. Am J Med 2003; 115:515–520
2. Guidelines for assessing and managing the perioperative risk from coronary artery disease associated with major noncardiac surgery: American College of Physicians. Ann Intern Med 1997; 127:309–312
3. ACC/AHA Guideline Update for Perioperative Cardiovascular Evaluation for Noncardiac Surgery-Executive Summary: a report of the American College of Cardiology/American Heart Association Task Force on Practice Guidelines (Committee to Update the 1996 Guidelines on Perioperative Cardiovascular Evaluation for Noncardiac Surgery). Anesth Analg 2002; 94:1052–1064
4. Goldman L, Caldera DL, Nussbaum SR, et al. Multifactorial index of cardiac risk in noncardiac surgical procedures N Engl J Med 1977; 297:845–850
5. Lee TH, Marcantonio ER, Mangione CM, et al. Derivation and prospective validation of a simple index for prediction of cardiac risk of major noncardiac surgery. Circulation 1999; 100:1043–1049
6. Mangano DT, Layug EL, Wallace A, et al. Effect of atenolol on mortality and cardiovascular morbidity after noncardiac surgery. N Engl J Med 1996; 335:1713–1720; Erratum in: N Engl J Med 1997; 336:1039
7. Poldermans D, Boersma E, Bax J, et al. The effect of bisoprolol on perioperative mortality and

myocardial infarction in high-risk patients undergoing vascular surgery. N Engl J Med 1999; 341: 1789–1794

8. Wijeysundera DN, Naik JS, Beattie WS. Alpha-2 adrenergic agonists to prevent perioperative cardiovascular complications: a meta-analysis. Am J Med 2003; 114:742–752

9. Heusch G, Schipke J, Thamer V. Clonidine prevents the sympathetic initiation and aggravation of poststenotic myocardial ischemia. J Cardiovasc Pharmacol 1985; 7:1176–1182

10. Lena P, Balarac N, Arnulf JJ, et al. Intrathecal morphine and clonidine for coronary artery bypass grafting. Br J Anaesth 2003; 90:300–303

11. McFalls EO, Ward HB, Moritz TE, et al. Coronary-artery revascularization before elective major vascular surgery. N Eng J Med 2004; 351:2795–2804

12 Heart Disease and Stroke Statistics-2003 Update. Dallas, TX: American Heart Association, 2003

13. Klatte K, Chaitman BT, Theroux P, et al. Increased mortality after coronary artery bypass graft surgery is associated with increased levels of postoperative creatine kinase-myocardial band isoenzyme release: results from the GUARDIAN trial. J Am Coll Cardiol 2001; 38:1070–1077

14. Lasocki S, Provenchere S, Benessiano J, et al. Cardiac troponin I is an independent predictor of in-hospital death after adult cardiac surgery. Anesthesiology 2002; 97:405–411

15. Hutfless R, Kazanegra R, Madani M, et al. Utility of B-type natriuretic peptide in predicting postoperative complications and outcomes in patients undergoing heart surgery. J Am Coll Cardiol 2004; 43:1873–1879

16. Cuthbertson BH, McKeown A, Croal BL, et al. Utility of B-type natriuretic peptide in predicting the level of peri and postoperative cardiovascular support required after coronary artery bypass grafting. Crit Care Med 2005; 33:437–442

17. Malmbe K, Ryden L, Efendic S. Randomized trial of insulin-glucose infusion followed by subcutaneous insulin treatment in diabetic patients with acute myocardial infarction (DIGAMI study): effects on mortality at 1 year. J Am Coll Cardiol 1995; 26:57–65

18. Corpus RA, George PB, House JA, et al. Optimal glycemic control is associated with a lower rate of target vessel revascularization in treated type II diabetic patients undergoing elective percutaneous coronary intervention. J Am Coll Cardiol 2004; 43:8–14

19. Khaw KT, Wareham N, Luben R, et al. Glycated haemoglobin, diabetes, and mortality in men in Norfolk cohort of European Prospective Investigation of Cancer and Nutrition (EPIC-Norfolk). BMJ 2001; 322:15–18

20. Lazar HL, Chipkin SR, Fitzgerald CA, et al. Tight glycemic control in diabetic coronary artery bypass graft patients improves perioperative outcomes and decreases recurrent ischemic events. Circulation 2004; 109:1497–1502

21. He J, Ogden LG, Bazzano LA, et al. Risk factors for congestive heart failure in US men and women: NHANES I epidemiologic follow-up study. Arch Intern Med 2001; 161:996–1002

22. Saydah SH, Fradkin J, Cowie CC. Poor control of risk factors for vascular disease among adults with previously diagnosed diabetes. JAMA 2004; 291:335–342

23. Bakris GL, Fonseca V, Katholi RE, et al. Metabolic effects of carvedilol vs metoprolol in patients with type 2 diabetes mellitus and hypertension. JAMA 2004; 292:2227–2236

24. Giugliano D, Acampora R, Marfella R, et al. Metabolic and cardiovascular effects of carvedilol and atenolol in non-insulin dependent diabetes mellitus and hypertension: a randomized, controlled trial. Ann Intern Med 1997; 126:955–959

25. Galletti F, Strazzullo P, Capaldo B, et al. Controlled study of the effect of angiotensin converting enzyme inhibition versus calcium-entry blockade on insulin sensitivity in overweight hypertensive patients: Trandolapril Italian Study (TRIS). J Hypertens 1999; 17:439–445

26. van den Berghe G, Wouters P, Weekers F, et al. Intensive insulin therapy in critically ill patients. N Engl J Med 2001; 345:1359–1367

27. Tight blood pressure control and risk of macrovascular and microvascular complications in type II diabetes: UKPDS 38; UK Prospective Diabetes Study Group. BMJ 1998; 317:703–713; Erratum in: BMJ 1999; 318:29

28. Yusuf S, Sleight P, Pogue J, et al. Effects of an angiotensin-converting-enzyme inhibitor, ramipril, on cardiovascular events in high-risk patients: the Heart Outcomes Prevention Evaluation Study Investigators. N Engl J Med 2000; 342:145–153; Erratum in: N Engl J Med 2000; 342:1376; N Engl J Med 2000; 342:748

29. Steinbrook R. Surgery for severe obesity. N Engl J Med 2004; 350:1075–1079

30. Wiener-Kronish JP, Niemann C. Anesthesia in patients with severe lung disease. Pulmonary and Critical Care Update (Online) 2003; 17(9):1–8. Available at: http://www.chestnet.org/education/online/pccu/vol17/lessons9_10/lesson9.php. Accessed April 2005
31. Morris RJ, Woodcock JP. Evidence-based compression: prevention of stasis and deep vein thrombosis. Ann Surg 2004; 239:162–171
32. Agnelli G. Prevention of venous thromboembolism in surgical patients. Circulation 2004; 110 (suppl IV)IV-4-IV-12
33. Geerts WH, Heit JA, Clagett GP, et al. Prevention of venous thromboembolism. Chest 2001; 119(suppl):132S–175S
34. Gutt CN, Oniu T, Wolkener F, et al. Prophylaxis and treatment of deep vein thrombosis in general surgery. Am J Surg 2005; 189:14–22
35. Raskob GE, Hirsh J. Controversies in timing of the first dose of anticoagulant prophylaxis against venous thromboembolism after major orthopedic surgery. Chest 2003; 124(suppl):379S–385S
36. Koch A, Ziegler S, Breitschwerdt H, et al. Low molecular weight heparin and unfractionated heparin in thrombosis prophylaxis: meta-analysis based on original patient data. Thromb Res 2001; 102:295–309
37. Eriksson BI, Agnelli G, Cohen AT, et al. The direct thrombin inhibitor melagatran followed by oral ximelagatran compared with enoxaparin for the prevention of venous thromboembolism after total hip or knee replacement: the EXPRESS study. J Thromb Haemost 2003; 1:2490–2496
38. Rao SV, Jollis JG, Harrington RA, et al. Relationship of blood transfusion and clinical outcomes in patients with acute coronary syndromes. JAMA 2004; 292:1555–1562
39. Hebert PC, Fergusson DA. Do transfusions get to the heart of the matter? JAMA 2004; 292:1610–1612
40. Wu WC, Rathore SS, Wang Y, et al. Blood transfusion in elderly patients with acute myocardial infarction. N Engl J Med 2001; 345:1230–1236
41. NKF-DOQI clinical practice guidelines for the treatment of anemia of chronic renal failure: National Kidney Foundation-Dialysis Outcomes Quality Initiative. Am J Kidney Dis 1997; 30(suppl 3): S192–S240
42. Engelfriet CP, Reesink HW, McCullough J, et al. Perioperative triggers for red cell transfusions. Vox Sang 2002; 82:215–226

UCSF Medical Center

Adult Venous Thromboembolism Prophylaxis Order Form

These recommendations are for prophylaxis only, not treatment of acute thromboembolic disease. DO NOT USE THESE GUIDELINES IF THE PATIENT IS RECEIVING THERAPEUTIC ANTICOAGULATION

DATE	TIME	ALLERGIES

1. ASSESSMENT   Check all pertinent risk factors (RFs)

RFs with value of 1 point
- ☐ Age 41-60 years
- ☐ Prior history of postoperative DVT
- ☐ Family history of DVT or PE
- ☐ Leg swelling, ulcers, stasis, varicose veins
- ☐ MI/CHF
- ☐ Stroke with paralysis
- ☐ Inflammatory bowel disease
- ☐ Central line
- ☐ Bed confinement / immobilization >12 hours
- ☐ General anesthesia time >2 hours

- ☐ Pregnancy, or postpartum < 1 month
- ☐ Obesity (>20% over IBW)
- ☐ Hyperviscosity syndromes
- ☐ Estrogen therapy

RFs with value of 2 points
- ☐ Age 61-70 years
- ☐ Prior h/o unprovoked/idiopathic DVT
- ☐ Major surgery
- ☐ Malignancy
- ☐ Multiple trauma
- ☐ Spinal cord injury with paralysis

RFs with value of 3 points
- ☐ Age over 70 years
- ☐ Prior history of PE
- ☐ Inherited thrombophilia
- ☐ Acquired thrombophilia

TOTAL RISK FACTOR **SCORE** (RFS) = _____   (see reverse side for abbreviations and thrombophilia definitions)

2. CONTRAINDICATIONS TO PHARMACOLOGIC PROPHYLAXIS

Relative (check if applicable)
- ☐ History of cerebral hemorrhage
- ☐ Craniotomy within 2 weeks
- ☐ GI, GU hemorrhage within the last 6 months
- ☐ Thrombocytopenia
- ☐ Coagulopathy (PT >18 sec)
- ☐ Active intracranial lesions/neoplasms/monitoring devices
- ☐ Proliferative retinopathy
- ☐ Vascular access/biopsy sites inaccessible to hemostatic control

Absolute (check if applicable)
- ☐ Active hemorrhage
- ☐ Heparin or warfarin use in active HIT
- ☐ Warfarin use in the first trimester of pregnancy
- ☐ Severe trauma to head, spinal cord or extremities with hemorrhage within the last 4 weeks
- ☐ Epidural/indwelling spinal catheter – placement or removal (see reverse side)

If contraindications exist to pharmacologic prophylaxis, consider sequential compression devices (SCDs).

3. REGIMENS FOR PROPHYLAXIS[a]

Low Risk (0 RFS)	Moderate Risk (1-2 RFS)	High Risk (3-4 RFS)	Very High Risk (>4 RFS)[b]
• Early ambulation	• LDUH (5000 U) q 8-12 h or • LMWH or • SCD	• LDUH (5,000 U) q 8h or • LMWH or • SCD	• LMWH or • Warfarin, INR 2-3 or • ADH

[a] See reverse side for dosing recommendations
[b] Consider consultation with the Comprehensive Hemostasis and Antithrombotic Service (CHAS) pager 719-4023
ADH = adjusted dose heparin, subcutaneous UFH to achieve aPTT at high range of normal (35 sec) six hours after dose.

ADDITIONAL CONSIDERATIONS
Renal impairment: Use low molecular weight heparins and fondaparinux with <u>caution</u> in patients with a Scr >2 or CrCL <30 mL/min.
Consider dose adjustments for pharmacologic prophylaxis in patients with a weight of < 50 kg. (Fondaparinux should not be used in patients < 50 kg.)
Obesity: Appropriate dosing for obese patients is not well established. Consider CHAS consult.

4. SELECTION OF THROMBOPROPHYLAXIS: (√ in box activates order)

A) *NON-PHARMACOLOGIC*
- ☐ **Early ambulation:** (Low Thromboembolic Risk)
- ☐ **SCD (Knee High):** (High Bleed Risk) – Send order to Materiel Services

B) *PHARMACOLOGIC* -- Send order to Pharmacy

☐	**Enoxaparin (LMWH)**	☐	30 mg SQ Q12H	☐	40 mg SQ Q24H
☐	**UFH** →	☐	5000 U SQ Q12H	☐	5000 U SQ Q8H

- ☐ **Other** _____

(Follow CBC with platelets QOD if heparin or LMWH is used. Follow daily INR if warfarin is used.)

Signature_____ M.D.#_____ Time_____ Date_____ Pager_____

FLAG CHART Checked by _____ R.N. Time_____ Date_____

P&T Approved June 2002; Revised 1/17/2003

Deep Venous Thrombosis Risk Factor Assessment

1. Abbreviations:

VTE	venous thromboembolism	**LMWH**	low molecular weight heparin
LDUH	low dose unfractionated heparin	**APLA**	antiphospholipid antibody
ADH	adjusted dose heparin	**CHAS**	Comprehensive Hemostasis & Antithrombotic Service
SCD	sequential compression device		(pager: 719-4023)
UFH	unfractionated heparin	**RFS**	risk factor score

2. ***Thrombophilia* includes:**

• Factor V Leiden	• Prothrombin variant G20210A
• APLA or lupus anticoagulant	• Antithrombin III deficiency
• Protein C or protein S deficiency	• Hyperhomocysteinemia
• Heparin induced thrombocytopenia	• Myeloproliferative disorders (polycythemia vera, essential thrombocytosis (ET))

3. *Recommendations for the use of antithrombotic prophylaxis in patients with epidural catheters.*

   For patients receiving low-dose SC unfractionated heparin (5000units Q12H)
   - Wait 4-6 hours after a prophylactic dose of UFH before placing or removing a catheter
   - Initiate UFH thromboprophylaxis 1-2 hours after placing or removing a catheter
   - Concurrent use of epidural or spinal catheter and SC low-dose unfractionated heparin is not contraindicated.

   For patients receiving prophylactic-dose LMWH
   - Wait 24 hours after a prophylactic dose of LMWH before placing a catheter or performing a neuraxial block
   - Wait 12-24 hours after a prophylactic dose of LMWH before removing a catheter
   - Initiate LMWH thromboprophylaxis 2-4 hours after removal of the catheter
   - Initiate LMWH thromboprophylaxis 24 hours after a "single shot" spinal procedure
   - Concurrent use of an epidural catheter and LMWH thromboprophylaxis needs to be approved by the pain service

   For patients receiving fondaparinux
   - Extreme caution is warranted given the sustained antithrombotic effect, early postoperative dosing, and "irreversibility".
   - Until further clinical experience is available, an alternate method of prophylaxis should be utilized.

4. Dosing recommendations for LMWH and fondaparinux (consider risk factors, caution in patients with renal insufficiency - CrCl < 30 ml/min):

Condition	*Recommended Dose
General Surgery	Enoxaparin 40 mg SQ q24h, 1st dose 2 h preop
Gynecologic Surgery	Enoxaparin 40 mg SQ q24h
Urologic Surgery	Enoxaparin 30 mg SQ q12h[c]
Major Orthopedic Surgery	Enoxaparin 30 mg SQ q12h, Enoxaparin 40 mg SQ q24h, *or* Fondaparinux 2.5 mg SQ q 24 h start 6 h post-op
Neurosurgery	Enoxaparin 40 mg SQ q24h If pharmacologic prophylaxis is the chosen intervention.
Trauma and acute spinal cord injury	Enoxaparin 30 mg SQ q12h If pharmacologic prophylaxis is the chosen intervention.
Medical Conditions (e.g. MI, CHF, malignancy)	Enoxaparin 40 mg SQ q24h

For low-risk procedures, early postoperative mobilization may be the prophylactic approach of choice. [c]High-risk patients include those undergoing more extensive, open procedures, including radical prostatectomy, cystectomy, or nephrectomy.

These recommendations are NOT intended to replace an individual clinician's judgment.

Notes

Notes

Severe Pneumonia

Michael S. Niederman, MD, FCCP

Objectives:

- To define the epidemiology of community-acquired pneumonia (CAP) and risk factors for mortality
- To discuss the common etiologic pathogens of severe CAP
- To review current treatment strategies for severe CAP
- To discuss the clinical relevance of atypical pathogens and penicillin-resistant pneumococci
- To describe the pathogenesis of ventilator-associated pneumonia (VAP)
- To discuss the organisms that cause VAP
- To outline therapies for VAP

Key words: antibiotic resistance; community-acquired pneumonia; drug-resistant pathogens; pneumonia; ventilator-associated pneumonia

Community-Acquired Pneumonia

Pneumonia and influenza together are the sixth leading cause of death in the United States and the number-one cause of mortality from infectious diseases. Community-acquired pneumonia (CAP) occurs in approximately 6 million people annually, with 20 to 30% requiring hospital admission.

Epidemiology and Risk Factors for Mortality

In a recent metaanalysis, the overall mortality for 33,148 patients reported on in 127 studies was 13.7%, ranging from 5.1% in a population that was both hospitalized and ambulatory to 13.6% for hospitalized patients. In the elderly, mortality was 17.6%, while among nursing home patients it was 30.8%; those admitted to the ICU had a mortality rate of 36.5%. When pneumococcus was responsible, the mortality rate was 12.3%, a rate similar to that seen when no pathogen could be identified (12.8%). Certain pathogens such as Pseudomonas aeruginosa, other Gram-negative organisms (such as Klebsiella pneumoniae), and Staphylococcus aureus had higher associated mortality rates.

A number of prognostic factors for mortality were identified; the most important were underlying neurologic disease, BUN >20 mg/dL, respiratory rate >20/min, systolic hypotension, hypothermia, bacteremia, multilobar disease, coexisting malignancy, and underlying congestive heart failure. The presence of a comorbid illness, more than specific bacteriology or patient age, is the major determinant of early and late mortality in patients with CAP. In one study, 16% of all hospitalized patients with CAP died, but an additional 32% of discharged patients died from all causes in the subsequent 2 years. Patients with CAP are at risk for recurrent infection, indicating the need to vaccinate all pneumonia patients before hospital discharge in an effort to avoid this complication, which has a very high mortality rate.

The British Thoracic Society rule uses certain clinical and laboratory features to identify certain high-risk patients who might have been unrecognized otherwise, but should be assessed on initial evaluation. It uses only three variables: respiratory rate ≥30/min, BUN >19.6 mg/dL, and diastolic BP ≤60 mm Hg. The presence of two of these three variables increases mortality 9- to 21-fold. More recently, confusion in the patient has been added as a fourth variable, and if two of four variables are present, there is a similar increased risk for death and need for ICU admission. When the four criteria are used, they are referred to as the "CURB" criteria, referring to confusion, elevated urea nitrogen, elevated respiratory rate, and low diastolic BP. One other modification is to use a fifth criterion, age >65, and, if at least three of these "CURB-65" criteria are present, the patient should be considered for ICU admission. Other factors that are associated with a poor outcome in CAP include age >65 years, the presence of comorbid illness, altered mental status, temperature >38.3°C, extrapulmonary sites of infection, extremes of white blood cell count, multilobar radiographic abnormalities, evidence of sepsis, respiratory failure, the presence of end organ dysfunction secondary to severe infection, delays in the initiation of appropriate antibiotic therapy, prolonged illness prior to therapy, and indistinct clinical features on presentation (*ie*, afebrile, absence of pleuritic chest pain). When multiple factors predicting a complicated course are present, hospitalization is indicated.

The PORT (Pneumonia Patient Outcomes Research Team) study has led to the development of a prediction rule for deciding who should be admitted to the hospital with CAP. This rule divides patients into five groups with different risks of death, and suggests that outpatient care be given for classes I and II, admission for classes IV and V, and individualized decision for class III. The system heavily weights age and comorbid illness. In a large prospective study, the rule was successful in increasing the number of low-risk patients who were discharged compared with situations when the rule was not used. However, even at sites that used the rule, 31% of low-risk patients were still admitted, emphasizing the fact that the admission decision remains an "art of medicine" decision that cannot easily be determined by a rule. The PORT criteria are not able to discriminate which patients need ICU admission, because in one study, 27% of all patients admitted to the ICU fell into risk classes I to III. In an ICU population, the rule could predict mortality, even though it could not define need for ICU care.

Need for ICU Admission

Although there is no uniformly accepted definition for severe community-acquired pneumonia, this term generally refers to any patient who is admitted to the ICU because of CAP. Most of these patients have "respiratory failure," defined by the presence of hypoxemia or hypercarbia, and not all such patients require mechanical ventilation. Bacteremia may not specifically correlate with more severe illness, and its presence alone is not always a predictor of a poor outcome, with most episodes of bacteremia being due to pneumococcus. However, in the elderly with pneumococcal pneumonia, bacteremia is present in one quarter of patients with CAP and is often associated with azotemia and multilobe involvement. When an infection, such as pneumonia, is complicated by severe sepsis or septic shock (not just bacteremia), outcome is adversely affected, with increases in mortality, length of stay, and costs for survivors.

In the 1993 American Thoracic Society (ATS) guidelines, 10 criteria from the literature were identified to define patients who needed ICU admission, with the presence of any one of these criteria defining severe illness. However, subsequent studies showed that 65% of all admitted patients with CAP (not needing ICU care) also had one of these criteria, and, thus, a more specific definition of the need for ICU admission was required. To better define the need of ICU care for CAP, Ewig and colleagues applied the 10 ATS criteria to 64 patients who were admitted to the ICU and compared the findings to the features present in 331 patients admitted to the hospital but not the ICU. With this approach, a better definition of severe CAP was derived, with a sensitivity of 78%, a specificity of 94%, a positive predictive value of 75%, and a negative predictive value of 95%. This definition required the presence of either two of three "minor criteria" present on admission, or one of two "major criteria" present on admission or later in the hospital course. The minor criteria were: systolic blood pressure <90 mm Hg, Pao_2/Fio_2 ratio <250, or multilobar infiltrates. The major criteria were need for mechanical ventilation or septic shock.

Pathogenesis

Most of the pathogens responsible for CAP reach the lung after first colonizing the oropharynx. Because patients with serious comorbidity have an increased risk of Gram-negative colonization of the oropharynx, those same patients appear to have an increased risk of pneumonia attributed to these types of pathogens. Community respiratory pathogens that can enter via inhalation without preceding oropharyngeal colonization include certain viruses, *Mycobacterium tuberculosis*, and Legionella.

One of the serious but infrequent complications of CAP is acute lung injury, presumably arising from activation of inflammatory mediators in the lung. Investigators have evaluated the normal host response to pneumonia in order to determine if the inflammatory response remains localized to the lung or if it enters into the systemic circulation, thereby creating the conditions that lead to lung injury and ARDS. In studies of unilateral pneumonia, the infected lung had enhanced production of tumor necrosis factor -α, interleukin-1β (IL-1β), IL-6, and IL-8 with little effect on the contralateral lung or systemic circulation. IL-8 may be a key mediator because it can recruit neutrophils to sites of infection, and alveolar levels of this cytokine correlate with the number of neutrophils in the alveolar space. The fact that the cytokine response to pneumonia is usually localized may explain why ARDS is an infrequent complication of CAP.

Pathogens

Bacteria, viruses, and "atypical pathogens" (*Mycoplasma pneumoniae* and *Chlamydia pneumoniae*) account for most cases of CAP, but in some 50% of patients a microbiologic diagnosis is not established, reflecting the limitations of current diagnostic testing, particularly in those patients who have received prior antibiotic therapy. In one recent study, transthoracic needle aspiration was performed in patients without a known diagnosis, and many of these patients were shown to have pneumococcal infection. Although this organism can account for many undiagnosed cases, it is also possible that not all pathogens causing CAP have been identified and studied, and new pathogens are commonly being described. The distribution of individual pathogens has also varied in studies, depending on the location of the study and the types of patients evaluated. For example, in a study of 385 patients at an inner-city US hospital, 205 of whom were HIV-negative, pneumococcus was found in 15%, *Haemophilus influenzae* in 7.3%, and atypical pathogens in 8%; in 37% of patients, no agent was identified. Most of these patients were older; 65% had a smoking history and 30% were classified as alcoholic. This distribution of etiologic agents contrasts with the results of a study done in Israel, in which 346 patients were evaluated and a diagnosis was established for 81%. Pneumococcus was found in 43%, *M pneumoniae* in 29%, *C pneumoniae* in 18%, Legionella in 16%, and viruses in 10%. Interestingly, in 38% of the patients, multiple organisms were present simultaneously. In a recent US study, 2,776 patients were studied and a possible etiologic diagnosis was made in 44.3%. In this group, *M pneumoniae* was most common (32.5%), followed by pneumococcus (12.6%), *C pneumoniae* (8.9%), influenza (7.4%), *H influenzae* (6.6%), and then Gram-negative bacilli and Legionella. In many of the more recent studies, atypical pathogen infections are common, often as coinfections with bacterial pathogens. In addition, the atypical organisms are seen not only in young and healthy adults, but also in older patients, particularly *C pneumoniae* and Legionella. When atypical pathogens occur as part of a mixed infection, the outcome may be more complex and the length of stay longer than if a single organism is causing infection. Studies of CAP in the ICU have shown that atypical pathogens are commonly present, accounting for up to 20% of all diagnosed etiologies of severe CAP. However, the identity of the responsible organism may change over time, with Legionella predominating in some years, and being replaced by Mycoplasma or Chlamydia at other times.

The elderly may have different pathogens than those seen in younger patients, with a higher incidence of infection with *H influenzae* and enteric Gram-negative organisms. Recent observations in ICU-admitted elderly patients coming from the nursing home, with aspiration risk factors, have shown that Gram-negative organisms are far more common than anaerobes. Although pneumococcus may also be seen in these patients, anaerobes are not only uncommon, even in the setting of suspected aspiration, but outcomes are not adversely affected if therapy does not cover anaerobic pathogens.

In general, the pathogens causing CAP vary in relation to specific patient factors (Table 1). The ATS has categorized inpatients into different groups, each with its own list of likely pathogens (Tables 2–3), by assessing several variables: the admission to the ICU or inpatient ward, the presence of cardiopulmonary disease, and/or the presence of modifying factors (including risk factors for *P aeruginosa*). Modifying factors (Table 1) are clinical conditions that put the patient at risk for infection with specific pathogens, such as drug-resistant pneumococci, enteric Gram-negative organisms, and *P aeruginosa*. For all groups, the most common pathogen is pneumococcus, and therapy for CAP should always provide adequate coverage for this organism. In the elderly and chronically ill, *H influenzae* (10 to 20% of cases) and enteric Gram-negative bacteria (20 to 40% of

Table 1. *Modifying Factors That Increase the Risk of Infection With Specific Pathogens*

Penicillin-Resistant and Drug-Resistant Pneumococci
    Age >65 yr
    β-lactam therapy within the past 3 mo
    Alcoholism
    Immune-suppressive illness (including therapy with corticosteroids)
    Multiple medical comorbidities
    Exposure to a child in a day care center
Enteric Gram-Negative Organisms
    Residence in a nursing home
    Underlying cardiopulmonary disease
    Multiple medical comorbidities
    Recent antibiotic therapy
P aeruginosa
    Structural lung disease (bronchiectasis)
    Corticosteroid therapy (>10 mg prednisone/d)
    Broad-spectrum antibiotic therapy for >7 days in the past month
    Malnutrition

Table 2. *Probable Organisms and Therapy in Hospitalized Patients With CAP*

With Cardiopulmonary Disease and/or Modifying Factors
Probable Organisms
- *S pneumoniae* (including DRSP*)
- *H influenzae*
- Atypical pathogens, such as *M pneumoniae* or *C pneumoniae*, alone or as mixed infection
- Aerobic Gram-negative bacilli
- *Legionella* spp
- Respiratory viruses
- Miscellaneous: *S aureus*, *Moraxella catarrhalis*, *M tuberculosis*, endemic fungi

Therapy
- Selected IV β-lactam with antipneumococcal activity (ceftriaxone, cefotaxime, ampicillin/sulbactam, high-dose ampicillin)

plus
- Macrolide (choose oral or IV) *or* doxycycline (choose oral or IV)

or
- IV antipneumococcal quinolone *alone*

With No Cardiopulmonary Disease and No Modifying Factors
Probable Organisms
- *S pneumoniae*
- *H influenzae*
- *M pneumoniae*
- *C pneumoniae*
- Mixed infection (bacteria plus atypical pathogen)
- Viruses
- *Legionella* spp
- Miscellaneous: *M tuberculosis*, endemic fungi, *P carinii*

Therapy
- IV azithromycin alone
- *If macrolide allergic or intolerant:* doxycycline and a β-lactam, *or* monotherapy with an antipneumococcal fluoroquinolone

*DRSP = drug-resistant *S pneumoniae*.

---

cases) are common organisms, but anaerobes must also be considered (although still not very common) in those at risk for aspiration because of impaired consciousness or altered swallowing reflexes. In severe CAP, pneumococcus is the most common organism, but studies have also found Legionella (as well as other atypical pathogens), *H influenzae*, and enteric Gram-negative organisms to be important. *P aeruginosa* has been identified from the respiratory tract cultures of 5 to 15% of all patients with severe CAP. In one study, risk factors for Gram-negative organisms were the following: probable aspiration (odds ratio [OR] = 2.3), previous hospital admission within 30 days of admission (OR = 3.5), previous antibiotics within 30 days of admission (OR = 1.9), and presence of pulmonary comorbidity (OR = 2.8). Risk factors for *P aeruginosa* were pulmonary comorbidity (OR = 5.8) and previous hospitalization (OR = 3.8). For those admitted to the ICU, patients are divided into those at risk for Pseudomonas and those who are not.

Although this categorization is useful in suspecting certain pathogens when other specific clues are absent, there are some epidemiologic findings that point to the presence of specific pathogens. *Legionella pneumophila* should be considered in the late summer and with exposure to contaminated water sources (cooling towers, air conditioning, saunas). *Coxiella burnetii* infection (Q fever) can follow exposure to infected cats, cattle, sheep, and goats. Exposure to turkeys, chicken, and psittacine birds can lead to infection with *Chlamydia psittaci*, while contaminated bat caves may lead to histoplasmosis. Immigrants from Asia, India, or Central America should always be evaluated for tuberculosis, and melioidosis should be considered in patients who have traveled to Southeast Asia. One recent consideration for those with travel to Asia is severe acute respiratory syndrome (SARS), which may cause pneumonia and rapidly progressive respiratory failure. Other epidemiologic associations with specific pathogens are listed in Table 4.

Table 3. *Hospitalized Patients With Severe CAP*

With No Pseudomonal Risk Factors
Probable Organisms
- *S pneumoniae* (including DRSP)
- *Legionella* spp
- *H influenzae*
- Enteric Gram-negative organisms
- *S aureus*
- *M pneumoniae* or *C pneumoniae*
- Respiratory viruses
- Miscellaneous: *M tuberculosis*, endemic fungi

Therapy
- Macrolide *or* antipneumococcal quinolone

plus
- Selected β-lactam with antipneumococcal activity (ceftriaxone, cefotaxime, ampicillin/sulbactam)

With Pseudomonal Risk Factors
Probable Organisms
- *S pneumoniae* (including DRSP)
- *Legionella* spp
- *H influenzae*
- Enteric Gram-negative organisms (including *P aeruginosa*)
- *S aureus*
- *M pneumoniae* or *C pneumoniae*
- Respiratory viruses
- Miscellaneous: *M tuberculosis*, endemic fungi

Therapy
- Ciprofloxacin *plus* antipseudomonal, antipneumococcal β-lactam (imipenem, meropenem, cefepime, piperacillin/tazobactam)

or
- Nonpseudomonal quinolone (levofloxacin, gatifloxacin, moxifloxacin) or macrolide

plus
- antipseudomonal, antipneumococcal β-lactam (imipenem, meropenem, cefepime, piperacillin/tazobactam) *plus* aminoglycoside

Comments About Specific Pathogens

Pneumococcus

A Gram-positive diplococcus, with 85% of cases caused by 23 of the 84 serotypes. Commonly preceded by viral illness; may cause lobar or bronchopneumonia. Common infection in those with asplenia, multiple myeloma, heart failure, alcoholism. Current vaccine includes 23 serotypes. Controversy about vaccine efficacy shows that it is safe, but may not be effective in the chronically ill. Case-control methodology has been used to show efficacy.

Penicillin-resistant *Streptococcus pneumoniae* (PRSP) is becoming a problem in some areas. In the United States, >40% of pneumococci are penicillin-resistant, with rates varying widely from region to region. Most have intermediate [penicillin minimum inhibitory concentration (MIC) ≥0.12 mg/mL but <2.0 mg/L] rather than high-level resistance (penicillin MIC ≥2 mg/L). The clinical relevance of *in vitro* resistance is debated, but there are data that show an increased risk of death if patients have organisms with a penicillin MIC of ≥4 mg/L, which is currently an uncommon occurrence. Resistance is rarely a *de novo* event and it is uncommon in low-risk patients; rather, it is seen in immunosuppressed and chronically ill patients, especially if they have received a beta-lactam antibiotic in the preceding 3 months, although cases of epidemic transmission of resistant organisms have been reported. Other risk factors for PRSP include age >60 years, alcoholism, and multiple medical comorbidity.

The mortality rate of hospitalized patients with pneumococcal CAP exceeds 20%, but is related to the status of the patient's immune defenses and overall health and not to whether the organism is penicillin-resistant. Although most studies have shown that patients with penicillin-resistant organisms have the same mortality rate as patients who are infected with penicillin-sensitive organisms, those with very high levels of resistance may have an increased risk of death. Penicillin resistance may mean multidrug resistance, and there is a high co-incidence of macrolide and trimethoprim-sulfa resistance among penicillin resistant pneumococci. There is not a direct correlation between all *in vitro* resistance and clinical outcomes, and treatment failure is infrequent with most antibiotics (β-lactams, macrolides, and quinolones) at current levels of resistance, even in the presence of *in vitro* resistance. Although quinolone resistance is uncommon for pneumococci, the less active agents ciprofloxacin and levofloxacin have been associated with failures of therapy due to resistance, especially if patients have received recent therapy with a quinolone.

Risk factors for mortality include the presence of bacteremia, the finding of bronchopneumonia rather than lobar consolidation, and the presence of multiple comorbid illnesses. Regardless of resistance pattern, therapy for pneumococcus with high-dose penicillin (2 million U q4h) or a third-generation cephalosporin (cefotaxime or

Table 4. Epidemiologic Conditions Related to Specific Pathogens in Patients With CAP

Condition	Commonly Encountered Pathogens
Alcoholism	*S pneumoniae* (including PRSP), anaerobes, Gram-negative bacilli
COPD/smoker	*S pneumoniae, H influenzae, M catarrhalis,* Legionella
Nursing home residency	*S pneumoniae,* Gram-negative bacilli, *H influenzae, S aureus,* anaerobes, *C pneumoniae*
Poor dental hygiene	Anaerobes
Epidemic Legionnaire's disease	Legionella spp
Exposure to bats	*Histoplasma capsulatum*
Exposure to birds	*C psittaci, Cryptococcus neoformans, H capsulatum*
Exposure to rabbits	*Francisella tularensis*
Travel to southwestern United States	Coccidioidomycosis
Exposure to farm animals or parturient cats	*C burnetii* (Q fever)
Influenza active in community	Influenza, *S pneumoniae, S aureus, H influenzae*
Suspected large-volume aspiration	Anaerobes, chemical pneumonitis, or obstruction
Structural disease of lung (bronchiectasis, cystic fibrosis, etc.)	*P aeruginosa, Burkholderia cepacia,* or *S aureus*
Injection drug use	*S aureus,* anaerobe, tuberculosis
Endobronchial obstruction	Anaerobes
Recent antibiotic therapy	Drug-resistant pneumococci, *P aeruginosa*
Sickle cell disease, asplenia	Pneumococccus, *H influenzae*
Suspected bioterrorism	Anthrax, tularemia, plague
Travel to Asia	SARS, tuberculosis, meliodoisis

ceftriaxone) is adequate for invasive pulmonary disease, provided that central nervous system involvement is not present. The incidence of penicillin resistance is rising in certain communities, and a knowledge of the frequency of the problem and of local antimicrobial susceptibilities is necessary to ensure adequate initial antibiotic therapy because some agents, such as trimethoprim-sulfamethoxazole, are increasingly ineffective against pneumococci. The new fluoroquinolones may represent appropriate empiric therapy for patients with suspected resistance. If they are used, there are differences in activity against pneumococci; the least to most active agents are, in order: levofloxacin less active than gatifloxacin or moxifloxacin.

L pneumophila

A weakly staining Gram-negative organism. Legionella is a waterborne organism, and should be suspected in all patients with severe CAP, and in other patients based on a careful epidemiologic evaluation. Increased risk is present in those who are immunocompromised, have a malignancy, smoke, have chronic lung disease, or older than 50 years. There is no constellation of clinical signs that is specific for Legionella infection. In addition to respiratory symptoms, patients may have confusion, diarrhea, elevated liver function tests, hyponatremia, and relative bradycardia.

Legionella is a commonly identified pathogen in patients with severe CAP, but its overall incidence is uncertain. Unless careful diagnostic testing is done, underestimation of its frequency is likely. Sputum samples that grow Legionella often have few polymorphonuclear cells and may be discarded by microbiology labs. Most cases cannot be diagnosed by a single immunofluorescent antibody titer (often negative at the time of the acute illness), and are only recognized if acute and convalescent serum titers are examined for a fourfold rise. The urinary antigen is a more sensitive single test, but it is specific only for infection with *L pneumophila* serogroup I.

M pneumoniae

Usually a mild illness, but can be severe, with complications of hemolytic anemia, myocarditis, hepatitis, cold agglutinins, or meningoencephalitis. Serologic diagnosis.

S aureus

Can cause CAP, particularly when bacterial pneumonia complicates influenza, or when right-sided endocarditis or cavitary lung lesions are present. *S aureus* is also seen after influenza, with chronic lung disease. May lead to cavities (pneumatoceles). Empyema is common.

C pneumoniae *(The TWAR Agent)*

A common pathogen in young adults with tracheobronchitis and/or pneumonia; often leads to a syndrome of "adult croup." The role of *C pneumoniae* as a respiratory pathogen is uncertain, with some studies suggesting that it functions as a copathogen more often than as a single agent. Confusion results because the organism can be isolated along with other pathogens, its clinical features cannot be differentiated from those of pneumonia caused by other organisms, and patients can recover without specific therapy. One recent study has shown that it can occur in the elderly, including those who reside in nursing homes, and it may spread from person to person. The mortality rate can be high in certain populations, and it may lead to severe forms of CAP.

Aspiration/Lung Abscess

Aspiration may involve acid (chemical pneumonitis), inert liquids or particulate matter (suffocation or postobstructive pneumonia), or oropharyngeal bacteria (aspiration pneumonia or lung abscess). Aspiration pneumonia often is polymicrobial, involving anaerobes; it may cavitiate, and can be an indolent infection that is confused with malignancy. If lung abscess is seen in an edentulous patient (no mouth anaerobes), consider lung malignancy, foreign body, or a GI source of chronic aspiration (esophageal diverticulum). The cavity usually has an air-fluid level and is >2 cm. Cavities from bacterial infection tend to be thick-walled and have a ragged inner lining. Lung abscess cavities usually have an air-fluid level. Tuberculosis cavities, by contrast, tend to be thin-walled and air-filled (without an air-fluid level), with a smooth inner wall. Aspiration pneumonia occurs in the superior segment of the lower lobe or the posterior segments of the upper lobe if aspiration occurs when supine, and in the lower lobe if aspiration occurs when upright. In patients who have aspiration risks together with poor dentition, a lower lobe infiltrate, and pleural or chest wall involvement, actinomycosis should be considered.

Influenza

Can be complicated by pneumonia. An RNA virus, with types A and B; type A infection is generally more severe. Vaccine is trivalent and directed at both types of influenza, and reduces mortality from respiratory illness. Amantadine and rimantadine are active only against type A. The new antivirals oseltamivir and zanamivir are active against both influenza A and B. Fall and early spring for epidemics. Attack rates are not increased in the elderly, but mortality is. Pneumonia may be viral or secondary bacterial. The latter occurs as the patient is improving from his initial infection, and is most commonly caused by pneumococcus, *S aureus*, *H influenzae*, or a Gram-negative organism. New interest in diagnosing influenza has come with the advent of the neuraminidase inhibitors zanamivir and oseltamivir. The former is given as a dry powder inhaler, and the latter as a pill.

HIV-Positive Patients

In HIV-positive patients, pneumococcus and *H influenzae* are common, but CAP with *P aeruginosa* has been reported. Infection with *Pneumocystis carinii* and *M tuberculosis* must always be considered.

Hantavirus

A newly described pathogen is the hantavirus, carried by rodents and first identified in the Four Corners area of New Mexico in May 1993. The hantavirus pulmonary syndrome is life-threatening and characterized by fulminant respiratory failure after a brief prodromal illness with symptoms of fever, myalgia, cough, dyspnea, GI symptoms, and headache. Patients are generally tachypneic and hypotensive with rapidly progressive pulmonary edema. Mortality is high, with only nonspecific and supportive therapy available.

Other Pathogens

Several Rickettsia can cause CAP, including the following: Q fever (*Coxiella burnetii*), which occurs worldwide; Rocky Mountain spotted fever

(RMSF); and scrub typhus (Rickettsia tsutsugamushi), which occurs in Asia and Australia. Transmission typically involves an intermediate vector, often ticks (Q fever, RMSF) or mites (scrub typhus), but also sheep, cows, and contaminated milk (Q fever). These infections have a variable incubation period, ranging from days to a few weeks and are characterized by a febrile syndrome that may have a pneumonic component and a maculopapular rash (Q fever and RMSF).

Severe Acute Respiratory Syndrome: In late 2003, a respiratory viral infection, caused by a coronavirus, emerged in parts of Asia and was termed *severe acute respiratory syndrome*, or *SARS*. The illness affected people from a variety of endemic areas in Asia, but was seen in North America when an outbreak occurred in Toronto, Canada. Importantly, worldwide, as many as 20% of affected patients were health-care workers, particularly those caring for patients admitted to the ICU. Transmission risk was greatest during emergent intubation and was also possible during noninvasive ventilation, making this latter modality of therapy contraindicated if SARS is suspected. Infection control may be quite effective in preventing the spread of SARS to health-care workers and includes the careful handling of respiratory secretions, ventilator circuits, and the use of N-95 respirator masks and careful use of gowns and gloves. Even more elaborate infection control measures, including personal air exchange units, are needed for health-care workers involved in high risk procedures, such as intubation.

Clinically, patients with SARS present after a 2 to 11 day incubation period with fever, rigors, chills, dry cough, dyspnea, malaise headache, and, frequently, pneumonia and ARDS. Laboratory data show not only hypoxemia, but also elevated liver function tests. In the Toronto experience, about 20% of hospitalized patients were admitted to the ICU, and 15% were mechanically ventilated. Respiratory involvement typically began on day 3 of the hospital stay, but respiratory failure was not until day 8. The mortality rate for ICU-admitted patients with SARS was over 30%, and, when patients died, it was generally from multiple-system organ failure and sepsis. There is no specific therapy, but anecdotal reports have suggested a benefit to the use of pulse doses of steroids and ribavirin.

Bioterrorism Considerations: Certain airborne pathogens can cause pneumonia as the result of deliberate dissemination by the aerosol route, in the form of a biological weapon, and present a clinical syndrome of CAP. The pathogens that are most likely to be used in this fashion and can lead to severe pulmonary infection are *Bacillus anthracis* (causes anthrax), *Yersinia pestis* (causes plague), and *Francisella tularensis* (causes tularemia)

To date, in the United States, anthrax is the only airborne respiratory agent that has been used in a bioterrorism attack. In the fall of 2001, a series of intentional attacks with anthrax led to 11 confirmed cases of inhalational illness. Anthrax is an aerobic, Gram-positive, spore-forming Bacillus that had rarely led to disease prior to 2001. Particle size is essential in determining the infectiousness of the spores, and a size of 1 to 5 microns is required for inhalation into the alveolar space, but, generally, infection requires an inoculum size of 8,000 to 40,000 spores. The organisms initially enter alveolar macrophages and are transported to mediastinal lymph nodes, where they can persist and germinate and produce two toxins (lethal toxin and edema toxin), and illness follows rapidly after germination. Although respiratory symptoms are often present, anthrax is not a typical pneumonic illness but rather a disease characterized by hemorrhagic thoracic lymphadenitis, hemorrhagic mediastinitis, and pleural effusion. While the incubation period of anthrax has varied from 2 to 43 days in prior outbreaks, in the October 2001 series, the incubation period was from 4 to 6 days. In the US experience, all patients had chills, fever, and sweats, and most had nonproductive cough, dyspnea, nausea, vomiting, and chest pain. Chest radiographs were abnormal in all of the first 10 patients, and 7 had mediastinal widening, 8 had pleural effusions (generally bloody), and 7 had pulmonary infiltrates. Blood culture results were positive in all eight patients in whom results were obtained prior to therapy, but sputum culture and Gram-stain results are unlikely to be positive. In the US attacks, 5 of 11 patients died.

Therapy includes supportive management and antibiotics, with possibly some role for corticosteroids if meningeal involvement or mediastinal edema are present. Recommended therapy is ciprofloxacin 400 mg intravenously bid or doxycycline 100 mg intravenously bid. Until the patient is clinically stable, one to two additional agents should be added, including clindamycin, vancomycin, imipenem, meropenem, chloramphenicol, penicillin, ampicillin, rifampin, and clarithromycin. Therapy should be continued after an initial response, with either ciprofloxacin or doxycycline for at least 60 days. Postexposure prophylaxis can be done with ciprofloxacin or, alternatively, doxycycline or amoxicillin for a total of 60 days.

Diagnostic Evaluation

Because of limited yield, extensive diagnostic testing is not indicated for most CAP patients. However, certain tests can help to determine the severity of illness and presence of extrapulmonary complications. Blood cultures are positive in only 15% of patients, but provide both therapeutic and prognostic information. Controversy about the value of sputum Gram stain and culture continues, but a sputum culture alone is not a reliable way to identify the etiologic pathogen for CAP. It is clear that if diagnostic testing is performed, it should be done promptly, as delaying antibiotic administration for >4 h after coming to the hospital is associated with increased mortality. Sputum culture should be reserved for situations in which an unusual or drug-resistant pathogen is suspected, particularly if the patient has not responded to initial empiric therapy. There are several limitations regarding the use of the Gram stain: Not all patients are able to produce an adequate specimen (>25 polys per low power field, <10 squames per low power field); the stain is often interpreted by technicians who are unfamiliar with the clinical circumstances; and results are often negative if the patient has taken antibiotics. In addition, a Gram stain can be either sensitive or specific, but not both; if used, it should probably be for its specificity. The finding of any Gram-positive diplococcus is very sensitive for finding samples that will grow pneumococcus, but the finding is not very specific. On the other hand, the finding of a predominance of Gram-positive diplococci, is more specific, but of course less sensitive.

An extensive diagnostic evaluation can also be useful when an unusual pathogen (*eg*, an endemic fungus, *C psittaci*) is suspected. Serologic testing is not routinely indicated, and should be reserved for nonresponding patients and for epidemiologic studies. Most serologic tests are positive when there is a fourfold rise in titer; this necessitates the collection of convalescent titers, as acute testing is rarely positive. Bronchoscopy and transtracheal aspirates are not usually indicated for CAP patients, but are of value in HIV-positive or other immunosuppressed patients. Patients with severe CAP often undergo an extensive diagnostic evaluation, but studies have not shown a benefit from having a specific etiologic diagnosis. When a patient with CAP is not responding to initial empiric therapy, a re-evaluation is needed, directed at identifying noninfectious processes that mimic pneumonia, unusual or drug-resistant organisms, and both infectious and noninfectious complications of pneumonia. Diagnostic studies in this setting may include bronchoscopy with cultures, CT scanning of the chest, and possibly open lung biopsy; the latter has its greatest value if a noninfectious process is suspected (bronchiolitis obliterans with organizing pneumonia, pulmonary vasculitis, etc).

The classification of the clinical presentation into "typical" and "atypical" patterns is generally of little use for predicting the microbial etiology. Not only are the clinical features caused by specific organisms not diagnostic, but infection with some organisms, such as Legionella, leads to a clinical picture that overlaps both patterns. Clinical features usually do not accurately predict etiology because certain patient populations, particularly the elderly and chronically ill, often have an inadequate response to infection. An elderly patient with a virulent bacterial CAP may present with confusion, incontinence, falling, or worsening of a comorbid illness, rather than with fever, respiratory symptoms, and other features of the "typical" pneumonia syndrome.

Therapy

Based on the likely organisms, therapy will differ for each of the patient subsets with CAP (Tables 2–3). Recent data show that atypical pathogen coinfection is common enough that all patients should be treated for these organisms, using either a quinolone alone or a macrolide added to a β-lactam. In general, trimethoprim-sulfamethoxazole is no longer a useful therapy because of the increased incidence of pneumococcal resistance to this agent. The new fluoroquinolones (levofloxacin, gatifloxacin, and moxifloxacin) are monotherapy options for complicated patients; they cover Gram-positive, Gram-negative, and atypical pathogens, and are active against penicillin-resistant or -sensitive pneumococci.

For hospitalized patients with nonsevere CAP, in the absence of cardiopulmonary disease and modifying factors (such patients are rarely admitted), an IV macrolide alone (such as azithromycin) (Table 2) should be used. For the hospitalized patient with cardiopulmonary disease and/or modifying factors, therapy should include a third-generation cephalosporin (cefotaxime, ceftriaxone) or ampicillin (ampicillin/sulbactam, high-dose ampicillin), combined with an oral or IV macrolide (or tetracycline) or, alternatively, with a new antipneumococcal quinolone alone (levofloxacin, gatifloxacin, moxifloxacin).

Patients with severe CAP (Table 3) should be considered for admission to an ICU, and they require a more aggressive therapeutic approach. Severe CAP has no uniform definition, but it is characterized by the presence of septic shock or the need for mechanical ventilation; alternatively, it is characterized by at least two of the following three: systolic BP < 90 mm Hg, Pao$_2$/fraction of inspired oxygen ratio <250, or multilobar pneumonia. Other criteria that suggest severe infection include respiratory rate >35/min, increase in the size of lung infiltrates by >50% in 48 h, oliguria, or acute renal failure. The role of the ICU in severe illness has been debated, but the ICU probably has its greatest value if used early in the course of severe disease.

Pathogens that lead to severe CAP are distinct, and slightly different from those seen in other populations; they include pneumococcus, Legionella, and enteric Gram-negative bacilli. Several studies have demonstrated that when initial empiric therapy was directed at these organisms and there was a prompt clinical response, outcome was better than if ineffective therapy was used. In these studies, identification of the pathogen has not led to an improved outcome, raising questions about the value of extensive diagnostic testing even in these critically ill patients. For patients with severe CAP, an IV macrolide or quinolone should be combined with additional agents, the type and number being dictated by the presence of pseudomonal risk factors (Table 3).

For hospitalized patients who improve with initial therapy, an early switch to oral antibiotics is appropriate, and may not only shorten length of stay, but also improve overall outcome. Criteria for early oral therapy include the absence of fever on at least two consecutive determinations, the absence of an unstable medical illness, a declining white blood cell count, improvement in cough and dyspnea, and the ability to take oral medications. In general, patients who receive effective therapy will improve in 48 to 72 h; the nonresponding patient should undergo an extensive diagnostic evaluation to identify unusual or drug-resistant pathogens, noninfectious mimics of pneumonia (vasculitis, bronchiolitis obliterans with organizing pneumonia), and complications of pneumonia. In the patient responding to therapy, radiographic resolution can be slow, with only 50% of a young, healthy population having radiographic clearing by 2 weeks. Slower resolution is seen in those with bacteremia, advanced age, multilobar involvement, or underlying chronic obstructive lung disease.

Vaccination

The mainstay of CAP prevention is vaccination with both the pneumococcal and influenza vaccines. Pneumococcal vaccine should be given to all patients over 65 years of age, and to patients, regardless of age, who have chronic heart, lung, or other medical illnesses. Patients who are asplenic, those who have a hematologic malignancy, and those with HIV infection should also be vaccinated. Hospital-based immunization with pneumococcal vaccine has been suggested for the majority of patients admitted for any diagnosis, because as many as 60% of all patients with CAP have been hospitalized for some reason in the preceding 4 years. The current Advisory Committee on Immunization Practices recommendation is to repeat pneumococcal vaccination after 5 years in patients who are likely to have had a rapid decline in antibody concentrations. These include patients with chronic renal failure, organ or bone marrow transplant recipients, and patients at risk for fatal infection, particularly those who are asplenic.

Influenza vaccination reduces hospital admissions and mortality rates if administered before an outbreak. Repeated influenza vaccination in elderly patients is both safe and effective in preventing influenza illness and its complications. In healthy adults, the influenza vaccine can reduce the incidence of upper respiratory illness; in a nursing home population, it can reduce hospitalization rates, pneumonia rates, and mortality. Antiviral therapy is used to supplement vaccination in immune-deficient patients; options include amantadine or rimantadine (active only against influenza A virus) and oseltamivir or zanamivir (active against influenza A and B). Antiviral therapy is indicated during an influenza outbreak in a closed environment (such as a nursing home) for all unvaccinated, high-risk persons for least 2 weeks after the late administration of vaccine. New studies with topical antiviral agents are promising, and these agents may have a role in the future.

Nosocomial Pneumonia

The incidence of nosocomial or hospital-acquired pneumonia (HAP) varies in relation to the concomitant comorbidity in a given patient population. While 10% of patients requiring ICU care after general surgery develop this infection, 20% of those who are intubated and up to 70% of those with ARDS will develop HAP. In critically ill, mechanically ventilated patients, the incidence of HAP is 1% per day during the first month of ventilation. However, because most patients are ventilated for short periods, up to half of all episodes of ventilator-associated pneumonia (VAP) occur within the first 4 days of ventilation (early-onset VAP). Recent data show that the risk of pneumonia is 3% per day in the first 5 days, 2% per day on days 5 to 10, and then 1% per day on days 10 to 15. The mortality rate of HAP can exceed 50% in mechanically ventilated patients, especially if the infection involves potentially resistant enteric Gram-negative organisms, such as P $aeruginosa$ and Acinetobacter organisms that are particularly common in patients who have received prior antibiotic therapy. Case-control studies in mechanically ventilated patients indicate that 50% of HAP patients die as a direct result of this infection, and not as a consequence of their underlying serious illness. One of the factors that adds to attributable mortality is the use of inadequate therapy, and this is more likely if patients are infected with antibiotic-resistant organisms.

Using the National Nosocomial Infections Surveillance system, the Centers for Disease Control and Prevention regularly collects data about nosocomial infections, and has reported the data collected between 1992 and 1997 in 112 medical ICUs in 97 hospitals throughout the United States, involving 181,993 patients. The most common infections by site were urinary tract (31%), pneumonia (27%), and primary bacteremia (19%), followed by all other infections. The common sites of infection were often device-related, with 87% of bacteremias associated with central lines, 86% of pneumonias with mechanical ventilation, and 95% of urinary tract infections with urinary catheters. The most common pathogens for primary bacteremia were coagulase-negative staphylococci (36%), enterococci (16%), and S $aureus$ (13%). Central-line infections were especially associated with coagulase-negative staphylococci. With nosocomial pneumonia, Gram-negative organisms predominated (64%); P $aeruginosa$ was most common (21%), followed by Enterobacter (9%), K $pneumoniae$ (8%), and Acinetobacter (6%). S $aureus$ was present in 20% of nosocomial pneumonia episodes. In VAP, Pseudomonas and Acinetobacter were most common, while $Escherichia$ $coli$ was more common in nonventilated patients. Many of the common Gram-negative and Gram-positive pathogens are antibiotic resistant, with as many as half of S $aureus$ being methicillin-resistant. Not surprisingly, the overall nosocomial infection rate correlated with average length of stay and device use. The pooled mean rate of VAP was 6.5 per 1,000 ventilator days. There was no association between device-associated infection rates and number of hospital beds, number of ICU beds, or length of stay.

Pathogenesis and Risk Factors

Patients usually develop HAP because of impaired host defenses and the consequent inability to contain encountered bacteria. In other patients, HAP develops because bacteria in the ICU environment are sufficiently numerous or virulent to overcome either normal or impaired host defenses. Recognized risk factors for HAP include patient-related conditions, therapeutic interventions, and factors related to infection control. Patient factors predisposing to HAP include the primary critical illness (shock, sepsis, extrapulmonary infection, respiratory failure) and underlying comorbid illness (diabetes, azotemia, COPD, central nervous system dysfunction, recent surgery).

Therapeutic interventions that increase HAP risk include sedatives, corticosteroids, cytotoxic agents, antacids, antibiotic therapy, enteral feeding, and especially endotracheal intubation. Patients can be exposed to large numbers of bacteria via the endotracheal tube, which itself can harbor a bacterial biofilm or serve as a conduit from a colonized oropharynx. In addition, secretions pooling above the endotracheal tube cuff often contain bacteria that can be aspirated into the lung. Proper attention to cuff pressure can minimize the leaking of secretions around the endotracheal tube cuff. Even though endotracheal tubes are often contaminated with organisms, they should not be routinely changed, as reintubation itself serves as a pneumonia risk. An exception may be replacement of a nasotracheal tube with an orotracheal tube; nasal tubes promote nosocomial sinusitis, a source of pathogens for HAP. The duration of mechanical ventilation is related to the risk of VAP, but that risk is greatest in the first 5 days of intubation and falls progressively as ventilation is continued. With the advent of noninvasive ventilation to manage respiratory failure, pneumonia has been less common in patients managed with this modality than with mechanical ventilation and endotracheal intubation.

Nosocomial sinusitis has been identified in the past as a risk factor for nosocomial pneumonia, and now an intervention study demonstrates that aggressive diagnosis and treatment of sinusitis can prevent pneumonia and mortality. In a study, 399 intubated patients, expected to be ventilated for >7 days, were enrolled and randomly assigned to an intervention group that had a systematic search for sinusitis when fever was present or to a control group that did not. Surprisingly, *all* patients were nasotracheally intubated, and all gastric tubes were nasally inserted, a practice that should be questioned given the data in this study and other before it. There were 199 patients in the intervention group, and whenever fever was present, the protocol required sinus CT scans at days 4 and 8 after intubation and then every 7 days. If radiographic sinusitis was present, a transnasal culture was obtained, and sinusitis was diagnosed if cultures showed >1,000 organisms/mL. Patients with sinusitis were treated with antibiotics and sinus lavage every 8 h. Nosocomial pneumonia was diagnosed in all patients by the finding of a new infiltrate and a positive culture from protected specimen brushing. The authors found that 110 of the 199 study patients had radiographic sinusitis, and 80 fulfilled microbiologic and clinical criteria for sinusitis. VAP occurred in 37 of 199 intervention patients (23 with sinusitis, 14 without) and 51 of 200 control patients (p = 0.02). Of the 23 patients with both VAP and sinusitis, the pneumonia occurred at the same time as the sinusitis or later in 16, and with the same organism in 43%. Interestingly, the mortality rate in the intervention group (36%) was significantly lower than the mortality in the control group (46%), suggesting that aggressive diagnosis and therapy of sinusitis can have a favorable impact on patient outcome. When the data are examined for the relationship between VAP and sinusitis, the finding was that VAP occurred in 29% of those with sinusitis (23/80) and in only 12% without sinusitis (14/119). One methodologic issue with the study is that nasal tubes were used, and if sinusitis was diagnosed, they were not removed. Therefore, it is unclear how valuable this protocol is for an ICU that does not use nasotracheal tubes.

The stomach's role in HAP pathogenesis is uncertain. Elevation of gastric pH by antacids, H_2 antagonists, or enteral feeding can lead to gastric overgrowth by enteric Gram-negative bacteria. However, the frequency with which these organisms lead to pneumonia is uncertain. Some, but not all, studies in critically ill patients show reduced HAP rates when sucralfate is used for intestinal bleeding prophylaxis instead of antacids or H_2 antagonists. Many factors influence whether gastric contents reach the lung, including increased reflux in the supine position or with enteral feeding tube placement in the stomach rather than the small bowel, gastric volume, and nasogastric tube diameter.

Infection-control risk factors for HAP include the failure to routinely use handwashing or isolation of resistant pathogens, and the use of contaminated respiratory therapy equipment. Respiratory therapy equipment does not commonly bring bacteria to the lung. Even if ventilator circuits are changed as infrequently as once a week, or are never changed, HAP risk is not increased.

Bacteriology

All HAP patients are at risk for infection with a core group of organisms, including nonresistant enteric Gram-negative organisms (Enterobacter, *E coli*, Klebsiella, Proteus, and *Serratia marcescens*), *H influenzae*, methicillin-sensitive *S aureus*, and *S pneumoniae*. These organisms are particularly likely if no unusual risk factors are present, and if the pneumonia begins within the first 5 days of hospitalization (early-onset HAP) (Table 5). When risk factors are present, or if the pneumonia begins on day 5 or later (late-onset HAP), the likely pathogens change. In addition to the core organisms, patients with witnessed aspiration are also at risk for anaerobes; those with coma, head injury, or diabetes are especially at risk for *S aureus* infection; those with a prolonged ICU stay, prior antibiotics, corticosteroids, malnutrition, or structural lung disease are at risk for *P aeruginosa* and Acinetobacter; and those who have had a prolonged ICU stay and prior antibiotics are also at risk for methicillin-resistant *S aureus* (MRSA) (Table 6). When HAP is severe, in the presence of risk factors, or if it is of late onset, resistant Gram-negative organisms and MRSA are particularly likely (Table 7).

In the setting of severe pneumonia, drug-resistant organisms are likely, particularly if the patient has been treated with antibiotics, corticosteroids, and prolonged ventilation. These resistant organisms include Gram-negative pathogens as well as MRSA. MRSA is an increasingly common pathogen causing VAP, and is more likely in patients who have received prolonged ventilation and prior antibiotics.

One group of organisms that is of unclear significance in VAP is anaerobes, and now a careful bronchoscopic study has found that these organisms almost never are involved in this infection. In this study, protected specimen brushing and BAL were performed in 143 patients with 185 episodes of suspected VAP, and in 25 patients with aspiration pneumonia who were receiving mechanical ventilation. A total of 63 of 185 suspected episodes and 12 of 25 aspiration patients met microbiologic criteria for pneumonia. The organisms included common Gram-negative and Gram-positive organisms, but an anaerobic organism was isolated from only one patient in the entire group. The authors concluded from these findings that routine anaerobic therapy is not needed in ventilated patients with VAP or aspiration pneumonia.

Diagnosis and Treatment

The clinical diagnosis of HAP is made when a patient has a new or progressive lung infiltrate plus at least two of the following: fever, purulent sputum, or leukocytosis. This clinical definition is

Table 5. *Initial Empiric Antibiotic Therapy for Hospital-Acquired Pneumonia in Patients With No Known Risk Factors for Multidrug-Resistant Pathogens*

Potential Pathogens	Recommended Therapy*
• *Streptococcus pneumoniae*[†]	Ceftriaxone
• *H influenzae*	OR
• Methicillin-sensitive *S aureus*	Levofloxacin, moxifloxacin
• Antibiotic-sensitive enteric Gram-negative bacilli	or ciprofloxacin
• *E coli*	OR
• *K pneumoniae*	Ampicillin/sulbactam
• Enterobacter species	OR
• Proteus species	Ertapenem
• *S marcescens*	

* Levofloxacin or moxifloxacin are preferred to ciprofloxacin, and the role of other new quinolones, such as gatifloxacin, is not established.
[†] The frequency of penicillin-resistant *S pneumoniae* (PRSP) and multidrug-resistant (MDR) *S pneumoniae* is increasing.

Table 6. *Initial Empiric Therapy for Hospital-Acquired Pneumonia, Ventilator-Associated Pneumonia, and Health-Care-Associated Pneumonia in Patients With Risk Factors for Multidrug-Resistant Pathogens*

Potential Pathogens	Combination Antibiotic Therapy
• Pathogens listed in Table 3 • *Legionella pneumophila** • MDR Pathogens 　• *P aeruginosa* 　• *K pneumoniae* (ESBL+)* 　• *Acinetobacter* species* 　• Methicillin-resistant *S aureus* (MRSA)	Antipseudomonal cephalosporin (cefepime, ceftazidime) OR Antipseudomonal carbapenem (imipenem or meropenem) OR β-lactam, β-lactamase inhibitor (piperacillin-tazobactam) PLUS Antipseudomonal fluoroquinolone* (ciprofloxacin or levofloxacin) OR Aminoglycoside (amikacin, gentamicin, or tobramycin) PLUS Linezolid or vancomycin (If MRSA risk factors are present or there is a high incidence locally)

* If an ESBL + strain, such as *K pneumoniae*, or an *Acinetobacter* species is suspected, a carbapenem is a reliable choice. If *L pneumophila* is suspected, the combination antibiotic regimen should include a macrolide (*eg*, azithromycin) or a fluoroquinolone (*eg*, ciprofloxacin or levofloxacin), rather than an aminoglycoside.

Table 7. *Risk Factors for Multidrug-Resistant Pathogens Causing Hospital-Acquired Pneumonia, Health-Care-Associated Pneumonia, and Ventilator-Associated Pneumonia*

- Prior antimicrobial therapy in preceding 90 days
- Current hospitalization of >5 days
- High frequency of antibiotic resistance in the community or in the specific hospital unit
- Presence of risk factors for HCAP:
  - Hospitalization for >2 days in the preceding 90 days
  - Residence in a nursing home or extended care facility
  - Home infusion therapy (including antibiotics)
  - Chronic dialysis within 30 days
  - Home wound care
  - Family member with multidrug-resistant pathogen
- Immunosuppressive disease and/or therapy

sensitive, but other disease processes may be misdiagnosed as HAP. The differential diagnosis includes congestive heart failure, atelectasis, pulmonary infarction, and inflammatory diseases (such as acute lung injury). In addition, many patients who have VAP can have coexisting infections including sinusitis, intra-abdominal infection, and central line infections.

The overdiagnosis of HAP is a particular concern in mechanically ventilated patients. Quantitative cultures of respiratory secretions, obtained bronchoscopically or with a blind catheter or brush insertion, have been used to define whether pneumonia is present. This approach is controversial because it relies on defining a microbiologic "threshold concentration" in respiratory secretions, above which pneumonia is diagnosed. Early forms of pneumonia may go undiagnosed with this approach, and there are technical problems involved in collecting samples and interpreting results, especially in patients who are concurrently receiving antibiotics. The impact of these procedures on the outcome of patients with VAP has been addressed by a number of studies. In these studies, bronchoscopy has not always had a benefit, but if a benefit was present, it was seen in populations that often received inadequate antibiotic therapy, due to a high frequency of drug-resistant organisms. Although bronchoscopy has been reported to lead to fewer patients getting antibiotics and to less antibiotic resistance than when management relies on clinical tools, not all studies have found this. In fact, in one study, similar benefits were seen when the clinical pulmonary infection score was used to decide whether to continue empiric antibiotic therapy after observing the patient's clinical course for 3 days during therapy. If quantitative cultures are not collected, the etiologic pathogen can still be identified in intubated patients (along with other colonizing, but not infecting, organisms), by collecting tracheal aspirates for culture. The role of expectorated or suctioned sputum cultures in nonintubated patients is controversial.

One thing that has become clear in studies of VAP is that initial antibiotic therapy must be accurate in order to assure the best possible outcome. If therapy is not accurate (and invasive methods may delay the initiation of therapy, and maybe even appropriate therapy), then outcome is poor, even if microbiologic data become available and explain why the initial therapy was incorrect. Thus, initial therapy is usually empiric and based upon the suspected etiologic pathogens (Tables 5–6). In the new guidelines for HAP, patients with VAP and health-care-related pneumonia are included. Therapy falls into two categories: patients at risk for multidrug-resistant pathogens and those who are not. The only patients not at risk are those who have early-onset infection and have not recently received antibiotics, hospitalization, or any exposure to a health-care environment (*eg*, dialysis, nursing home). Table 7 gives the definitions of health-care-related pneumonia. Many patients can be treated with a single broad-spectrum agent, but certain resistant organisms require combination therapy. Monotherapy can be used in patients with non-ICU HAP and in those who do not have special risk factors, and it can be used in the ICU patient with early-onset infection and no special risk factors. Combination therapy is superior to monotherapy for bacteremic *P aeruginosa* infection and should be used in this setting. For nonbacteremic *P aeruginosa* infection, combination therapy is often used to prevent the emergence of resistance during therapy, but the optimal combination regimen has not been defined, and the addition of an aminoglycoside to a β-lactam agent may have little benefit. However, current practice is to use combination therapy in an effort to prevent resistance in patients with severe, late-onset HAP, or in those who have severe, early-onset HAP in the presence of certain risk factors; however, more data supporting the efficacy of this approach are needed. Combination therapy can involve an antipseudomonal β-lactam with either an aminoglycoside or ciprofloxacin; the latter may be preferable because of its excellent penetration into respiratory secretions and because of the limited efficacy and enhanced renal toxicity associated with aminoglycosides. Stepdown to monotherapy may be appropriate if *P aeruginosa* or another highly resistant pathogen is not isolated from the tracheal aspirate of an intubated patient. This stepdown can be viewed as on type of de-escalation therapy—a strategy that involves initial empiric therapy with broad-spectrum agents but then focuses on a more narrow therapy, after the culture results and the clinical response to therapy are known. Agents that can be used as monotherapy for severe pneumonia not caused by a drug-resistant organism include ciprofloxacin (400 mg q8h), imipenem (1 g q8h), meropenem, cefepime, levofloxacin (750 mg), and piperacillin/tazobactam (P/T). If patients have risk factors for MRSA (see "Bacteriology," above), it may be necessary to add coverage for this organism pending the results of tracheal aspirate cultures. This is especially the case if the tracheal aspirate Gram stain shows Gram-positive organisms. Therapy for MRSA can involve vancomycin or one of its alternatives, such as linezolid or quinupristin/dalfopristin. Recent data have suggested that for proven MRSA as a cause of VAP, linezolid may be superior to vancomycin in reducing mortality.

In two recent studies, P/T was an effective monotherapy for HAP. In the first study, P/T (3 g/375 mg q4h) was compared with ceftazadime; each study arm was given tobramycin, which could be discontinued after respiratory culture results were known. A total of 300 patients were enrolled, with 136 clinically evaluable. The P/T group had a significantly higher clinical success rate (74% vs 50%), higher frequency of eradication of baseline pathogens (66% vs 38%), and lower mortality (7.7% vs 17%) than the ceftazadime group. The patients generally did not have severe illness (only 20% had severe illness), and the need to use antibiotics every 4 h is somewhat limiting. However in a second study a dose of 4.5 g of P/T three times daily was used, and approximately 50% of the study group were mechanically ventilated patients. The mean APACHE (acute physiology and chronic health evaluation) II score in this study was 14.7. P/T was compared with imipenem, and it was associated with significantly more success and fewer failures, greater success against P aeruginosa (90% vs 50%), and fewer episodes of P aeruginosa resistance during therapy, even when used as a monotherapy regimen. These data suggest that P/T can be used in mechanically ventilated patients as monotherapy for severe HAP, adding it to a list that includes a number of other agents.

One important trend in therapy is to reduce the duration of therapy to as short as 7 days. This may be possible in VAP if the patient has received an initially appropriate therapy, if there is a prompt clinical response (particularly improvement in the Pao_2/Fio_2 ratio), and if the infection is not due to P aeruginosa.

Prevention

Attention to pneumonia risk factors and infection-control efforts are the most effective preventive strategies. Recently, a specially adapted endotracheal tube that allows for the suction of subglottic secretions pooled above the endotracheal tube cuff has been shown to prevent some episodes of HAP. Prophylactic antibiotics, either as an aerosol or as part of a selective digestive decontamination strategy, do not lead to a reduction in mortality and raise concerns about the emergence of resistant pathogens. Such uses of antibiotics are experimental and should not be carried out in routine clinical practice.

Annotated References

CAP

Davidson R, Cavalcanti R, Brunton JL, et al. Resistance to levofloxacin and failure of treatment of pneumococcal pneumonia. N Engl J Med 2002; 346:747–750

Duchin JS, Koster FT, Peters CJ, et al. Hantavirus pulmonary syndrome: a clinical description of 17 patients with a newly recognized disease. N Engl J Med 1994; 330:949–955

This report describes the clinical and pathologic findings of the first 17 patients with the hantavirus pulmonary syndrome.

The mean age of patients was 32.2 years. The case fatality rate was 76%, with 88% developing rapidly progressive, noncardiogenic pulmonary edema. Most patients had fever, myalgias, cough, or dyspnea, along with GI symptoms and headache. Although hantavirus is not a new organism, this is the first description of a pulmonary syndrome resulting from this agent.

El-Solh AA, Pietrantoni C, Bhat A, et al. Microbiology of severe aspiration pneumonia in institutionalized elderly. Am J Respir Crit Care Med 2003; 167:1650–1654

Prospective microbiologic evaluation of elderly patients with severe CAP admitted to the ICU from a nursing home in the setting of risk factors for aspiration. The predominant organisms were Gram-negative and not anaerobes, and, even when anaerobes were identified, specific antibiotic therapy did not appear to be necessary.

Ewig S, Ruiz M, Mensa J, et al. Severe community-acquired pneumonia: assessment of severity criteria. Am J Respir Crit Care Med 1998; 158:1102–1108

Although the original ATS guidelines for CAP defined an entity termed "severe CAP," recent observations have suggested that this definition was overly inclusive, and that many patients who fit the definition did not actually need ICU admission. In this study of 395 patients, a modified rule for severe illness was derived from the ATS definition, because that definition (using only a single criterion for severe illness) had a specificity of only 32%. The modified rule defined the need for ICU admission as the presence of two of three "minor" criteria (systolic BP < 90 mm Hg, multilobar infiltrates, Pao_2/fraction of inspired oxygen ratio <250) or one of two "major" criteria (need for mechanical ventilation or septic shock). This modified definition had a sensitivity of 78% and a specificity of 94%, and a negative predictive value of 95%.

Feikin DR, Schuchat A, Kolczak M, et al. Mortality from invasive pneumococcal pneumonia in the era of antibiotic resistance, 1995–1997. Am J Public Health 2000; 90:223–229

Fine MJ, Auble TE, Yealy DM, et al. A prediction rule to identify low-risk patients with community-acquired pneumonia. N Engl J Med 1997; 336:243–250

Fine MJ, Smith MA, Carson CA, et al. Prognosis and outcomes of patients with community-acquired pneumonia: a meta-analysis. JAMA 1996; 275:134–141

A meta-analysis of factors predicting mortality in CAP was conducted, using 137 references and examining 33,148 patients in 127 study cohorts. The data provide an excellent view of the epidemiology of CAP, broken down into relevant outpatient and inpatient subsets. The predictors of mortality are identified and the impact of bacteriology on outcome is reported. By virtue of the number of patients examined, this report is a state-of-the-art summary of the mortality impact of CAP and its determinants.

Houck PM, MacLehose RF, Niederman MS, et al. Empiric antibiotic therapy and mortality among Medicare pneumonia inpatients in 10 Western states: 1993, 1995, 1997. Chest 2001; 119:1420–1426

Kauppinen MT, Saikku P, Kujala P, et al. Clinical picture of Chlamydia pneumoniae requiring hospital treatment: a comparison between chlamydial and pneumococcal pneumonia. Thorax 1996; 51:185–189

Leroy O, Santre C, Beuscart C. A 5-year study of severe community-acquired pneumonia with emphasis on prognosis in patients admitted to an ICU. Intensive Care Med 1995; 21:24–31

Lieberman D, Schlaeffer F, Boldur I, et al. Multiple pathogens in adult patients admitted with community-acquired pneumonia: a one year prospective study of 346 consecutive patients. Thorax 1996; 51:179–184

The authors of this prospective study of 346 hospitalized patients with CAP in Israel found a surprisingly high incidence of atypical pathogen infection in the context of identifying an etiologic diagnosis in 80.6% of all patients, a far greater number than in many similar studies. The most commonly identified pathogen was pneumococcus, but M pneumoniae was found in 29.2%, C pneumoniae in 17.9%, and Legionella in 16.2%. The high frequency of atypical pathogens can be explained by the careful serologic testing done and by the fact that more than one pathogen was identified in 38.4% of the patients. Atypical pathogens were seen in patients of all ages, and C pneumoniae was found more in older patients than in those <55 years of age. The implications of these findings for therapy are uncertain, as only about half of the patients with atypical pathogens received specific therapy. One possible role of atypical pathogens that the authors discuss is as agents that potentiate the role of bacterial organisms.

Mandell LA, Bartlett JG, Dowell SF, et al. Update of practice guidelines for the management of community-acquired pneumonia in immunocompetent adults. Clin Infect Dis 2003; 37:1405–1433 Marston BJ, Plouffe JF, File TM Jr, et al. Incidence of community-acquired pneumonia requiring hospitalization: results of a population-based active surveillance Study in Ohio; The Community-Based Pneumonia Incidence Study Group. Arch Intern Med 1997; 157:1709–1718

Metaly JP, Schulz R, Li Y-H, et al. Influence of age on symptoms at presentation in patients with community-acquired pneumonia. Arch Intern Med 1997; 157: 1453–1459

Mundy LM, Auwaerter PG, Oldach D, et al. Community-acquired pneumonia: impact of immune status. Am J Respir Crit Care Med 1995; 152:1309–1315

In a 1-year prospective study, 385 patients with CAP were evaluated at an inner-city hospital. The study is unique because both HIV-infected and nonimmunosuppressed patients were evaluated and the impact of immune status on bacteriology was examined. In the 205 patients not infected with HIV, pneumococcus was the most common pathogen, while H influenzae, Gram-negative bacilli, and atypical pathogens were the next most frequently identified causes of CAP; no diagnosis was found in 37%. The distribution of pathogens was such that the authors concluded that the ATS guidelines for CAP were appropriate for the population that they treated, and they endorsed the selective (rather than routine) use of macrolide therapy for hospitalized patients with CAP.

Neill AM, Martin IR, Weir R, et al. Community-acquired pneumonia: aetiology and usefulness of severity criteria on admission. Thorax 1996; 51:1010–1016

Niederman MS, Mandell LA, Anzueto A, et al. Guidelines for the management of adults with community-acquired lower respiratory tract infections: diagnosis, assessment of severity, antimicrobial therapy and prevention. Am J Respir Crit Care Med 2001; 163:1730–1754

This document reviews the literature relevant to the management of CAP and presents an empiric approach to management based on an assesment of severity of illness, place of therapy (inpatient or outpatient), and the presence of cardiopulmonary disease and/or modifying factors. There is also a discussion of the bacteriology of CAP, the recommended approach to diagnostic testing, criteria for hospitalization and for admission to the ICU, and an approach to evaluating the patient who has not responded to initial empiric therapy.

Pallares R, Linares J, Vadillo M, et al. Resistance to penicillin and cephalosporin and mortality from severe pneumococcal pneumonia in Barcelona, Spain. N Engl J Med 1995; 333:474–480

The authors present the results of a 10-year prospective study of 504 adults with invasive pneumococcal disease in Spain, reporting an incidence of penicillin resistance approaching 30%. Factors associated with mortality were examined, and the authors found that penicillin resistance per se was not associated with an enhanced risk of dying. Adequate outcome was achieved, even for resistant strains, with the use of high-dose penicillin or with the use of cefotaxime or ceftriaxone.

Plouffe JF, Breiman RF, Facklam RR, et al. Bacteremia with Streptococcus pneumoniae: implications for therapy and prevention. JAMA 1996; 275:194–198

Ruiz M, Ewig S, Torres A, et al. Severe community-acquired pneumonia: risk factors and follow-up epidemiology. Am J Respir Crit Care Med 160:923–929, 1999
In this single center study of severe CAP, the etiologic pathogens were defined in 2 consecutive decades. In both time periods, pneumococcus was the most common pathogen, and atypical organisms were also identified in nearly 20% of all patients. However, the identity of the specific atypical pathogens varied over time, with Legionella spp predominating in one period and being replaced by Mycoplasma and Chlamydia in the other period.

Nosocomial Pneumonia

Campbell GD, Niederman MS, Broughton WA, et al. Hospital-acquired pneumonia in adults: diagnosis, assessment of severity, initial antimicrobial therapy, and preventative strategies: a consensus statement. Am J Respir Crit Care Med 1996; 153:1711–1725

Chastre J, Wolff M, Fagon JY, et al. Comparison of 8 vs 15 days of antibiotic therapy for ventilator-associated pneumonia in adults: a randomized trial. JAMA 2003; 290:2588–2598

Cometta A, Baumgartner JD, Lew D, et al. Prospective randomized comparison of imipenem monotherapy with imipenem plus netilmicin for treatment of severe infections in nonneutropenic patients. Antimicrob Agents Chemother 1994; 38:1309–1313

Fagon JY, Chastre J, Vaugnat A, et al. Nosocomial pneumonia and mortality among patients in intensive care units. JAMA 1996; 275:866–869
The authors evaluated 1,978 consecutive patients admitted to the ICU to define the incidence of nosocomial pneumonia and its impact on mortality by using a logistic regression model. Among the 16.6% of patients in whom pneumonia developed, mortality was 52.4%, compared with a mortality of 22.4% in patients without pneumonia. These data led the authors to conclude that pneumonia does lead to the death of critically ill patients, having an "attributable mortality," but the findings are not in agreement with the conclusions of other investigators and the controversy associated with this issue is discussed.

Fagon JY, Chastre J, Wolff M, et al. Invasive and noninvasive strategies for management of suspected ventilator-associated pneumonia: a randomized trial. Ann Intern Med 2000; 132:621–630

Hatala R, Dinh T, Cook DJ. Once-daily aminoglycoside dosing in immunocompetent adults: a metaanalysis. Ann Intern Med 1996; 124:717–725

Hilf M, Yu VL, Sharp J, et al. Antibiotic therapy for *Pseudomonas aeruginosa* bacteremia: outcome correlations in a prospective study of 200 patients. Am J Med 1989; 87:540–546

Hoffken G, Niederman M. Nosocomial pneumonia: the importance of a de-escalating strategy for antibiotic treatment of pneumonia in the ICU. Chest 2002; 122:2183–2196

Holzapfel L, Chastang C, Demingeon G, et al. A randomized study assessing the systematic search for maxillary sinusitis in nasotracheally mechanically ventilated patients: influence of nosocomial maxillary sinusitis on the occurrence of ventilator-associated pneumonia. Am J Respir Crit Care Med 1999; 159: 695–701

Ibrahim EH, Ward S, Sherman G, et al. Experience with a clinical guideline for the treatment of ventilator-associated pneumonia. Crit Care Med 2001; 29:1109–1115

Jaccard C, Troillet N, Harbarth S, et al. Prospective randomized comparison of imipenem-cilastatin and piperacillin-tazobactam in nosocomial pneumonia or peritonitis. Antimicrob Agents Chemother 1998; 42:2966–2972

Joshi M, Bernstein J, Solomkin J, et al. Piperacillin/tazobactam plus tobramycin versus ceftazadime plus tobramycin for the treatment of patients with nosocomial lower respiratory tract infections. J Antimicrob Chemother 1999; 43:389–397

Kollef M. Inadequate antimicrobial treatment: an important determinant of outcome for hospitalized patients. Clin Infect Dis 2000; 31(suppl 4):S131–S138

Kollef M, Shapiro SD, Fraser VJ, et al. Mechanical ventilation with or without 7-day circuit changes: a randomized controlled trial. Ann Intern Med 1995; 123:168–174
A randomized controlled trial of 300 mechanicallly ventilated patients admitted to an ICU for more than 5 days evaluated the routine changing of ventilator circuits every 7 days vs no routine changes. VAP, diagnosed using clinical criteria, occurred in 24.5% of patients receiving no routine changes and in 28.8% of patients receiving routine changes. Mortality rates were comparable in both groups, but the failure to routinely change tubing was associated with substantial cost savings.

Kollef MH, Sherman G, Ward S, et al. Inadequate antimicrobial treatment of infections: a risk factor for hospital mortality among critically ill patients. Chest 1999; 115:462–474

Kollef MH, Silver P, Murphy DM, et al. The effect of late-onset ventilator-associated pneumonia in determining patient mortality. Chest 1995; 108:1655–1662

Lowenkron SE, Niederman MS. Definition and evaluation of the resolution of nosocomial pneumonia. Semin Respir Infect 1992; 7:271–281

Luna CM, Vujacich P, Niederman MS, et al. Impact of BAL data on the therapy and outcome of ventilator associated pneumonia. Chest 1997; 111:676–685

Luna CM, Banzaco D, Niederman MS, et al. Resolution of ventilator-associated pneumonia: prospective evaluation of the clinical pulmonary infection score as an early clinical predictor of outcome. Crit Care Med 2003; 31:676–682

Marik PE, Careau P. The role of anaerobes in patients with ventilator-associated pneumonia and aspiration pneumonia: a prospective study. Chest 1999; 115:178–183

Niederman MS, Craven DE, Bonten MJ, et al. Guidelines for the management of adults with hospital-acquired, ventilator-associated, and healthcare-associated pneumonia. Am J Respir Crit Care Med 2005; 171:388–416

Niederman MS, Torres A, Summer W. Invasive diagnostic testing is not needed routinely to manage suspected ventilator-associated pneumonia [editorial]. Am J Respir Crit Care Med 1994; 150:565–569

This editorial critically reviews the literature relevant to the use of invasive methods (bronchoscopic lavage and brushing) for the diagnosis of VAP. The authors conclude that invasive methods should not replace clinical judgment in deciding when to use antibiotics for supected nosocomial pneumonia. Problems with invasive methods include the possibility of overlooking early forms of infection and the inaccuracy of the methods in patients who are already receiving antibiotics. An opposing editorial opinion accompanies this article and argues in favor of invasive methods.

Prod'hom G, Leuenberger P, Koerfer J, et al. Nosocomial pneumonia in mechanically ventilated patients receiving antacid, ranitidine, or sucralfate as prophylaxis for stress ulcer: a randomized controlled trial. Ann Intern Med 1994; 120:653–662

In a randomized controlled trial, intubated ICU patients were given intestinal bleeding prophylaxis with antacids (n = 81), a continuous infusion of ranitidine (n = 80), or sucralfate (n = 83). Bleeding rates were identical with each regimen (p >0.2), and the rates of early-onset nosocomial pneumonia were also similar. However, patients who received sucralfate had a markedly reduced incidence (5%) of late-onset pneumonia compared with patients who received other regimens (p = 0.022). The distinction between early- and late-onset pneumonia that was made in this study had implications for prevention strategies and also had relevance to bacteriology, with the pathogens responsible for each type of pneumonia being dramatically different.

Rello J, Sa-Borges M, Correa H, et al. Variations in etiology of ventilator-associated pneumonia across four treatment sites: implications for antimicrobial prescribing practices. Am J Respir Crit Care Med 1999; 160:608–613

Richards MJ, Edwards JR, Culver DH, et al: Nosocomial infections in medical intensive care units in the United States. Crit Care Med 1999; 27:887–892

Rouby JJ, Laurent P, Gosnach M, et al. Risk factors and clinical relevance of nosocomial maxillary sinusitis in the critically ill. Am J Respir Crit Care Med 1994; 150:776–783

A prospective study of 162 patients mechanically ventilated for >7 days evaluated the incidence of nosocomial sinusitis and the influence of inserting tracheal and gastric tubes through the nose rather than through the mouth. In patients who did not start out with radiographic maxillary sinusitis, the use of oral or nasal tubes was selected randomly. Those who had nasal tubes inserted had a 95.5% incidence of sinusitis, while those who had oral tubes had a 22.5% incidence of radiographic sinusitis. The relevance of sinusitis was shown by the finding that 67% of patients with bacteriologically confirmed infectious sinusitis also developed nosocomial pneumonia.

Sachez-Nieto JM, Torres A, Garcia-Cordoba F, et al. Impact of invasive and noninvasive quantitative culture sampling on outcome of ventilator-associated pneumonia. Am J Respir Crit Care Med 1998; 157:371–376

Singh N, Rogers P, Atwood CW, et al. Short-course empiric antibiotic therapy for patients with pulmonary infiltrates in the intensive care unit: a proposed solution for indiscriminate antibiotic prescription. Am J Respir Crit Care Med 2000; 162:505–511

Vallés J, Artigas A, Rello J, et al. Continuous aspiration of subglottic secretions in preventing ventilator-associated pneumonia. Ann Intern Med 1995; 122:179–186

In a randomized, controlled, and blinded study, 76 patients were managed with an endotracheal tube that allowed for the continuous aspiration of subglottic secretions (CASS), while 77 were managed with conventional endotracheal tubes. The use of CASS was associated with a significant (p < 0.03) reduction in the incidence of nosocomial pneumonia and a reduction in the number of infections due to Gram-positive cocci and H influenzae, but no difference in the number of infections caused by P aeruginosa or other resistant Gram-negative organisms. When pneumonia developed, it occurred later in CASS patients than in control patients. The simplicity of this method for pneumonia prevention is very appealing, and contrasts with other more complex and less effective methods, as pointed out in the accompanying editorial.

Notes

Bleeding in the ICU

Aryeh Shander, MD, FCCP

Objectives:

- Understand the normal components of clotting
- Understand the elements of making the diagnosis of disseminated intravascular coagulation
- Understand the causes of acquired thrombocytopenia in adults
- Understand the diagnosis of the complex coagulopathies in adults
- Understand the remedies available to treat adults with iatrogenic coagulopathy

Key words: disseminated intravascular coagulation; fibrinolysis; heparin-induced thrombocytopenia; massive transfusion

Coagulation and Fibrinolysis or Clotting

The current understanding of the coagulation system has changed considerably over the past decade. The classic separation of clotting cascade into the intrinsic and extrinsic pathways is recognized as artificial, and the symphony of clotting is complex but well integrated *in vivo*. New directions in research of coagulation focus on cellular activation and signaling systems that regulate factor activation.

Under normal conditions, blood flows through vessels that are lined with endothelial cells (probably the largest organ in our body) that maintain a balance between clotting and clot dissolution (fibrinolysis). Injury to the vascular wall results in vasoconstriction that reduces blood flow and prevents loss of large volume of blood. The exposed subendothelial tissue releases collagen and tissue factor activating both platelets and the available circulating clotting factors.

Formation of a platelet plug is the first step of clot formation. First, platelets adhere to the vulnerable surface. Second, platelet surface proteins are activated, and the release of signaling proteins and molecules summon more platelets to aggregate and complete the plug. Simultaneous to platelet adhesion, activation, and aggregation is the activation of the clotting cascade.

A simplified approach to the cascade is described in this section. Tissue factor and collagen activate circulating factor VII. This then activates factor IX. Both activated forms of VII and IX activate factor X (tenase). Xa and Va form an enzyme complex on the platelet surface that activates prothrombin to thrombin. Thrombin is responsible for the conversion of fibrinogen to fibrin. Fibrin, cross-linked by factor XIIIa, forms a complex and strong matrix with the platelet plug. Left unchecked, this system will propagate clot to the areas that would compromise vascular flow and nutrient delivery. Those unharmed and healthy vascular beds must be able to destroy clot formation, and they do so via three mechanisms: (1) tissue factor pathway inhibitor; (2) antithrombin; and (3) activated protein C system. In addition to the above, tissue plasminogen activator, secreted by the endothelium, binds to fibrin and converts plasminogen to plasmin, which lysis the additional clot beyond the needed size for repair. Once bleeding has stopped, the platelets release growth factors to complete the healing of the damaged vessels.

History of Bleeding in Evaluation of the Bleeding Patient

Familial clotting disorders are rare. Most families with serious coagulopathies, such as hemophilia A and B and von Willebrand disease, are identified in childhood, so that adults with new, severe factor deficiencies have almost always acquired these disorders by virtue of having antibodies to a key factor. Histories of lesser bleeding tendencies may be useful for identifying families with inherited disorders of platelet function. Individual bleeding histories are important: immediate bleeding following a surgical or traumatic incident is usually associated with platelet insufficiency or severe dysfunction; in contrast, factor deficiency bleeding is usually characterized by delayed onset of bleeding. Surface bleeding of the skin or mucosal tissues is most often associated with platelet problems, and deep visceral bleeding with clotting factors deficiencies. Combined coagulopathies will produce both types of bleeding. Bleeding requiring transfusion is significant only if transfusion is typically rare during these surgeries, such as after elective uncomplicated GI, gynecologic, or oral surgery. Histories should also include adult disease associated with bleeding tendencies, including renal disease, diabetes, hematologic conditions, cancer, and liver disease. Drug histories and drug allergies are equally important in evaluating for acquired coagulopathy.

Common Sense Principles

The importance of positive history and clarification of laboratory abnormalities cannot be over emphasized. Understanding the coagulation defect before bleeding begins helps the clinician in directing appropriate therapy. In general, the goals of treatment are twofold: restoration of the capacity to form adequate clot, and abatement of the underlying condition causing the coagulopathy. Prophylaxis is usually reserved for specific situations: inherited disorders of coagulation such as hemophilia A, and elective surgical events in severe coagulopathy. In order to achieve the first goal, that of restoring the normal capacity to clot, targets for therapy (either pharmacologic agents or clotting factors) should be set and monitored at a frequency sufficient for the clinical situation. If transfusion of products is necessary, transfusion therapy should be as selective as possible in order to minimize risk and antibody formation. Prevention of common causes of bleeding in the ICU, mucosal bleeding, either gastric or pulmonary (aggressive suctioning) should be employed.

Severe Combined Coagulopathy: Disseminated Intravascular Coagulation

Dilutional Coagulopathy and Fibrinolysis

Acquired combined coagulopathies are the most complex to diagnose and manage in critically ill adults. The two most common entities are dilutional coagulopathy (DC) and disseminated intravascular coagulation (DIC). In DC, with loss of two to three blood volumes during active resuscitation with a cellular fluid, coagulation factors can be diluted to 15 and 5% of normal, respectively. Because of similarity of laboratory findings in both conditions, confusion is common when diagnosis is attempted. In both syndromes, factors are either consumed or lost and both activated prothrombin time (aPT) and activated partial thromboplastin time (APTT) are prolonged. Platelet counts are reduced, and fibrinogen levels fall below acceptable range. With these disorders, no single diagnostic test is available, so it is often difficult to have a definitive diagnosis.

DIC results when the delicate balance of clotting and unclotting is completely disturbed throughout the vascular tree, usually brought on by some supraphysiologic stress to the clotting system. Of note is the interruption of normal endothelial activity with resulting microangiopathic disease giving rise to damaged circulating RBCs with the characteristics appearance of schistocytes on the peripheral smear. The diseases with which DIC is associated are listed in Table 1. A subacute

Table 1. *Causes of Acute and Chronic DIC*

Shock, any cause
Hypotension
Hypoperfusion
Infectious
    Gram-negative sepsis
    Severe other bacterial sepsis
    Severe viral or rickettsial infections
SIRS
Traumatic
    Crush injury
    Brush
    Brain injury
Ischemia
Anaphylaxis
Heatstroke
Snakebite
Obstetric (can be confused with consumption coagulopathy)
    Abruptio placentae
    Fetal demise
    Amniotic fluid embolism
    Sever eclampsia
Hemolytic transfusion reaction
Allograft rejection
Glomerulonephritis
Malignancy
Intravascular abnormalities
    Vascular prostheses
    Kasabach-Merritt syndrome
    Extracorporeal circulation

form of DIC is frequently seen in ICU patients, but this disease is not generally associated with diffuse uncontrolled bleeding and persistent abnormalities are seen with the full-blown disease.

The consequences of DIC are notable. Patients who have DIC have a high mortality in the ICU: >90% in most studies. Whether this is a reflection of the severity of their underlying illness or whether DIC itself causes excess mortality, or both, is not clear. Generation of excess thrombin activity results in diffuse clotting, and current thinking is that demonstrating this activity may be diagnostic of DIC. This high thrombin activity results in microscopic clots that are found in multiple organs at autopsy in patients who have died with DIC. Roger Bone has argued that this is a significant contributor to multiorgan failure in the critically ill patient, although detailed clinical trials of this question have not been done. Ten percent of patients with DIC present with large-vessel thrombosis rather than bleeding, although this reported prevalence may be underestimated.

In the presence of diffuse bleeding, the diagnosis of DIC is made by recognizing that the patient has a condition that predisposes to DIC. In addition, one needs to assess the presence of factors that are consumed during the clotting process and may have reached abnormal values at the time diagnosis is made.

Platelets are consumed by diffuse intravascular platelet aggregation. Because platelet production by the marrow is relatively slow, the marrow lacks the capacity to replace platelets promptly, and thrombocytopenia is one of the hallmarks of DIC. Fibrinogen is being rapidly converted to fibrin monomers by the action of excess thrombin, and so fibrinogen is similarly depleted as an acute-phase reactant, late in the early stages of DIC. Newer scoring systems such as shown in Table 2 were derised by the Japanese Association for Acute Medicine and have eliminated fibrinogen and added systemic inflammatory response syndrome (SIRS) criteria. Either system is acceptable. Liver replacement of the entire supply of fibrinogen in the plasma takes <24 h in a normally functioning liver, and thus fibrinogen deficiency occurs uniformly in DIC. Although factors V and VIII are also consumed in clotting, measurements are less frequently performed because the tests are more expensive.

Excess thrombin activity generates fibrinogen deficiency, but it has other effects that may be measured during DIC. The generation of fibrinopeptide A, a fragment that is cleaved away from fibrinogen by thrombin, may be measured. Fibrin monomers are normally produced in high local concentrations in physiologic clotting, and they polymerize spontaneously and are thus unmeasurable in the peripheral blood. However, during DIC, fibrin monomers are being generated throughout the vascular tree and their levels are evaluated in the peripheral blood. The aPT and aPTT are elevated in DIC.

Finally, it is possible to measure the effect of enhanced plasmin activity in DIC. This may be done indirectly, by measuring the loss of plasma α_2-antiplasmin, or directly, by measuring the products of cleavage of fibrin molecules to plasmin. The test that is most often used for this purpose is the d-dimer assay, a specific radiommunoassay for the unique product of cleavage of end-to-end polymers and much more specific then the older "fibrin split products" assay.

The diagnosis of DIC must be made by using several of these tests, looking at different aspects of DIC. Platelets, fibrinogen, aPT/aPTT, and d-dimers make up the most widely available panel of tests for DIC. When only two of four tests are suggestive of DIC, the diagnosis is correct by only approximately 65% of the time. Three of four tests raises the accuracy to >75%, and four of four tests to >90%. The results of DIC testing may also evolve over time, so that a fibrinogen level that is high at the onset

Table 2. *Adopted Japanese Association for Acute Medicine Scoring System*

Variables	Score
SIRS criteria	Total of 1 point
≥3	
0–2	
Platelet count (×10⁹L) decrease	Total of 4 points
Prothrombin time (value of patient/ normal value), s	Total of 1 point
≥1.2	
<1.2	
Fibrin/fibrinogen degradation products vs fibrinogen level, mg/L	Total of 4 points
≥25	
≥10 and <25	
>10	
Diagnosis	
Four points or more	DIC

Table 3. *DIC Clinical Scoring System**

Variables	Points
Platelets, per μL	
>10,000	0
50,000–100,000	1
<50,000	2
Prothrombin prolongation, s	
<3	0
3–6	1
>6	2
Fibrinogen level, mg/dL	
>100	0
<100	1
Lysis/thrombin excess marker	
Normal	0
Moderate increase	1
Strong increase	2

*Appropriate clinical setting and score ≥5 has positive predictive value of >90%.

of DIC may not fall into the abnormal level for many hours, but rapidly falling fibrinogen level in the presence of the other indicators of DIC may be a clue to the diagnosis. An international committee of the Society for Hemostasis and Thrombosis has proposed a rapid clinical scoring system for making the diagnosis of DIC that is displayed in Table 3. Newer revised scoring systems test for the diagnosis of DIC have been published. Table 2 is an example of the addition of systemic inflammatory response syndrome (SIRS) to the score. In this system, fibrinogen has been omitted and replaced with fibrin split products (Table 2).

Treatment of DIC

The treatment of DIC requires attention to the two principles of therapy outlined at the beginning of this article: stopping the cause and treating the hemostatic deficiencies. DIC that has a readily reversible cause, such as hemolytic transfusion reaction or fetal demise, may require no other therapy than the reversal of the underlying condition if the patient is otherwise healthy. But in a critically ill patient, DIC can be protracted because the cause is not readily reversible and the patient is not able to restore hemostatic factors rapidly. Comparison of three complex coagulopathies including laboratory test differentiating one from another are listed in Table 4.

Treatment

The treatment of diffuse coagulopathy can be divided into three parameters: (1) treatment of the underlying disorder, a simple task that is not readily available in many ICU patients; (2) supportive management of bleeding complications; and (3) treatment of the coagulation process. DIC treatment aimed at suppressing the coagulation process has been tried in a number of nonrandomized trials. The most frequently used product has been heparin, which has the advantage of acting, with antithrombin III, directly on thrombin. Heparin is always used when DIC is manifested by thrombosis; heparin may be used, with or without other agents, when DIC is protracted or very severe. Heparin may increase bleeding; if this happens, it must be discontinued. Heparin prophylaxis was formerly used for induction therapy in patients with acute promyelocytic leukemia; its routine use in this high-risk setting is now very controversial, as bleeding risk may actually be increased. Heparin is the agent of the choice for the treatment of chronic DIC associated with cancer. The use of low-molecular-weight heparin for such purposes has been reported but has not been standardized.

Antithrombin III and tissue factor pathway inhibitors have failed to perform effectively in randomized clinical trials in DIC. Other newly developed antithrombins have not been subjected to formal clinical trials in this setting.

In patients with DIC, heparin is most commonly administered by continuous IV infusion at an hourly dose typical for a patient of the same size with thrombosis. Loading doses are usually modified—either greatly reduced or omitted—in order to avoid peak heparin levels that can completely compromise clotting. The aPTT target should remain two to three times normal aPTT, not the patient's baseline aPTT. The underlying DIC process may be monitored by checking fibrinogen or platelet levels, as the aPTT will be affected by heparin. Some physicians advocate the simultaneous use of heparin and lysine analogues such as epsilonaminocaproic acid or tranexamic acid. Both drugs are administered on multidose or infusion schedules to ensure continuous levels and are stopped when the heparin is stopped. These agents are the primary therapy of fibrinolysis.

Table 4. *Comparison of Four Complex Coagulopathies: Laboratory Diagnosis*

Disorder	aPT	Fibrinogen	Platelets	Fibrin Degradation Products	D-Dimer	Factor
DIC	High	Low Low	High	Very high	Normal to low	Normal to high
Liver failure	High	Normal or low	Normal to low	High	Slightly high	Normal to high
Consumptive coagulation	High	Low	Low	High	Normal	Normal
Fibrinolysis	High	Low	Normal to high	High	High	

Transfusion therapy for DIC usually relies on two components: platelets and fibrinogen. RBCs may be necessary in order to replace whole blood loss. Platelets are ordinarily used in groups of 5 or 6 U, and are administered with the goal of achieving a platelet count >50,000/µL. This may be difficult to sustain when DIC is very brisk, and repeated transfusion over a 24-h period may be necessary. Fibrinogen is usually administered as cryoprecipitate because large quantities may be administered in small volumes. Plasma is rarely needed, especially since cryoprecipitate also contains factor VIII. Repeated transfusion may also be needed; the goal of transfusion therapy is a fibrinogen level >100 mg/dL.

Treatment of massive transfusion (DC) requires blood bank supplementation. Several clinical studies show that platelet deficiency occurs earlier during the course of DC, often levels of 1.0 to 2.0 of the patient's blood volumes, than does soluble factor deficiency. aPTs may become elevated to levels of international normalized ratio (INR) >1.5 without symptomatic bleeding occurring. Replacement therapy should be entertained while or after the cause of bleeding has been stopped. Empiric therapy in this situation is discouraged since assessment of coagulation status can be obtained rapidly in most if not all hospitals. Indications for component therapy are as follows: (1) platelet count <80,000 to 100,000; fresh frozen plasma, aPT of 0.5 times normal; cryoppt, fibrinogen level <100 g/dL; and recombinant factor VIIa, unknown.

Liver Failure

Coagulopathy due to factor deficiency as a result of liver failure may be difficult to distinguish from DIC. Liver failure results in low levels of circulating procoagulants manufactured by the liver. Fibrinogen deficiency may result, for example, although this factor is often present in adequate levels even when multiple other factors are not. Platelet numbers may be low as a result of hypersplenism or the effects of alcohol on marrow production. And the results of less specific tests of fibrinolysis, such as old fibrin split products test, may be elevated.

Patients having liver failure may also be candidates for DIC owing to clinical circumstances such as shock or sepsis. There are several ways to distinguish DIC from liver failure: d-dimer assays may be mildly elevated, but usually not to levels seen in DIC; and factor VIII, which is consumed during DIC, may be helpful because this factor is not liver dependent.

Treatment for diffuse bleeding in liver failure emphasizes platelet and plasma replacement. One must keep in mind that when diffuse bleeding is a result of failing liver, replacement therapy is temporary; unless transplantation is in the patient's future, death is eminent.

Acquired Vitamin K Deficiency

Vitamin K, a mixture of compounds primarily found in green and leafy vegetables, is well absorbed and is important in the carboxylation of glutamate residues on preprocoagulant factors manufactured in the liver. Vitamin K-related substances are also produced by enteric bacteria, so that patients are not often deficient except under the special circumstances of the ICU. Patients at high risk for acquired vitamin K deficiency include patients who are eating poorly before admission to the hospital, who are ordered to have nothing by mouth in the hospital, who are administered parenteral nutrition, and who are treated with broad-spectrum antibiotic coverage. Because vitamin K is not stored, these patients may experience rapid depletion of factors II, VII, IX, and X, and resulting prolongation of the aPT, and to a lesser extent the aPTT. aPTs, if not rechecked and patients not supplemented enterally or parenterally, may result in bleeding and be a surprise to clinicians, occurring within a few days of normal coagulation test results at admission. Treatment is also rapidly effective; because of the presence of preprocoagulant proteins, carboxylation may occur within hours, and coagulation may be restored within 12 to 24 h. Slower rates of correction of the aPT may be achieved by the use of oral low-dose vitamin K. However, if patients are having active, life-threatening bleeding, the use of prothrombin complex or plasma repletion may be necessary.

Acquired Platelet Disorders

Platelet disorders are secondary to reduced production, destruction, or dysfunction. Platelet production by the marrow is normally slower than that of neutrophils: platelets are completely replaced in an average healthy person every 7 to 10 days, so daily production of new platelets is 10 to 15% of the total number of platelets. Platelet production may be reduced by a variety of diseases and situations, including drugs and marrow toxins, marrow diseases, acute infections, and autoimmune processes. These are summarized in Table 5.

When platelet production is low, platelet counts fall gradually, although not necessarily to zero. Platelet support from the blood bank is indicated when levels fall to <10,000/µL because of the risk of spontaneous intracerebral hemorrhage. When patients are bleeding or require surgery, platelets may be transfused to achieve levels of >50,000/µL. Recovery cannot occur until the underlying cause has been effectively treated.

Platelet destruction is characterized by peripheral loss of platelets produced in presumably adequate numbers by the bone marrow. This consumption may be immune mediated, as in idiopathic thrombocytopenic purpura (ITP) or posttransfusion purpura, or nonimmune, as in burns and intravascular devices. Antibodies against platelet membrane antigens may be produced in a variety of settings. Autoimmune disorders may be accompanied by antibody-medicated destruction of platelets; systemic lupus is the most common of these. Platelets may be destroyed as bystanders by the antibodies generated against homologous

Table 5. *Causes of Thrombocytopenia*

Diseases
    Uremia
    Primary cancers of the marrow (leukemia, myeloma, lymphoma)
    Secondary cancers in the marrow (breast, prostate, genitourinary, GI, melanoma)
    Myelodysplasia
    Inflammatory diseases in the marrow (tuberculosis, histoplasmosis, etc)
    Immunologic diseases
    Viral infections
    Chronic alcohol ingestion
Drugs (abbreviated list)
    Heparinoids
    Anticancer drugs, radiation
    Antimicrobials
    Antiinflammatroy drugs
    Cardiac medication including diuretics
    Antiepileptic drugs including benzodiazepines
    Histamine type 2 antagonists
    Antidepressant drugs
    Sulfa drugs
    Antihistamines
    Iodinated contrast media
    Illicit drugs

platelets after transfusion: the resulting thrombocytopenia is transient and resolves spontaneously but may be quite severe, and is called posttranfusion purpura. Neonates may have purpura as a consequence of maternal antibodies. Most drug-related autoimmune thrombocytopenias resolve with the removal of the drug, as the antibody binds to the platelet only in the presence of the drug.

An increasingly common platelet abnormality is drug-induced dysfunction by platelet-inhibiting drugs used to treat vascular disease. These drugs can be divided into either adenosine diphosphate-induced aggregation inhibition or glycoprotein IIb/IIIa receptor inhibition. Risk of bleeding in the presence of any of these agents can increase by two folds.

Clinical Platelet Disorders

ITP is a disorder in which the stimulus to platelet antibody formation is unknown. ITP may be transient, as it is most often in children, or chronic and relapsing. Platelets "labeled" with antibodies are destroyed by the reticuloendothelial system. Therefore, transfusions result in rapid consumption of homologous platelets and are of little benefit. However, both rapid treatment of the disease process, usually with steroids as the initial therapy, combined with the use of large doses if IV Ig, may permit transfusion of homologous platelets when necessary. Chronic ITP may be treated with variety of forms of immunosuppression; splenectomy is quite useful in patients who have responded to steroid therapy.

Thrombotic thrombocytopenic purpura (TTP) is a different disorder caused by the inborn or the acquired deficiency of a plasma protease, in which abnormal platelet aggregation is the basic mechanism of thrombocytopenia. The normal relationship between platelet and endothelial surface, which does not permit aggregation to occur, is disrupted and multimers of von Willebrand factor, which appear to mediate this platelet-endothelial interaction, disappear from the circulation. Microvascular platelet aggregation results in intravascular hemolysis. The other attributes of the TTP syndrome include CNS abnormalities, renal dysfunction, and fever. The mortality of untreated TTP is high: >80% in the early series.

Approximately one half of patients presenting with TTP have an underlying autoimmune disease (thrombocytopenic purpura); many acquire chronic relapsing TTP after the initial episode. TTP may be caused by drugs, particularly by ticlopidine and clopidogrel. The hemolytic-uremic syndrome has a similar presentation with the exception of very little CNS involvement; it is more common in children and is thought to be a consequence of exposure to endobacterial toxins in most cases. Patients with hypertensive emergencies and other systemic vasculopathy may have platelet consumption and renal insufficiency and be difficult to distinguish from TTP unless an assay for the plasma protease activity can be obtained.

Patients with active phase of TTP will need to be admitted to the ICU. The wide differential diagnosis of sepsis syndrome or other serious illness needs to be considered. Distinguishing features of the laboratory abnormalities will consist of thrombocytopenia, a microangiopathic anemia, and no evidence of excess thrombin activity or fibrinolysis. A DIC screen is usually sufficient to make the distinction. TTP therapy is unique, and consists of plasmapheresis and/or plasma exchange. Chronic TTP may occur after the remission of the acute episode, and may be treated with aspirin, steroids, and other immunosuppressing drugs.

Platelet Function Abnormalities

A variety of disorders and drugs may produce platelet function abnormalities. Most of these are accompanied by easy bruising and mucosal surface bleeding, if they have any clinical manifestations at all. Concerns about platelet function arise in the setting of the elective surgical procedures and mild thrombocytopenia, in which the severity of bleeding seems greater than the platelet count would predict.

Aspirin and other nonsteriodal anti-inflammatory drugs interfere with platelet cyclooxygenase, and thus platelets are affected permanently. However, assuming normal platelet production, most patients will resume normal platelet (clotting) function within 24 h of stopping aspirin, and can undergo routine elective surgery. For surgery that involves significant blood loss, such as major vascular surgery, bypass surgery, and prostate surgery, aspirin should be discontinued 1 week prior to surgery.

Inhibitors of the platelet surface receptor IIB/IIIA widely used after angioplasty for prevention of restenosis are associated with significant bleeding. Most such bleeding is due to iatrogenic interventions such as insertion of the angioplasty catheter. The half-life of some of these agents is short, and only local measures may be needed to arrest bleeding. However, in the presence of longer acting agents major bleeding occurs, platelet transfusion may be necessary.

Uremia produces platelet dysfunction that is remediable with more intensive dialysis. Persistent platelet dysfunction in the face of adequate dialysis may require treatment: desmopressin may be used to rapidly and temporarily raise von Willebrand factor levels and improve platelet aggregation; so may cryoprecipitate. Infusions of high doses of conjugated estrogens will produce a similar and more sustained effect.

Bleeding Due to Anticoagulation or Thrombolysis

Heparin and Bleeding

One of the major hazards of all heparin therapy is bleeding. This can occur as a result of inadvertent accidental drug overdose or spontaneously.

Most bleeding episodes are associated with peak doses and very high partial thromboplastin times. If heparin reversal is needed, 1 mg of protamine will bind and reverse the effect of approximately 100 U of heparin. For low-molecular-weight and fractionated heparins, the use of factor VIIa is a consideration if reversal is absolutely needed.

Heparin-Induced Thrombocytopenia

As many as 10% of all patients receiving heparin therapy acquire mild reduction in platelet numbers (type I heparin-induced thrombocytopenia [HIT]). This reduction occurs in the first 2 to 5 days of treatment and is not associated with increased risk of bleeding and is self-limited. While this mild syndrome may complicate the assessment of bleeding, it is not necessary to withdraw heparin therapy. The most feared complication of heparin occurs slightly later in the course of the therapy, and is caused when IgG antibodies to the heparin-platelet surface complex (platelet factor 4) develop. These cause platelet aggregation, resulting in either severe thrombocytopenia or major vessel thrombosis or both. HIT (type II), as it is called, is a highly morbid complication, occurring in 1 to 3% patients receiving heparin and is much more common with the bovine preparation than the porcine preparation. Other than prior exposure to heparin, there are no known predictors of this syndrome. HIT is associated with diffuse thrombosis 30 to 50% of the time, and mortality may be as high as 30%. HIT occurs 4 to 10 days after therapy initiation and abates 2 to 5 days after heparin discontinuation. In an ICU patient with a sudden drop in platelet count and signs of thrombosis or both within days of starting heparin therapy, type II HIT should be strongly suspected, although SIRS and sepsis can confuse this diagnosis. In any event, heparin must be discontinued, and low-molecular-weight heparin should not be considered an alternative. If warfarin therapy has been started at the onset of the heparin usage, such patients may already be adequately anticoagulated and no further intervention is needed.

The diagnosis of HIT can be difficult in the ICU setting. An enzyme-linked immunosorbent assay to detect the presence of serum anti-heparin PF4 IgG is 99% sensitive but only 90% specific. Heparin-induced platelet activation and serotonin release assays confirming the enzyme-linked immunosorbent assay are available and are more specific but are difficult to perform.

Management of HIT type II in patients requiring anticoagulation requires the use of thrombin inhibitors. A direct thrombin inhibitor, such as argatroban, dadaparoid, or recombinant hirudin (lepirudin), may be used. Thrombolysis or thrombectomy of major clots are also an option. If patients have severe thrombocytopenia without thrombosis and require cessation of anticoagulation, evidence suggests that argatroban and lepirudin may be useful in preventing new thrombotic events. Reexposure to heparin must be avoided.

Bleeding in the Presence of Warfarin Therapy

Bleeding is a common complication of warfarin therapy, although use of the INR to gauge warfarin levels has lessened the risks of bleeding. Patients who bleed while receiving warfarin may be segregated into two groups: those who bleed with therapeutic INRs, and those who bleed with supratherapeutic INRs. Studies of underlying causes of warfarin-associated bleeding suggest that high-risk patients are most often those who have focal localized bleeding with therapeutic INRs. These patients should be closely evaluated to determine the cause of the bleeding. In patients who bleed while receiving supratherapeutic doses of warfarin, the drug should be discontinued; the patients may be more acutely treated with vitamin K and life-threatening bleeding should be treated with vitamin K and either prothrombin complex or fresh frozen plasma (for dose calculation, see previous chapter). Rat poison consists of coumarols with extremely long half-lives, usually days to weeks, and thus vitamin K therapy to reverse the bleeding must be administered at a very high dose and sustained for a very long time. Acute, life-threatening bleeding in such patients should also be treated with prothrombin complex or fresh frozen plasma. Closed-space bleeding (cerebral bleed) will respond to a dose of rVIIa with minimum dose of 40 mics/kg. In a randomized and controlled blinded trial, the use of VIIa in the treatment of intracerebral bleeds resulted in significantly smaller size of hematoma and better function if the drug was used within 4 h of symptom onset in patients receiving warfarin.

Bleeding Due to Thrombolytic Agents

Thrombolysis may be associated with pathologic bleeding for two reasons: the dissolution of existing clots, and the inhibition of further clotting. Both streptokinase and alteplase (tissue plasminogen activator) produce clot dissolution. This problem is usually seen primarily at recent venipuncture sites, and is treated with local pressure with good results. Both drugs have very short half-lives, and therefore this effect does not last long. Streptokinase produces hypofibrinogenemia, sometimes to near zero levels, and thus further clotting may not occur until fibrinogen is given. The usual source for this is cryoprecipitate, which is empiric, first-line therapy for a patient with life-threatening bleeding due to streptokinase. Both drugs may raise plasma levels of fragments of fibrin clot, which may inhibit further clotting to a slight extent and may inhibit platelet function as well. Therefore, protracted, severe bleeding (after fibrinogen therapy in streptokinase-treated patients) may be further treated by platelet administration or plasma administration, although the clinical results are not clear. Administration of heparin following thrombolysis may be accompanied by a further bleeding tendency; the choice to discontinue heparin use depends on the severity and persistence of the bleeding problem.

Comments

Tests for coagulation in the nonbleeding patient are not predictive of bleeding. Clearly, the risk of bleeding increases with prolonged clotting *in vitro*, but a phenotypic presentation that increases the risk of thrombosis in patients results in prolongation of the INR. The use of bleeding time as a predictor of bleeding has also been abandoned. What seems to be emerging as a better quantitative test is the thromboelastograph, which allows for whole-blood determination of clotting and lysing activity of the sample. As mentioned previously, the clinical picture prevails and the laboratory testing adds a second dimension.

Additional Reading

American Society of Anesthesiologists Task Force on Perioperative Blood Transfusion and Adjuvant Therapies. Practice guidelines for perioperative blood transfusion and adjuvant therapies. Available at: www.asahq.org/publicationsAndservices/practiceparam.htm#blood

Dzik WH. Emily Cooley lecture 2002: transfusion safety in the hospital. Transfusion 2003; 43:1190–1199

Fowler RA, Berenson M. Blood conservation in the intensive care unit. Crit Care Med 2003; 31(12 suppl): S715–S720

Shander A, Goodnough LT. Consensus recommendations for the off-label use of recombinant human factor VIIa (novo seven) Therapy. P&T 2005; 30:11

Shander A, Popovsky, M. Understanding the consequences of transfusion-related acute lung injury. Chest 2005; 128:598S–604S

Spiess BD, Spence RK, Shander A. Perioperative transfusion medicine: second edition. Baltimore, MD: Lippincott, Williams & Wilkins, 2006

Notes

Antibiotic Therapy in Critical Illness

Michael S. Niederman, MD, FCCP

Objectives:

- Review antibiotic pharmacokintetics
- Review principles of antibiotic action
- Review proper dosing of antibiotics
- Use pneumonia to demonstrate the principles of using antibiotics effectively

Key words: antibiotic control; antibiotic dosing; antibiotic mechanisms; antibiotic penetration; pharmacodynamics; pharmacokinetics

The treatment of severe pneumonia can be used as a paradigm to demonstrate the principles of antibiotic therapy of critically ill patients. The focus of this discussion will be on empiric antibiotic therapy, but the principles of antibiotic penetration and concentration in the lung are summarized in Table 1.

Mechanisms of Action

Antibiotics interfere with the growth of bacteria by undermining the integrity of their cell wall or by interfering with bacterial protein synthesis or common metabolic pathways. The terms *bactericidal* and *bacteriostatic* are broad categorizations, and may not apply for a given agent against all organisms, with certain antimicrobials being bactericidal for one bacterial pathogen, but bacteriostatic for another. Bactericidal antibiotics kill bacteria, generally by inhibiting cell wall synthesis or by interrupting a key metabolic function of the organism. They include the penicillins, cephalosporins, aminoglycosides, fluoroquinolones, vancomycin, rifampin, and metronidazole. Bacteriostatic agents inhibit bacterial growth, do not interfere with cell wall synthesis, and rely on host defenses to eliminate bacteria. They include the macrolides, tetracycline, sulfa drugs, chloramphenicol, and clindamycin. The distinction between these two types of agents may not be important in the therapy of lung infections, as either can be effective. When neutropenia is present, or if there is accompanying endocarditis, meningitis, or osteomyelitis, then the use of a bactericidal agent may be advantageous.

Antimicrobial activity is often described by the terms *minimal inhibitory concentration* (MIC) and *minimal bactericidal concentration* (MBC). The term MIC defines the minimum concentration of an antibiotic that inhibits the growth of 90% of a standard-sized inoculum, leading to no visible growth in a broth culture. The term MBC refers to the minimum concentration needed to cause a 3-log drop (99.9% killing) in the size of the standard inoculum. These terms must be interpreted cautiously and, if pneumonia is the infection being treated, the clinician must consider MIC and MBC data with a knowledge of how well an agent can reach the lung. The MIC is used to define the "sensitivity" of a pathogen to a specific antibiotic, under the assumption that the concentration required for killing can be reached *in vivo*, but lung concentrations may be substantially lower than serum concentrations, the latter being the site that is generally used to define antimicrobial susceptibility patterns.

The relationship of the serum concentration of an antibiotic, relative to the MIC of the target organism, can be used to define the likelihood of

Table 1. *Penetration of Antibiotics Into Respiratory Secretions*

Lipid-Soluble, Concentrate Independent of Inflammation, Good Penetration
 Quinolones
 New macrolides: azithromycin, clarithromycin
 Tetracyclines
 Clindamycin
 Trimethoprim/sulfamethoxazole
 Linezolid

Relatively Lipid-Insoluble, Inflammation-Dependent for Concentration in the Lung, Poor Penetration
 Aminoglycosides
 β-lactams
  Penicillins
  Cephalosporins
  Monobactams
  Carbapenems

bacterial killing. For some agents (β-lactams), killing occurs in a time-dependent fashion and is optimized in relation to how long the concentration exceeds the MIC of the target organism, and a minimum of 40% of the dosing interval is required. If, for these agents, serum concentration is increased further, it may not optimize killing, although there may be some additive benefit for serum concentrations up to four times the MIC. In theory, continuous infusion of these agents could optimize their efficacy. For other agents (quinolones, aminoglycosides), killing is concentration-dependent and, thus, is optimized in relation to how high the serum peak concentration is, relative to the MIC, or how high the area is under the concentration-time curve, which is then divided by the MIC value (AUC/MIC). These agents are optimally dosed with the entire daily dose being given once daily.

Penetration Issues

The concentration of an antibiotic in the lung depends on the permeability of the capillary bed at the site of infection (the bronchial circulation), the degree of protein binding of the drug, and the presence or absence of an active transport site for the antibiotic in the lung. In the lung, the relevant site to consider for antibiotic penetration is controversial and not clearly defined. Sputum and bronchial concentrations are considered most relevant for bronchial infections, while concentrations in lung parenchyma, epithelial lining fluid, and in cells such as macrophages and neutrophils are probably more important for pneumonic infections. The localization of the pathogen may also be important, and intracellular organisms such as *Legionella pneumophila* and *Chlamydia pneumoniae* are probably best eradicated by agents that achieve high concentrations in macrophages. Although local concentration of an antibiotic is important, it is also necessary to consider the activity of an agent at the site that it reaches. For example, antibiotics can be inactivated by certain local conditions. Aminoglycosides have reduced activity at acidic pH levels, and some pneumonic areas of lung are acidic. Bacteria can produce β-lactamase enzymes that can render a number of common penicillins and cephalosporins inactive. In addition, bacteria can become resistant to an agent (requiring that higher concentrations than are possible to achieve be present in order to be killed), because they become impermeable to antibiotic entry or modify the site to which the antibiotic must bind in order to be active.

Specific Antibiotics

β-Lactam Antibiotics

These bactericidal antibiotics have in common the presence of a β-lactam ring, which is bound to a five-membered thiazolidine ring in the case of the penicillins and to a six-membered dihydrothiazine ring in the case of the cephalosporins. Modifications in the thiazolidine ring can lead to agents, such as the penems (imipenem and meropenem), while absence of the second ring structure characterizes the monobactams (aztreonam). These agents can also be combined with β-lactamase inhibitors such as sulbactam, tazobactam, or clavulanic acid, to create the β-lactam/β-lactamase inhibitor drugs. These agents extend the antimicrobial spectrum of the β-lactams by providing a substrate for the bacterial β-lactamases (sulbactam, clavulanic acid, tazobactam), thereby preserving the antibacterial activity of the parent compound. β-lactam antibiotics work by interfering with the synthesis of bacterial cell wall peptidoglycans by binding to bacterial penicillin binding proteins.

The penicillins used for respiratory tract infections include natural penicillins (penicillin G and V), the aminopenicillins (ampicillin, amoxicillin), the antistaphylococcal agents, the antipseudomonal agents, and the β-lactam/β-lactamase inhibitor combinations. The antipseudomonal penicillins include the older carboxypenicillins (ticarcillin) and the ureidopenicillins (piperacillin, azlocillin, mezlocillin), with piperacillin and azlocillin being the most active agents against *Pseudomonas aeruginosa*. The β-lactamase inhibitor combinations include clavulanic acid with either amoxicillin or ticarcillin; sulbactam with ampicillin; and tazobactam with piperacillin.

The cephalosporins span from first to fourth generation. The earlier agents were generally active against Gram-positive organisms, but did not have extended activity to the more complex Gram-negative organisms or anaerobes, and were susceptible to destruction by bacterial β-lactamases. The newer-generation agents are generally more specialized agents with broad-spectrum activity and with more mechanisms to resist breakdown by bacteria. The second-generation and newer agents are resistant to bacterial β-lactamases. The third-generation agents active against penicillin-resistant pneumococci include ceftriaxone and cefotaxime, while ceftazidime is active against *P aeruginosa*. The third-generation agents, as mentioned above, may induce β-lactamases among certain Gram-negative organisms, and thus promote the emergence of resistance during monotherapy. The fourth-generation agent, cefepime, is active against pneumococci and *P aeruginosa*, but is also less likely to induce resistance among the Enterobacteriaceae than the third-generation agents.

Imipenem and meropenem are the broadest-spectrum agents in this class, being active against Gram-positive organisms, anaerobes, and Gram-negative organisms including *P aeruginosa*. They have shown efficacy for patients with severe pneumonia, both community-acquired and nosocomial, and may be effective as monotherapy, taking into account the caveats discussed above. Aztreonam is a monobactam that is so antigenically different from the rest of the β-lactams that it can be used in penicillin-allergic patients. It is active only against Gram-negative organisms, having a spectrum very similar to the aminoglycosides.

Fluoroquinolones

These bactericidal agents act by interfering with bacterial DNA gyrase, leading to impaired DNA synthesis, repair, transcription, and other cellular processes, resulting in bacterial cell lysis. DNA gyrase is one form of bacterial topoisomerase enzyme that is inhibited by the quinolones, but activity against other similar enzymes is part of the effect of a variety of quinolones. Quinolones kill in a concentration-dependent fashion, related to the peak concentration/MIC ratio and to the area under the curve/MIC ratio of drug concentration relative to organism susceptibility.

There are two features of quinolones that make them well-suited to respiratory infections. First, they penetrate well into secretions and inflammatory cells within the lung, achieving concentrations that exceed serum levels in many instances. Thus, these agents may be clinically more effective than predicted by MIC values.

Secondly, these agents are highly bioavailable with oral administration, and thus similar levels can be reached if administered orally or IV. This allows for some "borderline" patients (such as nursing-home patients) with pneumonia to be managed with outpatient oral therapy and not be admitted solely for the purpose of IV therapy to achieve high serum levels of antibiotics. In addition, the high bioavailability of these agents permits an easy transition from IV to oral therapy of inpatients with pneumonia, facilitating early discharge when the patient is doing well, and permitting ongoing oral therapy with maintenance of high serum levels of antibiotics.

Currently, the quinolones fall into several "generations." The first-generation agents had Gram-negative activity only and were used for urinary tract infections, epitomized by the agent nalidixic acid. The second-generation agents had added Gram-positive activity and could be used for systemic infections; they included ciprofloxacin, ofloxacin, pefloxacin, fleroxacin, and lomefloxacin. These agents had limited value for respiratory infections because of relatively high MIC values among pneumococci, making it necessary to use high doses to achieve efficacy against this pathogen. The third-generation agents are characterized by better Gram-positive activity, particularly against pneumococcus. These agents include levofloxacin, gatifloxacin, gemifloxacin, and moxifloxacin, which are currently available. Among the third-generation agents, the most active against pneumococcus is gemifloxacin, then moxifloxacin, followed by gatifloxacin and then levofloxacin. These new agents also have long half-lives, allowing once-daily dosing with most of the third-generation agents. In addition, quinolones that are active against pneumococcus are likely to be effective regardless of penicillin susceptibility patterns, because penicillin and quinolone resistance do not generally occur together in the same organisms, and pneumococcal resistance rates to new quinolones are low. However, some coexistence of quinolone resistance with penicillin resistance has been reported, and the most active pneumococcal agents (on an MIC basis) are the least likely to develop resistance. With this in mind, it is not surprising that there have been reports of failures of therapy for pneumococcal community-acquired pneumonia (CAP) using levofloxacin. When quinolones are used for severe CAP, the current recommendation is not to use them as monotherapy.

Aminoglycosides

These bactericidal agents act by binding to the 30S ribosomal subunit of bacteria, thus interfering with protein synthesis. Aminoglycosides have primarily a Gram-negative spectrum of activity and are usually used in combination with other agents targeting difficult organisms such as *P aeruginosa* or other resistant Gram-negative organisms. When combined with certain β-lactam agents, they can achieve antibacterial synergy against *P aeruginosa*. Amikacin is the least susceptible to enzymatic inactivation by bacteria, while tobramycin is more active than gentamicin against *P aeruginosa*. Aminoglycosides penetrate poorly into lung tissue, and can be inactivated by the acid pH levels that are common in pneumonic lung tissue. Thus, in one clinical trial of nosocomial pneumonia therapy, the use of an aminoglycoside with a β-lactam was no more effective than a β-lactam alone, and the combination regimen was not more effective in preventing the emergence of pseudomonal resistance during therapy than was the monotherapy regimen with a β-lactam. In the treatment of bacteremic pseudomonal pneumonia, aminoglycoside combination therapy may be more effective than monotherapy. In spite of these findings, one recent metaanalysis reported no benefit with the addition of an aminoglycoside to a beta-lactam in the treatment of serious infections, including pneumonia, and including infections caused by *P aeruginosa*.

Aminoglycosides kill in a concentration-dependent fashion, and can be given once daily to optimize killing while minimizing toxicity. In clinical practice, this has not been proven to occur, and once-daily dosing is comparable in efficacy and nephrotoxicity to regimens using multiple daily doses. When aminoglycosides are used, it is necessary to monitor serum levels to minimize the occurrence of acute renal failure. Peak concentrations correlate with efficacy, but have meaning only with multiple daily doses, and their utility in once-daily regimens has not been established. Trough concentrations are monitored to minimize toxicity and probably should be followed regardless of dosing regimen.

Because of poor penetration into tissues, some investigators have used nebulized aminoglycosides for the therapy and/or prevention of Gram-negative pneumonia. This approach has been effective in the treatment of infectious exacerbations of cystic fibrosis, but has not been effective as adjunctive therapy to systemic antibiotics in patients with serious respiratory tract infections.

Oxazolidinones (Linezolid)

Linezolid is the first agent in a new class of antibiotics, the oxazolidinones, which act to inhibit bacterial protein synthesis. They work by binding to the 50S ribosomal subunit and preventing the binding of transfer RNA and preventing the formation of the 70S initiation complex. This is a unique mechanism and no cross-resistance to other agents is likely.

Linezolid is active against methicillin-resistant *Staphylococcus aureus* (MRSA), drug-resistant *Streptococcus pneumoniae*, and vancomycin-resistant enterococci (VRE) [both *Enterococcus faecium* and *Enterococcus faecalis*]. It is bacteriostatic, but bactericidal against some pneumococci. The kinetics suggest that the drug will be active at an MIC of ≤4 mg/L, and MRSA, penicillin-resistant *S pneumoniae*, and VRE all fall in this range. Dosing is 600 mg twice daily. The agent has high bioavailability, and thus serum levels are the same with oral or IV therapy. The half life is 4.5 to 5.5 h. Peak concentration is 18 mg/L after a 600-mg dose. Renal and nonrenal clearance occur, and dosing adjustment is not needed for patients with renal failure.

Efficacy has been shown for nosocomial pneumonia, CAP, complicated skin/soft tissue infections, and VRE. One recent analysis suggests that linezolid may be superior to vancomycin for the therapy of ventilator-associated pneumonia (VAP), which is proven to be caused by MRSA.

Side effects are not common and the agent is well tolerated. Nausea, diarrhea, anemia, and thrombocytopenia (with prolonged use, <1%) can occur. It is also a weak monoamine oxidase inhibitor.

Using Proper Dosing and Dosing Regimens

When an antimicrobial agent is used appropriately, it must be dosed in a manner that takes into account several factors, including its mechanism of action, its activity relative to the MIC of the target organism, and its penetration to the site of infection. Bactericidal antibiotics can kill bacteria in a time-dependent or concentration-dependent fashion. Time-dependent killing means that the organism is eradicated only as long as the concentration of antibiotic stays above the MIC of the target organism. The minimal time needed to exceed the MIC of the infecting pathogen is unknown, but most estimates are for at least 40% of the dosing interval. Drugs that kill in a concentration-dependent fashion are the β-lactams (penicillins and cephalosporins) and vancomycin. When time-dependent killing has been studied, the antibiotic concentration used to define the effect is the serum level, and this measurement may not account for the penetration of antibiotics to the site of infection. For example, some agents (quinolones, macrolides, and the oxazalidinone linezolid) penetrate well into sites of infection, such as the lung, achieving levels in lung tissue that exceed the serum level, while other agents (penicillins, cephalosporins, vancomycin) penetrate poorly, achieving levels in lung tissue below serum concentrations. Thus, for some drugs, serum concentrations may not accurately reflect time above MIC at the site of infection. In theory, with an antibiotic that kills in a time-dependent fashion, optimal killing, with minimal total dose of antibiotic, could be achieved by continuous infusion administration, but this approach has not been shown to have any beneficial effect on clinical success in the therapy of nosocomial pneumonia in trauma patients when ceftazidime has been administered in this fashion.

Antibiotics that kill in a concentration-dependent fashion are best administered as once-daily doses. This approach achieves high peak concentrations in the serum, thus maximizing efficacy, but with low trough concentrations, which may minimize the toxicity of agents, such as the aminoglycosides. For some agents, the concept of once-daily dosing not only takes advantage of concentration-dependent killing, but also relies on the postantibiotic effect of agents, meaning that they continue to kill even after the serum concentration falls below the MIC. Aminoglycosides have a good postantibiotic effect against enteric Gram-negative organisms, and thus have been used with once-daily dosing regimens without any significant impact on efficacy or toxicity. When concentration-dependent killing is present, the effect of the agent on the bacteria can be defined by examining the peak serum concentration relative to the MIC, or by looking at the area under the concentration time curve, divided by the MIC (the AUIC). For pneumococcus, quinolone killing is optimized by a peak concentration: MIC ratio of 12:1, or an AUIC of ≥30. For resistant Gram-negative organisms, the optimal AUIC for quinolones may be as high as 110 to 125. The recommended doses for commonly used antibiotics in the critically ill, with normal renal function, appear in Table 2.

Table 2. *Proper Doses of Common Antibiotics in The Critically Ill With Normal Renal Function*

β-Lactams
    Cefepime 1-2 g q8-12h
    Ceftazidime 2 g q8h
    Ceftriaxone 2 g qD
    Imipenem 1 g q8h or 500 mg q6h
    Meropenem 1 g q6-8h
    Piperacillin/tazobactam 4.5 g q6h

Aminoglycosides
    Gentamicin or tobramycin 7 mg/kg/d or amikacin 20 mg/kg/d

Antistaphylococcal agents (MRSA)
    Vancomycin 15 mg/kg q12h
    Linezolid 600 mg q12h

Quinolones
    Ciprofloxacin: 400 mg q8h
    Levofloxacin 750 mg qD

Streamlining Antimicrobial Therapy

As the importance of using broad-spectrum regimens when initiating empiric therapy has been stressed, it is equally important for clinicians to narrow or discontinue therapy when more data on the patient's clinical progress and the microbiologic data become available. This practice has been termed "deescalation" and can involve focusing from broad spectrum to narrow therapy, from multiple to single agents, and even discontinuing antibiotics if patients do not have proven infection. In the ICU, combination therapy may be needed for certain resistant pathogens, such as

P aeruginosa or mixed infections involving resistant Gram-positive and Gram-negative organisms. Once the clinical response has been observed and culture data are available, the patient's therapy can often be switched to fewer antibiotics, targeted to the cultures. Singh has shown that the duration of therapy can also be reduced in many patients based on clinical evaluation of signs and symptoms. One recent study documented that the use of a broad-spectrum empiric regimen for suspected VAP could be coupled with the intentional discontinuation of therapy after 7 days if further therapy was not absolutely necessary. With this protocol, the duration of antibiotic therapy was reduced with no significant impact on mortality, but a significant reduction in the incidence of respiratory superinfections. The ability to shorten duration of therapy for non-fermenting Gram-negative bacteria, like *P aeruginosa*, is uncertain.

Empiric Therapy of Pneumonia: An Example of Antibiotic Use

If the source of infection is unknown, or if it is known to be intraabdominal, empiric therapy can be given as in Table 3. Patients with severe pneumonia can be divided into three categories, each with its own list of likely pathogens, and from this list follow suggested antibiotic regimens. To decide which category a patient falls into, it is first necessary to determine if the pneumonia is community-acquired or hospital-acquired. Patients with severe CAP are likely to be infected with pneumococcus, Legionella, other atypical organisms, *S aureus*, and enteric Gram-negative organisms; they should receive the therapy directed to these pathogens. In the setting of severe hospital-acquired pneumonia (HAP), stratification is identical whether the patient is intubated or not, but patients are separated on the basis of whether or not they have risk factors for resistant pathogens. If no risk factors are present and if the pneumonia is early-onset (within the first 4 days of admission), then the patient is at risk for nonresistant Gram-negative organisms and *S aureus*, pneumococcus, and *Haemophilus influenzae*, and should receive therapy for these organisms. If the patient has late-onset HAP (day 5 or later) in the absence of risk factors, or pneumonia of any time of onset in the presence of risk factors, then the patient should be treated for potentially resistant Gram-positive and Gram-negative organisms.

Although all patients undergo some diagnostic testing, empiric antibiotic therapy must be initiated before the results of diagnostic testing become available. Empiric therapy is needed for CAP patients for several reasons: (1) even with extensive diagnostic testing, no diagnosis is found in up to half of all patients; (2) the bacteriology of severe CAP is predictable, making empiric therapy possible; and (3) in the setting of severe CAP, accurate empiric therapy has been shown to improve outcome. Similarly, empiric therapy, based on a clinical diagnosis of infection, is necessary for patients with severe HAP because (1) clinical criteria are sensitive to early and potentially treatable forms of pneumonia; (2) algorithms can be used to predict the likely pathogens and to guide therapy; and (3) empiric therapy can be modified once the results of tracheal aspirates or sputum cultures become available.

Severe CAP

Because the spectrum of likely pathogens is so broad and includes not only pneumococcus but also Legionella spp and enteric Gram-negative organisms, it is necessary to use multiple IV agents. This includes an IV macrolide or quinolone with the addition of other agents, the type and number being determined by whether risk factors for *P aeruginosa* are present. Macrolide monotherapy can be used in carefully selected CAP patients, but not in those with severe illness. Quinolone monotherapy is also not recommended for the treatment of severe CAP, since efficacy data are lacking.

Table 3. *Empiric Therapy for Sepsis*

Source Unknown
Organisms: *S aureus* (especially if IV line), Gram-negative organisms, fungi (steroids, prior antibiotics)
Therapy: Dual pseudomonal +/− oxacillin, vancomycin or alternatives (linezolid)

Intra-abdominal Source
Organisms: Gram-negative organisms, anaerobes, enterococci (latter two more with secondary vs primary infection)
Therapy: Ceftriaxone, ertapenem, ampicillin/sulbactam, +/− clindamycin/metronidazole *or* imipenem, meropenem, piperacillin/tazobactam +/− vancomycin, linezolid

The initial empiric regimen for severe CAP should be adequate for a penicillin-resistant pneumococcal infection. Recent studies have shown that most resistance is of the intermediate, and not high-level type. As many as 85 to 90% of penicillin-resistant organisms are still macrolide-sensitive, and high-dose β-lactam therapy, with a penicillin or third-generation cephalosporin, is also adequate for most resistant pneumococci. If penicillin resistance is especially likely, then cefotaxime or ceftriaxone should be used instead of an antipseudomonal third-generation cephalosporin. If a resistant pneumococcal infection is suspected and cultures of blood or sputum show high-level resistance to both cephalosporins and penicillin, then therapy should include either vancomycin or a new antipneumococcal quinolone.

One organism that is not well covered by the suggested empiric regimens is *S aureus*. This organism is not a common cause of severe CAP, but it is a concern when patients have diabetes mellitus or renal failure or after influenza infection. In these settings, the use of an antistaphylococcal penicillin or vancomycin should be considered, possibly in place of one of the antipseudomonal agents. Community-acquired methicillin-resistant *S aureus* is now being reported in some patients with severe CAP, especially after influenza, but optimal therapy is not defined and could include trimethoprim sulfa or linezolid.

Severe HAP

Patients with no risk factors for resistant pathogens and early onset of HAP are at risk for only the core pathogens, and they can often be treated with only a single antimicrobial agent. However, when patients are at risk for *P aeruginosa* or other resistant pathogens—because of the presence of risk factors such as prior antibiotics, corticosteroid use, or malnutrition, or because of prolonged mechanical ventilation (≥5 days) leading to late-onset pneumonia—combination therapy is necessary. Combination antipseudomonal therapy should be started in these patients, and continued if *P aeruginosa* or other resistant Gram-negative organisms (such as Enterobacter spp) are present. In immune-compromised patients, combination therapy can provide synergism against *P aeruginosa*, but this is not the usual reason for using combination regimens in other types of patients. The rationale for combination therapy is to prevent the emergence of resistance during treatment, a common event when only a single antimicrobial agent is used for these pathogens. In addition, there is evidence that dual-agent therapy can improve the outcome of patients with bacteremic *P aeruginosa* pneumonia.

The antimicrobials that are antipseudomonal (Table 4) are either β-lactams (penicillins, cephalosporins, monobactams, and carbapenems) or agents from other drug classes. These include penicillins such as piperacillin and mezlocillin; the β-lactam/β-lactamase inhibitor combination ticarcillin/clavulanate; the third-generation cephalosporins, ceftazidime and cefoperazone; the monobactam, aztreonam; the carbapenem, imipenem; a fluoroquinolone, ciprofloxacin; and the aminoglycosides. When these agents are combined, three general approaches can be used. The traditional combination includes a β-lactam and an aminoglycoside, which can achieve antibacterial synergy. This is rarely an important benefit for the nonneutropenic patient and it requires the use of an aminoglycoside, which has several limitations in the critically ill pneumonia patient. Aminoglycosides should be administered once daily, to take advantage of their enhanced killing when high peak levels are achieved, but even with this type of regimen, nephrotoxicity can occur. In addition, aminoglycosides penetrate poorly into the lung and may not be active at the acid pH levels that are common in pneumonic lung tissue.

Recently, Hatala and associates conducted a meta-analysis of once-daily aminoglycoside dosing studies and concluded that, compared with standard dosing regimens, bacteriologic cure rates are identical, but once-daily dosing regimens may have reduced toxicity. Given the ease of using

Table 4. *Antipseudomonal Antibiotics*

Quinolones: ciprofloxacin, high dose levofloxacin (750 mg)
Aminoglycosides: gentamicin, amikacin, tobramycin
β-lactams
  Antipseudomonal penicillins
  Cephalosporins: ceftazidime, cefepime
  Imipenem, meropenem
  Aztreonam
  β-lactam/β-lactamase inhibitor combinations:
  piperacillin/tazobactam, ticarcillin/clavulanate

these agents in a single daily dose and the associated reduced costs of this approach, the findings in this analysis may be sufficient to justify the widespread use of such dosing regimens.

An alternative type of combination regimen is to use two β-lactam agents, but this approach can lead to antagonism in the mechanism of action of the two drugs, and if one drug induces a bacterial β-lactamase, both drugs may be simultaneously inactivated. A third type of combination is to use ciprofloxacin with a β-lactam, thus avoiding a dual β-lactam regimen and avoiding the use of an aminoglycoside. This regimen also has the advantage of excellent respiratory tract penetration by the quinolone agent, ciprofloxacin.

In some patients with severe HAP, additional empiric therapy with vancomycin may be needed for possible MRSA infection, another organism seen in patients with late-onset pneumonia after prolonged intubation or prior antibiotic therapy. In the intubated patient, tracheal aspirates can be used to identify the pathogen(s) present, and therapy can be reduced to a single agent if P aeruginosa, other resistant Gram-negative organisms, and MRSA are not present. One recent multicenter trial showed that when such organisms were absent, patients with severe HAP could be successfully treated with a single agent such as ciprofloxacin or imipenem.

Antibiotic Resistance

There are four basic mechanisms of resistance:

1. Decreased permeability of microbial cell wall. This is an important mechanism for Gram-negative resistance and is caused by alteration of porin channels.

2. Production of destructive enzymes, such as β-lactamases. This is the major mechanism for Gram-negative resistance and can combine with altered permeability in specific organisms. β-lactamases can be type I or extended spectrum, and are commonly produced by organisms like P aeruginosa and the Enterobacteriaceae. Resistance to third-generation cephalosporins is often mediated by this mechanism.

3. Alteration of the target site of action, such as the penicillin-binding proteins, the DNA gyrase (quinolones), and RNA polymerase. This is an important mechanism for Gram-positive resistance. For pneumococcus, resistance can occur to beta-lactams by alteration of the penicillin-binding proteins and to macrolides by alteration of the ribosomal target of action. This type of macrolide resistance is coded by the *erm* gene and confers a high level of resistance, much higher than if resistance is caused by an efflux mechanism (below).

4. Active efflux of the antibiotic, which can occur in Gram-positive and Gram-negative organisms, but is an important mechanism of macrolide resistance in pneumococci, encoded for by the *mef* gene.

Antimicrobial Control Programs

Antimicrobial control programs, such as guidelines, standards, prior authorization policies, and performance measures, primarily focus on limiting antibiotic use. Several studies evaluating antibiotic control programs have not demonstrated reduced resistance rates. This may relate to the fact that other variables besides antibiotic use in ICUs determine the presence of resistance in the hospital. The type of antimicrobial control program that is used in a given hospital may be best dictated by a knowledge of local antibiotic usage and resistance patterns. If, for example, antibiotic usage is controlled and appropriate, and a single strain of a highly-resistant pathogen is present, then there may be a need for more intensive infection-control efforts. If, on the other hand, usage is high and inappropriate, and many strains of resistant pathogens are prevalent, control of antibiotic usage may be the most pressing need. Antibiotic rotation is another form of antibiotic control, but its benefit is uncertain.

Annotated References

Campbell GD, Niederman MS, Broughton WA, et al. Hospital-acquired pneumonia in adults: diagnosis, assessment of severity, initial antimicrobial therapy, and preventative strategies; a consensus statement. Am J Respir Crit Care Med 1996; 153:1711–1725

Chow JW, Fine MJ, Shlaes DM, et al. Enterobacter bacteremia: clinical features and emergence of antibiotic resistance during therapy. Ann Intern Med 1991; 115:585–590

Classic article showing that third-generation cephalosporins can promote the emergence of resistance during therapy of Enterobacter bacteremia, and are also a risk factor for resistance that is present prior to therapy.

Cometta A, Baumgartner JD, Lew D, et al. Prospective randomized comparison of imipenem monotherapy with imipenem plus netilmicin for treatment of severe infections in nonneutropenic patients. Antimicrob Agents Chemother 1994; 38:1309–1313

Addition of an aminoglycoside to imipenem for the therapy of nosocomial pneumonia was not associated with improved outcomes, but only with a higher rate of nephrotoxicity.

Craig W. Pharmacodynamics of antimicrobial agents as a basis for determining dosage regimens. Eur J Clin Microbiol Infect Dis 1993; 12:6–8

Craig WA. Pharmacokinetic/pharmacodynamic parameters: rationale for antimicrobial dosing of mice and men. Clin Infect Dis 1998; 26:1–12

Fink MP, Snydman DR, Niederman MS, et al. Treatment of severe pneumonia in hospitalized patients: results of a multicenter, randomized, double-blind trial comparing intravenous ciprofloxacin with imipenem-cilastatin. Antimicrob Agents Chemother 1994; 38:547–557

Multicenter randomized trial comparing ciprofloxacin 400 mg q8h to imipenem 1 g q8h and showing both to be effective monotherapy for severe VAP, provided no highly resistant organisms were present.

Forest A, Nix DE, Ballow CH, et al. Pharmacodynamics of intravenous ciprofloxacin in seriously ill patients. Antimicrob Agents Chemother 1993; 37:1073–1081

Landmark study showing that outcome in nosocomial pneumonia is improved if the AUIC of the drug used is ≥125, especially for Gram-negative infections.

Gold HS, Moellering RC. Antimicrobial-drug resistance. N Engl J Med 1996; 335:1445–1453

Hatala R, Dinh T, Cook DJ. Once-daily aminoglycoside dosing in immunocompetent adults: a metaanalysis. Ann Intern Med 1996; 124:717–725

Hilf M, Yu VL, Sharp J, et al. Antibiotic therapy for *Pseudomonas aeruginosa* bacteremia: outcome correlations in a prospective study of 200 patients. Am J Med 1989; 87:540–546

Study showing a mortality benefit for combination therapy vs monotherapy in patients with bacteremic P aeruginosa pneumonia.

Honeybourne D. Antibiotic penetration into lung tissues. Thorax 1994; 49:104–106

Mandell LA. Antibiotics for pneumonia therapy. Med Clin North Am 1994; 78:997–1014

Niederman MS. An approach to empiric therapy of nosocomial pneumonia. Med Clin North Am 1994; 78:1123–1141

Niederman MS. The principles of antibiotic use and the selection of empiric therapy for pneumonia. In: Fishman A, ed. Pulmonary diseases and disorders. 3rd ed. New York, NY: McGraw-Hill, 1997; 1939–1949

Paul M, Benuri-Silbiger I, Soares-Weiser K, et al. β-lactam monotherapy versus β-lactam – aminoglycoside combination therapy for sepsis in immunocompetent patients: systematic review and meta-analysis of randomized trials. BMJ 2004; 328:668

Preston SL, Drusano GL, Berman AL, et al. Pharmacodynamcis of levofloxacin: a new paradigm for early clinical trials. JAMA 1998; 279:125–129

Study that documents the need to achieve a peak concentration:MIC ratio of 10 to 12 to optimize outcomes in the therapy of CAP due to pneumococcus.

Prins JM, Van Deventer S, Kuijper EJ, et al. Clinical relevance of antibiotic-induced endotoxin release. Antimicrob Agents Chemother 1994; 38:1211–1218

Sieger B, Berman SJ, Geckler RW, et al. Empiric treatment of hospital-acquired lower respiratory tract infections with meropenem or ceftazidime with tobramycin: a randomized study. Crit Care Med 1997; 25:1663–1670

Wunderink, RG, J. Rello J, Cammarata SK, et al. 2003. Linezolid vs vancomycin: analysis of two double-blind studies of patients with methicillin-resistant *Staphylococcus aureus* nosocomial pneumonia. Chest 2003; 124:1789-1797

Notes

Head and Spinal Cord Trauma

Thomas P. Bleck, MD, FCCP

Objectives:

- Understand the role of primary and secondary injuries in head trauma
- Consider the controversies regarding hyperventilation, hypothermia, and cerebral perfusion pressure management in acute head trauma
- Recognize the potential importance of different means of blood pressure support in acute spinal cord injury
- Review the role of methylprednisolone and other agents in the management of acute spinal cord injury

Key words: cerebral blood flow; cerebral perfusion pressure; cerebral salt wasting; cerebral vasospasm; free radicals; head trauma; hyperventilation; hyponatremia; intracranial pressure; methylprednisolone; nosocomial pneumonia; pulmonary edema; seizures; spinal cord injury; tirilazad mesylate

---

Contemporary research into the optimal management of head and spinal cord trauma has generated considerable heat and very little light. This overview will touch on some accepted and some controversial aspects of management; in the interpretation of studies in this area, it is important to recall that most series use the National Institutes of Health's Traumatic Coma Data Bank (TCDB) of the 1970s as a benchmark.[1] One of the few solid statements one can make in this area is that everyone's outcomes will be better than the TCDB data, or their own historical controls. This probably reflects the decline of hypoxia and hypotension as causes of secondary injury, and generally higher standards of supportive medical and nursing care. A reasonable prognostic model is available for those inclined toward prognostication.[2]

The recently published guidelines for head trauma management[3] represent a very carefully performed evidence-based review of the available literature, and should be studied by anyone caring for these patients. Unfortunately, very few of the important questions about head injury management have been studied in randomized, double-blind trials, so very few actual standards could be developed. The following is a personal view of head injury management in the ICU.

One deplorable trend in this field is the increase in penetrating head injuries in urban areas,[4] as well as the continued epidemic of intoxicated drivers and failure to wear seat belts. The vast majority of severe head trauma in my institution would be easily preventable.

Pathophysiologic Considerations

Mass Lesions

Masses (in trauma, discrete masses are almost always hematomas) both distort normal structures (brain, cranial nerves, blood vessels, cerebrospinal fluid [CSF] pathways) and contribute to elevations in intracranial pressure (ICP). Epidural hematomas generally occur at sites of skull fractures that lacerate meningeal vessels; the bleeding forms a clot that requires a craniotomy for removal. Chronic subdural hematomas result from torn bridging veins in the subdural space; they are usually liquefied on presentation and can be evacuated via burr holes. In contrast, acute subdural hematomas almost always signify a deceleration injury with a substantial underlying cerebral contusion. The contusion itself swells and acts like a mass but is not separate from the brain substance.

Diffuse Axonal Injury

Older literature stressed the density difference between gray and white matter as the cause of shearing at the gray-white junction during deceleration injuries. While this does occur, and is probably responsible for the petechial and slit hemorrhages that occur in patients suffering this mechanism of injury, it does not appear to be the cause of diffuse axonal injury (DAI), which is a major cause of long-term disability in head-injured patients. In DAI, loss of the axon is an active process that begins with disruption of the microtubular structures at the initial segment and progresses (in humans) for about 24 h.[5] Current theories stress a connection between intracellular calcium toxicity, the resultant mitochondrial dysfunction, and DAI. Intrathecal cyclosporine (given prior to experimental injury) will attenuate or prevent these changes.[6]

Intracranial Pressure

Thirty years of research confirms that sustained elevation of ICP (>20 mm Hg) is associated with a poor outcome.[7] Beyond that, little has been proven regarding the role of ICP elevation itself in affecting prognosis. Patients with other conditions (eg, pseudotumor cerebri) commonly tolerate much higher ICPs for months.

The classic teaching (the Monro-Kellie hypothesis) states that the skull is a fixed volume in which brain, blood, and CSF are constrained. An increase in the volume of any one component must be balanced by movement of another component out of the skull. This relationship can be overcome by enlarging the skull, eg, by craniectomy.

In head trauma, the major causes of elevated ICP are mass lesions, hypercarbia, hypoxia, and hyperemia. The need to remove mass lesions that raise ICP or distort brain structures, and to prevent secondary injury due to hypoxia, seem well established. The importance of hyperemia remains debated, in part because of uncertainty about cerebral perfusion and substrate delivery.

Cerebral Perfusion Pressure

The concept of cerebral perfusion pressure [CPP; CPP = mean arterial pressure (MAP) − ICP] is used as a shorthand method to try to insure adequate substrate delivery at the tissue level, which is not usually measured directly. Recommendations to maintain CPP at a particular level are based in part on the effects of lowering CPP in normal subjects (eg, thresholds for clinical and EEG changes in people whose MAP is reduced, or in animals whose ICP is increased). One school of head-trauma management maintains the primacy of CPP, and ignores ICP (except for the removal of mass lesions) in favor of elevating MAP.[8] However, it appears that there is no utility to raising the CPP beyond about 60 mm Hg.[9]

The contention that increasing MAP produces compensatory cerebral vasoconstriction, and therefore lowers ICP by decreasing cerebral blood volume, depends on intact autoregulation. The degree to which autoregulation remains intact is uncertain, but when hyperemia is present, it would appear to be a sign that autoregulation has failed.

The CPP equation is commonly written as CPP = MAP − [the greater of ICP or jugular venous pressure (JVP)]. However, the JVP cannot be higher than the ICP, or jugular venous flow would be reversed until the ICP met the JVP.

Fluid administration should result in at least even fluid balance following adequate resuscitation.[9a]

A recently published parallel study in spinal cord injury patients suggests that aggressive volume and blood pressure support in this group will also improve outcome.[10] This study similarly investigates the problem of relying on historical control subjects rather than a concurrently randomized control group. It does suggest that vascular disorders affecting vessels from the microvasculature up to the anterior spinal artery may play an important role in secondary injury to the spinal cord, just as hypotension worsens outcome after head trauma. Because hypotension is a ubiquitous problem after cervical spinal cord injuries, there are many opportunities for this damage to be compounded.

A competing theory, espoused by the group in Lund, Sweden, holds that the arterial pressure in the head is the driving force for cerebral edema and thus should be lowered.[11] As with almost all post-TCDB studies, they claim improved outcome with respect to historical control subjects. At present, there is no randomized comparison of any of these strategies.

Cerebral Blood Flow

One important observation of the last several years is that a substantial minority of severe head injury patients (with a Glasgow Coma Score of 3 to 8) have regionally diminished cerebral blood flow (CBF) during the first 24 h.[12-14] Ischemic areas surrounding contusions may be particularly vulnerable.[15] Such observations led to a widely cited but rarely read study in which routine hyperventilation without respect to ICP or CPP had an apparently deleterious effect on outcome at 3 months, but not at 1 year.[16] The authors' conclusion should be reviewed by everyone who uses or eschews hyperventilation: "It is concluded that prophylactic hyperventilation is deleterious in head-injured patients with motor scores of 4–5."[16]

The effect of hyperventilation on CBF is not mediated by the $Paco_2$, but rather by the pH of the extracellular fluid bathing the arterioles. The CNS, in concert with the rest of the body, attempts to restore the pH after we perturb it. The commonly stated maxim that hyperventilation stops working is not strictly true. Rather, the effect of hyperventilation is counterbalanced by (1) continued evolution of the pathologic processes raising ICP in the first place; (2) active clearance of bicarbonate from the CSF by the choroid plexus, which lowers the pH despite a constant $Paco_2$; and occasionally (3) the increase in intrathoracic pressure produced by our attempts to further lower the $Paco_2$ below about 25 mm Hg.

A system for continuous direct CBF measurement by thermal diffusion is under investigation.[17] Other techniques, such as cold xenon CT, radioactive xenon scintigraphy, or positron emission tomography, provide data for only a narrow temporal window. Jugular venous oxygen measurements are certainly affected by CBF, but are also altered by many other factors.[18]

Glycolysis is also accelerated after severe head trauma,[19] although the relationships among this phenomenon, CBF, and outcome remain obscure.

Traumatic Subarachnoid Hemorrhage

Although trauma has long been recognized as the most common cause of subarachnoid hemorrhage (SAH), the influence of subarachnoid blood on head trauma prognosis and complications is only now becoming apparent.[20] Vasospasm does occur in trauma patients with SAH,[21] with the potential for delayed ischemic damage. Whether calcium channel manipulations will be helpful remains debated (but is still debated in aneurysmal SAH as well).[22]

Seizures

Acute seizures following head trauma are probably due to a combination of mechanical deformation of neurons and excessive extracellular concentrations of excitatory amino acids (eg, glutamate) and potassium. There is no clear relationship between early (first week) and later posttraumatic seizures; phenytoin prophylaxis decreases the early ones, but may not have much effect on later seizures.[23] Later seizures may relate to hemosiderin deposition in the cortex in addition to the factors producing early seizures.

Anatomic Considerations in Spinal Cord Injury

The susceptibility of the spinal cord to trauma arises from a combination of its relationship to the vertebral bodies, their processes, the intervertebral disks, and the blood vessels. In addition to direct cord trauma, vascular mechanisms should be considered. The patient with an anterior spinal artery infarction will lose motor strength and pain and temperature sensation below the lesion, but will typically retain proprioception.

An important, but commonly overlooked, critical care issue in the care of patients with spinal cord injuries is the role of the parasternal intercostal muscles in ventilation. Patients with lower cervical or upper thoracic cord lesions commonly present with adequate ventilatory parameters, but fail in a few days as they exhaust the ability of their accessory muscles to compensate for the loss of the stenting action of the parasternal intercostals. In some centers, these patients are routinely intubated on admission. We usually wait for an increase in rate and a decline in vital capacity, recognizing that by this time the patient is frequently in a halo vest and is difficult to intubate.

Free Radicals and Excitotoxins

Research into the mechanisms by which trauma damages the nervous system continues apace, with the role of free radicals and excitotoxins as final mediators of injury still appearing important. Trials of free radical scavengers, such as polyethylene glycol-superoxide dismutase, or PEG-SOD,[24] and tirilazad mesylate, have been disappointing in head trauma, as have a number of putative excitatory amino-acid antagonists.

In spinal cord injury, free-radical scavenging has a more established benefit. The high-dose methylprednisolone trial (National Acute Spinal

Cord Injury Study II, or NASCIS II) demonstrated a modest improvement in outcome in patients receiving the drug for 1 day at a dose of 30 mg/kg. More recently, NASCIS III demonstrated that high-dose methylprednisolone and tirilazad mesylate were equivalent in their beneficial effects.

Evaluation

Physical Examination

In addition to the general trauma surveys and the Glasgow Coma Score, patients with severe head trauma need careful observation for changes in their neurologic examination findings that may suggest the need for treatments beyond the "simple" management of ICP and CPP. In the sedated but unparalyzed patient, changes in eye movements, posturing, and the resting tone of the extremities provide clues regarding the actual consequences of ICP and CPP changes inside the skull. Neuromuscular junction blockade precludes performance of the physical examination except for pupillary responses, and should be avoided unless other measures are unable to keep the ICP and CPP in the desired ranges.

Signs of Herniation: Although the classical explanation of cerebral herniation is usually wrong, the observed signs remain extremely important. A third-nerve palsy initially develops when the diencephalon is displaced laterally, pulling the midbrain with it and stretching the ipsilateral third nerve between the cavernous sinus and the front of the midbrain. Early in this process, it is often easily reversed. At this time, the mesial temporal structures have not herniated over the tentorial edge; imaging studies show that the perimesencephalic cistern that is *larger* on the side of the lesion at that point. Later, the temporal lobe may herniate, producing the classic findings ascribed to herniation in earlier studies.

A change for the worse in the patient's examination findings should lead to consideration of acute interventions to lower ICP and raise CPP, and a repeat CT scan. Because a substantial, even life-threatening, degree of horizontal shift can occur before the ICP rises noticeably, one should not wait for the ICP to go up when the patient develops a third-nerve palsy, or a patient previously demonstrating flexor posturing becomes extensor. Although the mechanisms are uncertain, mannitol infusion or brief hyperventilation will often reverse these acute changes and allow time for consideration of more definitive treatment.

Serial examination of the patient with a spinal cord lesion is the only readily available monitor for change in function. The examiner should be familiar with the motor and sensory distributions of the spinal levels in order to detect changes in the extent of cord involvement.

ICP Monitoring and CSF Drainage: The best way to monitor and manage elevated ICP is largely a matter of personal preference. Centers that rely on ventriculostomies stress the ability to remove fluid as a means of ICP/CPP control, but keeping these catheters working is often difficult as the brain swells, and the risk of infection is substantial. Parenchymal pressure monitors—*eg*, the Camino (Integra NeuroSciences; Plainsboro, NJ) and Codman (Codman/Johnson & Johnson Professional, Inc; Randolph, MA) systems—are preferred in many centers, but begin to drift from the pressure monitored via ventriculostomy after about 5 days. This seems to reflect gliosis at the tip of the catheter; many physicians change the monitoring device at 5 days if it is still being used for clinical decisions. The older subarachnoid space monitoring devices (Richmond bolts, Philadelphia screws) are rarely used.

ICP monitoring is associated with better survival,[25] although the observational study demonstrating this did not reveal what aspects of management derived from the ICP data influenced the outcome.

CT Scanning: CT scanning is typically used in the initial evaluation of head injuries, and is certainly the current test of choice for the rapid exclusion of intracranial masses. Although MR imaging is more sensitive and may be a better prognosticator, CT will adequately reveal those lesions that require management. The scan merits repeating if physical examination or ICP changes suggest the possibility of a previously unsuspected mass.

It is important to recognize that all subsequent studies have shown improved outcome when compared with the TCDB data; nevertheless, these data demonstrate the relative percentages expected and the value of the CT classification scheme (Table 1[26]).

Table 1. *Marshall Classes of Head Injury by CT and Glasgow Outcome Scale From TCBD Data**

Category	Description	% of Patients	Glasgow Outcome Scale (%) Good/Moderate	Severe/Vegetative	Dead
No CT data	—	2.3	5.9	0.0	94.1
Diffuse injury I	No visible pathology on CT	7.0	61.6	28.8	9.6
Diffuse injury II	Cisterns visible, shift 0–5 mm, no high-or mixed-density lesion > 25 cm^3	23.7	34.5	52.0	13.5
Diffuse injury III (swelling)	Cisterns compressed or absent, shift 0–5 mm, no high- or mixed-density lesion > 25 cm^3	20.5	16.4	49.7	34.0
Diffuse injury IV (shift)	Shift > 5 mm, no high- or mixed-density lesion > 25 cm^3	4.3	6.2	37.6	56.2
Evacuated mass lesion	Any lesion surgically evacuated	37.0	22.8	38.4	38.8
Nonevacuated mass	High- or mixed-density lesion > 25 cm^3 not surgically evacuated	4.8	11.1	36.1	52.8
Brainstem injury	No brainstem reflexes by physical examination	0.4	0.0	33.3	66.7

*Data from Marshall et al.[26]

MRI: MRI has largely replaced myelography in the evaluation of spinal cord injury. It discloses information about the interior of the spinal cord (*eg*, contusion, hematomas, edema, ischemia) that is therapeutically and prognostically useful. If MRI is contraindicated, CT myelography is the next best choice.

MRI provides better prognostic information than CT,[27] but does not show other problems requiring acute management and is less well suited to detecting bony abnormalities; it is also more difficult to perform in trauma patients. CT remains the study of choice.

Jugular Venous Oxygen Saturation Monitoring: This continues to be an area of controversy. As a technique, it is supposed to measure the oxygen extraction of the brain in a manner analogous to mixed venous oxygen saturation measurements. The proponents of the technique believe that it can be used to determine what modes of therapy are most appropriate for ICP elevations—specifically, whether it is safe to increase the degree of CNS alkalosis by hyperventilation. Its opponents are concerned that a whole-hemi≠sphere measurement of oxygen extraction will be unable to detect focal areas of cerebral ischemia. A multivariate analysis of ICP, MAP, CPP, and jugular venous oxygen saturation revealed that jugular venous saturation did not have an independent effect on outcome.[28] It seems reasonable to assume that if increasing alkalosis increases oxygen extraction (or increases the cerebral venous lactate concentration), then the alkalosis should be reversed and another mode of therapy substituted. Whether it is safe to further increase the degree of alkalosis if the extraction does not increase is another matter.

More contemporary thinking about cerebral oxygen utilization in severe head trauma suggests that high jugular venous oxygen saturation values do not indicate hyperemia, but rather failure of oxygen utilization associated with hyperglycolysis.[29] This effect is underlined by the understanding that decreased oxygen extraction is itself a marker of poor outcome.[30]

Cortical Po_2 Monitoring: This is a relatively new technique in the clinical arena. It involves placing a Po_2-sensing electrode on the cerebral cortex at the time of a craniotomy. If jugular vein oxygen monitoring can be faulted for overlooking regional abnormalities in perfusion, this technique has the opposite problem: the volume of tissue sampled is very small. Initial reports suggest that it will be a useful technique.[31]

Transcranial Doppler Blood Flow Velocity Measurement: This technique is primarily of value for detecting vasospasm related to traumatic SAH. Vasospasm produces an increase in the flow velocity of RBCs in involved arteries: by Poiseuille's law, the velocity increases as the diameter of the vessel decreases. Because elevated ICP can also affect flow velocity, some recommend following the ratio of internal carotid to middle cerebral artery flow velocities.

EEG and Evoked Potentials: The role of EEG in the work-up of suspected seizures is relatively clear, but the utility and indications for continuous EEG monitoring remain to be established. Unsuspected, subclinical seizures have a deleterious effect on outcome in neuro-ICU patients.[32] Patients who develop refractory status epilepticus should have continuous EEG monitoring. Subclinical seizures occur in some head trauma patients, but the actual incidence of this problem is just coming into focus; Vespa et al[3] found that 20% of severely traumatized patients had at least brief subclinical seizures. Whether the breakdown product of atracurium (laudanosine) is epileptogenic in humans remains untested. In the head-trauma patient requiring neuromuscular junction blockade, EEG monitoring can be useful for assessing the degree of cortical function, and for determining whether sedation is needed (and the appropriate dose).

The degree of reactivity on a single EEG in the first 2 days after trauma is an excellent predictor of prognosis.[34]

Evoked-potential studies are very useful for prognostication in the first few hours following severe head trauma.[35] Somatosensory evoked potentials (SSEPs) have received the most study; prolongation or loss of the N20 potential (the first cortical component of the median nerve SSEP) is a powerful predictor of outcome. However, even the absence of SSEPs is not completely predictive of poor outcome.[36] A recent comprehensive review of this topic is available.[37]

Management

Resuscitation and Airway Management: The most important considerations in the prehospital and initial resuscitative phases in head or spinal cord trauma patients are to avoid hypoxia and hypotension.[38]

Head-trauma patients must be assumed to have a concomitant cervical spine injury until proven otherwise. Intubation is performed with in-line traction to prevent lateral movement. While fiberoptic oral intubation may be mechanically safest, the resulting delay in securing the airway is seldom worthwhile. Nasotracheal intubation is best avoided until basilar skull and cribriform plate fractures can be excluded, which generally means that orotracheal intubation has already been performed.

Intubation of patients with severe head trauma in the field (as opposed to the emergency department) was associated with higher mortality in one retrospective study.[39] While I suspect this means that the patients who had the most severe injury were chosen for field intubation, and that field intubation was more likely to be successful in the more severely injured patients, this bears further study.

Excluding cervical spine disorders often takes several days in the comatose patient who cannot indicate pain during flexion/extension views of the neck. When such patients are otherwise stable, we employ CT scanning with traction to exclude cervical spine instability.

Posture and Head Position: The standard recommendation, and our usual practice is to keep these patients sitting up between 30 and 60° above horizontal in hopes of improving their venous return and therefore lowering ICP.[40] It is important to remember that in such a patient, the CPP should be calculated based on the MAP *at the level of the ICP measurement*, generally estimated at the ear for parenchymal transducers.

The desirability of the head-up position is not universally accepted. The proponents of CPP-driven management attempt to keep the patient's head at the level of the heart to keep cerebral perfusion maximal. In other conditions associated with ICP elevation, such as hepatic failure, the ICP may actually increase as the head is raised. Thus, at a minimum, the decision to nurse the patient head-up depends on knowing the effect on ICP and CPP in the individual patient.

ICP, CCP, and CBF Management: Because these factors are so strongly interrelated, the modalities for their management will be discussed together.

Mannitol—Mannitol is usually the first-line drug for lowering ICP. The mechanism by which it works remains debated, but some combination of osmotic removal of extracellular fluid, improvement in RBC membrane deformability (and therefore, improved blood rheologic properties), free-radical scavenging, and increased cardiac output due to improved central filling pressures is probably involved. The initial dose is 0.25 g/kg q4h; although an upper limit for the increased osmolality often produced is often given (*eg*, 310 to 320 milliosmols per liter), there are few data upon which to base such a recommendation.

Hypertonic Saline Solution—Some investigators propose that small quantities of hypertonic saline solution be used in place of mannitol, claiming a prolonged ICP-lowering effect. This is a promising approach that deserves further study. A recent publication from Croatia suggests that cerebral salt wasting is unexpectedly common in patients with penetrating head trauma.[41]

Sedation—Sedative drugs, usually benzodiazepines (typically with a narcotic) or propofol, are frequently used in head-injury patients because they appear to be agitated, to lower ICP (either by relieving agitation or by decreasing cerebral metabolism, to which CBF is coupled under autoregulation), or to promote synchrony with the ventilator. Because of cost issues, midazolam and propofol are often eschewed in favor of lorazepam. The perceived advantage of midazolam as an agent whose effects will terminate rapidly is probably lost during infusions lasting days. Propofol is probably superior in this regard. However, the circumstances in which the ability to rapidly terminate sedative drug action is clinically important are quite rare. Propofol should not be abruptly terminated because of the risk of withdrawal seizures, even after only several hours of infusion.

Some members of the CPP camp attempt not to sedate patients, using the sympathetic nervous system effects of agitation to help raise MAP.

Although it is tempting to try to reverse the effects of benzodiazepines with flumazenil, the likelihood of seizures in this situation makes this process very dangerous.

Analgesia—Either morphine or fentanyl is an effective and inexpensive choice for sedation. We tend to favor fentanyl for reasons of less hypotension, less interference with gut motility, and more rapid clearance when the dose is reduced. When patients need "sedation" for a procedure, such as a CT scan, we typically use fentanyl because it can safely be reversed with naloxone if we need to return the patient to baseline for examination.

Mechanical Ventilation and Airway Management—If the ICP and CPP are easily maintained with normocarbia or only modest hypocarbia (*eg*, $Paco_2$ in the mid 30s), whatever ventilatory mode is best tolerated by the patient is adequate. We tend to use pressure support ventilation with a back-up rate in such patients not requiring sedation, or even a continuous positive airway pressure circuit, to prevent deconditioning. If sedation (or neuromuscular junction blockade) is required, then we choose synchronized intermittent mandatory ventilation or assist-control ventilation.

Although routine hyperventilation may be deleterious and is probably not useful, brief periods of hyperventilation may be life-saving during impending herniation. Hyperventilation works very rapidly, because CO_2 diffuses very rapidly across the blood-brain barrier.

The optimal ventilator-weaning strategy for head-trauma patients is not established. We decrease pressure support as tolerated, which works in most patients, some of whom are "rested on a rate" at night as they improve. Concurrent COPD, reactive airway disease, and pulmonary infections often delay or prolong weaning.

Positive end-expiratory pressure (PEEP) is acceptable as needed to maintain oxygenation.[42] ARDS and other conditions that stiffen the lung decrease the transmission of high alveolar pressures to the great veins by virtue of the poor lung compliance they produce. Thus, patients who need high levels of PEEP seldom experience further elevations in ICP when their airway pressures are high. However, patients with relatively normal lung mechanics may exacerbate their intracranial hypertension if one attempts to hyperventilate them profoundly for ICP control, regardless of whether hyperventilation is a performed by increasing the tidal volume (which raises mean intrathoracic pressure directly) or increasing the respiratory rate (which may generate unintended PEEP by stacking breaths).

When it is best to perform a tracheostomy in a head-injury patient remains to be established. We do so in patients who are ready to be weaned but who do not protect their airways adequately, or who are awakening and are uncomfortable with an endotracheal tube but who are not nearly ready to wean. Percutaneous tracheostomy is increasingly our method of choice.

We routinely perform early tracheostomy on patients with complete cervical cord lesions above the C5 level. Although this may delay a cervical fusion if one is required (due to concern about tracheal secretions infecting an anterior fusion wound), the risk of hypoxia or death with accidental extubation in these patients argues for an early surgical airway. Those with lesions between C5 and T5 often receive early tracheostomies as well.

Neuromuscular Junction Blockade—The mechanisms by which neuromuscular junction blockade decreases ICP in patients who are already deeply sedated are uncertain. Some improvement in thoracic compliance may play a role, but this often seems inadequate to explain the magnitude of the change.

CSF Drainage: Centers routinely placing ventriculostomy catheters for ICP measurement also use them for ICP control by withdrawing small amounts of CSF when ICP elevations occur. There is a learning curve for the ability to successfully and rapidly place a catheter in the small ventricles often found in head-injury patients. If the CT scan reveals hydrocephalus, then a ventriculostomy is the treatment of choice.

High-Dose Barbiturates: When ICP elevations fail to respond to the measures described above, many intensivists have used high-dose barbiturates in the past. This modality is still employed occasionally, although concerns about hypotension have diminished enthusiasm for it. A typical dose would be 5 to 12 mg/kg of pentobarbital as a loading dose, with an infusion starting at 1 mg/kg/h and increased as necessary for ICP control and as tolerated by the MAP. Although EEG burst suppression has been used as a marker for the depth of anesthesia (the pattern correlating with the maximal decrease in CBF, and therefore ICP, that can be achieved with barbiturates), we usually follow the ICP and the CPP rather than the EEG (although the neurosurgeons often ask for the EEG).

High-dose barbiturates are potent venodilators and myocardial depressants; these effects result in diminished cardiac output and hypotension. Because this runs counter to the goals of CPP management, these drugs are avoided by its practitioners.

Craniectomy: Craniectomy defeats the Monro-Kellie relationship by making more space for the swollen brain. This treatment was formally introduced in 1971 by Ransohoff and Kjellberg. Recently, Polin and colleagues[43] analyzed our results (but these data are not from a prospective, randomized trial): decompressive bifrontal craniectomy provides a statistical advantage over medical treatment of intractable posttraumatic cerebral hypertension and should be considered in the management of malignant posttraumatic cerebral swelling. If the operation can be accomplished before the ICP value exceeds 40 torr for a sustained period and within 48 h of the time of injury, the potential to influence outcome is greatest.[43]

Compared with hypothermia or high-dose barbiturates, craniectomy represents a more easily tolerated technique for managing ICP. The question of the added value of neuroprotection of the other methods remains to be studied.

Temperature Control: Hypothermia is emerging as a potentially useful modality to manage ICP and to improve outcome in severe head injury.[44,45] Unfortunately, the multicenter trial was stopped early and showed no benefit.[46] Fever control, however, should probably be approached aggressively, because it seems clear that fever raises ICP and cerebral energy expenditure,[47] and probably worsens outcome.

Antiseizure Drugs: Presently, most centers use antiseizure prophylaxis for the first week or so after severe head trauma. The available agents vary in their ability to prevent late epilepsy in experimental models, but to date this has not been translated into a successful clinical trial. We use phenytoin as the first agent. If this must be changed because of allergy (or, more commonly, part of an unexplained fever drill), we currently use gabapentin for patients able to absorb drugs from the GI tract. Those who cannot do so receive phenobarbital or valproate until they can. However, valproate may have deleterious consequences.[48]

Long-term phenytoin use appears to have negative cognitive and behavioral consequences in these patients,[49] and phenobarbital and the benzodiazepines carry theoretical risks.[50] Patients who have seizures after the first week should be treated chronically; we tend to use carbamazepine.

Free-Radical Scavengers: There has yet to be a free-radical scavenger of proven clinical benefit in humans with head injuries. In spinal cord injury, one unexpected finding of the NASCIS III trial was the benefit of 48 h of high-dose methylprednisolone in patients whose steroid regimen was started late.

Nutrition and GI Bleeding Prophylaxis: Despite all of our concerns about the need for nutrition in trauma patients, the optimal strategy remains unproven. We attempt to feed these patients enterally as soon as possible. All tubes are placed through the mouth to decrease the risk of sinusitis. If patients are candidates for tracheostomy, a percutaneous endoscopic gastrostomy is performed as well.

Patients who cannot be fed receive ulcer/gastritis prophylaxis, usually with an H_2 blocker.[51] If nonsteroidal anti-inflammatory agents are used, we add misoprostol.

Pulmonary Embolism and Venous Thromboembolism Prophylaxis: In head-trauma patients, we rely on sequential compression devices for prophylaxis. Spinal cord injury patients receive low-dose heparin initially, and are later converted to low-molecular-weight heparin.

Deterioration After Admission in Spinal Cord Injury Patients

A recent study examined this question in 182 patients with complete cervical spine injuries.[52] They categorized ascension of the injury into three discrete temporal subsets: early deterioration (<24 h) was typically related to traction and immobilization; delayed deterioration (24 h to 7 days) was associated with sustained hypotension in patients with fracture dislocations; late deterioration (>7 days) was observed in one patient with vertebral artery injuries.

References

1. Marshall LF, Becker DP, Bowers SA, et al. The National Traumatic Coma Data Bank: Part 1. Design, purpose, goals, and results. J Neurosurg 1983; 59:276–284
2. Signorini DF, Andrews PJ, Jones PA, et al. Predicting survival using simple clinical variables: a case study in traumatic brain injury. J Neurol Neurosurg Psychiatry 1999; 66:20–25
3. The Brain Trauma Foundation. The American Association of Neurological Surgeons. The Joint Section on Neurotrauma and Critical Care. Trauma systems. J Neurotrauma 2000; 17:457–627
4. Stone JL, Lichtor T, Fitzgerald LF, et al. Demographics of civilian cranial gunshot wounds: devastation related to escalating semiautomatic usage. J Trauma 1995; 38:851–854
5. Fitzpatrick MO, Dewar D, Teasdale GM, et al. The neuronal cytoskeleton in acute brain injury. Br J Neurosurg 1998; 12:313–317
6. Okonkwo DO, Povlishock JT. An intrathecal bolus of cyclosporin A before injury preserves mitochondrial integrity and attenuates axonal disruption in traumatic brain injury. J Cereb Blood Flow Metab 1999; 19:443–451
7. Signorini DF, Andrews PJ, Jones PA, et al. Adding insult to injury: the prognostic value of early secondary insults for survival after traumatic brain injury. J Neurol Neurosurg Psychiatry 1999; 66:26–31
8. Rosner MJ, Rosner SD, Johnson AH. Cerebral perfusion pressure: management protocol and clinical results. J Neurosurg 1995; 83:949–962
9. Juul N, Morris GF, Marshall SB, et al. Intracranial hypertension and cerebral perfusion pressure: influence on neurological deterioration and outcome in severe head injury; the Executive Committee of the International Selfotel Trial. J Neurosurg 2000; 92:1–6
9a. Clifton GL, Miller ER, Choi SC, et al. Fluid thresholds and outcome from severe brain injury. Crit Care Med 2002; 30:739-745
10. Vale FL, Burns J, Jackson AB, et al. Combined medical and surgical treatment after acute spinal cord injury: results of a prospective pilot study to assess the merits of aggressive medical resuscitation and blood pressure management. J Neurosurg 1997; 87:239–246
11. Eker C, Asgeirsson B, Grande PO, et al. Improved outcome after severe head injury with a new therapy based on principles for brain volume regulation and preserved microcirculation. Crit Care Med 1998; 26:1881–1886
12. Cold GE. Does acute hyperventilation provoke cerebral oligaemia in comatose patients after acute head injury? Acta Neurochir (Wien) 1989; 96:100–106
13. Bouma GJ, Muizelaar JP, Stringer WA, et al. Ultra-early evaluation of regional cerebral blood flow in severely head-injured patients using xenon-enhanced computerized tomography. J Neurosurg 1992; 77:360–368
14. Skippen P, Seear M, Poskitt K, et al. Effect of hyperventilation on regional cerebral blood flow in head-injured children. Crit Care Med 1997; 25:1402–1409

15. McLaughlin MR, Marion DW. Cerebral blood flow and vasoresponsivity within and around cerebral contusions. J Neurosurg 1996; 85:871–876
16. Muizelaar JP, Marmarou A, Ward JD, et al. Adverse effects of prolonged hyperventilation in patients with severe head injury: a randomized clinical trial. J Neurosurg 1991; 75:731–739
17. Carter LP. Thermal diffusion flowmetry. Neurosurg Clin N Am 1996; 7749–7754
18. Robertson CS, Cormio M. Cerebral metabolic management. New Horiz 1995; 3:410–422
19. Bergsneider M, Hovda DA, Shalmon E, et al. Cerebral hyperglycolysis following severe traumatic brain injury in humans: a positron emission tomography study. J Neurosurg 1997; 86:241–251
20. Taneda M, Kataoka K, Akai F, et al. Traumatic subarachnoid hemorrhage as a predictable indicator of delayed ischemic symptoms. J Neurosurg 1996; 84:762–768
21. Romner B, Bellner J, Kongstad P, et al. Elevated transcranial Doppler flow velocities after severe head injury: cerebral vasospasm or hyperemia? J Neurosurg 1996; 85:90–97
22. Murray GD, Teasdale GM, Schmitz H. Nimodipine in traumatic subarachnoid haemorrhage: a re-analysis of the HIT I and HIT II trials. Acta Neurochir (Wien) 1996; 138:1163–1167
23. Temkin NR, Dikmen SS, Wilensky AJ, et al. A randomized, double-blind study of phenytoin for the prevention of post-traumatic seizures. N Engl J Med 1990; 323:497–502
24. Young B, Runge JW, Waxman KS, et al. Effects of pegorgotein on neurologic outcome of patients with severe head injury: a multicenter, randomized controlled trial. JAMA 1996; 276:538–543
25. Lane PL, Skoretz TG, Doig G, et al. Intracranial pressure monitoring and outcomes after traumatic brain injury. Can J Surg 2000; 43:442–448
26. Marshall LF, Marshall SB, Klauber MR, et al. The diagnosis of head injury requires a classification based on computed axial tomography. J Neurotrauma 1992; 9 (suppl 1):S287–S292
27. Paterakis K, Karantanas AH, Komnos A, et al. Outcome of patients with diffuse axonal injury: the significance and prognostic value of MRI in the acute phase. J Trauma 2000; 49:1071–1075
28. Struchen MA, Hannay HJ, Contant CF, et al. The relation between acute physiological variables and outcome on the Glasgow Outcome Scale and Disability Rating Scale following severe traumatic brain injury. J Neurotrauma 2001; 18:115–125
29. Bergsneider M, Hovda DA, Shalmon E, et al. Cerebral hyperglycolysis following severe traumatic brain injury in humans: a positron emission tomography study. J Neurosurg 1997; 86:241–251
30. Macmillan CS, Andrews PJ, Easton VJ. Increased jugular bulb saturation is associated with poor outcome in traumatic brain injury. J Neurol Neurosurg Psychiatry 2001; 70:101–104
31. van Santbrink H, Maas AI, Avezaat CJ. Continuous monitoring of partial pressure of brain tissue oxygen in patients with severe head injury. Neurosurgery 1996; 38:21–31
32. Young GB, Jordan KG, Doig GS. An assessment of nonconvulsive seizures in the intensive care unit using continuous EEG monitoring: an investigation of variables associated with mortality. Neurology 1996; 47:83–89
33. Vespa PM, Nuwer MR, Nenov V, et al. Increased incidence and impact of nonconvulsive and convulsive seizures after traumatic brain injury as detected by continuous electroencephalographic monitoring. J Neurosurg 1999; 91:750–760
34. Gutling E, Gonser A, Imhof HG, et al. EEG reactivity in the prognosis of severe head injury. Neurology 1995; 45:915–918
35. Hutchinson DO, Frith RW, Shaw NA, et al. A comparison between electroencephalography and somatosensory evoked potentials for outcome prediction following severe head injury. Electroencephalogr Clin Neurophysiol 1991; 78:228–233
36. Schwarz S, Schwab S, Aschoff A, et al. Favorable recovery from bilateral loss of somatosensory evoked potentials. Crit Care Med 1999; 27:182–187
37. Carter BG, Butt W. Review of the use of somatosensory evoked potentials in the prediction of outcome after severe brain injury. Crit Care Med 2001; 29:178–186
38. Statham PF, Andrews PJ. Central nervous system trauma. Baillieres Clin Neurol 1996; 5:497–514
39. Murray JA, Demetriades D, Berne TV, et al. Prehospital intubation in patients with severe head injury. J Trauma 2000; 49:1065–1070
40. Meixensberger J, Baunach S, Amschler J, et al. Influence of body position on tissue-pO$_2$, cerebral perfusion pressure and intracranial pressure in patients with acute brain injury. Neurol Res 1997; 19:249–253

41. Bacic A, Gluncic I, Gluncic V. Disturbances in plasma sodium in patients with war head injuries. Mil Med 1999; 164:214–217
42. Cooper KR, Boswell PA, Choi SC. Safe use of PEEP in patients with severe head injury. J Neurosurg 1985; 63:552–555
43. Polin RS, Shaffrey ME, Bogaev CA, et al. Decompressive bifrontal craniectomy in the treatment of severe refractory posttraumatic cerebral edema. Neurosurgery 1997; 41:84–92
44. Metz C, Holzschuh M, Bein T, et al. Moderate hypothermia in patients with severe head injury: cerebral and extracerebral effects. J Neurosurg 1996; 85:533–541
45. Marion DW, Penrod LE, Kelsey SF, et al. Treatment of traumatic brain injury with moderate hypothermia. N Engl J Med 1997; 336:540–546
46. Clifton GL, Miller ER, Choi SC, et al. Lack of effect of induction of hypothermia after acute brain injury. N Engl J Med 2001; 344:556–563
47. Matthews DS, Bullock RE, Matthews JN, et al. Temperature response to severe head injury and the effect on body energy expenditure and cerebral oxygen consumption. Arch Dis Child 1995; 72:507–515
48. Temkin NR, Dikmen SS, Anderson GD, et al. Valproate therapy for prevention of posttraumatic seizures: a randomized trial. J Neurosurg 1999; 91:593–600
49. Dikmen SS, Temkin NR, Miller B, et al. Neurobehavioral effects of phenytoin prophylaxis of posttraumatic seizures. JAMA 1991; 265:1271–1277
50. Goldstein LB. Prescribing of potentially harmful drugs to patients admitted to hospital after head injury. J Neurol Neurosurg Psychiatry 1995; 58: 753–755
51. Tryba M, Cook D. Current guidelines on stress ulcer prophylaxis. Drugs 1997; 54:581–596
52. Harrop JS, Sharan AD, Vaccaro AR, et al. The cause of neurologic deterioration after acute cervical spinal cord injury. Spine 2001; 26:340–346

Notes

Seizures, Stroke, and Other Neurologic Emergencies

Thomas P. Bleck, MD, FCCP

Objectives:

- Improve the recognition, differential diagnosis, and management of seizures occurring in critically ill patients
- Understand the pharmacology and application of newer anticonvulsant drugs in the ICU
- Recognize and manage status epilepticus
- Understand the special diagnostic and management issues of refractory status epilepticus
- Improve recognition of patients with acute subarachnoid hemorrhage
- Recognize and manage the major CNS complications of subarachnoid hemorrhage
- Recognize the common systemic complications of subarachnoid hemorrhage
- Review the role of the critical care service in the management of stroke
- Briefly review other neurologic emergencies in the ICU setting

Key words: brain abscess; diazepam; encephalitis; Guillain-Barré syndrome; herpes simplex; ketamine; lorazepam; meningitis; myasthenia gravis; neurogenic respiratory failure; nonconvulsive status epilepticus; polymerase chain reaction; propofol; recombinant tissue-plasminogen activator; seizure; status epilepticus; stroke; subarachnoid hemorrhage

Seizures

Seizures complicate about 3% of adult ICU admissions for nonneurologic conditions. The medical and economic impact of these seizures confers importance on them out of proportion to their incidence. A seizure is often the first indication of a CNS complication; thus, their rapid etiologic diagnosis is mandatory. In addition, because epilepsy affects 2% of the population, patients with preexisting seizures occasionally enter the ICU for other problems. Because the initial treatment of these patients is the province of the intensivist, he or she must be familiar with seizure management as it affects the critically ill patient. Patients developing status epilepticus (SE) will often require the care of a critical care specialist in addition to a neurologist.

Seizures have been recognized at least since hippocratic times, their relatively high rate of occurrence in critically ill patients has only recently been recognized. Seizures complicating critical care treatments (eg, lidocaine) are also a recent phenomenon. Early attempts at treatment included bromide,[1] morphine,[2] and ice applications. Barbiturates were first employed in 1912, and phenytoin in the 1937.[3] Paraldehyde was popular in the next decades.[4] More recently, emphasis has shifted to the benzodiazepines, which were pioneered in the 1960s.[5]

Epidemiology

Limited data are available on the epidemiology of seizures the ICU. A 10-year retrospective study of all ICU patients with seizures at the Mayo Clinic found 7 patients per 1,000 ICU admissions.[6] Our 2-year prospective study of medical ICU patients identified 35 with seizures per 1,000 admissions.[7] These studies are not exactly comparable, as the patient populations and methods of detection differed. Seizures are probably even more frequent in pediatric ICUs.

Certain ICU patients are at higher risk for seizures, but the degree of that increase has not been quantified. Renal failure or an altered blood-brain barrier increases the seizure likelihood for patients receiving imipenem-cilastatin, but other patients receiving this antibiotic [or γ-aminobutyric acid (GABA) antagonists like penicillin] are also at risk. Transplant recipients, especially receiving cyclosporine, are also at increased risk, as are those who rapidly become hypo-osmolar from any etiology. Nonketotic hyperglycemia patients have an unusual predisposition toward partial seizures and partial SE.

Incidence estimates for generalized convulsive SE (GCSE) in the United States vary from 50,000 cases/yr[8] to 250,000 cases/yr.[9] Some portion of this difference derives from different definitions; the latter estimate represents the only population-based data available, however, and may be more accurate. Mortality estimates similarly vary from 1 to 2% in the former study to 22% in the latter. This disagreement follows from a conceptual discordance: the smaller number describes mortality that the authors directly attributed to SE, while the larger figure estimates the overall mortality rate, even though the cause of death was frequently the underlying disease rather than SE itself. For example, the study by DeLorenzo et al[9] included SE due to anoxia in its SE mortality estimate. In many of the reports surveyed in the earlier review, such patients would not have been counted.

Many risk factors emerged from the Richmond study. SE lasting >1 h carried a mortality of 32%, compared with 2.7% for a duration <1 h. SE caused by anoxia resulted in 70% mortality in adults, but <10% in children. The commonest cause of SE in adults was stroke, followed by withdrawal from antiepileptic drug therapy; cryptogenic SE; and SE related to alcohol withdrawal, anoxia, and metabolic disorders. Systemic infection was the commonest cause of childhood SE, followed by congenital anomalies, anoxia, metabolic problems, anticonvulsant withdrawal, CNS infections, and trauma.

The data in Table 1, based on 20 years of experience at the San Francisco General Hospital,[10-12] are of interest because almost all patients with SE in the city of San Francisco who begin to seize outside of a hospital are transported there. About 10% of epilepsy patients present with SE,[13] and nearly 20% of seizure patients experience an episode of SE within 5 years of their first seizure.[9]

Table 1. *Etiologies of SE at the San Francisco General Hospital**

Etiology	1970–1980 (%) (n = 98) Prior Seizures	1970–1980 (%) (n = 98) No Prior Seizures	1980–1989 (%) (n = 152) Prior Seizures	1980–1989 (%) (n = 152) No Prior Seizures
Ethanol-related	11	4	25	12
Anticonvulsant noncompliance	27	0	41	0
Drug toxicity	0	10	5	10
Refractory epilepsy	—	—	8	0
CNS infection†	0	4	2	10
Trauma	1	2	2	6
Tumor	0	4	2	7
Metabolic†	3	5	2	4
Stroke†	4	11	2	5
Anoxia†	0	4	0	6
Other	11	5	3	5

*Data from Lowenstein and Alldredge.[11]
†Indicates conditions most likely to result in ICU admission.

Classification

The most frequently used classification schema is that of the International League Against Epilepsy[14] (Table 2). This allows classification based on clinical criteria without inferring etiology. *Simple partial seizures* start focally in the cerebral cortex, without invading other structures. The patient is aware throughout the episode, and appears otherwise unchanged. Bilateral limbic dysfunction produces a *complex partial seizure;* awareness and ability to interact are diminished (but may not be completely abolished). *Automatisms* (movements that the patient makes without awareness) may occur. *Secondary generalization* results from invasion of the other hemisphere or subcortical structures.

Primary generalized seizures arise from the cerebral cortex and diencephalon at the same time; no focal phenomena are visible, and consciousness is lost at the onset. *Absence seizures* are

Table 2. *International Classification of Epileptic Seizures**

I. Partial seizures (seizures beginning locally)
   A. Simple partial seizures (SPS)—consciousness not impaired
      1. With motor symptoms
      2. With somatosensory or special sensory symptoms
      3. With autonomic symptoms
      4. With psychic symptoms
   B. Complex partial seizures—with impairment of consciousness
      1. Beginning as SPS and progressing to impairment of consciousness
         a. Without automatisms
         b. With automatisms
      2. With impairment of consciousness at onset
         a. With no other features
         b. With features of SPS
         c. With automatisms
   C. Partial seizures (simple or complex), secondarily generalized
II. Primary generalized seizures (bilaterally symmetric, without localized onset)
   A. Absence seizures
      1. True absence (*petit mal*)
      2. Atypical absence
   B. Myoclonic seizures
   C. Clonic seizures
   D. Tonic seizures
   E. Tonic-clonic seizures (grand mal; generalized tonic-clonic)
   F. Atonic seizures
III. Unclassified seizures

*Adapted from Bleck.[16]

frequently confined to childhood, consisting of the abrupt onset of a blank stare, usually lasting 5 to 15 s, from which the patient abruptly returns to normal. Atypical absence occurs in children with the Lennox-Gastaut syndrome. *Myoclonic seizures* start with brief synchronous jerking without initially altered consciousness, followed by a generalized convulsion. They frequently occur in the genetic epilepsies; in the ICU, they commonly follow anoxia or metabolic disturbances.[15] *Tonic-clonic seizures* start with tonic extension and evolve to bilaterally synchronous clonus, and conclude with a postictal phase. Clinical judgment is required to apply this system in the ICU. In patients whose consciousness has already been altered by drugs, hypotension, sepsis, or intracranial pathology, the nature of their partial seizures may be difficult to classify.

SE is classified by a similar system, altered to match observable clinical phenomena (Table 3).[16] *Generalized convulsive SE* (GCSE) is the commonest type encountered in the ICU, and poses the greatest risk to the patient. It may either be primarily generalized, as in the drug-intoxicated patient, or secondarily generalized, as in the brain abscess patient in whom GCSE develops. *Nonconvulsive SE* (NCSE) in the ICU frequently follows partially treated GCSE. Some use the term for all SE involving altered consciousness without convulsive movements; this blurs the distinctions among absence SE, partially treated GCSE, and *complex partial SE* (CPSE), which have different etiologies and treatments. *Epilepsia partialis continua* (a special form of partial SE in which repetitive movements affect a small area of the body) sometimes lasts for months or years.

Pathogenesis and Pathophysiology

The reported "causes" of SE can be divided into predispositions and precipitants. *Predispositions* are static conditions increasing the likelihood of SE in the presence of a precipitant. *Precipitants* are events that can produce SE in most, if not all, people, but tend to affect those with predispositions at lesser degrees of severity (*eg*, barbiturate withdrawal). The causes and effects of SE at the cellular, brain, and systemic levels are interrelated, but their individual analysis is useful for understanding them and their therapeutic implications. Longer SE durations produce more profound alterations with an increasing likelihood of permanence, and of becoming refractory to treatment. The processes involved in a single seizure and the transition to SE have recently been reviewed.[17]

The ionic events of a seizure follow the opening of ion channels coupled to excitatory amino acid (EAA) receptors. From the standpoint of the intensivist, three channels are particularly important because their activation may raise intracellular free calcium to toxic concentrations: alpha-amino-3-hydroxy-5-methyl-4-isoxazolepropionate (AMPA) channels, *N*-methyl-D-aspartate (NMDA) channels, and metabotropic channels. These EAA systems are crucial for learning and memory. Many drugs affect these systems but are too toxic for chronic use. The deleterious consequences of SE, and the brief period for which such agents would be needed, suggest that they may have a role in SE. Counterregulatory ionic events are triggered by the epileptiform discharge as well, such as the activation of inhibitory interneurons, which suppress excited neurons via GABA-A synapses.

The cellular effects of excessive EAA channel activity include (1) generating toxic concentrations of intracellular free calcium; (2) activating autolytic enzyme systems; (3) producing oxygen

Table 3. *Clinical Classification of Status Epilepticus**

I. Generalized seizures
   A. Generalized convulsive SE (GCSE)
      1. Primary generalized SE
         a. Tonic-clonic SE
         b. Myoclonic SE
         c. Clonic-tonic-clonic SE
      2. Secondarily generalized SE
         a. Partial seizure with secondary generalization
         b. Tonic SE
   B. Nonconvulsive SE (NCSE)
      1. Absence SE (*petit mal* status)
      2. Atypical absence SE
         (*eg*, in the Lennox-Gastaut syndrome)
      3. Atonic SE
      4. NCSE as a sequel of partially treated GCSE
II. Partial SE
   A. Simple partial SE
      1. Typical
      2. Epilepsia partialis continua
   B. Complex partial SE (CPSE)
III. Neonatal SE

*Adapted from Lothman.[17]

free radicals; (4) generating nitric oxide, which both enhances subsequent excitation and serves as a toxin; (5) phosphorylating enzyme and receptor systems, making seizures likely; and (6) increasing intracellular osmolality, producing neuronal swelling. If adenosine triphosphate production fails, membrane ion exchange ceases, and the neuron swells further. These events produce the neuronal damage associated with SE.

Many other biophysical and biochemical alterations occur during and after SE. The intense neuronal activity activates immediate-early genes and produces heat shock proteins, providing indications of the deleterious effects of SE and insight into the mechanisms of neuronal protection.[18] Wasterlain's group has summarized mechanisms by which SE damages the nervous system.[19] Absence SE is an exception among these conditions; it consists of rhythmically increased inhibition and does not produce clinical or pathologic abnormalities.

The mechanisms that terminate seizure activity are poorly understood. The leading candidates are inhibitory mechanisms, primarily GABAergic neuronal systems. Clinical observation supports the contention that human SE frequently follows withdrawal from GABA agonists (*eg*, benzodiazepines).

The electrical phenomena of SE at the whole brain level, as seen in the scalp EEG, reflect the seizure type that initiates SE, *eg*, absence SE begins with a 3-Hz wave-and-spike pattern. During SE, there is slowing of this rhythm, but the wave-and-spike characteristic remains. GCSE goes through a sequence of electrographic changes (Table 4).[20] The initial discharge becomes less well formed, implying that neuronal firing is losing synchrony. The sustained depolarizations that characterize SE alter the extracellular milieu, most importantly by raising extracellular potassium. The excess potassium ejected during SE exceeds the buffering ability of astrocytes. Raising extracellular potassium potentiates more seizures.

The increased cellular activity of SE elevates demand for oxygen and glucose, and blood flow initially increases. After about 20 min, however, energy supplies become exhausted. This causes local catabolism to support ion pumps (attempting to restore the internal milieu). This is a major cause of epileptic brain damage.

The brain contains systems to terminate seizure activity; GABAergic interneurons and inhibitory thalamic neurons are both important.

SE produces neuropathology even in patients who are paralyzed, ventilated, and maintained at normal temperature and blood pressure. The hippocampus, a crucial area for memory, contains the most susceptible neurons, but other regions are also vulnerable. In addition to damaging the CNS, GCSE produces life-threatening, systemic effects.[21] Systemic and pulmonary arterial pressures rise dramatically at seizure onset. Epinephrine and cortisol prompt further elevations and also produce hyperglycemia. Muscular work raises blood lactate. Breathing suffers from both airway obstruction and abnormal diaphragmatic contractions. CO_2 excretion falls while its production increases markedly. Muscular work accelerates heat production; skin blood flow falls concomitantly, sometimes raising core temperature dangerously.

After about 20 min, motor activity begins to diminish, and ventilation usually improves. Body temperature may rise further, however.

Table 4. *Electrographic-Clinical Correlations in GCSE**

Stage	Typical Clinical Manifestations	Electroencephalographic Features
1	Tonic-clonic convulsions; hypertension and hyperglycemia common	Discrete seizures with interictal slowing
2	Low- or medium-amplitude clonic activity, with rare convulsions	Waxing and waning of ictal discharges
3	Slight, but frequent, clonic activity, often confined to the eyes, face, or hands	Continuous ictal discharges
4	Rare episodes of slight clonic activity; hypotension and hypoglycemia become manifest	Continuous ictal discharges punctuated by flat periods
5	Coma without other manifestations of seizure activity	Periodic epileptiform discharges on a flat background

*Data from Treiman.[20]

Hyperglycemia diminishes; after 1 h, gluconeogenesis can fail, producing hypoglycemia. GCSE patients often aspirate oral or gastric contents, producing pneumonia. Rhabdomyolysis is common, and may lead to renal failure. Compression fractures, joint dislocations, and tendon avulsions are other sequelae.

Clinical Manifestations

Three problems occur in seizure recognition: (1) complex partial seizures in the setting of impaired awareness, (2) seizures in patients receiving pharmacologic paralysis, and (3) misinterpretation of other abnormal movements as seizures. ICU patients often have depressed consciousness in the absence of seizures, as a result of their disease, its complications (such as septic encephalopathy[22]), or drugs. A further decline in alertness may reflect a seizure; an EEG is required to diagnose one.

Patients receiving neuromuscular junction (NMJ) blocking agents do not manifest the usual signs of seizures. Because most such patients receive sedation with GABA agonists, the likelihood of seizures is small. Autonomic signs of seizures (hypertension, tachycardia, pupillary dilation) may also be the effects of pain or the response to inadequate sedation. Hence, in patients manifesting these findings who have a potential for seizures (*eg*, intracranial pathology), an EEG should be performed. The actual incidence of this problem is unknown.

Abnormal movements can occur in patients with metabolic disturbances or anoxia. Some can be distinguished from seizures by observation, but if doubt about their nature persists, an EEG should be performed. Psychiatric disturbances in the ICU occasionally resemble complex partial seizures. Prolonged EEG monitoring may be required if the problem is intermittent.

Manifestations of SE: The manifestations of SE depend on the type and, for partial SE, the cortical area of abnormality. Table 3 depicts the types of SE encountered. This focuses on those seen most in the ICU.

Primary GCSE begins as tonic extension of the trunk and extremities without preceding focal activity. No aura is reported and consciousness is immediately lost. After several seconds of tonic extension, the extremities start to vibrate, quickly giving way to clonic (rhythmic) extension of the extremities. This phase wanes in intensity over a few minutes. The patient may then repeat the cycle of tonus followed by clonic movements, or continue to have intermittent bursts of clonic activity without recovery. Less common forms of GCSE are *myoclonic SE* (bursts of myoclonic jerks increasing in intensity, leading to a convulsion) and *clonic-tonic-clonic SE* (clonic activity precedes the first tonic contraction). Myoclonic SE is usually seen in patients with anoxic encephalopathy or metabolic disturbances.

Secondarily generalized SE begins with a partial seizure and progresses to a convulsion. The initial focal clinical activity may be overlooked. This seizure type implies a structural lesion, so care must be taken to elicit evidence of lateralized movements.

Of the several forms of generalized NCSE, the one of greatest importance to intensivists is NCSE as a sequel of inadequately treated GCSE. When a patient with GCSE is treated with anticonvulsants (often in inadequate doses), visible convulsive activity may stop while the electrochemical seizure continues. Patients begin to awaken within 15 to 20 min after the successful termination of SE; many regain consciousness much faster. Patients who do not start to awaken after 20 min should be assumed to have entered NCSE. Careful observation may disclose slight clonic activity. NCSE is an extremely dangerous problem because the destructive effects of SE continue even without obvious motor activity. NCSE demands emergent treatment *under EEG monitoring* to prevent further cerebral damage, because there are no clinical criteria to indicate when therapy is effective.

Partial SE in ICU patients often follows a stroke or occurs with rapidly expanding brain masses. Clonic motor activity is most easily recognized, but the seizure takes on the characteristics of adjacent functional tissue. Therefore, somatosensory or special sensory manifestations occur, and the ICU patient may be unable to report such symptoms. Aphasic SE occurs when a seizure begins in a language area, and may resemble a stroke. *Epilepsia partialis continua* involves repetitive movements confined to a small region of the body. It may be seen with nonketotic hyperglycemia or with focal brain disease; anticonvulsant treatment is seldom useful. CPSE presents with diminished awareness. The diagnosis often comes as a surprise when an EEG is obtained.

Diagnostic Approach

When an ICU patient seizes, one has a natural tendency to try to stop the event. This leads to both diagnostic obscuration and iatrogenic complication. Beyond protecting the patient from harm, very little can be done rapidly enough to influence the course of the seizure. Padded tongue blades or similar items should not be placed in the mouth; they are more likely to obstruct the airway than to preserve it. Most patients stop seizing before any medication can reach the brain in an effective concentration.

Observation is the most important activity during a single seizure. This is the time to collect evidence of a partial onset, in order to implicate structural brain disease. The postictal examination is similarly valuable; language, motor, sensory, or reflex abnormalities after an apparently generalized seizure are evidence In the ICU patient, several potential seizure etiologies must be investigated. Drugs are a major cause of ICU seizures, especially in the setting of diminished renal or hepatic function, or when the blood-brain barrier is breached. Drug withdrawal is also a frequent offender. While ethanol withdrawal is common, discontinuing any hypnosedative agent may prompt convulsions 1 to 3 days later. A recent report suggests that narcotic withdrawal may produce seizures in the critically ill.[9]

The physical examination should emphasize the areas listed for the postictal examination. Evidence of cardiovascular disease or systemic infection should be sought, and the skin and fundi closely examined.

Illicit drug screening should be performed on patients with unexplained seizures. Cocaine is becoming a major cause of seizures.[23] Electrolytes and serum osmolality should also be measured. However, hypocalcemia rarely causes seizures beyond the neonatal period; its discovery must not end the diagnostic work-up. Hypomagnesemia has an equally unwarranted reputation as the cause of seizures in malnourished alcoholic patients.

The need for imaging studies in these patients has been an area of uncertainty. A prospective study of neurologic complications in medical ICU patients determined that 38 of 61 patients (62%) had a vascular, infectious, or neoplastic explanation for their fits. Hence, CT or MRI should be performed on most ICU patients with new seizures. Hypoglycemia and nonketotic hyperglycemia can produce seizures, and such patients might be treated for metabolic disturbances and observed if they lack other evidence of focal disease. With current technology, there are almost no patients who cannot undergo CT scanning. While MRI is preferable in most situations, the magnetic field precludes infusion pumps and other metallic devices. Whether to administer contrast for a CT depends on the clinical setting and on the appearance of the plain scan.

The EEG is a vital diagnostic tool for the seizure patient. Partial seizures usually have EEG abnormalities that begin in the area of cortex producing the seizures. Primary generalized seizures appear to start over the entire cortex simultaneously. Postictal slowing or depressed amplitude provide clues to the focal etiology of the seizures, and epileptiform activity helps to classify the type of seizure and guide treatment. In patients who do not begin to awaken soon after seizures have apparently been controlled, an emergent EEG is necessary to exclude NCSE.

Considering the etiologies of seizures in the ICU setting, patients who need cerebrospinal fluid (CSF) analysis usually require a CT scan first. When CNS infection is suspected, empiric antibiotic treatment should be started while these studies are being performed.

In contrast to the patient with a single seizure or a few seizures, the SE patient requires concomitant diagnostic and therapeutic efforts. Although 20 min of continuous or recurrent seizure activity usually define SE, one does not stand by waiting for this period to start treatment. Because most seizures stop within 2 to 3 min, it is reasonable to treat after 5 min of continuous seizure activity, or after the second or third seizure occurring without recovery between the spells.

GCSE can rarely be confused with decerebrate posturing, but observation usually makes the distinction straightforward. Tetanus patients are awake during their spasms, and flex their arms rather than extending them as seizure patients do.[18]

Treatment for SE should not be delayed to obtain an EEG. A variety of findings may be present on the EEG, depending on the type of SE and its duration (Table 4). CPSE patients often lack such organized discharges of GCSE, but instead have waxing and waning rhythmic activity in one or several head regions. A diagnostic trial of an IV benzodiazepine is often necessary to diagnose CPSE. Patients developing refractory SE or having seizures during NMJ blockade require continuous EEG monitoring.

Management Approach

Deciding to administer anticonvulsants to an ICU patient who experiences one seizure or a few seizures requires a provisional etiology, estimation of the recurrence likelihood, and recognition of the utility and limitations of anticonvulsants. For example, seizures during ethanol withdrawal do not indicate a need for chronic treatment, and giving phenytoin will not prevent more withdrawal convulsions. The patient may need prophylaxis against delirium tremens, but the few seizures themselves seldom require treatment. Patients who experience convulsions during barbiturate or benzodiazepine withdrawal, in contrast, should usually receive short-term treatment with lorazepam to prevent SE. Seizures related to drugs or metabolic disorders should also be treated briefly but not chronically.

The ICU patient with CNS disease who has even one seizure should usually start chronic anticonvulsant therapy, with review of this decision before discharge. Initiating this treatment after the first unprovoked seizure helps prevent subsequent epilepsy.[24] Starting after the first seizure in a critically ill patient at risk for seizure recurrence may be even more important, especially in conditions that would be seriously complicated by a convulsion. In the ICU setting, phenytoin is frequently selected for ease of administration and lack of sedation. The hypotension and arrhythmias that may complicate rapid administration can usually be prevented by slowing the infusion to <25 mg/min. Because of the rare occurrence of third-degree AV block, an external pacemaker should be available when patients with conduction abnormalities receive IV phenytoin. Fosphenytoin is safer to administer from an extravasation standpoint, but still carries risks of hypotension and arrhythmias. The phenytoin concentration should be kept in the "therapeutic" range of 10 to 20 μg/mL unless further seizures occur; the level may then be increased until signs of toxicity occur. Failure to prevent seizures at a concentration of 25 μg/mL is usually an indication to add phenobarbital.

Phenytoin is usually 90% protein-bound. Patients with renal dysfunction have lower total phenytoin levels at a given dose because the drug is displaced from binding sites, but the unbound level is not affected. Thus, renal failure patients, and perhaps others who are receiving highly protein-bound drugs (which compete for binding), may benefit from free-phenytoin level determination. Only the free fraction is metabolized, so the dose is not altered with changing renal function. The clearance half-time with normal liver function varies from about 12 to 20 h (IV form) to >24 h (extended-release capsules), so a new steady-state serum concentration occurs in 3 to 6 days. Phenytoin need not be given more frequently than every 12 h. Hepatic dysfunction mandates decreasing the maintenance dose.

Hypersensitivity is the major adverse effect of concern to the intensivist. This may manifest itself solely as fever, but commonly includes rash and eosinophilia. Adverse reactions to phenytoin and other anticonvulsants have been reviewed.[25]

Phenobarbital remains a useful anticonvulsant for those intolerant to phenytoin, or who have persistent seizures after adequate phenytoin. The target for phenobarbital in the ICU should be 20 to 40 μg/mL. Hepatic and renal dysfunction alter phenobarbital metabolism. Because its usual clearance half-time is about 96 h, give maintenance doses of this agent once a day. A steady-state level takes about 3 weeks to be established. Sedation is the major adverse effect; allergy occurs rarely.

Carbamazepine is seldom started in the ICU because its insolubility precludes parenteral formulation. Oral loading in conscious patients may produce coma lasting several days. This drug causes hyponatremia in patients receiving it chronically.

Management Issues in Acute Repetitive (Serial) Seizures

Despite the near-certainty that acute repetitive seizures not meeting a definition of SE must occur more frequently than SE itself, and that many cases of SE emerge from such a state, there has been little study of the issue of treatment. Although the use of IV benzodiazepines has become common in many inpatient settings, the choice of drug and the appropriate dose are uncertain. Many clinicians use IV diazepam, perhaps based more on tradition than pharmacokinetics. The anticonvulsant effect of a single dose of diazepam is very brief (about 20 min), while that of lorazepam is much longer (4 h or longer). Because the risk of serious adverse effects (*eg*, respiratory depression) is potentially greater for diazepam, lorazepam may represent a better choice.[26] If a shorter-acting agent is desired for diagnostic purposes when the diagnosis of a seizure is uncertain, midazolam may be a better choice. The role of other agents, such as intranasal or buccal midazolam or IV valproate, remain to be determined.[27]

Outside of the hospital setting, there is reasonably good evidence that rectal diazepam is effective and safe in the management of serial seizures, especially in children, at a dose of 0.2 to 0.5 mg/kg, with the dose repeated as necessary according to an age-based protocol.[28]

Management Issues in SE

Once the decision is made to treat the patient for SE, considerations for therapy should proceed on four fronts simultaneously (Table 5): (1) termination of SE; (2) prevention of seizure recurrence once SE is terminated; (3) management of potential precipitating causes for SE; and (4) management of the complications of SE and of underlying conditions.[29]

There is an implicit assumption here that the forms of SE that can produce neuronal damage should be terminated as rapidly as is safely possible. While there is no direct proof of this contention in humans, it appears to be the most reasonable approach.

The intensity of treatment for SE should reflect the risk that the patient experiences from the SE and its etiology. For example, GCSE puts the patient at risk for a panoply of neurologic, cardiac, respiratory, renal, hepatic, and orthopedic disorders, and should be terminated as rapidly one can safely accomplish the task, even if such termination requires the full support of a critical care unit. Typical absence SE, in contrast, probably poses a risk to the patient only if it occurs during a potentially dangerous activity (*eg*, driving an automobile), and initial attempts at its termination probably should not include agents likely to profoundly depress respiration and blood pressure. Treatment of CPSE, in which the risk of neurologic sequelae is considerable, should probably be similar to that recommended for GCSE. Simple partial SE appears to pose less risk to the patient than CPSE, and furthermore, attempts at therapy along the lines recommended for GCSE seldom result in prolonged seizure control. Therefore, therapy for simple partial SE is often pursued with somewhat less vigor that GCSE or CPSE.

The following recommendations were developed for patients in GCSE. There is very limited evidence regarding the optimal therapy for other types of SE. Because of the life-threatening nature of GCSE, and of the risks associated with its treatment, physicians caring for these patients must be constantly vigilant for respiratory and cardiovascular compromise, which may develop abruptly. Thus, neurologists and others caring for these patients should be adept at basic aspects of airway and blood pressure management. During the termination of SE, the patient should be constantly attended by personnel who can effectively perform bag-valve-mask ventilation, and plans for the rapid endotracheal intubation of such patients should be devised before intubation becomes necessary.

Termination of SE: The linchpin of treatment for SE is the rapid, safe termination of ictal activity. Numerous treatment modalities are available for this goal, and until recently there were few data to guide a decision among the various possible choices. The publication of the Veterans' Affairs (VA) cooperative trial allows a much greater degree of rational choice, and raises many new questions for study.[30]

Within the VA trial, patients were divided into the categories of "overt" and "subtle" SE. All patients were believed to have GCSE, which could be either primarily or secondarily generalized; the distinction between overt and subtle depended on the intensity of the clinically viewed convulsive activity. The subtle-SE patients were much

Table 5. *Suggested Management Protocol for Status Epilepticus*

I. Establish an airway. Whether to perform endotracheal intubation emergently depends primarily on the safety with which the airway can be maintained during the control of SE. Should NMJ blockade be needed, one must assume that the patient is still in SE despite the appearance of relaxation, unless EEG monitoring is available to demonstrate the actual state of brain function. Use a nondepolarizing agent (*eg*, vecuronium).

II. Determine the blood pressure. If the patient is hypotensive, begin volume replacement and/or vasoactive agents as clinically indicated. GCSE patients who present with hypotension will usually require admission to a critical care unit. (Hypertension should not be treated until SE is controlled, as terminating SE will usually substantially correct it, and many of the agents used to terminate SE can produce hypotension).

III. Rapidly determine the blood glucose. Unless the patient is known to be normo- or hyperglycemic, administer dextrose (1 mg/kg) and thiamine (1 mg/kg).

IV. Terminate SE. We recommend the following sequence:
  A. Lorazepam, 0.1 mg/kg at 0.04 mg/kg/min. This drug should be diluted in an equal volume of the solution being used for IV infusion, as it is quite viscous. Most adult patients who will respond will do so by a total dose of 8 mg. The latency of effect is debated, but lack of response after 5 min should be considered a failure.
  B. If SE persists after lorazepam, begin phenytoin 20 mg/kg at 0.3 mg/kg/min. If the patient tolerates this infusion rate, it may be increased to a maximum of 50 mg/min. Alternatively, administer fosphenytoin at the same dose, but at a rate of up to 150 mg/min. Hypotension and arrhythmias are the major concern. Many investigators believe that an additional 5-mg/kg dose of phenytoin or fosphenytoin should be administered before advancing to the next line of therapy.
  C. If SE persists, administer either midazolam or propofol. Midazolam can be given with a loading dose of 0.2 mg/kg, followed by an infusion of 0.1 to 2.0 mg/kg/h to achieve seizure control (as determined by EEG monitoring). Propofol can be given with a loading dose of 1 to 3 mg/kg, followed by an infusion of 1 to 15 mg/kg/h. We routinely intubate patients at this stage if this has not already been accomplished. Patients reaching this stage should be treated in a critical care unit.
  D. Should the patient not be controlled with propofol or midazolam, administer pentobarbital 12 mg/kg at 0.2 to 0.4 mg/kg/min as tolerated, followed by an infusion of 0.25 to 2.0 mg/kg/h as determined by EEG monitoring (with a goal of seizure suppression). Most patients will require systemic and pulmonary arterial catheterization, with fluid and vasoactive therapy as indicated to maintain blood pressure.
  E. Ketamine (1 mg/kg, followed by 10 to 50 µg/kg/min) is a potent NMDA antagonist[48] with intrinsic sympathomimetic properties that may be useful in patients who have become refractory to GABA-A agonists.

V. Prevent recurrence of SE. The choice of drugs depends greatly on the etiology of SE and the patient's medical and social situation. In general, patients not previously receiving anticonvulsants whose SE is easily controlled often respond well to chronic treatment with phenytoin or carbamazepine. In contrast, others (*eg*, patients with acute encephalitis) will require two or three anticonvulsants at "toxic" levels (*eg*, phenobarbital at greater than 100 µg/mL) to be weaned from midazolam or pentobarbital, and may still have occasional seizures.

VI. Treat complications.
  A. Rhabdomyolysis should be treated with a vigorous saline diuresis to prevent acute renal failure; urinary alkalinization may be a useful adjunct.
  B. Hyperthermia usually remits rapidly after termination of SE. External cooling usually suffices if the core temperature remains elevated. In rare instances, cool peritoneal lavage or extracorporeal blood cooling may be required. High-dose pentobarbital generally produces poikilothermia.
  C. The treatment of cerebral edema secondary to SE has not been well studied. When substantial edema is present, one should suspect that SE and cerebral edema are both manifestations of the same underlying condition. Hyperventilation and mannitol may be valuable if edema is life-threatening. Edema due to SE is vasogenic, so steroids may be useful as well.

---

more likely to have a serious underlying medical condition, and in general responded poorly to therapy. This discussion will concentrate on the overt-SE patients, because their results underlie the treatment paradigm developed herein.

In the study, 384 patients with overt SE were randomly divided into four treatment arms, which were chosen based on a survey of North American neurologists prior to the study's inception. These arms were (1) lorazepam, 0.1 mg/kg; (2) diazepam, 0.15 mg/kg, followed by phenytoin, 18 mg/kg; (3) phenytoin alone, 18 mg/kg; and (4) phenobarbital, 15 mg/kg. Successful treatment required both clinical and EEG termination of seizures within 20 min of the start of therapy, with no seizure recurrence within 60 min of the start of therapy. Patients in whom the first treatment failed received a second, and if necessary, a third study drug. These latter choices were not randomized, as this would have resulted in some patients

Table 6. *Treatment Results for First Agents in the VA Cooperative Study**

Agent	Overt SE Success Rate (%)	Subtle SE Success Rate (%)
Lorazepam	64.9	17.9
Phenobarbital	58.2	24.2
Diazepam/phenytoin	55.8	8.3
Phenytoin alone	43.6	7.7

*Data from Treiman and colleagues.[30]

receiving two loading doses of phenytoin, but the treating physician remained blinded to the treatments being given.

The overall success rates for patients whose diagnosis of overt SE was confirmed by subsequent review of clinical and EEG data are presented in Table 6. The results for patients with subtle SE are included for reference. Treatment with lorazepam demonstrated a statistically significant advantage over phenytoin (p = 0.002); there were no significant differences among the other agents. This differs from the intention-to-treat analysis, which showed similar trends but did not find a statistically significant difference among the treatment arms.

The results of this study may be compared to those of Leppik and colleagues,[31] who found lorazepam to be successful in about 85% of cases. However, this study used only clinical cessation of seizures as the criterion of success; preliminary data from the VA trial indicates that 20% of patients in whom SE appears to have been terminated actually remain in electrographic SE.

Preliminary analysis of the results of subsequent treatments in patients who did not respond to the first-line agents indicates that the aggregate response rate to the second-line drug regimen was 7.0%, and to the third-line treatment, 2.3% (Treiman DM; personal communication; 1998). These results call into question the common practice of using three conventional agents (*eg*, lorazepam, phenytoin, and phenobarbital) in the management of SE before using a more definitive approach.

Based on these results and the experience of many workers in the field, we recommend that treatment for GCSE begin with a single dose of lorazepam, 0.1 mg/kg. The limited data available do not suggest that administration of further conventional doses of lorazepam will be useful.[31] The drug should be administered after dilution with an equal volume of the IV solution through which it will be administered. If this fails to control SE within 5 to 7 min, a second agent should be chosen. The results of the VA trial suggest that a second conventional agent is unlikely to be successful. At this time, however, we still recommend the use of phenytoin (or fosphenytoin), 20 mg/kg, as the second drug. This approach carries the advantage that if it is effective, the patient may not require endotracheal intubation and extended critical care. However, it may delay the eventual termination of SE by more definitive treatment.

The introduction of the phenytoin prodrug fosphenytoin as a safer way of rapidly achieving an effective serum phenytoin concentration may prompt some reconsideration of the way in which this drug is used.[32] At its maximal rate of administration (150 mg phenytoin equivalent/min), and its 7-min half-time of conversion to phenytoin, a free-phenytoin level of about 2 μg/mL can be achieved with fosphenytoin in about 15 min, as opposed to about 25 min for phenytoin itself. Whether this greater speed of administration will produce a higher rate of SE control remains to be demonstrated. It is clear that fosphenytoin administration is safer, in that the risk of hypotension may be somewhat less, and the adverse effects of extravasation are nil with the newer drug. The much greater cost of fosphenytoin has discouraged many from using it, although pharmacoeconomic simulations suggest that its use may be cost-effective.[33]

Valproate is available in an IV form; its role in the termination of SE remains to be defined. Experimental data suggest that a serum valproate concentration of 250 μg/mL or greater may be necessary to control secondarily generalized SE.[34] We have limited experience using doses of 60 to 70 mg/kg to obtain such a concentration in patients, and have found the drug effective on occasion in situations where in was necessary to avoid the risks of hypotension and respiratory depression associated with other treatment modalities. However, more information is required before the role of this agent in SE becomes clear.

Patients who continue in SE after lorazepam and phenytoin have traditionally been treated with conventional doses of phenobarbital, but the results of the VA study suggest that this is very unlikely to result in the rapid termination of SE. At this point, we consider SE to be refractory, and go on to one of the more definitive forms of treatment.[35] These treatment modalities are very likely to result in termination of SE, but are also carry higher risks of respiratory depression, hypotension, and secondary complications such as infection. Patients who are to undergo one of these definitive therapies should be in a critical care unit and be endotracheally intubated if this has not yet been accomplished.

Discussion of the entire range of proposed definitive treatments for SE is beyond the scope of this paper. Three categories will be considered: high-dose barbiturates, high-dose benzodiazepines, and propofol.

It is our contention that patients reaching this stage in the treatment of SE should undergo continuous EEG monitoring. The technologic aspects of continuous EEG monitoring have been reviewed elsewhere.[36] What the goal regarding the activity on the EEG should be remains a matter of debate. There is no prospectively collected evidence that a burst-suppression EEG pattern is required for, or is efficacious for, the termination of SE. Many patients can achieve complete seizure control with a background of continuous slow activity, and do not thereby incur the greater risks associated with the higher doses of medication required to achieve a burst-suppression pattern. Conversely, a few patients will continue to have frequent seizures that emerge out of a burst-suppression background, and presumably need even higher doses of medication, which may result in very long periods of suppression or even a "flat" EEG. Without continuous EEG monitoring, one must rely on occasional samples of the EEG, which are thus associated with risks of under- and overtreatment.

Most of the published experience with high-dose barbiturates involves pentobarbital, although some of the earlier investigators used thiopental, and a few reports discuss phenobarbital. There are few data regarding efficacy rates and adverse effects of these drugs. Thiopental is the most rapidly acting of these drugs, but may produce more hypotension. Pentobarbital has emerged as one of the standard choices for refractory SE. A loading dose of 5 to 12 mg/kg is usually given IV, followed by an infusion of the drug at a dose chosen to achieve the desired effect on the EEG; this is usually in the range of 1 to 10 mg/kg/h. We usually increase the infusion rate, along with an additional 3- to 5-mg/kg loading dose, when a seizure occurs; almost all seizures at this stage of treatment are electrographic, probably as a consequence of the medications suppressing clinical seizure activity (twitchless electrical activity), and perhaps also as a consequence of the prolonged duration of SE by the time definitive treatment has commenced. After 12 h free of seizures, the pentobarbital infusion rate is decreased by 50%. If seizures recur, the patient again receives the smaller loading dose, and the infusion rate is raised to obtain another 12-h seizure-free period. Other medications (eg, phenytoin) are continued. Many patients reaching this point will require substantial maintenance anticonvulsant treatment in order to be weaned from the pentobarbital; we commonly maintain the serum phenytoin concentration in excess of 20 µg/mL, and load with phenobarbital to achieve a concentration in excess of 40 µg/mL (often, 100 µg/mL or an even higher concentration is required to successfully wean severely refractory patients, such as those with encephalitis, from their pentobarbital infusions). High doses of barbiturates are potently immunosuppressive, indicating extra care to avoid nosocomial infection and aggressive treatment if infection is suspected.

High-dose benzodiazepine strategies for SE usually employ either midazolam or lorazepam. Midazolam has the advantages of rapid onset of activity and greater water solubility, avoiding the problem of metabolic acidosis from the propylene glycol vehicle of the other benzodiazepines and the barbiturates. Its major disadvantage is tachyphylaxis; over 24 to 48 h, the dose of the drug must often be increased several-fold in order to maintain seizure control. A loading dose of 0.2 mg/kg is followed by an infusion of 0.1 to 2.0 mg/kg/h, titrated to produce seizure suppression by continuous EEG monitoring.[37] High-dose lorazepam, used in doses of up to 9 mg/h, was the subject of a report by Labar and colleagues.[38]

Propofol is a pharmacologically unique GABA-A agonist that may also have other mechanisms of anticonvulsant action. Soon after its introduction as a general anesthetic agent, concerns about a potential proconvulsant effect arose;

this apparently represented myoclonus rather than seizure activity. At the doses used to control SE, it has a very potent anticonvulsant action. A loading dose of 3 to 5 mg/kg is frequently administered, followed by an infusion of 1 to 15 mg/kg/h,[39] titrated to EEG seizure suppression. After 12 h of seizure suppression, we taper the dose as outlined above for pentobarbital. There is evidence that rapid discontinuation of propofol can induce withdrawal seizures.

In our experience, propofol is more likely than midazolam to provide rapid control of refractory SE, exhibits less tachyphylaxis than midazolam, and produces less hypotension than pentobarbital for an equivalent degree of seizure control.[40] However, a recent retrospective analysis of our patients suggests that those with APACHE (acute physiology and chronic health evaluation) II scores >20 may have better survival when treatment is started with midazolam.[41] There are few data addressing the immunosuppressive effects of the benzodiazepines or propofol[42]; clinically, these drugs appear associated with fewer nosocomial infections than high-dose pentobarbital. Although it is difficult to determine functionally equivalent doses of these agents because of differing rates of tachyphylaxis, in our institution the patient charge for midazolam appears to be about 10 times that for pentobarbital, and propofol about 2.5 times that for pentobarbital.

Many other agents have been employed for the control of refractory SE.[43] The information above represents a distillation of our experience; the available published data are inadequate to support more definite treatment recommendations.

Prevention of Seizure Recurrence Once SE Is Terminated: Once SE is controlled, attention turns to preventing its recurrence. The best regimen for an individual patient will depend on the cause of the patient's seizures and any previous history of anticonvulsant therapy. For example, a patient developing SE in the course of ethanol withdrawal may not need anticonvulsant therapy once the withdrawal phenomena have run their course. SE following changes in a previously effective anticonvulsant regimen will often mandate a return to the former successful mode of treatment. In contrast, patients with a new, ongoing epileptogenic stimulus (*eg*, encephalitis) may require extraordinarily high serum concentrations of anticonvulsant drugs to control their seizures as therapy for refractory SE is decreased.

Management of the Complications of SE and of Underlying Conditions: The major systemic complications of GCSE include rhabdomyolysis and hyperthermia. Patients presenting with GCSE should be screened at presentation for myoglobinuria (most effectively by a dipstick evaluation of the urine for occult blood; the reagent will react with myoglobin as well as hemoglobin, and if the reaction is present, a microscopic examination will determine whether red blood cells are present) and elevation of serum creatine kinase (CK). If myoglobinuria is present, or if the CK concentration is >10 times the upper limit of normal, one should consider instituting a saline diuresis as well as urinary alkalinization.

If the patient's core temperature exceeds 40°C, the patient should be cooled. The techniques available for managing hyperthermic patients have been reviewed elsewhere.[44]

Cerebral edema may complicate SE. Vasogenic edema may develop as a consequence of the seizures themselves, and the underlying cause of SE may also produce either vasogenic or cytotoxic edema. The management of secondary cerebral edema with increased intracranial pressure (ICP) depends on the etiology; edema due solely to seizures rarely causes problems with ICP.

Prognosis

Wijdicks and Sharbrough[6] report that 34% of patients experiencing a seizure died during that hospitalization. Our prospective study of neurologic complications in medical ICU patients found that having even one seizure if in the unit for a nonneurologic reason doubled in-hospital mortality.[7] This effect on prognosis primarily reflected the etiology of the seizure.

Three major factors determine outcome in SE: the type of SE, its etiology, and its duration. GCSE has the worst prognosis for neurologic recovery; in contrast, myoclonic SE that follows an anoxic episode carries a very poor prognosis for survival. CPSE can produce limbic system damage, usually manifested as a memory disturbance. Most studies of outcome concentrate on GCSE mortality. Hauser,[8] summarizing data available in

1990, suggested that mortality rates vary from 1 to 53%. Those studies attempting to distinguish mortality due to SE from that of the underlying disease have attributed mortality rates of 1 to 7% to SE and 2 to 25% to its cause. Population-based studies in Richmond, VA showed the mortality of SE lasting >1 h was increased 10-fold over SE lasting <1 h. Etiologies associated with increased mortality included anoxia, intracranial hemorrhages, tumors, infections, and trauma.

Limited data are available concerning the functional abilities of GCSE survivors, and none reliably permit a distinction between the effects of SE and of its etiologies. One review concluded that intellectual ability declined as a consequence of SE.[45] Survivors of SE frequently seem to have memory and behavioral disorders out of proportion to structural damage produced by the etiology of their seizures. A wealth of experimental data support this observation, arguing strongly for rapid and effective control of SE. Case reports of severe memory deficits following prolonged CPSE have also been published.[46] Whether treatment of SE reduces the risk of subsequent epilepsy remains uncertain. Recent experimental studies indicate that SE lowers the threshold for subsequent seizures.[47]

Subarachnoid Hemorrhage

The management of patients with acute aneurysmal subarachnoid hemorrhage (SAH) has changed substantially in the past two decades. Previously, patients were typically put on bed rest for 2 weeks, until the periods of maximal risk for rebleeding and vasospasm had passed; if they survived, they were then given the option of surgical treatment. Current management strategies recognize (1) improvements in surgical technique that make early, definitive obliteration of the aneurysm more feasible and safer; (2) the consequent ability to use induced hypertension and hypervolemia to treat cerebral vasospasm; (3) the introduction of nitrendipine-class calcium channel blockers to relieve or ameliorate the effects of vasospasm; (4) the development of interventional neuroradiologic techniques (*eg*, angioplasty and intra-arterial papaverine infusion) to treat symptomatic vasospasm; (5) the use of ventricular drainage to treat communicating hydrocephalus; and (6) the introduction in several countries, although not in North America, of a free-radical scavenger that appears to improve outcome in patients who present with high-grade SAH.

Future directions in the medical management of patients following SAH will probably depend primarily on the ability to recognize and manage cerebral vasospasm before it becomes symptomatic and before it produces cerebral infarction.

Epidemiology

The principal medical complications of aneurysmal SAH include rebleeding, cerebral vasospasm, and volume and osmolar disturbances. The risk of rebleeding from unsecured aneurysms varies with time after the initial hemorrhage: about 4% on the first postbleed day and about 1.5% per day up to day 28.[49] The mortality associated with rebleeding after the diagnosis of SAH exceeds 75%.[50] This complication is more frequent in patients with higher grades of SAH, in women, and in those with systolic blood pressures exceeding 170 mm Hg.[51] Cerebral vasospasm produces symptoms in up to 45% of patients,[52] but is noted angiographically in another 25% who appear asymptomatic.[53] Vasospasm usually starts to occur between postbleed days 4 and 6; the risk of its development is minimal after day 14. Volume and osmolar disturbances are reported in about 30% of patients.[54]

A number of other complications occur in this group of patients that are less directly related to the SAH itself.[52] Life-threatening cardiac arrhythmias are found 5%, with less ominous rhythm disturbances in 30%. Pulmonary edema is diagnosed in 23%, with 6% experiencing a severe form. Some degree of hepatic dysfunction is noted in 24% of patients, predominantly mild elevation of transaminase levels without symptoms; 4% experience severe hepatic dysfunction. Many of these patients are probably manifesting hepatic toxicity from anticonvulsants or other medications. Thrombocytopenia is reported in 4% of patients, usually related to sepsis or medications. Renal dysfunction is seen in 7%, but rarely requires dialysis.

Although this paper deals primarily with aneurysmal SAH, there are other causes of SAH, and their epidemiology is different. SAH following rupture of an arteriovenous malformation tends to occur at a younger age, with a peak incidence in the mid-20s. Traumatic SAH is a common accompaniment of severe head trauma, occurring in 15 to 40% of patients with severe head trauma. The incidence of the major complications of SAH in these patients appears to be lower than in patients with aneurysmal SAH, but data are scarce. After arteriovenous malformation rupture, the time course of angiographically diagnosable vasospasm is similar to that seen in aneurysmal SAH patients; it is usually asymptomatic,[55] except in rare cases.[56] The significance of vasospasm related to traumatic SAH continues to be debated, but in one series, 7 of 29 patients with large amounts of subarachnoid blood (detected by CT scanning) developed symptomatic vasospasm (detected angiographically) with subsequent infarction.[57] In patients with penetrating head trauma, the incidence (detected by transcranial Doppler [TCD] flow velocity measurements) may be as high as 40%.[58]

Pathophysiology

Rebleeding: Rebleeding of an aneurysm prior to its obliteration presumably reflects further leakage of blood at the site of the initial rupture. The tendency for this to occur appears to increase with arterial hypertension, which increases the stress on the aneurysm wall and the clot that occludes the original rupture site. Lowering the pressure in the subarachnoid space (*eg*, by lumbar puncture, or by allowing a ventriculostomy system to have a low pop-off pressure) similarly increases the pressure gradient across the aneurysm wall. Whether these procedures actually increase the risk of rebleeding is uncertain, and this theoretical concern does not militate against performing diagnostic lumbar punctures if needed either to prove the diagnosis of SAH or to exclude meningitis. Systemic factors that alter the balance between thrombosis and fibrinolysis (*eg*, disseminated intravascular coagulation) would presumably affect the risk of rebleeding as well.

Cerebral Vasospasm: Vasospasm appears to be a two-stage process, with an initial vasoconstrictive phase followed by a proliferative arteriopathy, associated with smooth-muscle-cell necrosis and fibrosis of the arterial wall.[59,60] Vasospasm appears to depend primarily on the presence of erythrocytes in the subarachnoid space,[61] but why it occurs more frequently and more symptomatically after aneurysmal SAH than after SAH due to other causes remains unexplained. The list of potential mediators contributing to the development of vasospasm is substantial, but the vasoconstrictor peptide endothelin-1 appears to be one of the most important.[62] Endothelin antagonists are promising experimental agents for the prevention and treatment of this condition.[63]

The maximal risk for vasospasm occurs from day 4 through day 14 after SAH, although about 10% of patients may have some angiographic signs of vasospasm at the time of the initial angiogram.[64]

The risk of developing vasospasm is related to the amount of blood in the subarachnoid space. Fisher and colleagues[65] reported that patients with thick subarachnoid clots were much more likely to develop vasospasm than those without such clots. Antifibrinolytic agents (*eg*, ε-aminocaproic acid, tranexamic acid) used to prevent rebleeding raise the risk of symptomatic vasospasm and delayed ischemic deficits,[66] but whether there is an actual increase in the rate of vasospasm, or an increase in the rate of occlusion of already spastic vessels, is uncertain.

Hyperglycemia probably worsens outcome in stroke patients,[67] and therefore presumably in SAH patients developing delayed ischemia. Plasma glucose concentrations exceeding 120 mg/dL in the first postbleed week are associated with poor outcome.[68] All of these studies suffer from the confounding effect of severity of illness on intrinsic plasma glucose regulation, but they do suggest that maintenance of normoglycemia is a reasonable goal.

Volume and Osmolar Disturbances: Although earlier studies attributed the hyponatremia and hypo-osmolality occurring after SAH to the syndrome of inappropriate antidiuretic hormone secretion (SIADH),[69] most investigators now believe that these disturbances are the result of cerebral salt wasting.[70] The pathophysiology of this condition remains to be completely elucidated, but probably begins with the release of atrial, brain, and C-type natriuretic factors from the brain.[71] These peptides produce isotonic volume loss by their renal effects, resulting in hypovolemia. This hypovolemic state then prompts an appropriate antidiuretic hormone response, causing a fall in free water clearance and thereby producing hyponatremia and hypo-osmolality. Hypovolemia appears to increase the risk of cerebral infarction (delayed ischemic deficits) in patients with vasospasm, and should therefore be prevented with prophylactic volume replacement.[72]

Physical signs of hypovolemia are rare in SAH patients, who are usually kept flat in bed, and in whom a putative increase in adrenal catecholamine secretion and increased sympathetic nervous system activity often produce hypertension. Overly vigorous treatment of this hypertension after the aneurysm is secured appears to worsen outcome.[73]

Seizures: Following SAH, patients may experience any of four patterns of seizures. About 6% of patients appear to suffer a seizure at the time of the hemorrhage,[74] although the distinction between a generalized convulsion and an episode of decerebrate posturing may be difficult to establish from the reports of nonmedical observers. Postoperative seizures occur in about 1.5% of SAH patients despite anticonvulsant prophylaxis (usually phenytoin).[75] Patients developing delayed ischemia from vasospasm may seize following reperfusion by angioplasty.[76] Late seizures occur in about 3% of patients over several years of follow-up.[75]

SAH patients are somewhat more likely to have a seizure at the time of presentation than are patients with other types of stroke.[77]

The mechanisms producing seizures in SAH patients are uncertain. Patients in whom aneurysmal rupture produces a concomitant intracerebral hematoma probably have a direct epileptogenic stimulus. Irritation from the aneurysm clipping appears to account for some postoperative seizures. Reperfusion injury accounts for a small percentage.[76] Late seizures may reflect the epileptogenic effects of iron on the cerebral cortex.[78]

Cardiovascular Complications: Cardiac arrhythmias and ECG signs of ischemia are frequent in SAH patients.[79] In one series, all 61 patients had at least one such abnormal finding.[80] The most serious of such problems is the development of ventricular tachycardia, typically of the *torsades de pointes* form.[81]

ECG changes resembling acute myocardial infarction, and elevation of the MB isoenzyme of CK (and, by inference, elevation of troponins) occur without evidence of coronary arterial occlusion. About 10% of patients will have an ECG suggesting acute myocardial infarction during the first 3 days post-SAH.[82] In one study, elevation of CK was associated with left ventricular wall motion abnormalities.[83] Histopathologically, these findings correspond to myocardial contraction band necrosis, which resembles the cardiomyopathic changes associated with pheochromocytomas.

Pulmonary edema occurring in SAH patients may be either cardiogenic or noncardiogenic in origin. Some patients have echocardiographic evidence of left ventricular dysfunction at the time their pulmonary edema is severe.[84] However, the majority of SAH patients have a defect in pulmonary gas exchange in the absence of evidence of cardiac dysfunction or aspiration, suggesting that neurogenic pulmonary edema is responsible.[85] This probably occurs as the consequence of a neurally mediated increase in extravascular lung water.[86]

CNS Infection: Excepting cases of ruptured mycotic aneurysms, CNS infections in SAH patients are almost always iatrogenic, either from organisms introduced during aneurysm clipping or, much more commonly, from ventriculostomy systems that become colonized with bacteria.

Other Infectious Complications: The non-CNS infectious complications of SAH patients vary with the severity of their illness. Patients remaining in Hunt and Hess grades 1 and 2 do not seem to be at particular risk for aspiration and may not need urinary catheters, feeding tubes, or central venous lines, which are the proximate causes of many ICU infections. Higher-grade patients are susceptible to the typical infectious complications of critical care. The contribution of corticosteroids in decreasing resistance to infection in these patients is unquantified. SAH patients in the trials of tirilazad mesylate,[87] a steroid free-radical scavenger without glucocorticoid effects, were not given glucocorticoids either before or after procedures to secure their aneurysms; they did not appear to suffer ICP problems. Although this question has not been formally tested, it raises the possibility that routine dexamethasone administration may not be necessary in this population.

Withholding this agent would be expected to decrease both infectious and metabolic complications in these patients.

Higher-grade patients may need feeding tubes for nutritional support, or larger-bore gastric tubes should an ileus develop. Placing these tubes via the nasal route appears to increase the risk of nosocomial sinusitis, and probably of pneumonia as well.[88]

Deep Venous Thrombosis and Pulmonary Embolism: SAH patients are at risk for the development of deep venous thromboses and subsequent pulmonary embolism by virtue of immobilization. Whether the use of antifibrinolytic agents increases the risk of deep venous thrombosis has long been debated; the use of these agents for 2 weeks in patients undergoing late aneurysm surgery probably does increase these risks.[89] Brief use of these agents to decrease the risk of rebleeding prior to early surgery probably carries a lower risk.[90] Although the concentration of circulating fibrinogen complexes is increased in SAH patients (and other stroke patients) compared with controls,[91] the role of this finding in the genesis of venous thrombosis remains speculative.

Nutrition

Although standard critical care practice emphasizes the early institution of nutritional support to maintain muscle mass and gut integrity, the importance of nutritional support for SAH patients remains unproven. Starvation prior to experimental ischemia may result in a shift to the metabolism of fuels other than glucose, even in the brain, and potentially result in an improved outcome after delayed ischemia.[92] However, the balance between risks and benefits of this approach remains to be established. SAH patients are markedly catabolic, and may have a defect in the utilization of amino acids[93]; the mechanism of this defect is unknown.

Management

The higher-grade SAH patient may require all of the skills a critical care team can muster. The sickest of these patients can still attain a good functional outcome despite what appear to be overwhelming difficulties. Thus, attention to all of the details of care in these patients is essential. Guidelines for the care of SAH patients have recently been published by the American Heart Association[94] and the Canadian Neurosurgical Society.[95]

Rebleeding: Although aneurysm obliteration is the most important method of preventing rebleeding, antihypertensive drugs and antifibrinolytic agents may be valuable prior to surgery or interventional radiologic approaches. Preoperative blood pressures are typically elevated; we strive to maintain systolic pressures below 150 mm Hg and mean arterial pressures below 100 mm Hg in these patients. Nimodipine, which is used to try to prevent delayed ischemic deficits, often lowers the blood pressure to a modest degree. Labetolol (Table 7), which has both α- and β-adrenergic blocking effects when given IV, is commonly the first drug employed for blood pressure control. Hydralazine is also commonly used, although there is a theoretical concern about the use of pure vasodilators in preoperative SAH

Table 7. *Selected Drugs Useful in the Management of SAH Patients*

Agent	Dose	Comments
Enalaprilat	0.625 to 1.25 mg q6h	May decrease renal plasma flow and raise creatinine
Esmolol	250 to 500 μg/kg, then 50 to 200 μg/kg/min	May produce congestive heart failure
Hydralazine	10 to 20 mg q3-4h	Theoretical risk of increasing shear forces
Labetolol	10 mg q10min, up to 300 mg	Oral form lacks significant β-adrenergic blocking effect
Nicardipine	0.075 to 0.15 mg/kg/h	May produce congestive heart failure
Nimodipine	60 mg q4h for 14 to 21 days	Duration of therapy uncertain
Nitroprusside	0.25 to 10 μg/kg/min	Rarely necessary
Phenytoin	15 to 20 mg/kg loading dose, then 5 to 8 mg/kg/day maintenance (q12h for suspension, q24h for Dilantin* capsules	Duration of therapy uncertain; maintain serum concentration between 10 and 20 μg/mL. Hold tube feeding 1 h before and after dose.

*Dilantin; Parke-Davis; Morris Plains, NJ.

patients (increasing pulse pressure may increase stress on the aneurysm wall). Enalaprilat may be useful for patients who do not respond to these agents. We tend to avoid nitrates because of the potential for increased ICP, but rarely nitroprusside may be the only effective drug. Pain relief with acetaminophen, codeine, or fentanyl is often necessary, and is frequently helpful in lowering blood pressure as well.

Postoperatively, the blood pressure may be allowed to rise to higher levels. Patients at risk for vasospasm may require higher blood pressures for adequate cerebral perfusion. In patients with more than one aneurysm, the risk of producing a new SAH from a previously unruptured aneurysm appears to be small (but not absent[96]) during the first few postbleed weeks.

Cerebral Vasospasm: Delayed ischemic deficits from vasospasm have emerged as the major cause of morbidity and mortality in patients undergoing early aneurysm obliteration. Management approaches attempt to prevent both spasm and its consequences, although it is not clear that any of the currently used techniques actually prevent vasospasm. Rather, most attempt to preserve either perfusion or neuronal survival in areas affected by vasospasm.

Vasospasm is definitively diagnosed angiographically, although spasm in vessels below the resolution of angiography probably occurs in patients whose symptoms suggest vasospasm. The initial symptom of vasospasm is typically decreased interaction with the unit staff and the patient's family and visitors. The patient may then progress to an abulic state, or appear to have bilateral frontal lobe dysfunction. The etiology of these symptoms is uncertain, as they do not appear to depend on the location of the aneurysm, the localization of subarachnoid blood, or the development of complications such as hydrocephalus. At this point, the TCD velocity measurements are usually elevated (*eg*, mean velocities >120 cm/s). Xenon-CT blood flow studies suggest that TCD may underestimate the incidence and severity of vasospasm.[97] Lateralized motor findings suggest the development of delayed ischemic lesions.

Nimodipine, a voltage-sensitive calcium channel blocker, was introduced with the expectation that it would prevent vasospasm. Angiographic studies did not confirm this effect, at least in vessels visible by radiologic techniques, but clinical trials did confirm its utility in improving outcome.[98] Nicardipine, a related agent, does appear to decrease angiographically diagnosed vasospasm.[99] The outcome of patients treated with nicardipine did not differ statistically from that in patients receiving placebo, but the placebo patients received rescue hypertensive-hypervolemic therapy (HHT) more frequently.

Volume replacement and expansion, usually practiced by attempts to maintain either a fixed, relatively high saline solution intake (*eg*, 3 to 6 L/d of normal or mildly hypertonic saline solution) or a positive fluid balance, is relatively standard in centers caring for SAH patients. While this usually prevents volume contraction due to cerebral salt wasting, it is unlikely that it prevents vasospasm *per se*. However, it appears to be very useful in preventing or decreasing the extent of symptomatic vasospasm and delayed ischemic deficits.

The free-radical scavenger tirilazad may be effective in improving outcome in SAH patients, primarily those in higher grades. A European-Australian trial showed efficacy at a dose of 6 mg/kg/d only in men,[100] presumably because the drug is more rapidly metabolized in women. A parallel North American trial did not achieve a statistically significant result.[87] This appears at least in part to reflect a higher percentage of North American patients receiving phenytoin, which accelerates the metabolism of tirilazad.[101] Higher-dose trials have been concluded, but the results have not yet been published. This agent has been licensed for SAH in men in 13 countries. The drug has poor blood-brain barrier penetration; more lipophilic derivatives have been synthesized,[102] and await clinical trials.

Treatment for Vasospasm: Two approaches are currently used for the management of vasospasm. The first is volume expansion, usually accompanied by induced hypertension (by means of HHT).[103] Although some consider hemodilution (to hemoglobin concentrations between 10 and 11 g/dL) to be part of this treatment as well, in the hope that decreasing blood viscosity will improve perfusion, this is the least consistently practiced part of this approach. HHT has not been subjected to a randomized clinical trial, and substantial debate persists regarding its utility.[104,105] If it is to be employed, careful patient monitoring is necessary, involving an arterial line and either a central venous line or, preferably, a pulmonary artery catheter to guide vasopressor and volume management. Angiographic confirmation of the diagnosis of vasospasm is usually obtained before instituting vasopressor therapy.

Because SAH patients appear to have low thresholds for the development of hydrostatic pulmonary edema, we try to maintain the pulmonary capillary wedge pressure (PCWP) between 15 and 18 mm Hg. In some patients, this volume expansion alone is adequate to produce an increase in cardiac index and mean arterial pressure. What mixture of colloid and crystalloid to use for volume expansion in this setting is the subject of endless debate and absent data. If the patient's examination does not improve, we next raise the mean arterial pressure using phenylephrine, dopamine, norepinephrine, epinephrine, or a combination of phenylephrine and dobutamine, as suggested by the patient's heart rate, the cardiac index produced, and evidence of ectopy, cardiac ischemia, or renal dysfunction. None of these medications has a proven advantage over the others in this setting, and each case provides individual challenges. Hypertensive encephalopathy can apparently complicate overly vigorous therapy.[106]

The second approach to vasospasm patient management involves interventional radiologic techniques, either angioplasty or papaverine infusion.[107] We use both hemodynamic and radiologic techniques. Intraventricular infusion of nitroprusside may be useful in the future.[108]

Volume and Osmolar Disturbances: Volume deficits are prevented or corrected as discussed above. If SAH patients receive adequate saline solution replacement, hypo-osmolality is an infrequent occurrence.

Evaluation of the SAH patient whose laboratory results indicate a low serum sodium concentration requires both clinical and laboratory evaluation. Prior to intervention, serum and urine osmolality measurements should be obtained. This will prevent the inadvertent treatment of the patient for hypo-osmolality when the real problem is, for example, a factitious hyponatremia due to hyperglycemia or pseudohyponatremia from hyperlipidemia. Truly hypo-osmolar SAH patients require careful thought, rather than just salt administration. Unless the patient has developed pulmonary edema or other signs suggesting congestive heart failure, one should not assume that hyponatremia is due to combined salt and water excess. The likely occurrence of cerebral salt wasting favors a diagnosis of salt loss with water retention. Osmolality measurements will usually indicate that the patient's urine is inappropriately concentrated for a patient with hypotonic serum. While this combination may suggest SIADH in many circumstances, this condition should rarely be diagnosed during the first 2 weeks postbleed. Attempts to treat the patient with volume restriction will likely lead to greater problems with delayed ischemic deficits. One potentially useful biochemical assay is the serum uric acid level, which tends to be low in SIADH but normal in cerebral salt wasting.

Management of hypo-osmolar states depends critically on their rate of development.[109] Rapidly developing (*eg*, over hours) hypo-osmolality produces neuronal swelling, and is associated with elevated ICP and seizures. More slowly developing (over days) hypo-osmolality is accompanied by solute shifts out of neurons, which prevent ICP increases and are unlikely to produce seizures; the patient may become confused, lethargic, and weak, but seldom experiences any life-threatening complications from the osmolality itself. However, these are the patients at risk for central and extrapontine myelinolysis if their osmolalities are raised too rapidly.

Patients who became rapidly hypo-osmolar may be treated with small doses of hypertonic saline solution (*eg*, 100 mL of 3N) to begin correcting this problem. They usually respond quickly with lower ICP and resolution of seizures. Those who became hypo-osmolar more slowly must be corrected more slowly; a goal of 6 milliosmols/L/day increases appears safe. Because these patients should not be allowed to become volume-depleted, this is best performed by replacement of their urine output and insensible loss by mildly hypertonic solutions, or, in patients receiving enteral feeding, addition of salt to their food. Attempts to decrease the urine osmolality with loop diuretics are seldom sufficiently successful to be useful.

Cardiovascular Complications: Prevention of electrolyte disturbances and magnesium replacement are probably useful for the prevention of arrhythmias. α- and β-adrenergic blockade may decrease or prevent myocardial contraction band necrosis, but this has not been tested.

Cardiac arrhythmias in SAH are seldom life-threatening. Sinus tachycardia and other supraventricular tachycardias should lead to a reassessment of electrolytes, volume status, pain control, infection, and endocrine (especially thyroid) function. Depending on the arrhythmia and its hemodynamic consequences, treatment with adenosine, calcium antagonists, β-blocking agents, or digoxin may be indicated. Ventricular arrhythmias frequently reflect adrenergic drug administration (*eg*, dopamine) or electrolyte disorders; alternatively, they may represent signs of myocardial ischemia. If possible, dopamine-induced rhythm disorders indicate switching to another agent. Lidocaine or procainamide may be required if runs of ventricular tachycardia appear. *Torsades de pointes* may respond to supplemental magnesium, or may require overdrive pacing.

SAH patients with heart failure who develop signs suggesting vasospasm will usually require pulmonary artery catheterization for volume and hemodynamic management.

CNS Infection: Infection is a major problem for SAH patients, because fever may increase the degree of damage produced by delayed ischemia. Another problem is the diagnosis of the etiology of fever in these patients. A preliminary analysis in our unit suggests that about 20% of SAH patients experience fever without evidence of infection on retrospective review, suggesting that they have developed "central fever."[110] These patients frequently receive antibiotics, putting them at risk for drug reactions and increasing expense, because it is difficult to prove that they do not have an infection. Drug-induced fevers are a major problem in all ICU patients, and SAH patients are no exception. Commonly implicated drugs include phenytoin, antibiotics, and, less frequently, agents such as histamine$_2$-antagonists and stool softeners.

Whether patients with ventriculostomies or lumbar drains should receive antibiotic prophylaxis is an open question. If prophylaxis is to be given, a cephalosporin with activity against *Staphylococcus aureus* (*eg*, cefazolin) is probably the most reasonable choice. Activity against coagulase-negative staphylococci does not seem important; nor do the brain or CSF penetration characteristics of the drug. A risk-benefit analysis suggests that ventriculostomy catheters probably should be changed every 5 days.[111]

Treatment of ventriculostomy infections should be based initially on a Gram stain of CSF. If staphylococcal infection is suspected, initial treatment with vancomycin is appropriate pending culture and sensitivity results. Patients with Gram-negative rods in the CSF should receive either a cephalosporin with antipseudomonal activity (*eg*, cefepime) or meropenem until microbiologic results are available. If the CSF contains increasing numbers of white cells but the Gram stain is negative, a combination of vancomycin and either meropenem or cefepime seems reasonable, although some of these patients will have an aseptic postoperative meningitis.

Other Infectious Complications: The question of routine changes of central venous catheters and pulmonary artery catheters is beyond the scope of this discussion. Whatever local practices control these policies for other critically ill patients should apply to SAH patients.

We attempt to place all tracheal and gastric tubes through the mouth, rather than the nose, to decrease the incidence of sinusitis[112] (see above).

Seizures: Because seizures in patients with unsecured aneurysms may promote rebleeding, it is a common, although by no means universal, practice to administer anticonvulsants to SAH patients.

The standard agent for prophylaxis in North America is phenytoin. Fosphenytoin, a water-soluble prodrug, is safer to administer IV, and may be given IM if necessary. An adequate loading dose should be given.

Should seizures occur in an SAH patient, one should obtain a CT scan to look for new intracranial pathology. At the same time, one should give an additional dose of phenytoin to raise the serum concentration. If seizures recur, and the phenytoin has been pushed to the point of symptomatic toxicity (in the responsive patient) or a level of about 24 μg/mL (in patients with impaired ability to respond), adding either phenobarbital or carbamazepine have been standard approaches. The recent introductions of gabapentin and an IV form of valproate increase the number of therapeutic options. This choice must be individualized.

Phenytoin is frequently implicated as a cause of drug-induced fever. When a rash and fever appear in a patient taking this drug, it is typically discontinued. Because of its long half-life, several days will elapse before it is cleared from the patient. Substitution of another anticonvulsant (*eg*, gabapentin) without sedative effects and without cross-sensitivity is a reasonable approach. Suspected allergy is the only circumstance in which most anticonvulsants should be stopped abruptly.

Deep Venous Thrombosis and Pulmonary Embolism: Before securing the aneurysm, many physicians are reluctant to give prophylactic doses of heparin, and instead rely on sequential compression devices to prevent deep venous thrombosis. These devices are effective in many circumstances, but have not been formally tested in SAH patients. Interestingly, sequential compression devices accelerate *in vitro* measurements of fibrinolysis,[113] and part of their effectiveness probably stems from this mechanism. We continue to use these devices for prophylaxis in bed-bound patients after the aneurysm has been secured.

Deep venous thrombosis or pulmonary embolism in patients with either unsecured aneurysms or fresh craniotomies pose difficult management problems. Our approach is usually to place an inferior vena cava filter, and not to give anticoagulant therapy until at least 1 week after surgery. The filter is generally held to be safer than immediate anticoagulation.[114]

Nutrition and GI Bleeding Prophylaxis: Despite strongly held opinions, there are few data on which to base recommendations for nutrition in SAH patients. In view of the likely deleterious effect of hyperglycemia on outcome after delayed ischemia, whatever nutritional approach is taken should include frequent measurements of blood glucose, and probably its tight control. So-called "trophic" feeding, in which a small volume (*eg*, 5 mL/h) of an enteral nutrition formula is constantly infused via a gastric or jejunal feeding tube, may maintain the structure of the intestinal villi and help to prevent both bacterial translocation and the subsequent incidence of diarrhea when full feedings are instituted.

If patients are npo, some form of prophylaxis against GI bleeding seems reasonable. Clinically important GI bleeding occurs in up to 6% of SAH patients.[115] Histamine$_2$-blocking agents such as ranitidine or nizatidine are commonly used. These agents are occasionally associated with neutropenia or thrombocytopenia; in this circumstance, sucralfate or omeprazole may be substituted. The use of nonsteroidal anti-inflammatory agents appears to increase the risk of GI bleeding; we routinely administer misoprostol with these agents. Once patients are fully fed, these prophylactic agents may no longer be necessary.

When feedings begin, patients frequently develop diarrhea. Because a large percentage of patients are receiving antibiotics, the possibility of antibiotic-induced *Clostridium difficile* infection must be considered. After sending specimens for fecal leukocyte, cytotoxin, and *C difficile* cultures, we use kaolin and pectin to attempt to decrease the diarrhea. Some patients appear to have diarrhea induced by sorbitol, used in many solutions of drugs for tube administration.

Intracerebral Hemorrhage

The major causes of intracerebral hemorrhage (ICH) include chronic hypertension, coagulation disturbances, and underlying vascular lesions. Hypertensive ICH occurs where small penetrating arteries arise from large arterial trunks. There is reasonable evidence demonstrating that it is safe to acutely lower blood pressure in an attempt to decrease hematoma formation, but it is not known whether this is useful. A recent phase II study of recombinant factor VIIa shows that it will limit hematoma growth and improve functional outcome; a phase III study is in progress.[115a] This has only been studied in patients without coagulation disturbances.

Stroke

Stroke is the most common neurologic cause for hospital admission in the United States. About 80% of strokes are ischemic, with the remainder divided between intracerebral hemorrhage and SAH. The incidence of stroke is declining, coincident with and probably in part reflecting improvement in the treatment of hypertension. The association of stroke with hypertension, particularly intracerebral hemorrhage, has been slightly overstated in the past (blood pressures were often measured when the patient presented with the stroke, rather than seeking a documented history of hypertension; the same is true of many studies of hyperglycemia in stroke). Other risk factors include diabetes, cardiac disease, previous cerebrovascular disease (transient ischemic attack or stroke), age, sex, lipid disorders, excessive ethanol ingestion, elevated hematocrit, elevated fibrinogen, and cigarette smoking. Smoking is the most powerful risk factor for aneurysmal SAH. In younger patients (usually defined as those <55 years old), one should consider abnormalities of antithrombin III, protein S, protein C, or antiphospholipid antibodies. Young stroke patients with marfanoid habitus should be worked up for homocysteinuria; the heterozygous state is associated with stroke, and many patients respond to pyridoxine treatment.

The intensivist most commonly encounters potential stroke patients in the settings of (1) suspected carotid artery disease, and (2) cardiac disturbances that are potentially emboligenic. Patients with *asymptomatic* carotid bruits have approximately a 2% annual risk of stroke, but the side of the bruit does not predict the side of the stroke. There are no data on which to base the selection of patients for further work-up. I tend to start an aspirin regimen (80 to 325 mg/d) in these people, but not investigate them further. If studies (noninvasive or angiographic) have already been obtained, I would *consider* endarterectomy for *otherwise healthy* patients who have >70% stenosis or a large area of ulceration. The common practice of "prophylactic" endarterectomy before other vascular surgical procedures lacks validation; from the poor data available, the risk of stroke related to such procedures does not seem to exceed the risks related to endarterectomy itself. The results of the Asymptomatic Carotid Artery Stenosis (ACAS) trial suggest that men with asymptomatic carotid stenosis of >70% derive greater benefit from carotid endarteractomy than from medical therapy alone. Endarterectomy of the vertebral arteries and angioplasty of any cerebral vessel remain experimental techniques.

About 30% of untreated patients with new-onset transient ischemic attacks will suffer a stroke in the next 2 years. If the patient has 70 to 99% stenosis in the relevant carotid artery, endarterectomy reduces the risk of stroke or death to about 10%. Patients not appropriate candidates for surgery should probably receive ticlopidine 250 mg bid (with appropriate monitoring of the WBC count); this drug appears effective in both men and women (aspirin has not been universally efficacious in women).

If a cardiac source of embolism is suspected, anticoagulation with warfarin is usually indicated. For patients with nonvalvular atrial fibrillation, a prothrombin time of 1.3 to 1.7 times control (or an international normalized ratio of about 3.0; should be >2.0 and <5.0) is probably adequate and has few side effects (in three recent studies of prophylaxis, minor bleeding was more common in the warfarin groups than in the control group, but intracerebral hemorrhage or other major bleeding was not). One study suggested that aspirin also reduced stroke rates; it could be used in patients who are poor risks for warfarin. In patients with suspected embolism from other cardiac disorders (*eg*, cardiomyopathies, left ventricular aneurysms), low-dose warfarin has not been well studied. The aortic arch is a hitherto underrecognized source of emboli; management of this condition remains to be established.

Transesophageal echocardiography can detect clots and other lesions that escape detection by transthoracic echocardiography. In some series, the rate of detection of cardiac lesions is so high that their significance is uncertain.

In patients 6 h or more into acute ischemic stroke, no treatment has been proven useful. Heparin may be indicated to prevent subsequent embolic strokes, but does not affect either a completed stroke or so-called stroke-in-evolution. If the patient is to receive anticoagulant therapy because of a suspected source of embolism, some investigators feel that patients with large infarcts should not be given anticoagulants for several days because of a presumed risk of hemorrhage into the infarct. Other data suggest that the greatest risk of re-embolization occurs in the first few days after the initial stroke, which argues for early anticoagulation of this group. I favor the latter approach.

Patients who follow a stuttering course may benefit from induced hypertension to improve flow through stenotic vessels until collateral vessels can open. Spontaneous hypertension in these patients should be considered a compensatory response, and should not be treated in the first few poststroke days unless evidence of end-organ damage develops. We avoid treating blood pressure unless the *mean* pressure exceeds 160 mm Hg. After the patient has stabilized neurologically, a course of chronic antihypertensive treatment can be instituted.

The role of hyperglycemia in worsening stroke outcome seems established, but no studies have been done to determine whether tight control of blood sugar will improve prognosis.

The National Institute of Neurological Disorders and Stroke rt-PA Stroke Study Group (NINDS) trial[116] showed that thrombolysis was safe and effective if performed within 3 h of stroke onset (this does not mean 3 h after waking up with a new stroke; the time of stroke onset must be known). The recombinant tissue-plasminogen activator dose in this study was 0.9 mg/kg, with 10% of the dose as a bolus and the remainder over 1 h. The treated patients had a very significant improvement in functional outcome. There were more intracerebral hemorrhages in the treated group, but their mortality was actually lower (this did not reach statistical significance).

Patients who develop serious increases in ICP during the first 3 to 4 days poststroke are at risk for herniation and death. The earliest sign is usually diminished consciousness, often followed by an ipsilateral third-nerve palsy. Corticosteroids do not decrease the cytotoxic edema associated with strokes, and should not be used (unless the cause of the stroke is vasculitic). Although the routine use of hyperventilation in stroke patients is not indicated, this technique is appropriate to prevent herniation. Mannitol can also be used. If more drastic therapy is contemplated (*eg*, high-dose barbiturates), an ICP monitor should be inserted. We now use hemicraniectomy to reduce ICP in these patients, with surprisingly good functional outcomes; this has not become the standard of care. Experimental results suggest that the skull should be removed before swelling occurs, in order to protect the cortex from loss of pial collaterals.

Intracerebral hemorrhage produces much more rapid rises in ICP because of the volume of the hematoma. The major concerns for the internist are (1) exclusion or treatment of a bleeding diathesis, which should always be considered, and (2) management of ICP. Although the edema around an intracerebral hemorrhage is vasogenic, it does not respond to steroids. Three controlled studies have documented poorer outcome in steroid-treated patients, owing to the side effects of the steroids. In older patients, especially those with more than one episode of hemorrhage and without a history of hypertension, amyloid angiopathy becomes a diagnostic consideration (about 15% of all intracerebral hemorrhages). In younger patients, intracerebral hemorrhage related to sympathomimetic agents (including cocaine) is becoming an increasingly frequent problem.

Although neurogenic pulmonary edema may occur in any acute intracranial condition, SAH patients seem particularly prone to it; about 40% of our SAH patients have some degree of oxygenation difficulty not explained by other conditions. In neurogenic pulmonary edema, the PCWP is normal, and the edema fluid has a high protein content; this reflects the presumed pathogenic mechanism of pulmonary venoconstriction. One must then attempt to balance the need to expand volume in patients with the need to keep their lungs dry. We tend to keep the PCWP around 10 mm Hg, and use vasopressors to improve cerebral perfusion if necessary.

Nervous System Infections

Meningitis

The consensus of opinion seems to favor presumptive treatment for suspected meningitis in any situation in which lumbar puncture (LP) is delayed. This includes even delays to obtain CT scans, because the commonest causes of meningitis in adults (pneumococcal and meningococcal) can kill the patient while waiting for the scan. I believe that patients who are alert and have normal fundi and neurologic exams can undergo LP without scanning, because the possibility of a patient in that setting herniating soon after LP is infinitesimally small, but presumptive treatment is clearly more important than intellectual purity. With the increasing prevalence of penicillin-resistant pneumococci, cefotaxime (2 g q4h) or ceftriaxone (2 *g* q12h) should be used for empiric therapy. A few pneumococci with significant resistance to third-generation cephalosporins have emerged, prompting some to add vancomycin until results of sensitivity testing are available. Cefuroxime is inferior to these third-generation cephalosporins and should no longer be used. Because ampicillin-resistant *Haemophilus influenzae* infections are common, children should also receive the third-generation agents. Chloramphenicol is often recommended for truly penicillin-allergic (*eg*, anaphylactic) patients, although clinical failures have been reported in patients with penicillin-resistant pneumococci. In most cases, the initial dose of antibiotics will not sterilize the CSF within 30 to 60 min; even if this occurs, testing for bacterial antigens will reveal the etiology in the majority of cases. Blood cultures should be obtained before antibiotics are given. Further treatment decisions can be made based on the Gram stain and antigen results. If listeriosis is suspected (immune-compromised host, or negative Gram stain and bacterial antigen tests), ampicillin or sulfamethoxazole-trimethoprim should be added until an organism is isolated or blood and CSF cultures have been negative for at least 3 days. Because of its epileptogenic effects, imipenem should usually be avoided in CNS infections.

In infants and children, pretreatment with steroids (dexamethasone, 0.15 mg/kg q6h for 4 days) appears to decrease neurologic dysfunction after recovery from meningitis (predominantly that due to *H influenzae*). This is presumed to reflect a decrease in inflammation from lysis of organisms, with the subsequent host elaboration of tumor necrosis factor and other inflammatory mediators. The use of steroids in adult meningitides remains controversial, but does not appear to be deleterious in the few patients so far studied. I think that the evidence favors its use in adults as well, but this is still debated. A recent study in children suggests that 2 days of dexamethasone is as useful as 4 days. The issue is clouded when vancomycin is used for potential penicillin-resistant pneumococci, because steroids may decrease vancomycin penetration into the CSF (this is debated in humans).

Increased ICP in meningitis patients is treated as described above. Cerebral edema in children appears to respond to steroids; it is probably appropriate to treat adults in the same fashion if elevated ICP is a problem. Hyponatremia is common, and may exacerbate vasogenic cerebral edema; it usually responds to fluid restriction. Whether this increases the rate of cerebral venous thrombosis is not clear. However, it is important not to let the cerebral perfusion pressure fall below about 60 mm Hg; this is more important that fluid restriction. Seizures are initially managed with benzodiazepines and phenytoin; the treatment of SE is covered above.

Encephalitis

As in meningitis, the weight of expert opinion is shifting (albeit more slowly) to the "shoot first and ask questions later" approach. When encephalitis is suspected, acyclovir (10 to 15 mg/kg q8h) is begun while the work-up is in progress; adequate hydration is necessary to prevent renal toxicity. The most sensitive test is CSF–polymerase chain reaction; MRI with gadolinium is second, with EEG third. Even though brain biopsy has a low rate of complications (3%, most of which are minor), the relative safety of acyclovir has encouraged many physicians to treat presumptively, and perform a biopsy only in patients who do not respond or in whom the work-up raises the possibility of another diagnosis. The commonly quoted list of "treatable disorders that mimic herpes simplex encephalitis" from the National Institute of Allergy and Infectious Diseases cooperative studies is not relevant in the MRI era. Seizures and elevated ICP are common.

Brain Abscess

Unless there is a strong suspicion of the etiology of a brain abscess (*eg*, the patient had a proven bacteremia prior to developing the abscess), empiric treatment for suspected brain abscess should include a third-generation cephalosporin, vancomycin, and metronidazole. Vancomycin is probably adequate treatment for Listeria, but if there is a reason to suspect this organism, one usually adds ampicillin or sulfamethoxazole-trimethoprim. Although some surgeons have tried to avoid aspiration, biopsy, or resection of these patients on the grounds that empiric medical treatment seems effective, this contention is based on small numbers of patients. Furthermore, it is often difficult to be certain that a particular lesion is an abscess and not a high-grade astrocytoma.

Surgery also offers some direct relief of ICP problems. For these reasons, I recommend early aspiration of suspected abscesses, with possible later debulking or resection.

Neurogenic Respiratory Failure

Myasthenia Gravis

Although the standard teaching about myasthenia gravis stresses fatigability with exercise, this is rarely what brings the patient to medical attention. The usual complaints are diplopia, ptosis, difficulty with speech and secretions, proximal limb weakness, and ventilatory dysfunction. The condition preferentially affects young women and older men. There is overrepresentation of human leukocyte antigen-A1 (HLA-A1), HLA-B8, and HLA-DRw3 (another instance in which HLA testing is not clinically useful). This is a true autoimmune disease, in which antibodies directed at myoid cells in the thymus [which express acetylcholine receptors (AChR)] attack the NMJ. There is a greater than expected incidence of other autoimmune diseases, including systemic lupus erythematosus, Sjögren's syndrome, polymyositis, and autoimmune thyroid disease. About 70% of patients have thymic hyperplasia, and 15% have thymomas. Anti-AChR antibodies are present in most patients with generalized myasthenia, and about 60% of those with ocular myasthenia. Antistriated muscle antibodies are a marker for thymoma.

Diagnostic studies include the edrophonium test (for which change in ptosis is the only truly objective bedside parameter to follow), measurement of anti-AChR antibodies, electromyography with repetitive stimulation, and chest CT to evaluate the thymus. Patients with generalized myasthenia who are developing ventilatory failure should be followed with vital capacity and negative inspiratory force (maximal inspiratory pressure) measurements; hypercapnia is a late finding. We usually intubate and ventilate patients when the vital capacity falls below about 12 mL/kg; some will require intubation because of upper airway problems but not need mechanical ventilation. Sometimes we will permit hypercapnia if the upper airway is intact and the patient is in the ICU. Edrophonium testing to distinguish myasthenic crisis from cholinergic crisis (too much anticholinesterase) is dangerous and should rarely be performed.

Treatment includes anticholinesterases (pyridostigmine), immunosuppressives (steroids, azathioprine, cyclophosphamide, sometimes cyclosporine), and thymectomy. Plasma exchange or IVIg can be dramatically effective, but each is only a short-term measure, primarily used for patients in crisis or to prepare them for thymectomy. Patients with purely ocular symptoms and normal thymic size on CT can be treated with anticholinesterases alone, but most other patients should be treated for the progressive autoimmune disease they have.

A large number of drugs have been reported to exacerbate myasthenia. The most important ones to remember are aminoglycosides, macrolides, lidocaine, propranolol, and quinidine. The effects of neuromuscular blocking agents is usually quite prolonged. Steroids often worsen the weakness before the patient improves.

Other Conditions

Respiratory failure due to diseases of the nervous system is predominantly hypercapnic, except in the case of neurogenic pulmonary edema. The diagnosis of neuromuscular respiratory failure is usually straightforward if one considers it as a possibility. Many of these conditions will be apparent at presentation, but on occasion a diagnosis of amyotrophic lateral sclerosis is made only when the patient has difficulty weaning from the ventilator. Critical illness polyneuropathy is a relatively recently described entity in which critically ill patients (most of whom have been septic) cannot be weaned from mechanical ventilation. Electromyographic studies show an axonal neuropathy; the prognosis for eventual recovery is very good, but these patients commonly require 4 to 6 months of mechanical ventilation.

Roelofs and coworkers,[117] Zochodne and colleagues,[118] and others described a unique peripheral neuropathy in patients who fail to wean from mechanical ventilation after an episode of critical illness, usually involving bacteremia. In a prospective study, Witt and colleagues[119] identified 43 patients with sepsis and multiple organ failure; electrophysiologic studies revealed sensorimotor axonal neuropathy in 70% of these patients, and 15 (35%) experienced difficulty in weaning from ventilatory support after improvement in their underlying conditions. Such patients display limb weakness on examination, with diminished or absent deep tendon reflexes. In the study by Witt and colleagues,[119] 23 of the patients (53%) survived; although all of the neuropathic patients improved, three with very severe neuropathy made incomplete recoveries. The authors suggested that the decrements in peripheral nerve function were related to hyperglycemia and hypoalbuminemia. They speculated that the likely etiologies of this neuropathy include the metabolic stresses that accompany sepsis, as well as the microcirculatory abnormalities. A study of other neurologic causes of failure to wean from ventilatory support has been reported, and emphasizes the high frequency of neuromuscular diseases in ICU patients with respiratory failure.[120] Interestingly, in general ICU patients, failure to wean from a neurologic cause carries a better prognosis than does similar failure due to a pulmonary cause.[121]

Patients who have flaccid paralysis after the use of NMJ blockers have received considerable attention in recent years. One group, with a relatively brief duration of paralysis, represents patients who have accumulated large amounts of these agents and take days to clear them. A second group, most commonly including asthmatics and other patients treated with steroids in addition to NMJ blockade, appears to have a myopathy, and the patients may take a very long time to recover. While earlier reports emphasized a relationship with the steroid-based NMJ-blocking drugs, this condition has been seen with atracurium as well.

Plasmapheresis is well established as a treatment for acute idiopathic polyneuritis (Guillain-Barré syndrome) if it is started in the first 2 weeks after onset. Usually, five treatments are given over 10 days. Ventilatory support is initiated as described above for myasthenia gravis. Autonomic instability may appear in the second week of the illness, and has become a leading cause of death. Thus, patients need careful observation until they are clearly improving. IVIg is also commonly used for both acute idiopathic polyneuritis and myasthenia gravis.

Neuroleptic Malignant Syndrome

The neuroleptic malignant syndrome (NMS) was recognized in the late 1950s.[122] It occurs in <1% of patients exposed to these agents, but may be more frequent in patients requiring higher than normal doses or multiple agents.[123] Although some agents have been more frequently associated with NMS than others (most prominently haloperidol, fluphenazine, and the thioxanthines), it has been reported with almost every neuroleptic agent and mixed dopamine-serotonin agents. Long-acting forms of haloperidol may result in more cases in the next several years. It may also occur in parkinsonian patients from whom either dopaminergic agonists or anticholinergic agents are abruptly withdrawn,[124] although the epidemiology of this problem is uncertain. Early studies cite a mortality rate of up to 20%,[123] although more recent work suggests approximately 4% to be correct.[125]

The condition appears to stem from central dopaminergic blockade in the majority of cases;[126] the few reports of parkinsonian patients who develop the condition when dopaminergic therapy is terminated suggest that lack of dopamine effect alone, rather than some other effect on the receptor, is necessary and sufficient to produce NMS. Drugs with stronger D_2-receptor antagonist effects are more likely to produce NMS. A patient with a mutation in the D_2 receptor has been reported.[127] Dopaminergic blockade may also affect thermoregulation by altering the hypothalamic set-point for temperature.

Most cases occur within a few weeks of either a dosage increase or, less commonly, the start of neuroleptic treatment.[128] Reported predispositions include strenuous exercise, dehydration, other CNS disorders, and the use of fluphenazine decanoate.[129] States of diminished osmolality may contribute to the pathogenesis of NMS.[130]

The major diagnostic findings of NMS include fever, severe rigidity (usually, but not always, accompanied by tremor), obtundation, and autonomic dysfunction (diaphoresis, pallor, unstable blood pressure, tachycardia, tachypnea, and pulmonary congestion).[131] Kurlan and colleagues[128] reviewed 52 published cases, summarized in Table 8.

NMS patients typically have a mild to marked leukocytosis.[132] The combination of sustained

Table 8. *Clinical Findings in NMS**

Feature	% Affected
Systemic findings	
Fever	100
Tachycardia	79
Diaphoresis	60
Labile blood pressure	54
Tachypnea	25
Movement-related findings	98
Tremor	56
Dystonia	33†
Chorea	15
Other neurologic findings	
Dysphagia	40
Akinetic mutism	38
Stupor	27
Coma	27

*Data from Kurlan and colleagues.[128]
†Includes 6% with oculogyric crises.

muscular contraction and immobility predisposes these patients to rhabdomyolysis; in combination with volume depletion, this often produces acute renal failure. The differential diagnosis of rhabdomyolysis in association with acute CNS dysfunction is extensive; Table 9 is adapted from the review by Bertorini.[44]

Other common systemic complications include disseminated intravascular coagulation and pulmonary embolism. Thrombocytopenia has recently been reported.[133]

The major differential diagnostic concerns are malignant hyperthermia (MH), the serotonin syndrome, and lethal catatonia.

Once NMS is suspected, neuroleptic drugs should be withdrawn and the patient adequately hydrated. Whether to administer dopaminergic agonists (*eg*, bromocriptine) or a direct muscle relaxant[134] (dantrolene) remains the subject of debate. Dantrolene relaxes muscle contraction by decreasing Ca^{2+} release from the sarcoplasmic reticulum. Electroconvulsive therapy has also been proposed as a treatment,[135] blurring the distinction between NMS and lethal catatonia. Neuroleptic medications should not be resumed for at least 2 weeks because of the risk of recurrence.[136]

Malignant Hyperthermia

MH was recognized as an anesthetic complication in the 1960s.[137] It is an autosomal-dominant

Table 9. *Differential Diagnosis of Rhabdomyolysis in Association With Acute CNS Dysfunction**

Myofiber Metabolic Exhaustion
    Seizures
    Delirium
    Tetanus
    Strychnine intoxication
    Extremes of environmental temperature
    Malignant hyperthermia
    Neuroleptic malignant syndrome
    Diabetic ketoacidosis
    Electric shock
Infectious Myositides
    Influenza
    HIV
    Toxic shock
    Clostridial myonecrosis (*Clostridium perfringens* bacteremia)
Toxins and Abused Drugs
    Alcohol
    Cocaine and other central stimulants
    LSD
    Narcotics
    Phencyclidine
    Envenomations (wasps, bees, spiders, snakes, etc)
    Medications
    Salicylate overdose
    Theophylline
    Lithium
Fluid and Electrolyte Disturbances
    Hyperosmolar states
    Hypo-osmolar states
    Severe hypophosphatemia
    Trauma

Adapted from Bertorini.[44]

disorder that most typically follows exposure to anesthetic agents. A porcine model and several clinical studies have implicated abnormally high levels of Ca^{2+} release from a sarcoplasmic calcium channel (also known as the ryanodine receptor). This results in Ca^{2+}-induced Ca^{2+} release, which lowers the threshold for sustained muscle contracture.[138] (Most human cases are associated with a defect on chromosome 19, although a few cases are not associated with the defined ryanodine-receptor abnormality.[139]) The drugs that induce MH do so by triggering this Ca^{2+} release; the sustained contraction produced by Ca^{2+} release causes excessive oxygen consumption and heat production. High-energy phosphate stores are quickly depleted, resulting in failure of Ca^{2+} reuptake. As in other cells, sustained excessive elevation of free intracellular Ca^{2+} produces membrane lysis, and consequently myoglobin leaks from muscle cells.

Table 10. *Triggering Agents in Malignant Hyperthermia*

Recognized Agents	
Inhalational anesthetics	Desflurane
	Enflurane
	Halothane (most common)
	Isoflurane
	Sevoflurane
Depolarizing NMJ blockers	Decamethonium
	Succinylcholine (most common)
	Suxamethonium
Possible Agents	
Calcium	
Catecholamines	
Ketamine	
Monoamine oxidase inhibitors	
Phenothiazines	
Potassium	
"Safe Agents"	
Barbiturates	
β-Blockers	
Benzodiazepines	
Local anesthetics	
Nitrous oxide	
Nondepolarizing NMJ blockers	
Propofol	

MH begins with muscle contraction (classically, although not always, in the masseters) in response to a triggering agent (Table 10).

In a typical anesthetic-induced case, a rise in end-tidal CO_2 often signifies MH onset.[140] Quickly thereafter, rapidly rising temperature, metabolic acidosis, hypoxemia, and cardiac arrhythmias may follow. The combination of muscle breakdown and acidosis results in hyperkalemia. On rare occasions, the condition may not arise until after the operation is over, or may occur in other situations of metabolic stress, such as exercise.

A personal or appropriate family history of anesthetic complications is usually sufficient reason to suspect MH, and to consider *in vitro* muscle testing where it is available. A muscle biopsy specimen (obtained under local anesthesia) is electrically stimulated during exposure to varying concentrations of caffeine or halothane. Patients with other muscle diseases, such as central core disease, dystrophinopathies, and several others, may be at risk for MH-like reactions. Muscle biopsies from MH patients are frequently abnormal, but not specifically so.[44]

The major management issues in MH involve termination of exposure to the triggering agent and the use of dantrolene.

Serotonin Syndrome

In 1955, a patient died after taking a combination of iproniazid and meperidine.[141] By 1960, the serotonin syndrome (SS) was well described.[142] Most patients with SS are receiving more than one serotonergic agent (or a monoamine oxidase inhibitor, raising extracellular serotonin concentrations), although overdoses of single agents may trigger the syndrome.[143] The newer reversible monoamine oxidase inhibitors, such as moclobemide, may be less likely to precipitate SS[144] but are not devoid of this potential.[145] SS resembles NMS, but is frequently associated with myoclonus, and less frequently involves muscle rigidity.[146] Autonomic instability is common in both conditions.[147] The duration of SS is usually shorter than that of NMS. A case of SS also involving stroke in a young patient suggests that the spectrum of this disorder may involve precipitation of complicated migraine.[148] Treatment is supportive.

Lethal Catatonia

Lethal catatonia was described by Stauder in 1934, almost half a decade before the introduction of neuroleptic agents. The presentation of lethal catatonia is essentially indistinguishable from NMS, although published case reports of the two syndromes indicate differences in mode of onset, signs and symptoms, and outcome.[149] Lethal catatonia often begins with extreme psychotic excitement, which leads to fever, exhaustion, and death. In contrast, NMS begins with severe muscle rigidity. Lethal catatonia may require neuroleptic treatment, although electroconvulsive therapy is more commonly employed. Occasional reports of cases "requiring" treatment with both electroconvulsive therapy and dantrolene serve to blur the distinction between lethal catatonia and NMS.[150] The underlying pathophysiology of lethal catatonia remains unknown.

References

1. Wilks S. Bromide and iodide of potassium in epilepsy. Med Times Gaz (Lond) 1861; 2:635–636

2. Gowers WR. Epilepsy and other chronic convulsive diseases: their causes, symptoms, and treatment. London, UK: J. and A. Churchill, 1881
3. Bleck TP, Klawans HL. Mechanisms of epilepsy and anticonvulsant action. In: Klawans HL, Goetz CG, Tanner CM, eds. Textbook of clinical neuropharmacology. New York, NY: Raven Press, 1992; 23–30
4. Weschler IS. Intravenous injection of paraldehyde for control of convulsions. JAMA 1940; 114:2198
5. Gastaut H, Naquet R, Poiré R, et al. Treatment of status epilepticus with diazepam (Valium). Epilepsia 1965; 6:167–182
6. Wijdicks EFM, Sharbrough FW. New-onset seizures in critically ill patients. Neurology 1993; 43:1042–1044
7. Bleck TP, Smith MC, Pierre-Louis JC, et al. Neurologic complications of critical medical illnesses. Crit Care Med 1993; 21:98–103
8. Hauser WA. Status epilepticus: epidemiologic considerations. Neurology 1990; 40(suppl 2):9–13
9. DeLorenzo RJ, Towne AR, Pellock JM, et al. Status epilepticus in children, adults, and the elderly. Epilepsia 1992; 33(suppl 4):S15–S25
10. Aminoff MJ, Simon RP. Status epilepticus: causes, clinical features and consequences in 98 patients. Am J Med 1980; 69:657–666
11. Lowenstein DH, Alldredge BK. Status epilepticus in an urban public hospital in the 1980s. Neurology 1993; 42:483–488
12. Bleck TP. Status epilepticus. University Reports on Epilepsy 1992; 1:1–7
13. Ettinger AB, Shinnar S. New-onset seizures in an elderly hospitalized population. Neurology 1993; 43:489–492
14. Proposal for revised clinical and electroencephalographic classification of epileptic seizures: from the Commission on Classification and Terminology of the International League Against Epilepsy. Epilepsia 1981; 22:489–501
15. Bleck TP. Metabolic encephalopathy. In: Weiner WJ, ed. Emergent and urgent neurology. Philadelphia, PA: Lippincott, 1991; 27–57
16. Bleck TP. Status epilepticus. In: Klawans HL, Goetz CG, Tanner CM, eds. Textbook of clinical neuropharmacology. 2nd ed. New York, NY: Raven Press, 1992; 65–73
17. Lothman EW. The biochemical basis and pathophysiology of status epilepticus. Neurology 1990; 40(suppl 2):13–23
18. Lowenstein DH, Simon RP, Sharp FR. The pattern of 72-kDa heat shock protein-like immunoreactivity in the rat brain following fluothyl-induced status epilepticus. Brain Res 1990; 531:173–182
19. Wasterlain CG, Fujikawa DG, Penix L, et al. Pathophysiological mechanisms of brain damage from status epilepticus. Epilepsia 1993; 34(suppl 1):S37–S53
20. Treiman DM. Generalized convulsive status epilepticus in the adult. Epilepsia 1993; 34(suppl 1):S2–S11
21. Walton NY. Systemic effects of generalized convulsive status epilepticus. Epilepsia 1993; 34(suppl 1):S54–S58
22. Bolton CF, Young GB, Zochodne DW. The neurologic complications of sepsis. Ann Neurol 1993; 33:94–100
23. Rowbotham MC; Lowenstein DH. Neurologic complications of cocaine use. Annu Rev Med 1990; 41:417–422
24. Randomized clinical trial of the efficacy of antiepileptic drugs in reducing the risk of relapse after a first unprovoked tonic-clonic seizure: First Seizure Trial Group (FIR.S.T. Group). Neurology 1993; 43:478–483
25. Smith MC, Bleck TP. Toxicity of anticonvulsants. In: Klawans HL, Goetz CG, Tanner CM, eds. Textbook of clinical neuropharmacology. 2nd ed. New York, NY: Raven Press, 1992; 45–64
26. Mitchell WG. Status epilepticus and acute repetitive seizures in children, adolescents, and young adults: etiology, outcome, and treatment. Epilepsia 1996; 37(suppl 1):S74–S80
27. Bebin EM. Additional modalities for treating acute seizures in children: overview. J Child Neurol 1998; 13(suppl 1):S23–S26
28. Dreifuss FE, Rosman NP, Cloyd JC, et al. A comparison of rectal diazepam gel and placebo for acute repetitive seizures. N Engl J Med 1998; 338:1869–1875
29. Chang CWJ, Bleck TP. Status epilepticus. Neurol Clin 1995; 13:529–548
30. Treiman DM, Meyers PD, Walton NY, et al. A comparison of four treatments for generalized convulsive status epilepticus: Veterans Affairs Status Epilepticus Cooperative Study Group. N Engl J Med 1998; 339:792–798
31. Leppik IE, Derivan AT, Homan RW, et al. Double-blind study of lorazepam and diazepam in status epilepticus. JAMA 1983; 249:1452–1454
32. Bebin M, Bleck TP. New anticonvulsant drugs. Drugs 1994; 48:153–171

33. Graves N. Pharmacoeconomic considerations in treatment options for acute seizures. J Child Neurol 1998; 13(suppl 1):S27–S29
34. Walton NY, Treiman DM. Valproic acid treatment of experimental status epilepticus. Epilepsy Res 1992; 12:199–205
35. Bleck TP. Refractory status epilepticus in 2001. Arch Neurol 2002; 59:188–189
36. Bleck TP. Electroencephalographic monitoring. In: Tobin MR, ed. Principles and practice of intensive care monitoring. New York, NY: McGraw Hill, 1998; 1035–1046
37. Kumar A, Bleck TP. Intravenous midazolam for the treatment of refractory status epilepticus. Crit Care Med 1992; 20:483–488
38. Labar DR, Ali A, Root J. High-dose intravenous lorazepam for the treatment of refractory status epilepticus. Neurology 1994; 44:1400–1403
39. Stecker MM, Kramer TH, Raps EC, et al. Treatment of refractory status epilepticus with propofol: clinical and pharmacokinetic findings. Epilepsia 1998; 39: 18–26
40. Huff JS, Bleck TP. Propofol in the treatment of refractory status epilepticus. Acad Emerg Med 1996; 3:179
41. Prasad A, Worrall BB, Bertram EB, et al. Propofol and midazolam in the treatment of refractory status epilepticus. Epilepsia 2001; 42:380–386
42. Galley HF, Dubbels AM, Webster NR. The effect of midazolam and propofol on interleukin-8 from human polymorphonuclear leukocytes. Anesth Analg 1998; 86:1289–1293
43. Weise KL, Bleck TP. Status epilepticus in children and adults. Crit Care Clin 1997; 14:629–646
44. Bertorini TE. Myoglobinuria, malignant hyperthermia, neuroleptic malignant syndrome and serotonin syndrome. Neurol Clin 1997; 15:649–671
45. Dodrill CB, Wilensky AJ. Intellectual impairment as an outcome of status epilepticus. Neurology 1990; 40(suppl 2):23–27
46. Treiman DM, Delgado-Escueta AV. Complex partial status epilepticus. Adv Neurol 1983; 34:69–81
47. Lothman EW, Bertram EH. Epileptogenic effects of status epilepticus. Epilepsia 1993; 34(suppl 1): S59–S70
48. Borris DJ, Bertram EH, Kapur J. Ketamine controls prolonged status epilepticus. Epilepsy Res 2000; 42:117–122
49. Kassell NF, Torner JC. Aneurysmal rebleeding: a preliminary report from the Cooperative Aneurysm Study. Neurosurgery 1983; 13:479–481
50. Nishioka H, Torner JC, Graf CJ, et al. Cooperative study of intracranial aneurysms and subarachnoid hemorrhage: a long-term prognostic study. II. Ruptured intracranial aneurysms managed conservatively. Arch Neurol 1984; 41:1142–1146
51. Torner JC, Kassell NF, Wallace RB, et al. Preoperative prognostic factors for rebleeding and survival in aneurysm patients receiving antifibrinolytic therapy: a report of the cooperative aneurysm study. Neurosurgery 1981; 9:506–513
52. Solenski NJ, Haley EC Jr, Kassell NF, et al. Medical complications of aneurysmal subarachnoid hemorrhage: a report of the multicenter, cooperative aneurysm study. Crit Care Med 1995:23:1007–1017
53. Biller J, Godersky JC, Adams HP Jr. Management of aneurysmal subarachnoid hemorrhage. Stroke 1988; 19:1300–1305
54. Hasan D, Wijdicks EF, Vermeulen M. Hyponatremia is associated with cerebral ischemia in patients with aneurysmal subarachnoid hemorrhage. Ann Neurol 1990; 27:106–108
55. von Holst H, Ericson K, Haberbeck-Modesto M, et al. Angiographic investigation of cerebral vasospasm in subarachnoid haemorrhage due to arteriovenous malformation. Acta Neurochir (Wien) 1988; 94:129–132
56. Kothbauer K, Schroth G, Seiler RW, et al. Severe symptomatic vasospasm after rupture of an arteriovenous malformation. AJNR Am J Neuroradiol 1995; 16:1073–1075
57. Taneda M, Kataoka K, Akai F, et al. Traumatic subarachnoid hemorrhage as a predictable indicator of delayed ischemic symptoms. J Neurosurg 1996; 84:762–768
58. Kordestani RK, Counelis GJ. McBride DQ, et al. Cerebral arterial spasm after penetrating craniocerebral gunshot wounds: transcranial Doppler and cerebral blood flow findings. Neurosurgery 1997; 41:351–359
59. Macdonald RL, Weir B. Cerebral vasospasm: prevention and treatment. In: Batjer HH, ed. Cerebrovascular disease. Philadelphia, PA: Lippincott-Raven, 1997; 1111–1121
60. Vorkapic P, Bevan JA, Bevan RD. Longitudinal *in vivo* and in vitro time-course study of chronic cerebrovasospasm in the rabbit basilar artery. Neurosurg Rev 1991; 14:215–219
61. Macdonald RL, Weir BKA. A review of hemoglobin and the pathogenesis of cerebral vasospasm. Stroke 1991; 22:971–982

62. Pluta RM, Boock RJ, Afshar JK, et al. Source and cause of endothelin-1 release into cerebrospinal fluid after subarachnoid hemorrhage. J Neurosurg 1997; 87:287–293
63. Kwan AL, Bavbek M, Jeng AY, et al. Prevention and reversal of cerebral vasospasm by an endothelin-converting enzyme inhibitor, CGS 26303, in an experimental model of subarachnoid hemorrhage. J Neurosurg 1997; 87:281–286
64. Qureshi AI, Sung GY, Suri MA, et al. Prognostic value and determinants of ultraearly angiographic vasospasm after aneurysmal subarachnoid hemorrhage. Neurosurgery 1999; 44:967–973
65. Fisher CM, Kistler JP, Davis JM. Relation of cerebral vasospasm to subarachnoid hemorrhage visualized by computerized tomographic scanning. Neurosurgery 1980; 6:1–9
66. Haley EC Jr, Torner JC, Kassell NF. Antifibrinolytic therapy and cerebral vasospasm. Neurosurg Clin N Am 1990; 1:349–356
67. Wass CT, Lanier WL. Glucose modulation of ischemic brain injury: review and clinical recommendations. Mayo Clin Proc 1996; 71:801–812
68. Lanzino G, Kassell NF, Germanson T, et al. Plasma glucose levels and outcome after aneurysmal subarachnoid hemorrhage. J Neurosurg 1993; 79:885–891
69. Doczi T, Bende J, Huszka E, et al. Syndrome of inappropriate secretion of antidiuretic hormone after subarachnoid hemorrhage. Neurosurgery 1981; 9:394–397
70. Harringan MR. Cerebral salt wasting syndrome: a review. Neurosurgery 1996; 38:152–160
71. Wijdicks EF, Schievink WI, Burnett JC Jr. Natriuretic peptide system and endothelin in aneurysmal subarachnoid hemorrhage. J Neurosurg 1997; 87:275–280
72. Wijdicks EF, Vermeulen M, ten Haaf JA, et al. Volume depletion and natriuresis in patients with a ruptured intracranial aneurysm. Ann Neurol 1985; 18:211–216
73. Hasan D, Vermeulen M, Wijdicks EF, et al. Effect of fluid intake and antihypertensive treatment on cerebral ischemia after subarachnoid hemorrhage. Stroke 1989; 20:1511–1515
74. Pinto AN, Canhao P Ferro JM. Seizures at the onset of subarachnoid haemorrhage. J Neurol 1996; 243:161–164
75. Baker CJ, Prestigiacomo CJ, Solomon RA. Short-term perioperative anticonvulsant prophylaxis for the surgical treatment of low-risk patients with intracranial aneurysms. Neurosurgery 1995; 37:863–870
76. Schoser BG, Heesen C, Eckert B, et al. Cerebral hyperperfusion injury after percutaneous transluminal angioplasty of extracranial arteries. J Neurol 1997; 244:101–104
77. Talavera JO, Wacher NH, Laredo F, et al. Predictive value of signs and symptoms in the diagnosis of subarachnoid hemorrhage among stroke patients. Arch Med Res 1996; 27:353–357
78. Kabuto H, Yokoi I, Habu H, et al. Reduction in nitric oxide synthase activity with development of an epileptogenic focus induced by ferric chloride in the rat brain. Epilepsy Res 1996; 25:65–68
79. Lanzino G, Kongable G, Kassell N. Electrographic abnormalities after nontraumatic subarachnoid hemorrhage. J Neurosurg Anesth 1994; 6:156–162
80. Brouwers PJ, Wijdicks EF, Hasan D, et al. Serial electrocardiographic recording in aneurysmal subarachnoid hemorrhage. Stroke 1989; 20:1162–1167
81. Provencio JJ, Bleck TP. Cardiovascular disorders related to neurologic and neurosurgical emergencies. In: Cruz J, ed. Neurologic and neurosurgical emergencies. Philadelphia, PA: WB Saunders, 1997; 39–50
82. Zaroff JG, Rordorf GA, Newell JB, et al. Cardiac outcome in patients with subarachnoid hemorrhage and electrocardiographic abnormalities. Neurosurgery 1999; 44:34–39
83. Mayer SA, Lin J, Homma S, et al. Myocardial injury and left ventricular performance after subarachnoid hemorrhage. Stroke 1999; 30:780–786
84. Mayer SA. LiMandri G. Sherman D, et al. Electrocardiographic markers of abnormal left ventricular wall motion in acute subarachnoid hemorrhage. J Neurosurg 1995; 83:889–896
85. Vespa P, Bleck TP, Brock DG, et al. Impaired oxygenation after acute aneurysmal subarachnoid hemorrhage [abstract]. Neurology 1994; 44(suppl 1):A344
86. Touho H, Karasawa J, Shishido H, et al. Neurogenic pulmonary edema in the acute stage of hemorrhagic cerebrovascular disease. Neurosurgery 1989; 25:762–768
87. Haley EC Jr, Kassell NF, Apperson-Hansen C, et al. A randomized, double-blind, vehicle-controlled trial of tirilazad mesylate in patients with aneurysmal subarachnoid hemorrhage: a cooperative

study in North America. J Neurosurg 1997; 86: 467–474
88. Rouby JJ, Laurent P, Gosnach M, et al. Risk factors and clinical relevance of nosocomial maxillary sinusitis in the critically ill. Am J Respir Crit Care Med 1994; 150:776–783
89. Sundt TM Jr, Kobayashi S, Fode NC, et al. Results and complications of surgical management of 809 intracranial aneurysms in 722 cases: related and unrelated to grade of patient, type of aneurysm, and timing of surgery. J Neurosurg 1982; 56: 753–765
90. Leipzig TJ, Redelman K, Horner TG. Reducing the risk of rebleeding before early aneurysm surgery: a possible role for antifibrinolytic therapy. J Neurosurg 1997; 86:220–225
91. Fletcher AP, Alkjaersig N, Davies A, et al. Blood coagulation and plasma fibrinolytic enzyme system pathophysiology in stroke. Stroke 1976; 7: 337–348
92. Kirsch JR, D'Alecy LG. Effect of altered availability of energy-yielding substrates upon survival from hypoxia in mice. Stroke 1979; 10:288–291
93. Hersio K, Vapalahti M, Kari A, et al. Impaired utilization of exogenous amino acids after surgery for subarachnoid haemorrhage. Acta Neurochir (Wien) 1990; 106:13–17
94. Mayberg MR, Batjer HH, Dacey R, et al. Guidelines for the management of aneurysmal subarachnoid hemorrhage: a statement for healthcare professionals from a special writing group of the Stroke Council, American Heart Association. Stroke 1994; 25:2315–2328
95. Findlay JM. Current management of aneurysmal subarachnoid hemorrhage guidelines from the Canadian Neurosurgical Society. Can J Neurol Sci 1997; 24:161–170
96. Levy M, Giannotta S. Cardiac performance indices during hypervolemic therapy for cerebral vasospasm. J Neurosurg 1991; 75:27–31
97. Clyde BL, Resnick DK, Yonas H, et al. The relationship of blood velocity as measured by transcranial doppler ultrasonography to cerebral blood flow as determined by stable xenon computed tomographic studies after aneurysmal subarachnoid hemorrhage. Neurosurgery 1996; 38:896–904
98. Adams HP Jr. Calcium antagonists in the management of patients with aneurysmal subarachnoid hemorrhage: a review. Angiology 1990; 41(11 pt 2):1010–1016
99. Haley EC Jr, Kassell NF, Torner JC. A randomized trial of nicardipine in subarachnoid hemorrhage: angiographic and transcranial Doppler ultrasound results; a report of the Cooperative Aneurysm Study. J Neurosurg 1993; 78:548–553
100. Kassell NF, Haley EC Jr, Apperson-Hansen C, et al. Randomized, double-blind, vehicle-controlled trial of tirilazad mesylate in patients with aneurysmal subarachnoid hemorrhage: a cooperative study in Europe, Australia, and New Zealand. J Neurosurg 1996; 84:221–228
101. Fleishaker JC, Fiedler-Kelly J, Grasela TH. Population phamacokinetics of tirilazad: effects of weight, gender, concomitant phenytoin, and subarachnoid hemorrhage. Pharm Res 1999; 16:575-583
102. Hall ED, Andrus PK, Smith SL, et al. Pyrrolopyrimidines: novel brain-penetrating antioxidants with neuroprotective activity in brain injury and ischemia models. J Pharmacol Exp Ther 1997; 281:895–904
103. Kassell NF, Peerless SJ, Durward QJ, et al. Treatment of ischemic deficits from vasospasm with intravascular volume expansion and induced arterial hypertension. Neurosurgery 1982; 11:337–343
104. Oropello JM, Weiner L, Benjamin E. Hypertensive, hypervolemic, hemodilutional therapy for aneurysmal subarachnoid hemorrhage: is it efficacious? No. Crit Care Clin 1996; 12:709–730
105. Ullman JS, Bederson JB. Hypertensive, hypervolemic, hemodilutional therapy for aneurysmal subarachnoid hemorrhage: is it efficacious? Yes. Crit Care Clin 1996; 12:697–707
106. Amin-Hanjani S, Schwartz RB, Sathi S, et al. Hypertensive encephalopathy as a complication of hyperdynamic therapy for vasospasm: report of two cases. Neurosurgery 1999; 44:1113–1116
107. Firlik KS, Kaufmann AM, Firlik AD, et al. Intraarterial papaverine for the treatment of cerebral vasospasm following aneurysmal subarachnoid hemorrhage. Surg Neurol 1999; 51:66–74
108. Thomas JE, Rosenwasser RH. Reversal of severe cerebral vasospasm in three patients after aneurysmal subarachnoid hemorrhage: initial observations regarding the use of intraventricular sodium nitroprusside in humans. Neurosurgery 1999; 44:48–57
109. Bleck TP. Metabolic encephalopathy. In: Weiner WJ, Shulman LM, eds. Emergent and urgent neurology. 2nd ed. Philadelphia, PA: Lippincott, 1999; 223–253

110. Bleck TP, Henson S. Sources of fever in patients after surgery for aneurysmal subarachnoid hemorrhage. Crit Care Med 1992; 20(suppl):S31
111. Paramore CG, Turner DA. Relative risks of ventriculostomy infection and morbidity. Acta Neurochir (Wien) 1994; 127:79–84
112. Deutschman CS, Wilton PB, Sinow J, et al. Paranasal sinusitis: a common complication of nasotracheal intubation in neurosurgical patients. Neurosurgery 1985; 17:296–299
113. Jacobs DG, Piotrowski JJ, Hoppensteadt DA, et al. Hemodynamic and fibrinolytic consequences of intermittent pneumatic compression: preliminary results. J Trauma 1996; 40:710–716
114. Swann KW, Black PM, Baker MF. Management of symptomatic deep venous thrombosis and pulmonary embolism on a neurosurgical service. J Neurosurg 1986; 64:563–567
115. Takaku A, Tanaka S, Mori T, et al. Postoperative complications in 1,000 cases of intracranial aneurysms. Surg Neurol 1979; 12:137–144
115a. Mayer SA, Brun NC, Begtrup K, et al. Recombinant activated factor VII for acute intracerebral hemorrage. N Engl J Med 2005; 352:777–785
116. Tissue plasminogen activator for acute ischemic stroke: The National Institute of Neurological Disorders and Stroke rt-PA Stroke Study Group. N Engl J Med 1995; 333:1581–1587
117. Roelofs RI, Cerra F, Bielka N, et al. Prolonged respiratory insufficiency due to acute motor neuropathy: a new syndrome. Neurology 1983; 33(suppl 2):240
118. Zochodne W, Bolton CF, Wells GA, et al. Critical illness polyneuropathy: a complication of sepsis and multiple organ failure. Brain 1987; 110:819–842
119. Witt NJ, Zochodne DW, Bolton CF, et al. Peripheral nerve function in sepsis and multiple organ failure. Chest 1991; 99:176–184
120. Spitzer AR, Giancarlo T, Maher L, et al. Neuromuscular causes of prolonged ventilator dependency. Muscle Nerve 1992; 15:682–686
121. Kelly BJ, Luce JM. The diagnosis and management of neuromuscular diseases causing respiratory failure. Chest 1991; 99:1485–1494
122. Preston J. Central nervous system reaction to small doses of tranquilizers: report of one death. American Practitoner and Digest of Treatment 1959; 10:627–630
123. Caroff SN, Mann SC. The neuroleptic malignant syndrome. J Clin Psychiatr 1908; 41:79–83
124. Keyser DL, Rodnitzky RL. Neuroleptic malignant syndrome in Parkinson's disease after withdrawal or alteration of dopaminergic therapy. Arch Intern Med 1977; 86:794–796
125. Addonizio G, Susman VL, Roth SD. Neuroleptic malignant syndrome: review and analysis of 115 cases. Biol Psychiatr 1987; 22:1004–1020
126. Henderson VM, Wooten GF. Neuroleptic malignant syndrome: a pathogenetic role for dopamine receptor blockade? Neurology 1981; 31:132–137
127. Ram A, Cao Q, Keck PE Jr, et al. Structural change in dopamine D_2 receptor gene in a patient with neuroleptic malignant syndrome. Am J Med Genet 1995; 60:228–230
128. Kurlan R, Hamill R, Shoulson I. Neuroleptic malignant syndrome. Clin Neuropharmacol 1984; 7:109–120
129. Guzé BH, Baxter LR. Neuroleptic malignant syndrome. N Engl J Med 1985; 313:163–166
130. Wedzicha JA, Hoffbrand BI. Neuroleptic malignant syndrome and hyponatraemia. Lancet 1984; 1:963
131. Weiner WJ, Lang AE. Movement disorders: a comprehensive survey. Mount Kisco, NY: Futura Publishing Co, 1989; 617
132. Keyser DL, Rodnitzky RL. Neuroleptic malignant syndrome in Parkinson's disease after withdrawal or alteration of dopaminergic therapy. Arch Intern Med 1991; 151:794-796
133. Ray JG. Neuroleptic malignant syndrome associated with severe thrombocytopenia. J Intern Med 1997; 241:245–247
134. Buckley PF, Hutchinson M. Neuroleptic malignant syndrome. J Neurol Neurosurg Psychiatr 1995; 58:271–278
135. Addonizio G, Susman VL. ECT as a treatment alternative for patients with symptoms of neuroleptic malignant syndrome. J Clin Psychiatry 1987; 48:102–105
136. Susman VL, Addonizio G. Recurrence of neuroleptic malignant syndrome. J Nerv Ment Dis 1988; 176:234–241
137. Denborough MA, Lovell RRH. Anaesthetic deaths in a family. Lancet 1960; 2:45–46
138. El-Hayek R, Yano M, Antonui B, et al. Altered E-C coupling in trials isolated from malignant hyperthermia-susceptible porcine muscle. Am J Physiol 1995; 268(6 pt 1):C1831
139. Gronert GA, Mott J, Lee J. Aetiology of malignant hyperthermia. Br J Anaesth 1988; 60:253–260

140. Struebing VL. Differential diagnosis of malignant hyperthermia: a case report. AANA J 1995; 63: 455–460
141. Mitchell RS. Fatal toxic encephalitis occurring during iproniazid therapy in pulmonary tuberculosis. Ann Intern Med 1955; 42:417–419
142. Oates JA, Sjoerdsma A. Neurotoxic effects of tryptophan in patients receiving a monoamine oxidase inhibitor. Neurology 1960:10:1076–1080
143. Kolecki P. Isolated venlafaxine-induced serotonin syndrome. J Emerg Med 1997; 15:491–493
144. Hilton SE, Maradit H, Moller HJ. Serotonin syndrome and drug combinations: focus on MAOI and RIMA. Eur Arch Psychiatry Clin Neurosci 1997; 247:113–119
145. Singer PP, Jones GR. An uncommon fatality due to moclobemide and paroxetine. J Anal Toxicol 1997; 21:518–520
146. Kam PC, Chang GW. Selective serotonin reuptake inhibitors: pharmacology and clinical implications in anaesthesia and critical care medicine. Anaesthesia 1997; 52:982–988
147. Halman M, Goldbloom DS. Fluoxetine and neuroleptic malignant syndrome. Biol Psychiatry 1990; 28:518–522
148. Molaie M. Serotonin syndrome presenting with migrainelike stroke. Headache 1997; 37: 519–521
149. Castillo E, Rubin RT, Holsboer-Trachsler E. Clinical differentiation between lethal catatonia and neuroleptic malignant syndrome. Am J Psychiatry 1989; 146:324–328
150. Nolen WA, Zwaan WA. Treatment of lethal catatonia with electroconvulsive therapy and dantrolene sodium: a case report. Acta Psychiatr Scand 1990; 82:90–92

Notes

Notes

Notes